W9-ACV-079

The GALE ENCYCLOPEDIA of SURGERY AND MEDICAL TESTS

SECOND EDITION

TECHNICAL COLLEGE OF THE LOWCOUNTRY
LEARNING RESOURCES CENTER
POST OFFICE BOX 1288
BEAUFORT, SOUTH CAROLINA 29901-1288

The GALE
ENCYCLOPEDIA *of*
SURGERY AND
MEDICAL TESTS

SECOND EDITION

VOLUME

3

L–P

BRIGHAM NARINS, EDITOR

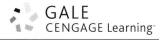

GALE
CENGAGE Learning

Detroit • New York • San Francisco • New Haven, Conn • Waterville, Maine • London

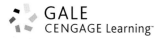

Gale Encyclopedia of Surgery and Medical Tests, Second Edition

Project Editor: Brigham Narins

Editorial: Donna Batten, Amy Kwolek, Jeffrey Wilson

Product Manager: Kate Hanley

Editorial Support Services: Andrea Lopeman

Indexing Services: Katherine Jensen, Indexes, etc.

Rights Acquisition and Management: Margaret Chamberlain-Gaston, Kelly A. Quin, and Robyn V. Young

Composition: Evi Abou-El-Seoud

Manufacturing: Wendy Blurton

Imaging: Lezlie Light

Product Design: Pam Galbreath

© 2009 Gale, Cengage Learning

ALL RIGHTS RESERVED. No part of this work covered by the copyright herein may be reproduced, transmitted, stored, or used in any form or by any means graphic, electronic, or mechanical, including but not limited to photocopying, recording, scanning, digitizing, taping, Web distribution, information networks, or information storage and retrieval systems, except as permitted under Section 107 or 108 of the 1976 United States Copyright Act, without the prior written permission of the publisher.

For product information and technology assistance, contact us at
Gale Customer Support, 1-800-877-4253.
For permission to use material from this text or product,
submit all requests online at **www.cengage.com/permissions.**
Further permissions questions can be emailed to
permissionrequest@cengage.com

While every effort has been made to ensure the reliability of the information presented in this publication, Gale, a part of Cengage Learning, does not guarantee the accuracy of the data contained herein. Gale accepts no payment for listing; and inclusion in the publication of any organization, agency, institution, publication, service, or individual does not imply endorsement of the editors or publisher. Errors brought to the attention of the publisher and verified to the satisfaction of the publisher will be corrected in future editions.

Library of Congress Cataloging-in-Publication Data

The Gale encyclopedia of surgery and medical tests : a guide for patients and caregivers / Brigham Narins, editor. -- 2nd ed.
    p. cm.
Includes bibliographical references and index.
ISBN-13: 978-1-4144-4884-8 (set : alk. paper)
ISBN-13: 978-1-4144-4885-5 (vol. 1 : alk. paper)
ISBN-13: 978-1-4144-4886-2 (vol. 2 : alk. paper)
ISBN-13: 978-1-4144-4887-9 (vol. 3 : alk. paper)
[etc.]
    1. Surgery--Encyclopedias. 2. Diagnosis--Encyclopedias. I. Narins, Brigham, 1962-.

RD17.G342 2008
617.003--dc22   2008020207

Gale
27500 Drake Rd.
Farmington Hills, MI, 48331-3535

ISBN-13: 978-1-4144-4884-8 (set)   ISBN-10: 1-4144-4884-8 (set)
ISBN-13: 978-1-4144-4885-5 (vol. 1)   ISBN-10: 1-4144-4885-6 (vol. 1)
ISBN-13: 978-1-4144-4886-2 (vol. 2   ISBN-10: 1-4144-4886-4 (vol. 2)
ISBN-13: 978-1-4144-4887-9 (vol. 3)   ISBN-10: 1-4144-4887-2 (vol. 3)
ISBN-13: 978-1-4144-4888-6 (vol. 4)   ISBN-10: 1-4144-4888-0 (vol. 4)

This title is also available as an e-book.
ISBN-13: 978-1-4144-4889-3 ISBN-10: 1-4144-4889-9
Contact your Gale, Cengage Learning sales representative for ordering information.

Printed in China
1 2 3 4 5 6 7 12 11 10 09 08

CONTENTS

LIST OF ENTRIES

H

Hair transplantation
Hammer, claw, and mallet toe surgery
Hand surgery
Health care proxy
Health history
Health Maintenance Organization (HMO)
Heart surgery for congenital defects
Heart transplantation
Heart-lung machines
Heart-lung transplantation
Heller myotomy
Hemangioma excision
Hematocrit
Hemispherectomy
Hemoglobin test
Hemoperfusion
Hemorrhoidectomy
Hepatectomy
Hiatal hernia
HIDA Scan
Hip osteotomy
Hip replacement
Hip revision surgery
Home care
Hospice
Hospital services
Hospital-acquired infections
Human leukocyte antigen test
Hydrocelectomy
Hypophysectomy
Hypospadias repair
Hysterectomy
Hysteroscopy

I

Ileal conduit surgery
Ileoanal anastomosis
Ileoanal reservoir surgery
Ileostomy
Immunoassay tests

Immunologic therapies
Immunosuppressant drugs
Implantable cardioverter-defibrillator
In vitro fertilization
Incision care
Incisional hernia repair
Informed consent
Inguinal hernia repair
Intensive care unit
Intensive care unit equipment
Intestinal obstruction repair
Intra-Operative Parathyroid Hormone Measurement
Intravenous rehydration
Intussusception reduction
Iridectomy
Islet cell transplantation

K

Kidney dialysis
Kidney function tests
Kidney transplantation
Knee arthroscopic surgery
Knee osteotomy
Knee replacement
Knee revision surgery
Kneecap removal

L

Laceration repair
Laminectomy
Laparoscopy
Laparoscopy for endometriosis
Laparotomy, exploratory
Laryngectomy
Laser in-situ keratomileusis (LASIK)
Laser iridotomy
Laser posterior capsulotomy
Laser skin resurfacing
Laser surgery
Laxatives

LDL cholesterol test
Leg lengthening or shortening
Length of hospital stay
Limb salvage
Lipid profile
Lipid tests
Liposuction
Lithotripsy
Liver biopsy
Liver function tests
Liver transplantation
Living will
Lobectomy, pulmonary
Long-term care insurance
Lumpectomy
Lung biopsy
Lung transplantation
Lymphadenectomy

M

Magnetic resonance angiogram
Magnetic resonance imaging
Magnetic resonance venogram
Mammography
Managed care plans
Mantoux test
Mastectomy
Mastoidectomy
Maze procedure for atrial fibrillation
Mechanical circulation support
Mechanical ventilation
Meckel's diverticulectomy
Mediastinoscopy
Medicaid
Medical charts
Medical co-morbidities
Medical errors
Medicare
Medication Monitoring
Meningocele repair
Mental health assessment
Mentoplasty
Microsurgery

Sedimentation rate
Segmentectomy
Sentinel lymph node biopsy
Septoplasty
Serum chloride level
Serum creatinine level
Serum glucose level
Sestamibi scan
Sex reassignment surgery
Shoulder joint replacement
Shoulder resection arthroplasty
Sigmoidoscopy
Simple mastectomy
Skin grafting
Skull x rays
Sling procedure
Smoking cessation
Snoring surgery
Sphygmomanometer
Spinal fusion
Spinal instrumentation
Spirometry tests
Splenectomy
Stapedectomy
Stereotactic radiosurgery
Stethoscope
Stress test
Sulfonamides
Surgical instruments
Surgical mesh
Surgical oncology
Surgical risk
Surgical team
Surgical training
Surgical triage
Sympathectomy
Syringe and needle

T

Talking to the doctor
Tarsorrhaphy
Telesurgery
Temperature measurement
Tendon repair
Tenotomy
Tetracyclines
Thermometer
Thoracic surgery
Thoracotomy
Thrombolytic therapy
Thyroidectomy
Tonsillectomy
Tooth extraction
Tooth replantation
Trabeculectomy
Tracheotomy
Traction
Transfusion
Transplant surgery
Transurethral bladder resection
Transurethral resection of the
  prostate
Trocars
Tubal ligation
Tube enterostomy
Tube-shunt surgery
Tumor marker tests
Tumor removal
Tympanoplasty
Type and screen

U

Ultrasound
Umbilical hernia repair

Upper GI exam
Ureteral stenting
Ureterosigmoidoscopy
Ureterostomy, cutaneous
Urinalysis
Urinary anti-infectives
Urine culture
Urologic surgery
Uterine stimulants

V

Vagal nerve stimulation
Vagotomy
Vascular surgery
Vasectomy
Vasovasostomy
Vein ligation and stripping
Venous thrombosis
  prevention
Ventricular assist device
Ventricular shunt
Vertical banded gastroplasty
Vital signs

W

Webbed finger or toe
  repair
Weight management
Whipple procedure
White blood cell count and
  differential
Wound care
Wound culture
Wrist replacement

LIST OF ENTRIES BY BODY SYSTEM

Cardiovascular

Angiography
Angioplasty
Aortic aneurysm repair
Aortic valve replacement
Arteriovenous fistula
Balloon valvuloplasty
Cardiac catheterization
Cardiac event monitor
Cardiac marker tests
Cardiac monitor
Cardiopulmonary resuscitation
Cardioversion
Carotid endarterectomy
Coronary artery bypass graft surgery
Coronary stenting
Defibrillation
Echocardiography
Electrocardiogram
Electrocardiography
Electrophysiology study of the heart
Endovascular stent surgery
Femoral hernia repair
Heart surgery for congenital defects
Heart transplantation
Heart-lung machines
Heart-lung transplantation
Hemangioma excision
Implantable cardioverter-defibrillator
Magnetic resonance angiogram

Magnetic resonance venogram
Maze procedure for atrial fibrillation
Mechanical circulation support
Minimally invasive heart surgery
Mitral valve repair
Mitral valve replacement
Multiple-gated acquisition (MUGA) scan
Myocardial resection
Pacemakers
Pericardiocentesis
Peripheral endarterectomy
Peripheral vascular bypass surgery
Portal vein bypass
Sclerotherapy for varicose veins
Stress test
Vascular surgery
Vein ligation and stripping
Venous thrombosis prevention
Ventricular assist device
Ventricular shunt

Endocrine

Adenoidectomy
Adrenalectomy
Endoscopic retrograde cholangiopancreatography
Hypophysectomy
Intra-Operative Parathyroid Hormone Measurement
Islet cell transplantation
Oral glucose tolerance test

Pancreas transplantation
Pancreatectomy
Parathyroidectomy
Sestamibi scan
Thyroidectomy
Whipple procedure

Gastrointestinal

Antrectomy
Appendectomy
Artificial sphincter insertion
Barium enema
Biliary stenting
Bowel preparation
Bowel resection
Bowel resection, small intestine
Cholecystectomy
Colonic stent
Colonoscopy
Colorectal surgery
Colostomy
Defecography
Diverticulitis
Endoscopic ultrasound
Esophageal atresia repair
Esophageal function tests
Esophageal resection
Esophagogastrectomy
Esophagogastroduodenoscopy
Gastrectomy
Gastric acid inhibitors
Gastric bypass
Gastroduodenostomy

Gastroenterologic surgery

Gastroesophageal reflux scan

Gastroesophageal reflux surgery

Gastrostomy

Glossectomy

Heller myotomy

Hemorrhoidectomy

Hepatectomy

HIDA Scan

Ileoanal anastomosis

Ileoanal reservoir surgery

Ileostomy

Intestinal obstruction repair

Intussusception reduction

Liver biopsy

Liver transplantation

Laxatives

Parotidectomy

Pyloroplasty

Rectal prolapse repair

Rectal resection

Sclerotherapy for esophageal varices

Sigmoidoscopy

Tube enterostomy

Upper GI exam

Vagotomy

Vertical banded gastroplasty

Hematological

ABO blood typing

Alanine aminotransferase test

Albumin Test, Blood

Anticoagulant and antiplatelet drugs

Arterial blood gases (ABG)

Aspartate aminotransferase test

Autologous blood donation

Blood Ca (calcium) level

Blood carbon dioxide level

Blood culture

Blood donation and registry

Bloodless surgery

Blood phosphate level

Blood potassium level

Blood pressure measurement

Blood salvage

Blood sodium level

Blood type test

Blood urea nitrogen test

Bone marrow aspiration and biopsy

Bone marrow transplantation

BUN-creatinine ratio

Chemistry screen

Cholesterol and triglyceride tests

Complete blood count

Creatine phosphokinase (CPK)

Electrolyte tests

Enhanced external counterpulsation

Hematocrit

Hemoglobin test

Hemoperfusion

Human leukocyte antigen test

LDL cholesterol test

Lipid profile

Lipid tests

Liver function tests

Meckel's diverticulectomy

Partial thromboplastin time

Phlebography

Phlebotomy

Photocoagulation therapy

Prothrombin time

Pulse oximeter

Red blood cell indices

Rh blood typing

Rheumatoid factor testing

Sedimentation rate

Serum chloride level

Serum creatinine level

Serum glucose level

Sphygmomanometer

Thrombolytic therapy

Transfusion

Type and screen

White blood cell count and differential

Integumentary

Bedsores

Blepharoplasty

Cleft lip repair

Debridement

Dermabrasion

Face lift

Fasciotomy

Forehead lift

Laceration repair

Laser skin resurfacing

Mohs surgery

Skin grafting

Webbed finger or toe repair

Musculoskeletal

Abdominal wall defect repair

Abdominoplasty

Amputation

Arthrography

Arthroplasty

Arthroscopic surgery

Bankart procedure

Bone grafting

Bone x rays

Bunionectomy

Club foot repair

Craniofacial reconstruction

Disk removal

Eye muscle surgery

Finger reattachment

Fracture repair

Ganglion cyst removal

Hammer, claw, and mallet toe surgery

Hand surgery

Hiatal hernia

Hip osteotomy

Hip replacement

Hip revision surgery

Incisional hernia repair
Inguinal hernia repair
Knee arthroscopic surgery
Knee osteotomy
Knee replacement
Knee revision surgery
Kneecap removal
Laminectomy
Leg lengthening or shortening
Limb salvage
Mastoidectomy
Mentoplasty
Orthopedic surgery
Pectus excavatum repair
Rotator cuff repair
Shoulder joint replacement
Shoulder resection arthroplasty
Skull x rays
Spinal fusion
Spinal instrumentation
Tendon repair
Tenotomy
Traction
Umbilical hernia repair
Wrist replacement

Neurological

Anterior temporal lobectomy
Bispectral index
Carpal tunnel release
Cerebral aneurysm repair
Cerebrospinal fluid (CSF)
  analysis
Corpus callosotomy
Craniotomy
Deep brain stimulation
Electroencephalography
Hemispherectomy
Meningocele repair
Myelography
Neurosurgery
Pallidotomy
Rhizotomy
Stereotactic radiosurgery
Sympathectomy
Vagal nerve stimulation

Reproductive, Female

Abortion, induced
Amniocentesis
Breast biopsy
Breast implants
Breast reconstruction
Breast reduction
Cervical cerclage
Cervical cryotherapy
Cesarean section
Colporrhaphy
Colposcopy
Colpotomy
Cone biopsy
Dilatation and curettage
Episiotomy
Fallopian tube implants
Fetal surgery
Fetoscopy
Hysterectomy
Hysteroscopy
In vitro fertilization
Laparoscopy for endometriosis
Lumpectomy
Mammography
Mastectomy
Modified radical mastectomy
Myomectomy
Obstetric and gynecologic surgery
Oophorectomy
Quadrantectomy
Salpingo-oophorectomy
Salpingostomy
Simple mastectomy
Tubal ligation
Uterine stimulants

Reproductive, Male

Circumcision
Hydrocelectomy
Hypospadias repair

Open prostatectomy
Orchiectomy
Orchiopexy
Penile prostheses
Transurethral resection of the
  prostate
Vasectomy
Vasovasostomy

Respiratory

Bronchoscopy
Chest tube insertion
Cricothyroidotomy
Endoscopic sinus surgery
Endotracheal intubation
Laryngectomy
Lobectomy, pulmonary
Lung biopsy
Lung transplantation
Mantoux test
Mechanical ventilation
Mediastinoscopy
Pharyngectomy
Pneumonectomy
Septoplasty
Snoring surgery
Spirometry tests
Tracheotomy

Sensory

Cochlear implants
Corneal transplantation
Cryotherapy for cataracts
Cyclocryotherapy
Endolymphatic shunt
Enucleation, eye
Extracapsular cataract extraction
Goniotomy
Iridectomy
Laser in-situ keratomileusis
  (LASIK)
Laser iridotomy
Laser posterior capsulotomy
Myringotomy and ear tubes

Ophthalmologic surgery
Ophthalmoscopy
Otoplasty
Phacoemulsification for
cataracts
Photorefractive keratectomy
(PRK)
Retinal cryopexy
Scleral buckling
Sclerostomy
Stapedectomy
Tarsorrhaphy
Trabeculectomy
Tube-shunt surgery
Tympanoplasty

Urinary

Bladder augmentation
Catheterization, female
Catheterization, male
Collagen periurethral injection
Cystectomy
Cystocele repair
Cystoscopy
Gallstone removal
Ileal conduit surgery
Kidney dialysis
Kidney function tests
Kidney transplantation
Lithotripsy
Needle bladder neck suspension
Nephrectomy
Nephrolithotomy, percutaneous
Nephrostomy
Patent urachus repair
Retropubic suspension
Sacral nerve stimulation
Sling procedure
Transurethral bladder
resection
Ureteral stenting
Ureterosigmoidoscopy
Ureterostomy, cutaneous
Urinalysis
Urinary anti-infectives

Urine culture
Urologic surgery

Other Surgeries

Abscess incision and drainage
Axillary dissection
Curettage and electrosurgery
Ear, nose, and throat surgery
Elective surgery
Emergency surgery
Essential surgery
Exenteration
General surgery
Gingivectomy
Laparoscopy
Laparotomy, exploratory
Laser surgery
Lymphadenectomy
Microsurgery
Necessary surgery
Omphalocele repair
Outpatient surgery
Pediatric surgery
Plastic, reconstructive, and
cosmetic surgery
Radical neck dissection
Rhinoplasty
Robot-assisted surgery
Root canal treatment
Scar revision surgery
Second-look surgery
Segmentectomy
Sex reassignment surgery
Splenectomy
Telesurgery
Thoracic surgery
Thoracotomy
Tonsillectomy
Tooth extraction
Tooth replantation
Trabeculectomy
Transplant surgery
Tumor removal

Other Tests & Procedures

Abdominal ultrasound
Anaerobic bacteria culture
Antibody tests, immunoglobulins
Biofeedback
Chest x ray
Cryotherapy
CT scans
Dental implants
Epidural therapy
Glucose tests
Hair transplantation
Immunoassay tests
Immunologic therapies
Intravenous rehydration
Liposuction
Magnetic resonance imaging
Medication Monitoring
Mental health assessment
Oxygen therapy
Paracentesis
Parentage testing
Pelvic ultrasound
Peritoneovenous shunt
pH monitoring
Physical examination
Positron emission tomography
(PET)
Sentinel lymph node biopsy
Temperature measurement
Tumor marker tests
Ultrasound
Weight management

Drugs

Acetaminophen
Adrenergic drugs
Analgesics
Analgesics, opioid
Anesthesia evaluation
Anesthesia, general
Anesthesia, local

PLEASE READ—IMPORTANT INFORMATION

The *Gale Encyclopedia of Surgery and Medical Tests, 2ⁿᵈ Edition* is a health reference product designed to inform and educate readers about a wide variety of surgeries, tests, diseases and conditions, treatments and drugs, equipment, and other issues associated with surgical and medical practice. Cengage Learning believes the product to be comprehensive, but not necessarily definitive. It is intended to supplement, not replace, consultation with physicians or other healthcare practitioners. While Cengage Learning has made substantial efforts to provide information that is accurate, comprehensive, and up-to-date, Cengage Learning makes no representations or warranties of any kind, including without limitation, warranties of merchantability or fitness for a particular purpose, nor does it guarantee the accuracy, comprehensiveness, or timeliness of the information contained in this product. Readers should be aware that the universe of medical knowledge is constantly growing and changing, and that differences of opinion exist among authorities. Readers are also advised to seek professional diagnosis and treatment for any medical condition, and to discuss information obtained from this book with their healthcare provider.

INTRODUCTION

The *Gale Encyclopedia of Surgery and Medical Tests, 2nd Edition* is a unique and invaluable source of information. This collection of 535 entries provides in-depth coverage of various issues related to surgery, medical tests, diseases and conditions, hospitalization, and general health care. These entries generally follow a standard format, including a definition, purpose, demographics, description, diagnosis/preparation, aftercare, precautions, risks, side effects, interactions, morbidity and mortality rates, alternatives, normal results, questions to ask your doctor, and information about who performs the procedures and where they are performed. Topics of a more general nature related to surgical hospitalization and medical testing round out the set. Examples of this coverage include entries on Adult day care, Ambulatory surgery centers, Death and dying, Discharge from the hospital, Do not resuscitate (DNR) order, Exercise, Finding a surgeon, Hospice, Hospital services, Informed consent, Living will, Long-term care insurance, Managed care plans, Medicaid, Medicare, Patient rights, Planning a hospital stay, Power of attorney, Private insurance plans, Second opinion, Talking to the doctor, and others.

Scope

The *Gale Encyclopedia of Surgery and Medical Tests, 2nd Edition* covers a wide variety of topics relevant to the user. Entries follow a standardized format that provides information at a glance. Rubrics include the following (not every entry will make use of all of them):

- Definition
- Description
- Purpose
- Demographics
- Diagnosis/preparation
- Aftercare
- Precautions
- Risks
- Side effects
- Interactions
- Morbidity and mortality rates
- Alternatives
- Normal results
- "Questions to ask the doctor"
- "Who performs the procedure and where is it performed?"
- Resources
- Key Terms

Inclusion criteria

A preliminary list of topics was compiled from a wide variety of sources, including health reference books, general medical encyclopedias, and consumer health guides. The advisory board evaluated the topics and made suggestions for inclusion. Final selection of topics to include was made by the advisory board in conjunction with the editor.

About the contributors

The essays were compiled by experienced medical writers, including medical doctors, pharmacists, and registered nurses. The advisers reviewed the completed essays to ensure that they are appropriate, up-to-date, and accurate.

How to use this book

The *Gale Encyclopedia of Surgery and Medical Tests, 2nd Edition* has been designed with ready reference in mind.

- Straight **alphabetical arrangement** of topics allows users to locate information quickly.
- **Bold-faced terms** within entries direct the reader to related articles.
- **Cross-references** placed throughout the encyclopedia direct readers from alternate names and related topics to entries.
- A list of **Key terms** is provided where appropriate to define terms or concepts that may be unfamiliar to the user. A **glossary** of key terms in the back of the fourth volume contains a concise list of terms arranged alphabetically.
- The **Resources** section directs readers to additional sources of information on a topic.
- Valuable **contact information** for health organizations is included with most entries. An Appendix of **organizations** in the back of the fourth volume contains an extensive list of organizations arranged alphabetically.
- A comprehensive **general index** guides readers to significant topics mentioned in the text.

Graphics

The *Gale Encyclopedia of Surgery and Medical Tests, 2nd Edition* is also enhanced by color photographs, illustrations, and tables.

Acknowledgements

The editor wishes to thank all of the people who contributed to this encyclopedia. There are too many names to list here, so the reader is urged to review the Advisory board and Contributors pages for the list of writers, physicians, and health-care experts to whom he is indebted. Special thanks must go to Rosalyn Carson-DeWitt for all the writing, updating, and advising she did; the project could not have been completed without her. L. Fleming Fallon provided invaluable assistance at every step of the way; his writing, advice, and good humor made this project a pleasure. Laurie Cataldo's expertise in so many areas helped make this book as good as it is. And Maria Basile provided not only many beautifully written entries, but she performed some last-minute review work for which the editor is most grateful. To all of you, my deepest thanks.

ADVISORS

A number of experts in the medical community provided invaluable assistance in the formulation of this encyclopedia. Our advisory board performed a myriad of duties, from defining the scope of coverage to reviewing individual entries for accuracy and accessibility. The editor would like to express his appreciation to them.

Rosalyn Carson-DeWitt, MD
Medical Writer
Durham, NC

Laura Jean Cataldo, RN, EdD
Nurse, Medical Consultant,
Educator
Germantown, MD

L. Fleming Fallon, Jr, MD, DrPH
Professor of Public Health

Bowling Green State University
Bowling Green, OH

Chitra Venkatasubramanian, MD
Clinical Assistant Professor,
Neurology and Neurological
Sciences
Stanford University School of
Medicine
Palo Alto, CA

CONTRIBUTORS

Laurie Barclay, MD
Neurological Consulting
  Services
Tampa, FL

Jeanine Barone
Nutritionist, Exercise Physiologist
New York, NY

Julia Barrett
Science Writer
Madison, WI

Donald G. Barstow, RN
Clinical Nurse Specialist
Oklahoma City, OK

Maria Basile, PhD
Neuropharmacologist
Roselle, NJ

Mary Bekker
Medical Writer
Willow Grove, PA

**Mark A. Best, MD, MPH,
  MBA**
Associate Professor of Pathology
St. Matthew's University
Grand Cayman, BWI

Randall J. Blazic, MD, DDS
Oral and Maxillofacial Surgeon
Goodyear, AZ

Robert Bockstiegel
Medical Writer
Portland, OR

Maggie Boleyn, RN, BSN
Medical Writer
Oak Park, MN

Susan Joanne Cadwallader
Medical Writer
Cedarburg, WI

Diane M. Calabrese
*Medical Sciences and Technology
  Writer*
Silver Spring, MD

Richard H. Camer
Editor
International Medical News Group
Silver Spring, MD

Rosalyn Carson-DeWitt, MD
Medical Writer
Durham, NC

Laura Jean Cataldo, RN, EdD
*Nurse, Medical Consultant,
  Educator*
Germantown, MD

Lisa Christenson, Ph.D.
Science Writer
Hamden, CT

Rhonda Cloos, RN
Medical Writer
Austin, TX

Constance Clyde
Medical Writer
Dana Point, CA

Angela M. Costello
Medical writer
Cleveland, OH

L. Lee Culvert, PhD
Health writer
Alna, ME

Tish Davidson, AM
Medical Writer
Fremont, CA

Lori De Milto
Medical Writer
Sicklerville, NJ

Victoria E. DeMoranville
Medical Writer
Lakeville, MA

Altha Roberts Edgren
Medical Writer
Medical Ink
St. Paul, MN

Lorraine K. Ehresman
Medical Writer
Northfield, Quebec, Canada

Abraham F. Ettaher, MD

**L. Fleming Fallon, Jr, MD,
  DrPH**
Professor of Public Health
Bowling Green State
  University
Bowling Green, OH

Paula Ford-Martin
Medical Writer
Warwick, RI

Janie F. Franz
Journalist
Grand Forks, ND

Rebecca J. Frey, PhD
Medical Writer
New Haven, CT

Debra Gordon
Medical Writer
Nazareth, PA

Jill Granger, MS
Sr. Research Associate
Dept. of Pathology
University of Michigan Medical
  Center
Ann Arbor, MI

Peter Gregutt
Medical Writer
Asheville, NC

Laith Farid Gulli, MD, MS
Consultant Psychotherapist in Private Practice
Lathrup Village, MI

Stephen John Hage, AAAS, RT(R), FAHRA
Medical Writer
Chatsworth, CA

Maureen Haggerty
Medical Writer
Ambler, PA

Robert Harr
Associate Professor and Chair
Department of Public and Allied Health
Bowling Green State University
Bowling Green, OH

Dan Harvey
Medical Writer
Wilmington, DE

Katherine Hauswirth, APRN
Medical Writer
Deep River, CT

Caroline A. Helwick
Medical Writer
New Orleans, LA

Lisette Hilton
Medical Writer
Boca Raton, FL

Fran Hodgkins
Medical Writer
Sparks, MD

René A. Jackson, RN
Medical Writer
Port Charlotte, FL

Nadine M. Jacobson, RN
Medical Writer
Takoma Park, MD

Randi B. Jenkins, BA
Copy Chief
Fission Communications
New York, NY

Michelle L. Johnson, MS, JD
Patent Attorney
ZymoGenetics, Inc.
Seattle, WA

Paul Johnson
Medical Writer
San Diego, CA

Cindy L. A. Jones, PhD
Biomedical Writer
Sagescript Communications
Lakewood, CO

Linda D. Jones, BA, PBT (ASCP)
Medical Writer
Asheboro, NY

Crystal H. Kaczkowski, MSc
Health writer
Chicago, IL

Beth A. Kapes
Medical Writer
Bay Village, OH

Mary Jeanne Krob, MD, FACS
Physician, writer
Pittsburgh, PA

Monique Laberge, PhD
Sr. Res. Investigator
Dept. of Biochemistry & Biophysics, School of Medicine
University of Pennsylvania
Philadelphia, PA

Richard H. Lampert
Senior Medical Editor
W.B. Saunders Co.
Philadelphia, PA

Renee Laux, MS
Medical Writer
Manlius, NY

Victor Leipzig, PhD
Biological Consultant
Huntington Beach, CA

Lorraine Lica, PhD
Medical Writer
San Diego, CA

John T. Lohr, PhD
Assistant Director, Biotechnology Center
Utah State University
Logan, UT

Jennifer Lee Losey, RN
Medical Writer
Madison Heights, MI

Nicole Mallory, MS, PA-C
Medical Student, Wayne State University
Detroit, MI

Jacqueline N. Martin, MS
Medical Writer
Albrightsville, PA

Nancy McKenzie, PhD
Public Health Consultant
Brooklyn, NY

Mercedes McLaughlin
Medical Writer
Phoenixville, CA

Miguel A. Melgar, MD, PhD
Neurosurgeon
New Orleans, LA

Christine Miner Minderovic, BS, RT, RDMS
Medical Writer
Ann Arbor, MI

Mark Mitchell, MD, MPH, MBA
Medical Writer
Bothell, WA

Alfredo Mori, MD, FACEM, FFAEM
Emergency Physician
The Alfred Hospital
Victoria, Australia

Bilal Nasser, MD, MS
Senior Medical Student, Wayne State University
Detroit, MI

Erika J. Norris
Medical Writer
Oak Harbor, WA

Teresa Norris, RN
Medical Writer
Ute Park, NM

Debra Novograd, BS, RT(R)(M)
Medical Writer
Royal Oak, MI

Jane E. Phillips, PhD
Medical Writer
Chapel Hill, NC

J. Ricker Polsdorfer, MD
Medical Writer
Phoenix, AZ

Elaine R. Proseus, MBA/TM, BSRT, RT(R)
Medical Writer
Farmington Hills, MI

Robert Ramirez, BS
Medical Student
University of Medicine &
    Dentistry of New Jersey
Stratford, NJ

Esther Csapo Rastegari, RN, BSN, EdM
Medical Writer
Holbrook, MA

Martha Reilly, OD
*Clinical Optometrist, Medical
    Writer*
Madison, WI

Toni Rizzo
Medical Writer
Salt Lake City, UT

Richard Robinson
Medical Writer
Sherborn, MA

Nancy Ross-Flanigan
Science Writer
Belleville, MI

Belinda Rowland, PhD
Medical Writer
Voorheesville, NY

Laura Ruth, PhD
*Medical, Science, & Technology
    Writer*
Los Angeles, CA

Uchechukwu Sampson, MD, MPH, MBA

Kausalya Santhanam, PhD
Technical Writer
Branford, CT

Joan M. Schonbeck
Medical Writer
Nursing
Massachusetts Department of
    Mental Health
Marlborough, MA

Stephanie Dionne Sherk
Medical Writer
University of Michigan
Ann Arbor, MI

Lee A. Shratter, MD
Consulting Radiologist
Kentfield, CA

Jennifer E. Sisk, MA
Medical Writer
Havertown, PA

Allison Joan Spiwak, MSBME
Circulation Technologist
The Ohio State University
Columbus, OH

Kurt Richard Sternlof
Science Writer
New Rochelle, NY

Margaret A Stockley, RGN
Medical Writer
Boxborough, MA

Dorothy Elinor Stonely
Medical Writer
Los Gatos, CA

Bethany Thivierge
Biotechnical Writer and Editor
Technicality Resources
Rockland, ME

Carol A. Turkington
Medical Writer
Lancaster, PA

Samuel D. Uretsky, PharmD
Medical Writer
Wantagh, NY

Chitra Venkatasubramanian, MD
*Clinical Assistant Professor,
    Neurology and Neurological
    Sciences*
Stanford University School of
    Medicine
Palo Alto, CA

Ellen S. Weber, MSN
Medical Writer
Fort Wayne, IN

Barbara Wexler
Medical Writer
Chatsworth, CA

Abby Wojahn, RN, BSN, CCRN
Medical Writer
Milwaukee, WI

Kathleen D. Wright, RN
Medical Writer
Delmar, DE

Mary Zoll, PhD
Science Writer
Newton Center, MA

Michael Zuck, PhD
Medical Writer
Boulder, CO

L

Laceration repair

Definition

Laceration repair includes all the steps required to treat a wound in order to promote healing and minimize the risks of infection, premature splitting of sutures (dehiscence), and poor cosmetic result.

Purpose

A laceration is a wound caused by a sharp object producing edges that may be jagged, dirty, or bleeding. Lacerations most often affect the skin, but any tissue may be lacerated, including subcutaneous fat, tendon, muscle, or bone.

A laceration should be repaired if it:

- Continues to bleed after application of pressure for 10–15 minutes.
- Is more than one-eighth (0.125 in, or 0.3 cm) to one-fourth inch (0.25 in, or 0.6 cm) deep.
- Exposes fat, muscle, tendon, or bone.
- Causes a change in function surrounding the area of the laceration.
- Is dirty or has visible debris in it.
- Is located in an area where an unsightly scar is undesirable.

Lacerations are less likely to become infected if they are repaired soon after they occur. Many physicians will not repair a laceration that is more than eight hours old because the risk of infection is too great.

Description

Laceration repair mends a tear in the skin or other tissue. The four goals of laceration repair are to stop bleeding, prevent infection, preserve function, and restore appearance.

The laceration is cleaned by removing any foreign material or debris. Removing foreign objects from penetrating wounds can sometimes cause bleeding, so this type of wound must be cleaned very carefully. The wound is then irrigated with saline solution and a disinfectant. The disinfecting agent may be mild soap or a commercial preparation. An antibacterial agent may be applied.

Once the wound has been cleansed, the physician anesthetizes the area of the repair. Most lacerations are anesthetized by local injection of lidocaine, with or without epinephrine, into the wound edges. Lidocaine without epinephrine is used in areas with limited blood supply such as fingers, toes, ears, penis, and nose, because epinephrine could cause constriction of blood vessels (vasoconstriction) and interfere with the supply of blood to the laceration site. Alternatively, a topical anesthetic combination such as lidocaine, epinephrine, and tetracaine may also be used.

The physician may trim edges that are jagged or extremely uneven. Tissue that is too damaged to heal must be removed (**debridement**) to prevent infection. If the laceration is deep, several absorbable **stitches** (sutures) are placed in the tissue under the skin to help bring the tissue layers together. Suturing also helps eliminate any pockets where tissue fluid or blood can accumulate. The skin wound is closed with sutures. Suture material used on the surface of a wound is usually non-absorbable and will have to be removed later. A light dressing or an adhesive bandage is applied for 24–48 hours. In areas where a dressing is not feasible, an antibiotic ointment can be applied. If the laceration is the result of a human or animal bite, if it is very dirty, or if the patient has a medical condition that alters wound healing, a broad-spectrum antibiotic may be prescribed.

Newer types of laceration repair do not require sutures. Materials such as **staples** or dermabond **glue**

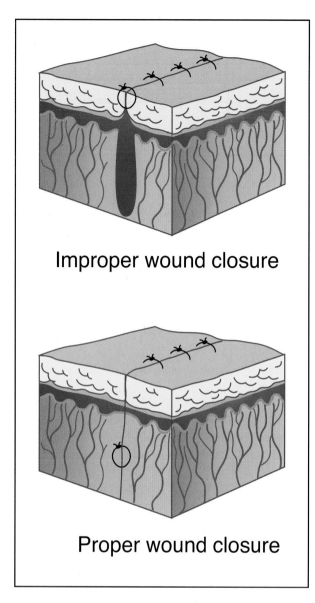

Improper wound closure

Proper wound closure

A laceration is a traumatic break in the skin caused by a sharp object producing edges that may be jagged, dirty or bleeding. The underlying tissue may also be severed. In such instances, the physician may place absorbable sutures in the tissue to help bring the edges together before the skin is sutured closed. *(Illustration by Electronic Illustrators Group. Cengage Learning, Gale.)*

may be used to hold the edges of a laceration together, allowing the edges to knit together.

Diagnosis/Preparation

Preparation for laceration repair involves inspecting the wound and the underlying tendons or nerves to evaluate the risk of infection, the degree of tissue damage, the need for debridement, and its complexity. If hair is located in or around the wound, it is usually removed to minimize contamination and allow for good visibility of the wound. If nerves or tendons have been injured, a surgeon may be needed to complete the repair.

Aftercare

The laceration is kept clean and dry for at least 24 hours after the repair. Light bathing is generally permitted after 24 hours if the wound is not soaked. The physician will provide directions for any special **wound care**. Sutures are removed three to 14 days after the repair is completed. Timing of suture removal depends on the location of the laceration and physician preference.

The repair should be examined frequently for signs of infection, which include redness, swelling, tenderness, drainage from the wound, red streaks in the skin surrounding the repair, chills, or fever. If any of these occur, the physician should be contacted immediately.

Risks

The most serious risk associated with laceration repair is infection. Risk of infection depends on the nature of the wound and the type of injury sustained. Infection risks are increased in wounds that are contaminated with soil or fecal matter, are the result of bites, have been open longer than one hour, or are located on the extremities or on the region between the thighs, genitalia, or other areas where opposing skin surfaces touch and may rub.

Normal results

All lacerations will heal with a scar. Wounds that are repaired with sutures are less likely to develop scars that are unsightly, but it cannot be predicted how wounds will heal and who will develop unsightly scars. **Plastic surgery** can improve the appearance of many scars.

Alternatives

The only alternative to laceration repair is to leave the wound without medical treatment. This increases the risk of infection, poor healing, and an undesirable cosmetic result.

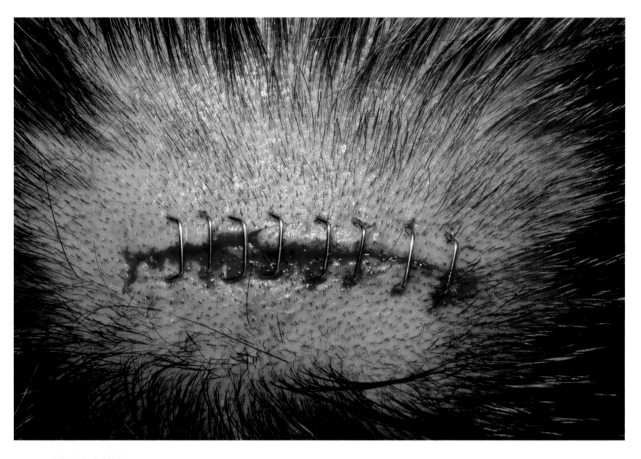

Close-up view of scalp laceration, closed with staples. *(Scott Camazine/Phototake. Reproduced by permission.)*

KEY TERMS

Debridement—The act of removing any foreign material and damaged or contaminated tissue from a wound to expose surrounding healthy tissue.

Dehiscence—A premature bursting open or splitting along natural or surgical suture lines. A complication of surgery that occurs secondary to poor wound healing.

Laceration—A torn, ragged, mangled wound.

Sutures—Materials used in closing a surgical or traumatic wound.

Vasoconstriction—The diminution of the diameter of blood vessels, leading to decreased blood flow to a part of the body.

Resources

BOOKS

Marx, John A., et al. Rosen's Emergency Medicine.6th ed. St. Louis, MO: Mosby, Inc., 2006.

PERIODICALS

Beredjiklian, P. K. "Biologic Aspects of Flexor Tendon Laceration and Repair." The Journal of Bone and Joint Surgery 85-A (March 2003): 539–550.

Gordon, C. A. "Reducing Needle-stick Injuries with the Use of 2-octyl Cyanoacrylates for Laceration Repair." Journal of the American Academy of Nurse Practitioners 13 (January 2001): 10–12.

Klein, E. J., D. S. Diekema, C. A. Paris, L. Quan, M. Cohen, and K. D. Seidel. "A Randomized, Clinical Trial of Oral Midazolam Plus Placebo Versus Oral Midazolam Plus Oral Transmucosal Fentanyl for Sedation during Laceration Repair." Pediatrics 109 (May 2002): 894–897.

Pratt, A. L., N. Burr, and A. O. Grobbelaar. "A Prospective Review of Open Central Slip Laceration Repair and Rehabilitation." The Journal of Hand Surgery: Journal of the British Society for Surgery of the Hand 27 (December 2002): 530–534.

Singer, A. J., J. V. Quinn, H. C. Thode Jr., and J. E. Hollander. "Determinants of Poor Outcome after Laceration and Surgical Incision Repair." Plastic and Reconstructive Surgery 110 (August 2002): 429–437.

ORGANIZATIONS

The Association of Perioperative Registered Nurses, Inc. (AORN). 2170 South Parker Rd, Suite 300, Denver, CO 80231-5711. (800) 755-2676. http://www.aorn.org/.

WHO PERFORMS THE
PROCEDURE AND WHERE IS IT
PERFORMED?

Primary care physicians, emergency room physicians, and surgeons usually repair lacerations. All physicians are trained in the basics of wound assessment, cleansing, and anesthesia. They are also familiar with the basic suturing techniques and have the experience required to attend to the details of wound repair, such as proper selection and preparation of equipment, careful wound preparation, appropriate use of specific closure methods, and effective patient education, required to avoid wound infection and excessive scarring.

Laceration repair is routinely performed in hospitals and clinics on an outpatient basis.

QUESTIONS TO ASK THE
DOCTOR

- How will my wound be repaired?
- Will the procedure hurt?
- How can I avoid infection after surgery?
- Will I be able to wash the wound?
- What are the possible complications?
- How long will it take to heal?
- Will there be a scar?
- When can the sutures be removed?

OTHER

"Cuts and Scrapes." Mayo Clinic Online. http://www.mayo clinic.com/invoke.cfm?objectid = FDEFD23A-F29F-47FB-9A7CD4CF4427D590.

"A Systematic Approach to Laceration Repair." Postgraduate Medicine Page. http://www.postgradmed.com/issues/2000/04_00/wilson.htm.

"Wound Repair." Family Practice Notebook. http://www.fpnotebook.com/SUR18.htm.

Mary Jeanne Krob, MD, FACS
Monique Laberge, PhD
Rosalyn Carson-DeWitt, MD

Lactate dehydrogenase isoenzymes test *see*
Liver function tests

Laminectomy

Definition

A laminectomy is a surgical procedure in which the surgeon removes a portion of the bony arch, or lamina, on the dorsal surface of a vertebra, which is one of the bones that make up the human spinal column. It is done to relieve back pain that has not been helped by more conservative treatments. In most cases a laminectomy is an elective procedure rather than **emergency surgery**. A laminectomy for relief of pain in the lower back is called a lumbar laminectomy or an open decompression.

Purpose

Structure of the spine

In order to understand why removal of a piece of bone from the arch of a vertebra relieves pain, it is helpful to have a brief description of the structure of the spinal column and the vertebrae themselves. In humans, the spine comprises 33 vertebrae, some of which are fused together. There are seven vertebrae in the cervical (neck) part of the spine; 12 vertebrae in the thoracic (chest) region; five in the lumbar (lower back) region; five vertebrae that are fused to form the sacrum; and four vertebrae that are fused to form the coccyx, or tailbone. It is the vertebrae in the lumbar portion of the spine that are most likely to be affected by the disorders that cause back pain.

The 24 vertebrae that are not fused are stacked vertically in an S-shaped column that extends from the tailbone below the waist up to the back of the head. This column is held in alignment by ligaments, cartilage, and muscles. About half the weight of a person's body is carried by the spinal column itself and the other half by the muscles and ligaments that hold the spine in alignment. The bony arches of the laminae on each vertebra form a canal that contains and protects the spinal cord. The spinal cord extends from the base of the brain to the upper part of the lumbar spine, where it ends in a collection of nerve fibers known as the cauda equina, which is a Latin phrase meaning "horse's tail." Other nerves branching out from the spinal cord pass through openings formed by adjoining vertebrae. These openings are known as foramina (singular, foramen).

Between each vertebra is a disk that serves to cushion the vertebrae when a person bends, stretches, or twists the spinal column. The disks also keep the foramina between the vertebrae open so that the spinal nerves can pass through without being pinched or

Laminectomy

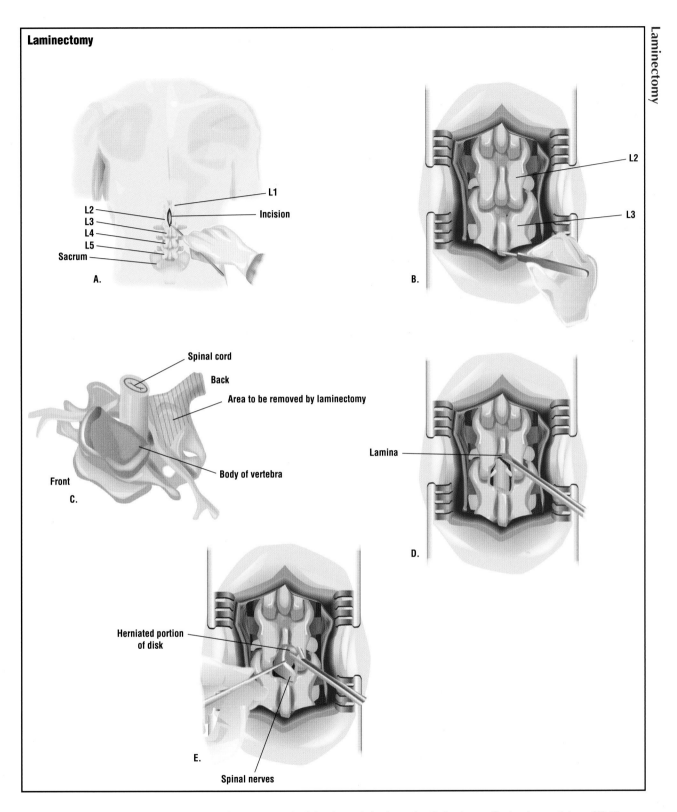

In this posterior (from the back) lumbar laminectomy, an incision is made in the patient's back over the lumbar vertebrae (A). The wound is opened with retractors to expose the L2 and L3 vertebrae (B). A piece of bone at the back of the vertebrae is removed (C and D), allowing a damaged disk to be repaired (E). *(Illustration by GGS Information Services. Cengage Learning, Gale.)*

KEY TERMS

Cauda equina—The collection of spinal nerve roots that lie inside the spinal column below the end of the spinal cord. The name comes from the Latin for "horse's tail."

Cauda equina syndrome (CES)—A group of symptoms characterized by numbness or pain in the legs and/or loss of bladder and bowel control, caused by compression and paralysis of the nerve roots in the cauda equina. CES is a medical emergency.

Chiropractic—A system of therapy based on the notion that health and disease are related to the interactions between the brain and the nervous system. Treatment involves manipulation and adjustment of the segments of the spinal column. Chiropractic is considered a form of alternative medicine.

Decompression—Any surgical procedure done to relieve pressure on a nerve or other part of the body. A laminectomy is sometimes called an open decompression.

Dorsal—Referring to a position closer to the back than to the stomach. The laminae in the spinal column are located on the dorsal side of each vertebra.

Dura—A tough fibrous membrane that covers and protects the spinal cord.

Foramen (plural, foramina)—The medical term for a natural opening or passage. The foramina of the spinal column are openings between the vertebrae for the spinal nerves to branch off from the spinal cord.

Laminae (singular, lamina)—The broad plates of bone on the upper surface of the vertebrae that fuse together at the midline to form a bony covering over the spinal canal.

Laminotomy—A less invasive alternative to a laminectomy in which a hole is drilled through the lamina.

Ligamenta flava (singular, ligamentum flavum)—A series of bands of tissue that are attached to the vertebrae in the spinal column. They help to hold the spine straight and to close the spaces between the laminar arches. The Latin name means "yellow band(s)."

Lumbar—Pertaining to the part of the back between the chest and the pelvis.

Myelogram—A special type of x ray study of the spinal cord, made after a contrast medium has been injected into the space surrounding the cord.

Osteopathy—A system of therapy that uses standard medical and surgical methods of diagnosis and treatment while emphasizing the importance of proper body alignment and manipulative treatment of musculoskeletal disorders. Osteopathy is considered mainstream primary care medicine rather than an alternative system.

Pain disorder—A psychiatric disorder in which pain in one or more parts of the body is caused or made worse by psychological factors. The lower back is one of the most common sites for pain related to this disorder.

Retractor—An instrument used during surgery to hold an incision open and pull back underlying layers of tissue.

Sciatica—Pain in the lower back, buttock, or leg along the course of the sciatic nerve.

Somatization disorder—A chronic condition in which psychological stresses are converted into physical symptoms that interfere with work and relationships. Lower back pain is a frequent complaint of patients with somatization disorder.

Spinal stenosis—Narrowing of the canals in the vertebrae or around the nerve roots, causing pressure on the spinal cord and nerves.

Vertebra (plural, vertebrae)—One of the bones of the spinal column. There are 33 vertebrae in the human spine.

damaged. As people age, the intervertebral disks begin to lose moisture and break down, which reduces the size of the foramina between the vertebrae. In addition, bone spurs may form inside the vertebrae and cause the spinal canal itself to become narrower. Either of these processes can compress the spinal nerves, leading to pain, tingling sensations, or weakness in the lower back and legs. A lumbar laminectomy relieves pressure on the spinal nerves by removing the disk, piece of bone, tumor, or other structure that is causing the compression.

Causes of lower back pain

The disks and vertebrae in the lower back are particularly vulnerable to the effects of aging and daily wear and tear because they bear the full weight of the upper body, even when one is sitting quietly in a chair. When a person bends forward, 50% of the motion occurs at the hips, but the remaining 50% involves the lumbar spine. The force exerted in bending is not evenly divided among the five lumbar vertebrae; the segments between the third and fourth lumbar vertebrae (L3-L4) and the fourth and fifth (L4-L5) are most likely to break down over time. More than 95% of spinal disk operations are performed on the fourth and fifth lumbar vertebrae.

Specific symptoms and disorders that affect the lower back include:

- Sciatica. Sciatica refers to sudden pain felt as radiating from the lower back through the buttocks and down the back of one leg. The pain, which may be experienced as weakness in the leg, a tingling feeling, or a "pins and needles" sensation, runs along the course of the sciatic nerve. Sciatica is a common symptom of a herniated disk.

- Spinal stenosis. Spinal stenosis is a disorder that results from the narrowing of the spinal canal surrounding the spinal cord and eventually compressing the cord. It may result from hereditary factors, from the effects of aging, or from changes in the pattern of blood flow to the lower back. Spinal stenosis is sometimes difficult to diagnose because its early symptoms can be caused by a number of other conditions and because the patient usually has no history of back problems or recent injuries. Imaging studies may be necessary for accurate diagnosis.

- Cauda equina syndrome (CES). Cauda equina syndrome is a rare disorder caused when a ruptured disk, bone fracture, or spinal stenosis put intense pressure on the cauda equina, the collection of spinal nerve roots at the lower end of the spinal cord. CES may be triggered by a fall, automobile accident, or penetrating gunshot injury. It is characterized by loss of sensation or altered sensation in the legs, buttocks, or feet; pain, numbness, or weakness in one or both legs; difficulty walking; or loss of control over bladder and bowel functions. *Cauda equina syndrome is a medical emergency requiring immediate treatment.* If the pressure on the nerves in the cauda equina is not relieved quickly, permanent paralysis and loss of bladder or bowel control may result.

- Herniated disk. The disks between the vertebrae in the spine consist of a fibrous outer part called the annulus and a softer inner nucleus. A disk is said to herniate when the nucleus ruptures and is forced through the outer annulus into the spaces between the vertebrae. The material that is forced out may put pressure on the nerve roots or compress the spinal cord itself. In other cases, the chemicals leaking from the ruptured nucleus may irritate or inflame the spinal nerves. More than 80% of herniated disks affect the spinal nerves associated with the L5 vertebra or the first sacral vertebra.

- Osteoarthritis (OA). OA is a disorder in which the cartilage in the hips, knees, and other joints gradually breaks down, allowing the surfaces of the bones to rub directly against each other. In the spine, OA may result in thickening of the ligaments surrounding the spinal column. As the ligaments increase in size, they may begin to compress the spinal cord.

Factors that increase a person's risk of developing pain in the lower back include:

- Hereditary factors. Some people are born with relatively narrow spinal canals and may develop spinal stenosis fairly early in life.

- Sex. Men are at greater risk of lower back problems than women, in part because they carry a greater proportion of their total body weight in the upper body.

- Age. The intervertebral disks tend to lose their moisture content and become thinner as people get older.

- Occupation. Jobs that require long periods of driving (long-distance trucking; bus, taxi, or limousine operation) are hard on the lower back because of vibrations from the road surface transmitted upward to the spine. Occupations that require heavy lifting (nursing, child care, construction work, airplane maintenance) put extra stress on the lumbar vertebrae. Other high-risk occupations include professional sports, professional dance, assembly line work, foundry work, mining, and mail or package delivery.

- Lifestyle. Wearing high-heeled shoes, carrying heavy briefcases or shoulder bags on one side of the body, or sitting for long periods of time in one position can all throw the spine out of alignment.

- Obesity. Being overweight, particularly if the extra pounds are concentrated in the abdomen, adds to the strain on the muscles and ligaments that support the spinal column.

- Trauma. Injuries to the back from contact sports, falls, criminal assaults, or automobile accidents may lead to misalignment of the vertebrae or a ruptured disk. Traumatic injuries may also trigger the onset of cauda equina syndrome.

Demographics

Pain in the lower back is a chronic condition that has been treated in various ways from the beginnings of human medical practice. The earliest description of disorders affecting the lumbar vertebrae was written in 3000 B.C. by an ancient Egyptian surgeon. In the modern world, back pain is responsible for more time lost from work than any other cause except the common cold. Between 10% and 15% of workers' compensation claims are related to chronic pain in the lower back. It is estimated that the direct and indirect costs of back pain to the American economy range between $75 and $80 billion per year.

In the United States, about 13 million people seek medical help each year for the condition. According to the Centers for Disease Control, 14% of all new visits to primary care doctors are related to problems in the lower back. The CDC estimates that 2.4 million adults in the United States are chronically disabled by back pain, with another 2.4 million temporarily disabled. About 80% of people will experience pain in the lower back at some point in their lifetime; on a yearly basis, one person in every five will have some kind of back pain.

Back pain primarily affects the adult population, most commonly people between the ages of 45 and 64. It is more common among men than women, and more common among Caucasians and Hispanics than among African Americans or Asian Americans.

Description

A laminectomy is performed with the patient under **general anesthesia**, usually positioned lying on the side or stomach. The surgeon begins by making a small straight incision over the damaged vertebra.

The surgeon next uses a retractor to spread apart the muscles and fatty tissue overlying the spine. When the laminae have been reached, the surgeon cuts away part of the bony arch in order to expose the ligamentum flavum, which is a band of yellow tissue attached to the vertebra that helps to support the spinal column and closes in the spaces between the vertebral arches. The surgeon then cuts an opening in the ligamentum flavum in order to reach the spinal canal and expose the compressed nerve. At this point the cause of the compression (herniated disk, tumor, bone spur, or a fragment of the disk that has separated from the remainder) will be visible.

Bone spurs, if any, are removed in order to enlarge the foramina and the spinal canal. If the disk is herniated, the surgeon uses the retractor to move the compressed nerve aside and removes as much of the disk as necessary to relieve pressure on the nerve. The space that was occupied by the disk will be filled eventually by new connective tissue.

If necessary, a **spinal fusion** is performed to stabilize the patient's lower back. A small piece of bone taken from the hip is grafted onto the spine and attached with metal screws or plates to support the lumbar vertebrae.

Following completion of the spinal fusion, the surgeon closes the incision in layers, using different types of sutures for the muscles, connective tissues, and skin. The entire procedure takes one to three hours.

Diagnosis/Preparation

Diagnosis

The differential diagnosis of lower back pain is complicated by the number of possible causes and the patient's reaction to the discomfort. In many cases the patient's perception of back pain is influenced by poor-quality sleep or emotional issues related to occupation or family matters. A primary care doctor will begin by taking a careful medical and occupational history, asking about the onset of the pain as well as its location and other characteristics. Back pain associated with the lumbar spine very often affects the patient's ability to move, and the muscles overlying the affected vertebrae may feel sore or tight. Pain resulting from heavy lifting usually begins within 24 hours of the overexertion. Most patients who do not have a history of chronic pain in the lower back feel better after 48 hours of bed rest with pain medication and either a heating pad or ice pack to relax muscle spasms.

If the patient's pain is not helped by rest and other conservative treatments, he or she will be referred to an orthopedic surgeon for a more detailed evaluation. An orthopedic evaluation includes a **physical examination**, neurological workup, and imaging studies. In the physical examination, the doctor will ask the patient to sit, stand, or walk in order to see how these functions are affected by the pain. The patient may be asked to cough or to lie on a table and lift each leg in turn without bending the knee, as these maneuvers can help to diagnose nerve root disorders. The doctor will also palpate (feel) the patient's spinal column and the overlying muscles and ligaments to determine the external location of any tender spots, bruises, thickening of the ligaments, or other structural abnormalities. The neurological workup will focus on the patient's reflexes and the spinal nerves that affect the functioning of the legs. Imaging studies for lower back pain typically include an x-ray study and CT scan of the lower spine, which will reveal bone deformities, narrowing of the intervertebral disks, and loss of cartilage. An MRI may be ordered if spinal stenosis is suspected. In some cases the doctor may order a myelogram, which is an x ray or CT scan of the lumbar spine performed after a special dye has been injected into the spinal fluid.

Lower back pain is one of several common general medical conditions that require the doctor to assess the possibility that the patient has a concurrent psychiatric disorder. Such diagnoses as somatization disorder or pain disorder do not mean that the patient's physical symptoms are imaginary or that they should not receive surgical or medical treatment. Rather, a psychiatric diagnosis indicates that the patient is allowing the back pain to become the central focus of life or responding to it in other problematic ways. Some researchers in Europe as well as North America think that the frequency of lower back problems in workers' disability claims reflect emotional dissatisfaction with work as well as physical stresses related to specific jobs.

Preparation

Most hospitals require patients to have the following tests before a laminectomy: a complete physical examination; **complete blood count** (CBC); an **electrocardiogram** (EKG); a urine test; and tests that measure the speed of blood clotting.

Aspirin and arthritis medications should be discontinued seven to 10 days before a laminectomy because they thin the blood and affect clotting time. Patients should provide the surgeon and anesthesiologist with a complete list of all medications, including over-the-counter and herbal preparations, that they take on a regular basis.

The patient is asked to stop smoking at least a week before surgery and to take nothing by mouth after midnight before the procedure.

Aftercare

Aftercare following a laminectomy begins in the hospital. Most patients will remain in the hospital for one to three days after the procedure. During this period the patient will be given fluids and antibiotic medications intravenously to prevent infection. Medications for pain will be given every three to four hours, or through a device known as a PCA (patient-controlled anesthesia). The PCA is a small pump that delivers a dose of medication into the IV when the patient pushes a button. To get the lungs back to normal functioning, a respiratory therapist will ask the patient to do some simple breathing exercises and begin walking within several hours of surgery.

Aftercare during the hospital stay is also intended to lower the risk of a venous thromboembolism (VTE), or blood clot in the deep veins of the leg.

Prevention of VTE involves medications to thin the blood and wearing compression stockings or boots.

Most surgeons prefer to see patients one week after surgery to remove **stitches** and check for any postoperative complications. Patients should not drive or return to work before their checkup. A second follow-up examination is usually done four to eight weeks after the laminectomy.

Patients can help speed their recovery by taking short walks on a daily basis; avoiding sitting or standing in the same position for long periods of time; taking brief naps during the day; and sleeping on the stomach or the side. They may take a daily bath or shower without needing to cover the incision. The incision should be carefully patted dry, however, rather than rubbed.

Risks

Risks associated with a laminectomy include:

- bleeding
- infection
- damage to the spinal cord or other nerves
- weakening or loss of function in the legs
- blood clots
- leakage of spinal fluid resulting from tears in the dura, the protective membrane that covers the spinal cord
- worsening of back pain

Normal results

Normal results depend on the cause of the patient's lower back pain; most patients can expect considerable relief from pain and some improvement in functioning. There is some disagreement among surgeons about the success rate of laminectomies, however, which appears to be due to the fact that the operation is generally done to improve quality of life—cauda equina syndrome is the only indication for an emergency laminectomy. Different sources report success rates between 26% and 99%, with 64% as the average figure. According to one study, 31% of patients were dissatisfied with the results of the operation, possibly because they may have had unrealistic expectations of the results.

Morbidity and mortality rates

The mortality rate for a lumbar laminectomy is between 0.8% and 1%. Rates of complications depend partly on whether a spinal fusion is performed as part of the procedure; while the general rate of complications following a lumbar laminectomy is given as 6–7%, the rate rises to 12% of a spinal fusion has been done.

Alternatives

Conservative treatments

Surgery for lower back pain is considered a treatment of last resort, with the exception of cauda equina syndrome. Patients should always try one or more conservative approaches before consulting a surgeon about a laminectomy. In addition, most health insurers will require proof that the surgery is necessary, since the average total cost of a lumbar laminectomy is $85,000.

Some conservative approaches that have been found to relieve lower back pain include:

- Analgesic or muscle relaxant medications. Analgesics are drugs given to relieve pain. The most commonly prescribed pain medications are aspirin or NSAIDs. Muscle relaxants include methocarbamol, cyclobenzaprine, or diazepam.

- Epidural injections. Epidural injections are given directly into the space surrounding the spinal cord. Corticosteroids are the medications most commonly given by this route, but preliminary reports indicate that epidural injections of indomethacin are also effective in relieving recurrent pain in the lower back.

- Rest. Bed rest for 48 hours usually relieves acute lower back pain resulting from muscle strain.

- Appropriate exercise. Brief walks are recommended as a good form of exercise to improve blood circulation, particularly after surgery. In addition, there are several simple exercises that can be done at home to strengthen the muscles of the lower back. A short pamphlet entitled *Back Pain Exercises* may be downloaded free of charge from the American Academy of Orthopaedic Surgeons (AAOS) web site.

- Losing weight. People who are severely obese may wish to consider weight reduction surgery to reduce the stress on their spine as well as their heart and respiratory system.

- Occupational modifications or change. Lower back pain related to the patient's occupation can sometimes be eased by taking periodic breaks from sitting in one position; by using a desk and chair proportioned to one's height; by learning to use the muscles of the thighs when lifting heavy objects rather than the lower back muscles; and by maintaining proper posture when standing or sitting. In some cases the patient may be helped by changing occupations.

- Physical therapy. A licensed physical therapist can be helpful in identifying the patient's functional back problems and planning a course of treatment to improve flexibility, strength, and range of motion.

> ## WHO PERFORMS THE PROCEDURE AND WHERE IS IT PERFORMED?
>
> A lumbar laminectomy is performed by an orthopedic surgeon or a neurosurgeon. It is performed as an inpatient procedure in a hospital with a department of orthopedic surgery. Minimally invasive laminotomies and microdiscectomies are usually performed in outpatient surgery facilities.

- Osteopathic manipulative treatment (OMT). Osteopathic physicians (DOs) receive the same training in medicine and surgery as MDs; however, they are also trained to evaluate postural and spinal abnormalities and to perform several different manual techniques for relief of back pain. An article published in the *New England Journal of Medicine* in 1999 reported that OMT was as effective as physical therapy and standard medication in relieving lower back pain, with fewer side effects and lower health care costs. OMT is recommended in the United Kingdom as a very low-risk treatment that is more effective than bed rest or mild analgesics.

- Transcutaneous electrical nerve stimulation (TENS). TENS is a treatment technique developed in the late 1960s that delivers a mild electrical current to stimulate nerves through electrodes attached to the skin overlying a painful part of the body. It is thought that TENS works by stimulating the production of endorphins, which are the body's natural painkilling compounds.

Surgical alternatives

The most common surgical alternative to laminectomy is a minimally invasive laminotomy and/or microdiscectomy. In this procedure, which takes about an hour, the surgeon makes a 0.5-in (1.3-cm) incision in the lower back and uses a series of small dilators to separate the layers of muscle and fatty tissue over the spine rather than cutting through them with a scalpel. A tube-shaped retractor is inserted to expose the part of the lamina over the nerve root. The surgeon then uses a power drill to make a small hole in the lamina to expose the nerve itself. After the nerve has been moved aside with the retractor, a small grasping device is used to remove the herniated portion or fragments of the damaged spinal disk.

The advantages of these minimally invasive procedures are fewer complications and a shortened

QUESTIONS TO ASK THE DOCTOR

- What conservative treatments would you recommend for my lower back pain?
- How much time should I allow for conservative therapies to demonstrate effectiveness before considering surgery?
- Am I a candidate for a laminotomy and microdiscectomy?
- How many laminectomies have you performed?

recovery time for the patient. The average postoperative stay is three hours. In addition, 90% of patients are pleased with the results.

Complementary and alternative (CAM) approaches

Two alternative methods of treating back disorders that have been shown to help many patients are acupuncture and chiropractic. Chiropractic is based on the belief that the body has abilities to heal itself provided that nerve impulses can move freely between the brain and the rest of the body. Chiropractors manipulate the segments of the spine in order to bring them into proper alignment and restore the nervous system to proper functioning. Many are qualified to perform acupuncture as well as chiropractic adjustments of the vertebrae and other joints. Several British and Swedish studies have reported that acupuncture and chiropractic are at least as effective as other conservative measures in relieving pain in the lower back.

Movement therapies, including yoga, tai chi, and gentle stretching exercises, may be useful in maintaining or improving flexibility and range of motion in the spine. A qualified yoga instructor can work with the patient's doctor before or after surgery to put together an individualized set of beneficial stretching and breathing exercises. The Alexander technique is a type of movement therapy that is often helpful to patients who need to improve their posture.

Resources

BOOKS

Browner BD et al. Skeletal Trauma: Basic science, management, and reconstruction. 3rd ed. Philadelphia: Elsevier, 2003.

Canale, ST, ed. Campbell's Operative Orthopaedics. 10th ed. St. Louis: Mosby, 2003.

DeLee, JC and D. Drez. DeLee and Drez's Orthopaedic Sports Medicine. 2nd ed. Philadelphia: Saunders, 2005.

Harris ED et al. Kelley's Textbook of Rheumatology. 7th ed. Philadelphia: Saunders, 2005.

PERIODICALS

Aldrete, J. A. "Epidural Injections of Indomethacin for Postlaminectomy Syndrome: A Preliminary Report." Anesthesia and Analgesia 96 (February 2003): 463–468.

Braverman, D. L., J. J. Ericken, R. V. Shah, and D. J. Franklin. "Interventions in Chronic Pain Management. 3. New Frontiers in Pain Management: Complementary Techniques." Archives of Physical Medicine and Rehabilitation 84 (March 2003) (3 Suppl 1): S45–S49.

Harvey, E., A. K. Burton, J. K. Moffett, and A. Breen. "Spinal Manipulation for Low-Back Pain: A Treatment Package Agreed to by the UK Chiropractic, Osteopathy and Physiotherapy Professional Associations." Manual Therapy 8 (February 2003): 46–51.

Hurwitz, E. L., H. Morgenstern, P. Harber, et al. "A Randomized Trial of Medical Care With and Without Physical Therapy and Chiropractic Care With and Without Physical Modalities for Patients with Low Back Pain: 6-Month Follow-Up Outcomes from the UCLA Low Back Pain Study." Spine 27 (October 15, 2002): 2193–2204.

Nasca, R. J. "Lumbar Spinal Stenosis: Surgical Considerations." Journal of the Southern Orthopedic Association 11 (Fall 2002): 127–134.

Pengel, H. M., C. G. Maher, and K. M. Refshauge. "Systematic Review of Conservative Interventions for Subacute Low Back Pain." Clinical Rehabilitation 16 (December 2002): 811–820.

Sleigh, Bryan C., MD, and Ibrahim El Nihum, MD. "Lumbar Laminectomy." eMedicine. August 8, 2002 [cited May 3, 2003]. http://www.emedicine.com/aaem/topic500.htm.

Wang, Michael Y., Barth A. Green, Sachin Shah, et al. "Complications Associated with Lumbar Stenosis Surgery in Patients Older Than 75 Years of Age." Neurosurgical Focus 14 (February 2003): 1–4.

ORGANIZATIONS

American Academy of Neurological and Orthopaedic Surgeons (AANOS). 2300 South Rancho Drive, Suite 202, Las Vegas, NV 89102. (702) 388-7390. http://www.aanos.org.

American Academy of Neurology. 1080 Montreal Avenue, Saint Paul, MN 55116. (800) 879-1960 or (651) 695-2717. http://www.aan.com.

American Academy of Orthopaedic Surgeons (AAOS). 6300 North River Road, Rosemont, IL 60018. (847) 823-7186 or (800) 346-AAOS. http://www.aaos.org.

American Chiropractic Association. 1701 Clarendon Blvd., Arlington, VA 22209. (800) 986-4636. http://www.amerchiro.org.

American Osteopathic Association (AOA). 142 East Ontario Street, Chicago, IL 60611. (800) 621-1773 or (312) 202-8000. http://www.aoa-net.org.

American Physical Therapy Association (APTA). 1111 North Fairfax Street, Alexandria, VA 22314. (703)684-APTA or (800) 999-2782. http://www.apta.org.

National Institute of Arthritis and Musculoskeletal and Skin Diseases (NIAMS) Information Clearinghouse. National Institutes of Health, 1 AMS Circle, Bethesda, MD 20892. (301) 495-4484. TTY: (301) 565-2966. http://www.niams.nih.gov.

OTHER

American Academy of Orthopaedic Surgeons (AAOS). Back Pain Exercises. March 2000 [cited May 5, 2003]. http://www.orthoinfo.aaos.org.

American Physical Therapy Association. Taking Care of Your Back. 2003 [cited May 4, 2003]. http://www.apta.org/Consumer/ptandyourbody/back.

Waddell, G., A. McIntosh, A. Hutchinson, et al. Clinical Guidelines for the Management of Acute Low Back Pain. London, UK: Royal College of General Practitioners, 2000.

Rebecca Frey, Ph.D.

Laparoscopic cholecystectomy *see*
Cholecystectomy

Laparoscopy

Definition

Laparoscopy is a minimally invasive procedure used as a diagnostic tool and surgical procedure that is performed to examine the abdominal and pelvic organs, or the thorax, head, or neck. Tissue samples can also be collected for biopsy using laparoscopy and malignancies treated when it is combined with other therapies. Laparoscopy can also be used for some cardiac and vascular procedures.

Purpose

Laparoscopy is performed to examine the abdominal and pelvic organs to diagnose certain conditions and—depending on the condition—can be used to perform surgery. Laparoscopy is commonly used in gynecology to examine the outside of the uterus, the fallopian tubes, and the ovaries—particularly in pelvic pain cases where the underlying cause cannot be determined using diagnostic imaging (**ultrasound** and computed tomography). Examples of gynecologic conditions diagnosed using laparoscopy include endometriosis, ectopic pregnancy, ovarian cysts, pelvic inflammatory disease [PID], infertility, and cancer. Laparoscopy is used in **general surgery** to examine the abdominal organs, including the gallbladder, bile ducts, the liver, the appendix, and the intestines.

During the laparoscopic surgical procedure, certain conditions can be treated using instruments and devices specifically designed for laparoscopy. Medical devices that can be used in conjunction with laparoscopy include surgical lasers and electrosurgical units. Laparoscopic surgery is now preferred over open surgery for several types of procedures because of its minimally invasive nature and its association with fewer complications.

Microlaparoscopy can be performed in the physician's office using smaller laparoscopes. Common clinical applications in gynecology include pain mapping (for endometriosis), sterilization, and fertility procedures. Common applications in general surgery include evaluation of chronic and acute abdominal pain (as in appendicitis), basic trauma evaluation, biopsies, and evaluation of abdominal masses.

Laparoscopy is commonly used by gynecologists, urologists, and general surgeons for abdominal and pelvic applications. Laparoscopy is also being used by orthopedic surgeons for spinal applications and by cardiac surgeons for **minimally invasive heart surgery**. Newer video-assisted laparoscopic procedures include **thyroidectomy** and **parathyroidectomy**.

Demographics

At first, laparoscopy was only been performed on young, healthy adults, but the use of this technique has greatly expanded. Populations on whom laparoscopies are now performed include infants, children, the elderly, the obese, and those with chronic disease states, such as cancer. The applications of this type of surgery have grown considerably over the years to include a variety of patient populations, and will continue to do so with the refinement of laparascopic techniques.

Description

Laparoscopy is typically performed in the hospital under **general anesthesia**, although some laparoscopic procedures can be performed using local anesthetic agents. Once under anesthesia, a urinary catheter is inserted into the patient's bladder for urine collection. To begin the procedure, a small incision is made just below the navel and a cannula or trocar is inserted into the incision to accommodate the insertion of the laparoscope. Other incisions may be made in the abdomen to allow the insertion of additional laparoscopic instrumentation. A laparoscopic insufflation device is used to inflate the abdomen

Laparoscopy

A.
Incision

Incision

B.
Lung
Pneumoperitoneum
Bladder
CO₂
Uterus

C.
gallbladder
To video monitor
Camera
Laparoscope
Intestines
Lung
Liver
Cystic duct of gallbladder
Spine

D.
Gallbladder
Pneumoperitoneum
Stomach
Rib
Spleen
Liver
Kidney
Spine

The surgeon has a choice of incision options for laparoscopy, depending on the needs of the procedure (A). In this abdominal procedure, carbon dioxide is pumped into the cavity to create a condition called pneumoperitoneum, which allows the surgeon easier access to internal structures. The laparoscope is connected to a video monitor, and special forceps are used to carry out any necessary procedure (C and D) *(Illustration by GGS Information Services. Cengage Learning, Gale.)*

with carbon dioxide gas to create a space in which the laparoscopic surgeon can maneuver the instruments. After the laparoscopic diagnosis and treatment are completed, the laparoscope, cannula, and other instrumentation are removed, and the incision is sutured and bandaged.

Laparoscopes have integral cameras for transmitting images during the procedure, and are available in various sizes depending upon the type of procedure performed. The images from the laparoscope are transmitted to a viewing monitor that the surgeon uses to visualize the internal anatomy and guide any surgical procedure. Video and photographic equipment are also used to document the surgery, and may be used postoperatively to explain the results of the procedure to the patient.

Robotic systems are available to assist with laparoscopy. A robotic arm, attached to the operating table may be used to hold and position the laparoscope. This serves to reduce unintentional camera movement that is common when a surgical assistant holds the laparoscope. The surgeon controls the robotic arm movement by foot pedal with voice-activated command, or with a handheld control panel.

Microlaparoscopy has become more common over the past few years. The procedure involves the use of smaller laparoscopes (that is, 2 mm compared to 5–10 mm for hospital laparoscopy), with the patient undergoing **local anesthesia** with **conscious sedation** (during which the patient remains awake but very relaxed) in a physician's office. Video and photographic equipment, previously explained, may be used.

KEY TERMS

Ascites—Accumulation of fluid in the abdominal cavity; laparoscopy may be used to determine its cause.

Cholecystitis—Inflammation of the gallbladder, often diagnosed using laparoscopy.

Electrosurgical device—A medical device that uses electrical current to cauterize or coagulate tissue during surgical procedures; often used in conjunction with laparoscopy.

Embolism—Blockage of an artery by a clot, air or gas, or foreign material. Gas embolism may occur as a result of insufflation of the abdominal cavity during laparoscopy.

Endometriosis—A disease involving occurrence of endometrial tissue (lining of the uterus) outside the uterus in the abdominal cavity; often diagnosed and treated using laparoscopy.

Hysterectomy—Surgical removal of the uterus; often performed laparoscopically.

Insufflation—Inflation of the abdominal cavity using carbon dioxide; performed prior to laparoscopy to give the surgeon space to maneuver surgical equipment.

Oophorectomy—Surgical removal of the ovaries; often performed laparoscopically.

Pneumothorax—Air or gas in the pleural space (lung area) that may occur as a complication of laparoscopy and insufflation.

Subcutaneous emphysema—A pathologic accumulation of air underneath the skin resulting from improper insufflation technique.

Trocar—A small sharp instrument used to puncture the abdomen at the beginning of the laparoscopic procedure.

Laparoscopy has been explored in combination with other therapies for the treatment of certain types of malignancies, including pelvic and aortic lymph node dissection, ovarian cancer, and early cervical cancer. Laparoscopic radiofrequency ablation is a technique whereby laproscopy assists in the delivery of radiofrequency probes that distribute pulses to a tumor site. The pulses generate heat in malignant tumor cells and destroys them.

The introduction of items such as temperature-controlled instruments, **surgical instruments** with greater rotation and articulation, improved imaging systems, and multiple robotic devices will expand the utility of laparoscopic techniques in the future. The skills of surgeons will be enhanced as well, with further development of training simulators and computer technology.

Diagnosis/Preparation

Before undergoing laparoscopic surgery, the patient should be prepared by the doctor for the procedure both psychologically and physically. It is very important that the patient receive realistic counseling before surgery and prior to giving **informed consent**. This includes discussion about further open abdominal surgery (laparotomy) that may be required during laparoscopic surgery, information about potential complications during surgery, and the possible need for blood transfusions. In the case of diagnostic laparoscopy for chronic pelvic pain, the procedure may simply indicate that all organs are normal and the patient should be prepared for this possibility. The surgery may be explained using pictures, models, videotapes, and movies. It is especially important for the patient to be able to ask questions and express concerns. It may be helpful, for the patient to have a family member or friend present during discussions with the doctor. Such conversations could understandably cause anxiety, and information relayed may not be adequately recalled under such circumstances.

There is usually a presurgical exam two weeks before the surgery to gather a medical history and obtain blood and urine samples for laboratory testing. It is important that the patient inform the doctor completely about any prior surgeries, medical conditions, or medications taken on a regular basis, including **nonsteroidal anti-inflammatory drugs** (NSAIDs), such as **aspirin**. Patients taking blood thinners, like Coumadin or Heparin (generic name: warfarin) should not adjust their medication themselves, but should speak with their prescribing doctors regarding their upcoming surgery. (Patients should never adjust dosage without their doctors' approval. This is especially important for elderly patients, asthmatics, those with hypertension, or those who are on ACE inhibitors.) If a tubal dye study is planned during the procedure, the patient may also be required to provide information on menstrual history. For some procedures, an autologous (self) **blood donation** may be suggested prior to the surgery to replace blood that may be lost during the procedure. Chest x rays may also be required. For some obese patients, weight loss may be necessary prior to surgery.

Immediately before to surgery, there are several pre-operative steps that the patient may be advised to take. The patient should shower at least 24 hours prior to the surgery, and gently but thoroughly cleanse the umbilicus (belly button) with antibacterial soap and water using a cotton-tipped swab. Because laparoscopy requires general anesthesia in most cases, the patient may be asked to eat lightly 24 hours prior to surgery and fast at least 12 hours prior to surgery. Bowel cleansing with a laxative may also required, allowing the it to be more easily visualized and to prevent complications in the unlikely event of bowel injury. Those who are have diabetes or have hypoglycemia may wish to schedule their procedures early in the morning to avoid low blood sugar reactions. The patient should follow the directions of the hospital staff, arriving early on the day of surgery to sign paperwork and to be screened by the anesthesiology staff. Questions will be asked regarding current medications and dosages, allergies to medication, previous experiences with anesthesia (that is, allergic reactions, and previous experiences regarding time-to-consciousness), and a variety of other questions. It is often helpful for the patient to make a list of this information beforehand so that the information can be easily retrieved when requested by the hospital staff.

Aftercare

Following laparoscopy, patients are required to remain in a recovery area until the immediate effects of anesthesia subside and until normal voiding is accomplished (especially if a urinary catheter was used during the surgery). **Vital signs** are monitored to ensure that there are no reactions to anesthesia or internal injuries present. There may be some nausea and/or vomiting, which may be reduced by the use of the propofol anesthetic for healthy patients undergoing elective procedures such as **tubal ligation**, diagnostic laparoscopy, or hernia repair. Laparoscopy is usually an outpatient procedure and patients are discharged from the recovery area within a few hours after the procedure. For elderly patients and those with other medical conditions, recovery may be slower. Patients with more serious medical conditions, or patients undergoing emergency laparoscopy, an overnight hospital stay or a stay of several days may be required.

Discharged patients will receive instructions regarding activity level, medications, postoperative dietary modifications, and possible side effects of the procedure. It may be helpful to have a friend or family member present when these instructions are given, as the aftereffects of anesthesia may cause some temporary confusion. Postoperative instructions may include information on when one might resume normal activities such as bathing, housework, and driving. Depending on the nature of the laparoscopic procedure and the patient's medical condition, daily activity may be restricted for a few days and strenuous during administration of anesthesia may cause some soreness. Additionally, shoulder pain may persist as long as 36 hours after surgery. Pain-relieving medications and **antibiotics** may be prescribed for several days postoperatively.

Patients will be instructed to watch for signs of a urinary tract infection (UTI) or unusual pain; either may indicate organ injury. It is important to understand the difference between normal discomfort and pain, because pain may indicate a problem. Patients may also experience an elevated temperature, and occasionally "postlaparoscopy syndrome"; this condition is similar in appearance to peritonitis (marked by abdominal pain, constipation, vomiting, and fever) that disappears shortly after surgery without antibiotics. However, any postoperative symptoms that cause concern for the patient should be discussed with the doctor, so that any fears can be alleviated and recovery can be accomplished. Due to the after-effects of anesthesia, patients should not drive themselves home.

It is advisable for someone to stay with the patient for a few hours following the procedure, in case complications arise. Injury to an organ might not be readily apparent for several days after the procedure. The physical signs that should be watched for and reported immediately include:

- fever and chills
- abdominal distension
- vomiting
- difficulty urinating
- sharp and unusual pain in the abdomen or bowel
- redness at the incision site, which indicates infection
- discharge from any places where tubes were inserted or incisions were made

Additional complications may include a urinary tract infection (resulting from catheterization) and minor infection of the incision site. An injury to the ureter may be indicated by abdominal distention or a pain in the flank. Additional testing may be required if a complication is suspected.

Risks

Complications may be associated with the laparoscopy procedure in general, or may be specific to the type of operation that is performed. Patients should consult with their doctors regarding the types of risks that are specific for their procedures. The most serious complication that can occur during laparoscopy is laceration of a major abdominal blood vessel resulting from improper positioning, inadequate insufflation (inflation) of the abdomen, abnormal pelvic anatomy, and too much force exerted during scope insertion. Thin patients with well-developed abdominal muscles are at higher risk, since the aorta may only be an inch or so below the skin. Obese patients are also at higher risk because more forceful and deeper needle and scope penetration is required. During laparoscopy, there is also a risk of bleeding from blood vessels, and adhesions may require repair by open surgery if bleeding cannot be stopped using laparoscopic instrumentation. In laparoscopic procedures that use electrosurgical devices, burns to the incision site are possible due to passage of electrical current through the laparoscope caused by a fault or malfunction in the equipment.

Complications related to insufflation of the abdominal cavity include gas inadvertently entering a blood vessel and causing an embolism, pneumothorax, or subcutaneous emphysema. One common but not serious side effect of insufflation is pain in the shoulder and upper chest area for a day or two following the procedure.

Any abdominal surgery, including laparoscopy, carries the risk of unintentional organ injury (punctures and perforations). For example, the bowel, bladder, ureters, or fallopian tubes may be injured during the laparoscopic procedure. Many times these injuries are unavoidable due to the patient's anatomy or medical condition. Patients at higher risk for bowel injury include those with chronic bowel disease, PID, a history of pervious abdominal surgery, or severe endometriosis. Some types of laparoscopic procedures have a higher risk of organ injury. For instance, during laparoscopic removal of endometriosis adhesions or ovaries, the ureters may be injured due to their proximity to each other.

Several clinical studies have shown that the complication rate during laparoscopy is associated with inadequate surgeon experience. Surgeons who are more experienced in laparoscopic procedures have fewer complications than those performing their first 100 cases.

Normal results

In diagnostic laparoscopy, the surgeon will be able to see signs of a disease or condition (for example, endometriosis adhesions; ovarian cysts; diseased gallbladder) immediately, and can either treat the condition surgically or proceed with appropriate medical management. In

WHO PERFORMS THE PROCEDURE AND WHERE IS IT PERFORMED?

Laparoscopy may be performed by a gynecologist, general surgeon, gastroenterologist, or other physician—depending upon the patient's condition. An anesthesiologist is required during the procedure to administer general and/or local anesthesia and to perform patient monitoring. Nurses and surgical technicians/assistants are needed during the procedure to assist with scope positioning, video system adjustments and image recording, and laparoscopic instrumentation.

diagnostic laparoscopy, biopsies may be taken of tissue in questionable areas, and laboratory results will govern medical treatment. In therapeutic laparoscopy, the surgeon performs a procedure that rectifies a known medical problem, such as hernia repair or appendix removal. Because laparoscopy is minimally invasive compared to open surgery, patients may experience less trauma and postoperative discomfort, have fewer procedural complications, have a shorter hospital stay, and return more quickly to daily activities. The results will vary, however, depending on the patients's condition and type of treatment.

Morbidity and mortality rates

Laparoscopic surgery, like most surgeries, is not without risk. Risks should be thoroughly explained to the patient. Complications from laparoscopic surgeries arise in 1–5% of the cases, with a mortality of about 0.05%. Complications may arise from the laparoscopic entry during procedure, and the risks vary depending on the elements specific to a particular procedure. For example, the risk of injury to the common bile duct in laparoscopic biliary surgery is 0.3–0.6% of cases. The factors that contribute to morbidity are currently under study and debate. Injury may occur to blood vessels and internal organs. Some studies examining malpractice data indicate that trocar injury to the bowel or blood vessels may account up to one-fourth of laparoscopic medical claims. It has been suggested that these injuries can be reduced by alterations in the placement and use of the Verses needle, or by using an open technique of trocar insertion in which a blunt cannula (non-bladed) is inserted into the abdominal cavity through an incision. The insertion of secondary **trocars** may be of particular interest as a risk factor. There is still some debate,

QUESTIONS TO ASK THE DOCTOR

- Will this surgery be covered by my insurance? Will any postsurgical care that I require also be covered?

- What do I need to do to prepare for the surgery? Are there any restrictions on diet, fluid intake, or other measures?

- Are there any medications that should be stopped prior to the surgery?

- Does my medical history pose any potential problems that need to be considered before undergoing this procedure?

- What is your (the doctor's) training in performing this surgery? Will you perform the actual surgery or will a trainee?

- What aftereffects can I expect?

- Are there any post-surgical symptoms that might indicate a complication that I should report, and to whom should these questions be directed? What post-surgical symptoms should be considered "normal" and how might discomfort be relieved?

- What is the expected recovery period from this procedure?

- What special care or self-care is required following this surgery?

however, as to which method of trocar insertion is most appropriate in a particular situation, as no technique is without risk. The most commonly cited injury in laparoscopic malpractice claims has been injury to the bile duct (66%). Proper identification of this structure by an experienced surgeon, or by a cholangiogram, may reduce this type of injury. Other areas of the body may be injured during access including the stomach, bladder, and liver. Hemorrhages may also occur during the operation.

Laparoscopic entry injuries have been the subject of recent study. Data collected from insurance companies and medical device regulation indicate that bowel and vascular injuries may account for 76% of the injuries that occur when a primary port is created. Delayed recognition of bowel injuries was noted to be an important factor in mortality. The risk of possible injury or **death** in laparoscopy depends on such factors as the anatomy of the patient, the force of entry, and the type operative procedure being performed.

Alternatives

The alternatives to laparoscopy vary, depending on the medical condition being treated. Laparotomy (open abdominal surgery with larger incision) may be pursued when further visualization is needed to treat the condition, such as in the case of pain of severe endometriosis with deeper lesions. For those female patients with pelvic masses, transvaginal sonography may be a helpful technique in obtaining information about whether such masses are malignant, assisting in the choice between laparoscopy or laparotomy.

Resources

BOOKS

Gabbe, SG et al. Obstetrics: Normal and Problem Pregnancies. 5th ed. London: Churchill Livingstone, 2007.

Katz VL et al. Comprehensive Gynecology. 5th ed. St. Louis: Mosby, 2007.

Khatri, VP and JA Asensio. Operative Surgery Manual. 1st ed. Philadelphia: Saunders, 2003.

Townsend, CM et al. Sabiston Textbook of Surgery. 17th ed. Philadelphia: Saunders, 2004.

PERIODICALS

Abu-Rustum, Nadeem R. "Laparoscopy 2003: Oncologic Perspective." Clinical Obstetrics and Gynecology 46, no.1 (March 2003): 61-69.

Bieber, Eric. "Laparoscopy: Past, Present, and Future." Clinical Obstetrics and Gynecology 46, no. 1 (March 2003): 3-14.

ORGANIZATIONS

American College of Obstetricians and Gynecologists. 409 12th Street SW, P.O. Box 96920, Washington, DC 20090-6920. http://www.acog.org.

Society of American Gastrointestinal Endoscopic Surgeons(SAGES). 2716 Ocean Park Boulevard, Suite 3000, Santa Monica, CA 90405. (310) 314-2404. http://www.endoscopy-sages.com.

Society of Laparoendoscopic Surgeons. 7330 SW 62nd Place, Suite 410, Miami, FL 33143-4825. (305) 665-9959. http://www.sls.org.

OTHER

Agency for Healthcare Research And Quality. http://www.webmm.ahrq.gov/cases.aspx?ic = 3.

"Diagnostic Laparoscopy." Society of Gastrointestinal Endoscopic Surgeons. http://www.sages.org/pi_diaglap.html.

"Laparoscopy." WebMD.com. October 24, 2002. <http://my.webmd.com/content/healthwise/21/5199.htm?last selectedguid = {5FE84E90-BC77-4056-A91C-9531713CA348>.

Jennifer E. Sisk, M.A.
Jill Granger, M.S.

Laparoscopy for endometriosis

Definition

Laparoscopy is a surgical procedure in which a laparoscope, a telescope-like instrument, is inserted into the abdomen through a small incision and used to diagnose or treat various diseases. Specifically, laparoscopy may be used to diagnose and treat endometriosis, a condition in which the tissue that lines the uterus grows elsewhere in the body, usually in the abdominal cavity.

Purpose

The endometrium is the inner lining of the uterus; it is where a fertilized egg will implant during the early days of pregnancy. The endometrium normally sheds during each menstrual cycle if the egg released during ovulation has not been fertilized. Endometriosis is a condition that occurs when cells from the endometrium begin growing outside the uterus. The outlying endometrial cells respond to the hormones that control the menstrual cycle, bleeding each month the way the lining of the uterus does. This causes irritation of the surrounding tissue, leading to pain and scarring.

Endometrial growths are most commonly found on the pelvic organs, including the ovaries (the most common site), fallopian tubes, bladder, rectum, cervix, vagina, and the outer surface of the uterus. Growths are also sometimes found in other areas of the body, including the skin, lungs, brain, or surgical scars. There are numerous theories as to the cause of endometriosis; these include retrograde menstruation (movement of menstrual blood up through the fallopian tubes), movement of endometrial tissue through the blood or lymph system, or surgical transplantation (when endometriosis is found in surgical scars).

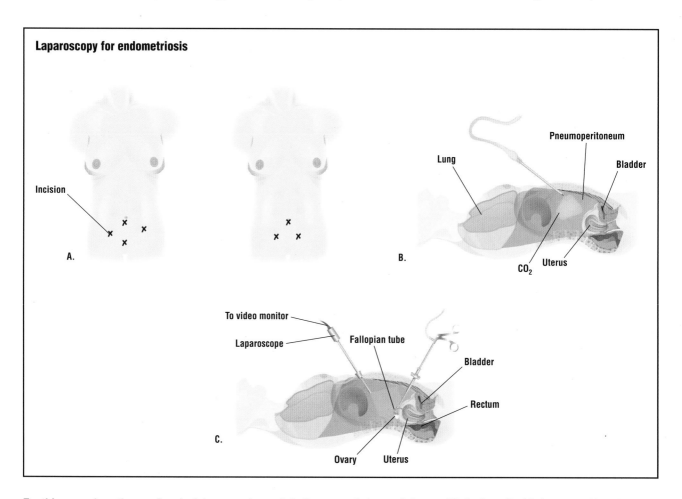

Laparoscopy for endometriosis

Incision

A.

Lung
Pneumoperitoneum
Bladder
CO_2
Uterus

B.

To video monitor
Laparoscope
Fallopian tube
Bladder
Rectum
Ovary
Uterus

C.

For this procedure, three or four incisions may be made in the woman's lower abdomen (A). Carbon dioxide is pumped into the abdomen to create a condition called pneumoperitoneum, which allows the surgeon to work easier in the abdomen (B). A laparoscope with video monitor is used to view the internal structures, while endometrial growths are removed with other tools (C). *(Illustration by GGS Information Services. Cengage Learning, Gale.)*

KEY TERMS

Acupuncture—The insertion of tiny needles into the skin at specific spots on the body for curative purposes.

Fallopian tubes—The structures that carry a mature egg from the ovaries to the uterus.

Ovulation—A process in which a mature female egg is released from one of the ovaries (egg-shaped structures located to each side of the uterus) every 28 days.

Sub-fertility—A decreased ability to become pregnant.

There are a number of reasons why laparoscopy is used to treat endometriosis. It is useful as both a diagnostic tool (to visualize structures in the abdominal cavity and examine them for endometrial growths) and as an operative tool (to excise or destroy endometrial growths). A patient's recovery time following laparoscopic surgery is shorter and less painful than following a traditional laparotomy (a larger surgical incision into the abdominal cavity). A disadvantage to laparoscopy is that some growths may be too large or extensive to remove with laparoscopic instruments, necessitating a laparotomy.

Demographics

Endometriosis has been estimated to affect up to 10% of women. Approximately four out of every 1,000 women are hospitalized as a result of endometriosis each year. Women ages 25–35 are most affected, with 27 being the average age at diagnosis. The incidence of endometriosis is higher among white women and among women who have a family history of the disease.

Description

The patient is given anesthesia before the procedure commences. The method of anesthesia depends on the type and duration of surgery, the patient's preference, and the recommendation of the physician. **General anesthesia** is most common for operative laparoscopy, while diagnostic laparoscopy is often performed under regional or **local anesthesia**. A catheter is inserted into the bladder to empty it of urine; this is done to minimize the risk of injury to the bladder.

A small incision is first made into the patient's abdomen in or near the belly button. A gas such as carbon dioxide is used to inflate the abdomen to allow the surgeon a better view of the surgical field. The laparoscope is a thin, lighted tube that is inserted into the abdominal cavity through the incision. Images taken by the laparoscope may be seen on a video monitor connected to the scope.

The surgeon will examine the pelvic organs for endometrial growths or adhesions (bands of scar tissue that may form after surgery or trauma). Other incisions may be made to insert additional instruments; this would allow the surgeon to better position the internal organs for viewing. To remove or destroy endometrial growths, a laser or electric current (electrocautery) may be used. Alternatively, implants may be cut away with a scalpel (surgical knife). After the procedure is completed, any incisions are closed with **stitches**.

Diagnosis/Preparation

Some of the symptoms of endometriosis include pelvic pain (constant or during menstruation), infertility, painful intercourse, and painful urination and/or bowel movements during menstruation. Such symptoms, however, are also exhibited by a number of other diseases. A definitive diagnosis of endometriosis may only be made by laparoscopy or laparotomy.

Prior to surgery, the patient may be asked to refrain from eating or drinking after midnight on the day of surgery. An intravenous (IV) line will be placed for administration of fluids and/or medications.

Aftercare

After the procedure is completed, the patient will usually spend several hours in the **recovery room** to ensure that she recovers from the anesthesia without complication. After leaving the hospital, she may experience soreness around the incision, shoulder pain from the gas used to inflate the abdomen, cramping, or constipation. Most symptoms resolve within one to three days.

Risks

Risks that are associated with laparoscopy include complications due to anesthesia, infection, injury to organs or other structures, and bleeding. There is a risk that endometriosis will reoccur or that not all of the endometrial implants will be removed with surgery.

WHO PERFORMS THE PROCEDURE AND WHERE IS IT PERFORMED?

Laparoscopy for endometriosis is performed by a surgeon or gynecologist who has been trained in laparoscopic techniques. A gynecologist is a medical doctor who has completed specialized training in the areas of women's general and reproductive health, pregnancy, labor and delivery, and prenatal testing. Laparoscopy is usually performed in a hospital on an outpatient basis.

QUESTIONS TO ASK THE DOCTOR

- Why is laparoscopic surgery recommended for my particular case?
- Will operative laparoscopy be performed if endometriosis is diagnosed?
- What options do I have in terms of anesthesia and pain relief?
- What are the risks if I decide against surgical treatment?
- What alternatives to laparoscopy are available to me?

Normal results

After laparoscopy for endometriosis, a woman should recover quickly from the surgery and experience a significant improvement in symptoms. Some studies suggest that surgical treatment of endometriosis may improve a sub-fertile woman's chance of getting pregnant.

Morbidity and mortality rates

The overall rate of risks associated with laparoscopy is approximately 1–2%, with serious complications occurring in only 0.2% of patients. The rate of reoccurrence of endometrial growths after laparoscopic surgery is approximately 19%. The mortality rate associated with laparoscopy is less than five per 100,000 cases.

Alternatives

While laparoscopy remains the definitive approach to diagnosing endometriosis, some larger endometrial growths may be located by **ultrasound**, a procedure that uses high-frequency sound waves to visualize structures in the human body. Ultrasound is a non-invasive technique that may detect endometriomas (cysts filled with old blood) larger than 0.4 in (1 cm).

A physician may recommend noninvasive measures to treat endometriosis before resorting to surgical treatment. Over-the-counter or prescription pain medications may be recommended to relieve pain-related symptoms. Oral contraceptives or other hormone drugs may be prescribed to suppress ovulation and menstruation. Some women seek alternative medical therapies such as acupuncture, management of diet, or herbal treatments to reduce pain.

Severe endometriosis may need to be treated by more extensive surgery. Conservative surgery consists of excision of all endometrial implants in the abdominal cavity, with or without removal of bowel that is involved by the disease. Semi-conservative surgery involves removing some of the pelvic organs; examples are **hysterectomy** (removal of the uterus) and **oophorectomy** (removal of the ovaries). Radical surgery involves removing the uterus, cervix, ovaries, and fallopian tubes (called a total hysterectomy with bilateral **salpingo-oophorectomy**).

Resources

BOOKS

Gabbe, SG et al. Obstetrics: Normal and Problem Pregnancies. 5th ed. London: Churchill Livingstone, 2007.

Katz VL et al. Comprehensive Gynecology. 5th ed. St. Louis: Mosby, 2007.

Khatri, VP and JA Asensio. Operative Surgery Manual. 1st ed. Philadelphia: Saunders, 2003.

Townsend, CM et al. Sabiston Textbook of Surgery. 17th ed. Philadelphia: Saunders, 2004.

ORGANIZATIONS

American Association of Gynecologic Laparoscopists. 13021 East Florence Ave., Sante Fe Springs, CA 90670-4505. (800) 554-AAGL. http://www.aagl.com.

Endometriosis Association. 8585 North 76th Place, Milwaukee, WI 53223. (414) 355-2200. http://www.endometriosisassn.org.

OTHER

"Endometriosis." UC Davis Health System. 2002 [cited March 22, 2003]. http://www.ucdmc.ucdavis.edu/ucdhs/health/a-z/74Endometriosis__/.

Hurd, William W., and Janice M. Duke. "Gynecologic Laparoscopy." eMedicine. November 27, 2002 [cited March 22, 2003]. http://www.emedicine.com/med/topic3299.htm.

Kapoor, Dharmesh. "Endometriosis." eMedicine. September 17, 2002 [cited March 22, 2003]. http://www.emedicine.com/med/topic3419.htm.

"What is Endometriosis?" Endometriosis Association. 2002 [cited March 22, 2003]. http://www.endometriosisassn. org/endo.html.

Stephanie Dionne Sherk

Laparotomy, exploratory

Definition

A laparotomy is a large incision made into the abdomen. Exploratory laparotomy is used to visualize and examine the structures inside of the abdominal cavity.

Purpose

Exploratory laparotomy is a method of abdominal exploration, a diagnostic tool that allows physicians to examine the abdominal organs. The procedure may be recommended for a patient who has abdominal pain of unknown origin or who has sustained an injury to the abdomen. Injuries may occur as a result of blunt trauma (e.g., road traffic accident) or penetrating trauma (e.g., stab or gunshot wound). Because of the nature of the abdominal organs, there is a high risk of infection if organs rupture or are perforated. In addition, bleeding into the abdominal cavity is considered a medical emergency. Exploratory laparotomy is used to determine the source of pain or the extent of injury and perform repairs if needed.

Laparotomy may be performed to determine the cause of a patient's symptoms or to establish the extent of a disease. For example, endometriosis is a disorder in which cells from the inner lining of the uterus grow elsewhere in the body, most commonly on the pelvic and abdominal organs. Endometrial growths, however, are difficult to visualize using standard imaging techniques such as x ray, **ultrasound** technology, or computed tomography (CT) scanning. Exploratory laparotomy may be used to examine the abdominal and pelvic organs (such as the ovaries, fallopian tubes, bladder, and rectum) for evidence of endometriosis. Any growths found may then be removed.

Exploratory laparotomy plays an important role in the staging of certain cancers. Cancer staging is used to describe how far a cancer has spread. A laparotomy enables a surgeon to directly examine the abdominal organs for evidence of cancer and remove samples of tissue for further examination. When laparotomy is used for this use, it is called staging laparotomy or pathological staging.

Some other conditions that may be discovered or investigated during exploratory laparotomy include:

- cancer of the abdominal organs
- peritonitis (inflammation of the peritoneum, the lining of the abdominal cavity)
- appendicitis (inflammation of the appendix)
- pancreatitis (inflammation of the pancreas)
- abscesses (a localized area of infection)
- adhesions (bands of scar tissue that form after trauma or surgery)
- diverticulitis (inflammation of sac-like structures in the walls of the intestines)
- intestinal perforation
- ectopic pregnancy (pregnancy occurring outside of the uterus)
- foreign bodies (e.g., a bullet in a gunshot victim)
- internal bleeding

Demographics

Because laparotomy may be performed under a number of circumstances to diagnose or treat numerous conditions, no data exists as to the overall incidence of the procedure.

Description

The patient is usually placed under **general anesthesia** for the duration of surgery. The advantages to general anesthesia are that the patient remains unconscious during the procedure, no pain will be experienced nor will the patient have any memory of the procedure, and the patient's muscles remain completely relaxed, allowing safer surgery.

Incision

Once an adequate level of anesthesia has been reached, the initial incision into the skin may be made. A scalpel is first used to cut into the superficial layers of the skin. The incision may be median (vertical down the patient's midline), paramedian (vertical elsewhere on the abdomen), transverse (horizontal), T-shaped, or curved, according to the needs of the surgery. The incision is then continued through the subcutaneous fat, the abdominal muscles, and finally, the peritoneum. Electrocautery is often used to cut through the subcutaneous tissue as it has the ability to stop bleeding as it cuts. Instruments called retractors may be used to hold the incision open once the abdominal cavity has been exposed.

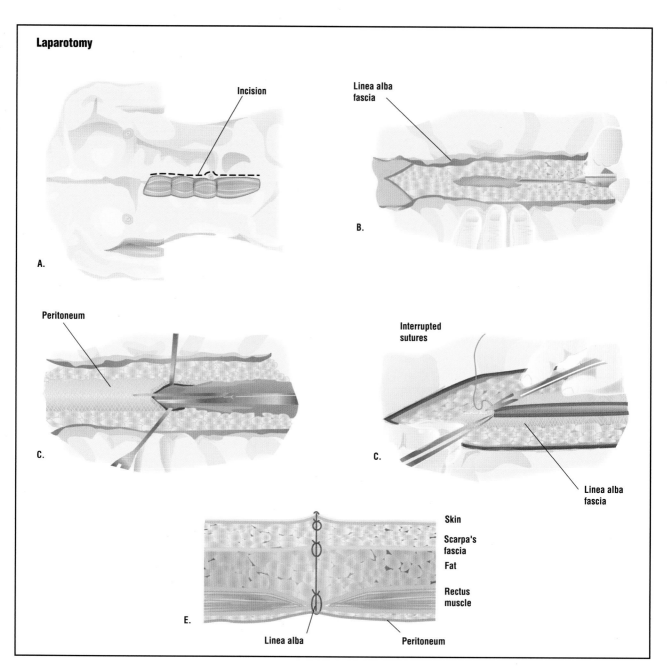

During a laparotomy, and an incision is made into the patient's abdomen (A). Skin and connective tissue called fascia is divided (B). The lining of the abdominal cavity, the peritoneum, is cut, and any exploratory procedures are undertaken (C). To close the incision, the peritoneum, fascia, and skin are stitched (E). *(Illustration by GGS Information Services. Cengage Learning, Gale.)*

Abdominal exploration

The surgeon may then explore the abdominal cavity for disease or trauma. The abdominal organs in question will be examined for evidence of infection, inflammation, perforation, abnormal growths, or other conditions. Any fluid surrounding the abdominal organs will be inspected; the presence of blood, bile, or other fluids may indicate specific diseases or injuries. In some cases, an abnormal smell encountered upon entering the abdominal cavity may be evidence of infection or a perforated gastrointestinal organ.

If an abnormality is found, the surgeon has the option of treating the patient before closing the wound or initiating treatment after exploratory surgery. Alternatively, samples of various tissues and/or fluids may be removed for further analysis. For example, if cancer is suspected, biopsies may be obtained so that the tissues can be examined microscopically for

KEY TERMS

Intestinal perforation—A hole in the intestinal wall.

Subcutaneous—Under the skin.

evidence of abnormal cells. If no abnormality is found, or if immediate treatment is not needed, the incision may be closed without performing any further surgical procedures.

During exploratory laparotomy for cancer, a pelvic washing may be performed; sterile fluid is instilled into the abdominal cavity and washed around the abdominal organs, then withdrawn and analyzed for the presence of abnormal cells. This may indicate that a cancer has begun to spread (metastasize).

Closure

Upon completion of any exploration or procedures, the organs and related structures are returned to their normal anatomical position. The incision may then be sutured (stitched closed). The layers of the abdominal wall are sutured in reverse order, and the skin incision closed with sutures or **staples**.

Diagnosis/Preparation

Various diagnostic tests may be performed to determine if exploratory laparotomy is necessary. Blood tests or imaging techniques such as x ray, computed tomography (CT) scan, and **magnetic resonance imaging** (MRI) are examples. The presence of intraperitoneal fluid (IF) may be an indication that exploratory laparotomy is necessary; one study indicated that IF was present in nearly three-quarters of patients with intra-abdominal injuries.

Directly preceding the surgical procedure, an intravenous (IV) line will be placed so that fluids and/or medications may be administered to the patient during and after surgery. A Foley catheter will be inserted into the bladder to drain urine. The patient will also meet with the anesthesiologist to go over details of the method of anesthesia to be used.

Aftercare

The patient will remain in the postoperative **recovery room** for several hours where his or her recovery can be closely monitored. **Discharge from the hospital** may occur in as little as one to two days after the procedure, but may be later if additional procedures were performed or complications were encountered. The patient

WHO PERFORMS THE PROCEDURE AND WHERE IS IT PERFORMED?

Depending on the reason for performing an exploratory laparotomy, the procedure may be performed by a general or specialized surgeon in a hospital operating room. In the case of trauma to the abdomen, laparotomy may be performed by an emergency room physician.

will be instructed to watch for symptoms that may indicate infection, such as fever, redness or swelling around the incision, drainage, and worsening pain.

Risks

Risks inherent to the use of general anesthesia include nausea, vomiting, sore throat, fatigue, headache, and muscle soreness; more rarely, blood pressure problems, allergic reaction, heart attack, or stroke may occur. Additional risks include bleeding, infection, injury to the abdominal organs or structures, or formation of adhesions (bands of scar tissue between organs).

Normal results

The results following exploratory laparotomy depend on the reasons why it was performed. The procedure may indicate that further treatment is necessary; for example, if cancer was detected, chemotherapy, radiation therapy, or more surgery may be recommended. In some cases, the abnormality is able to be treated during laparotomy, and no further treatment is necessary.

Morbidity and mortality rates

The operative and postoperative complication rates associated with exploratory laparotomy vary according to the patient's condition and any additional procedures performed.

Alternatives

Laparoscopy is a relatively recent alternative to laparotomy that has many advantages. Also called minimally invasive surgery, laparoscopy is a surgical procedure in which a laparoscope (a thin, lighted tube) and other instruments are inserted into the abdomen through small incisions. The internal operating field may then be visualized on a video monitor that is connected to the scope. In some patients, the technique may be used for abdominal exploration in place of a

QUESTIONS TO ASK THE DOCTOR

- Why is exploratory laparotomy being recommended?
- What diagnostic tests will be performed to determine if exploratory laparotomy is necessary?
- Are any additional procedures anticipated?
- What type of incision will be used and where will it be located?

laparotomy. Laparoscopy is associated with faster recovery times, shorter hospital stays, and smaller surgical scars.

Resources

BOOKS

Khatri, VP and JA Asensio. Operative Surgery Manual. 1st ed. Philadelphia: Saunders, 2003.

Marx, John A., et al. Rosen's Emergency Medicine. 6th ed. St. Louis, MO: Mosby, Inc., 2006.

Townsend, CM et al. Sabiston Textbook of Surgery. 17th ed. Philadelphia: Saunders, 2004.

PERIODICALS

Hahn, David D., Steven R. Offerman, and James F. Holmes. "Clinical Importance of Intraperitoneal Fluid in Patients with Blunt Intra-abdominal Injury." American Journal of Emergency Medicine 20, no. 7 (November 2002).

OTHER

Awori, Nelson, et al. "Laparotomy." Primary Surgery. [cited April 6, 2003]. http://www.meb.uni-bonn.de/dtc/primsurg/index.html.

"Surgery by Laparotomy." Stream OR. 2001 [cited April 6, 2003]. http://www.streamor.com/opengyn/openindex.html.

Stephanie Dionne Sherk

Large bowel resection *see* **Bowel resection**

Laryngectomy

Definition

A laryngectomy is the partial or complete surgical removal of the voice box (larynx).

Purpose

Because of its location, the voice box, or larynx, plays a critical role in breathing, swallowing, and speaking. The larynx is located above the windpipe (trachea) and in front of the food pipe (esophagus). It contains two small bands of muscle called the vocal cords that close to prevent food from entering the lungs and vibrate to produce the voice. If cancer of the larynx develops, a laryngectomy is performed to remove tumors or cancerous tissue. In rare cases, the procedure may also be performed when the larynx is badly damaged by gunshot, automobile injuries, or other traumatic accidents.

Demographics

The American Cancer Society estimates that, in 2007, about 11,300 people in the United States will be found to have laryngeal cancer; 8,960 cases will occur in men and 2,340 cases will occur in women. Tobacco smoking is by far the greatest risk factor for laryngeal cancer. Others include alcohol abuse, radiation exposure, asbestos exposure, and genetic factors.

Description

Laryngectomies may be total or partial. In a total laryngectomy, the entire larynx is removed. If the cancer has spread to other surrounding structures in the neck, such as the lymph nodes, they are removed at the same time. If the tumor is small, a partial laryngectomy is performed, by which only a part of the larynx, usually one vocal chord, is removed. Partial laryngectomies are also often performed in conjunction with other cancer treatments, such as radiation therapy or chemotherapy.

During a laryngectomy, the surgeon removes the larynx through an incision in the neck. The procedure also requires the surgeon to perform a **tracheotomy**, because air can no longer flow into the lungs. He makes an artificial opening called a stoma in the front of the neck. The upper portion of the trachea is brought to the stoma and secured, making a permanent alternate way for air to get to the lungs. The connection between the throat and the esophagus is not normally affected, so after healing, the person whose larynx has been removed (called a laryngectomee) can eat normally.

Diagnosis/Preparation

A laryngectomy is performed after cancer of the larynx has been diagnosed by a series of tests that allow the otolaryngologist (a physician often called an ear, nose and throat, or ENT specialist) to examine the throat and take tissue samples (biopsies) to confirm and stage the cancer. People need to be in good general health to undergo a laryngectomy, and will have

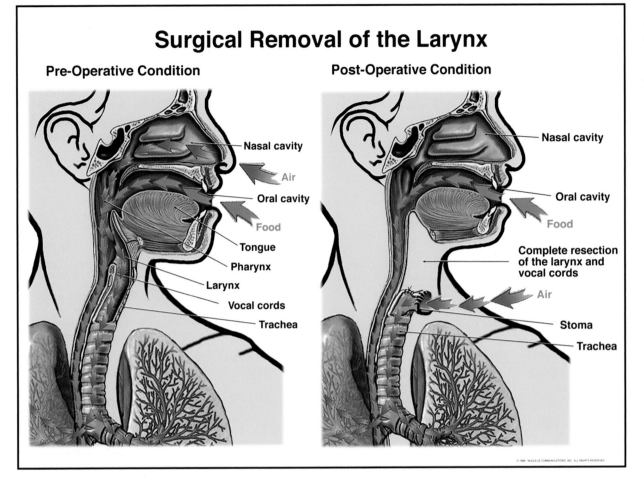

Surgical Removal of the Larynx

Pre-Operative Condition

- Nasal cavity
- Air
- Oral cavity
- Food
- Tongue
- Pharynx
- Larynx
- Vocal cords
- Trachea

Post-Operative Condition

- Nasal cavity
- Oral cavity
- Food
- Complete resection of the larynx and vocal cords
- Air
- Stoma
- Trachea

© 1998 NUCLEUS COMMUNICATIONS, INC. ALL RIGHTS RESERVED

The surgical removal of the larynx. *(Nucleus Medical Art, Inc./Alamy)*

standard pre-operative blood work and tests to make sure they are able to safely withstand the operation.

As with any surgical procedure, the patient is required to sign a consent form after the procedure is thoroughly explained. Blood and urine studies, along with **chest x ray** and EKG may be ordered as required. If a total laryngectomy is planned, the patient meets with a speech pathologist for discussion of post-operative expectations and support.

Aftercare

A person undergoing a laryngectomy spends several days in intensive care (ICU) and receives intravenous (IV) fluids and medication. As with any major surgery, blood pressure, pulse, and respiration are monitored regularly. The patient is encouraged to turn, cough, and deep-breathe to help mobilize secretions in the lungs. One or more drains are usually inserted in the neck to remove any fluids that collect. These drains are removed after several days.

It takes two to three weeks for the tissues of the throat to heal. During this time, the laryngectomee cannot swallow food and must receive nutrition through a tube inserted through the nose and down the throat into the stomach. Normal speech is also no longer possible and patients are instructed in alternate means of vocal communication by a speech pathologist.

When air is drawn in normally through the nose, it is warmed and moistened before it reaches the lungs. When air is drawn in through the stoma, it does not have the opportunity to be warmed and humidified. In order to keep the stoma from drying out and becoming crusty, laryngectomees are encouraged to breathe artificially humidified air. The stoma is usually covered with a light cloth to keep it clean and to keep unwanted particles from accidentally entering the lungs. Care of the stoma is extremely important, since it is the person's only way to get air to the lungs. After a laryngectomy, a health-care professional will teach the laryngectomee and his or her caregivers how to care for the stoma.

KEY TERMS

Larynx—Also known as the voice box, the larynx is composed of cartilage that contains the apparatus for voice production. This includes the vocal cords and the muscles and ligaments that move the cords.

Lymph nodes—Accumulations of tissue along a lymph channel, which produce cells called lymphocytes that fight infection.

Tracheotomy—A surgical procedure in which an artificial opening is made in the trachea (windpipe) to allow air into the lungs.

There are three main methods of vocalizing after a total laryngectomy. In esophageal speech, patients learn how to "swallow" air down into the esophagus and create sounds by releasing the air. Tracheoesophageal speech diverts air through a hole in the trachea made by the surgeon. The air then passes through an implanted artificial voice. The third method involves using a hand-held electronic device that translates vibrations into sounds. The choice of vocalization method depends on several factors including the age and health of the laryngectomee, and whether other parts of the mouth, such as the tongue, have also been removed (**glossectomy**).

Risks

Laryngectomy is often successful in curing early-stage cancers. However, it requires major lifestyle changes and there is a risk of severe psychological stress from unsuccessful adaptations. Laryngectomees must learn new ways of speaking, they must be constantly concerned about the care of their stoma. Serious problems can occur if water or other foreign material enters the lungs through an unprotected stoma. Also, women who undergo partial laryngectomy or who learn some types of artificial speech will have a deep voice similar to that of a man. For some women this presents psychological challenges. As with any major operation, there is a risk of infection. Infection is of particular concern to laryngectomees who have chosen to have a voice prosthesis implanted, and is one of the major reasons for having to remove the device.

Normal results

Ideally, removal of the larynx will remove all cancerous material. The person will recover from the operation, make lifestyle adjustments, and return to an active life.

WHO PERFORMS THE PROCEDURE AND WHERE IS IT PERFORMED?

A laryngectomy is usually performed by an otolaryngologist in a hospital operating room. In the case of trauma to the throat, the procedure may be performed by an emergency room physician.

Morbidity and mortality rates

The American Cancer Society estimates that 3,660 people will die of laryngeal cancer in 2007. Of these, 2,900 will be men and 760 will be women.

Alternatives

There are two alternatives forms of treatment:

• Radiation therapy, a treatment that uses high-energy rays (such as x rays) to kill or shrink cancer cells.

• Chemotherapy, a treatment that uses drugs to kill cancer cells. Usually the drugs are given into a vein or by mouth. Once the drugs enter the bloodstream, they spread throughout the body to the cancer site.

Resources

BOOKS

Abeloff, MD et al. Clinical Oncology. 3rd ed. Philadelphia: Elsevier, 2004.

Cummings, CW, et al. Otolayrngology: Head and Neck Surgery. 4th ed. St. Louis: Mosby, 2005.

PERIODICALS

King, A. I., B. E. Stout, and J. K. Ashby. "The Stout prosthesis: an alternate means of restoring speech in selected laryngectomy patients." Ear Nose and Throat Journal 82 (February 2003): 113–116.

Landis, B. N., R. Giger, J. S. Lacroix, and P. Dulguerov. "Swimming, snorkeling, breathing, smelling, and motorcycling after total laryngectomy." American Journal of Medicine 114 (March 2003): 341–342.

Nakahira, M., K. Higashiyama, H. Nakatani, and T. Takeda. "Staple-assisted laryngectomy for intractable aspiration." American Journal of Otolaryngology 24 (January-February 2003): 70–74.

ORGANIZATIONS

American Academy of Otolaryngology - Head and Neck Surgery. One Prince Street, Alexandria, VA 22314. (703) 806-4444. http://www.entnet.org.

American Cancer Society. National Headquarters. 1599 Clifton Road NE, Atlanta, GA 30329. (800) ACS-2345.http://www.cancer.org.

Cancer Information Service. National Cancer Institute. Building 31, Room 10A19, 9000 Rockville Pike, Bethesda, MD 20892. (800)4-CANCER. http://www.nci.nih.gov/cancerinfo/index.html.

QUESTIONS TO ASK THE DOCTOR

- Is laryngectomy my only viable treatment option?
- How will drinking and eating be affected?
- How will I talk without my larynx?
- How will my breathing be affected?
- What about my usual activities?
- Is there a support group in the area that can assist me after surgery?
- How long will it be until I can verbally communicate? What are my options?
- What is the risk of recurring cancer?

International Association of Laryngectomees (IAL). http://www.larynxlink.com/.

National Institute on Deafness and Other Communication Disorders. National Institutes of Health. 31 Center Drive, MSC 2320, Bethesda, MD 20892-2320. http://www.nidcd.nih.gov.

The Voice Center at Eastern Virginia Medical School. Norfolk, VA 23507. http://www.voice-center.com.

OTHER

"Laryngectomy: The Operation." The Voice Center. http://www.voice-center.com/laryngectomy.html.

Kathleen Dredge Wright
Tish Davidson, A.M.
Monique Laberge, Ph.D.
Rosalyn Carson-DeWitt, MD

Larynx removal *see* **Laryngectomy**

Laser coagulation therapy *see* **Photocoagulation therapy**

Laser in-situ keratomileusis (LASIK)

Definition

Laser in-situ keratomileusis (LASIK) is a non-reversible refractive procedure performed by ophthalmologists to correct myopia, hyperopia, or astigmatism. The surgeon uses an excimer laser to cut or reshape the cornea so that light will focus properly on the retina.

Purpose

LASIK is an **elective surgery** for patients who want to permanently correct myopia (nearsightedness), hyperopia (farsightedness), or astigmatism without eyeglasses, contact lenses, or refractive surgical procedures. The goal for most patients is to be free of any type of corrective lenses. Some patients may find wearing eyeglasses or contact lenses interferes with their careers or hobbies. Many professional athletes have chosen LASIK to improve their performance. However, patients with higher degrees of refractive error will still need some type of corrective lens.

LASIK is most commonly performed on myopes. For myopia, the surgeon flattens the cornea; for hyperopia, the surgeon steepens the cornea. Surgeons correct astigmatism by creating a normally shaped cornea with the excimer laser.

A new type of LASIK also can treat contrast sensitivity as well as refractive error. Custom LASIK incorporates new eye mapping technology into standard LASIK. The surgeon measures the eye from front to back creating a three dimensional corneal map. This much-more detailed map gives surgeons more specific information for the excimer laser and enables them to correct other abnormalities besides refractive error.

Demographics

LASIK candidates have myopia, hyperopia, or astigmatism; are 18 or older; and have had stable vision for at least two years. The American Academy of Ophthalmology (AAO) estimated that 1.3 million refractive surgery procedures were performed in 2002. LASIK was estimated to account for 95% of those procedures.

The first LASIK patients in the late 1990s were in the upper class, or upper middle class, and in their early 30s to mid-40s. The market was limited for the elective procedure that at first could range as expensive as $5,000 per eye. The number of younger patients receiving LASIK (in their early to mid-20s) was expected to rise in 2003 and beyond. The number of procedures also was expected to increase as prices continued to stabilize, and surgery centers and physicians offered payment plans.

Description

LASIK is a relatively new procedure. In April 1985, German physician Theo Seiler was the first to use an excimer laser to attempt to correct astigmatism in blind eyes. Experiments with excimer lasers on blind eyes were also completed in the United States in the mid-1980s. The term LASIK was invented by Greek ophthalmologist Ioannis Pallikari, the first surgeon to

Laser in situ keratomileusis

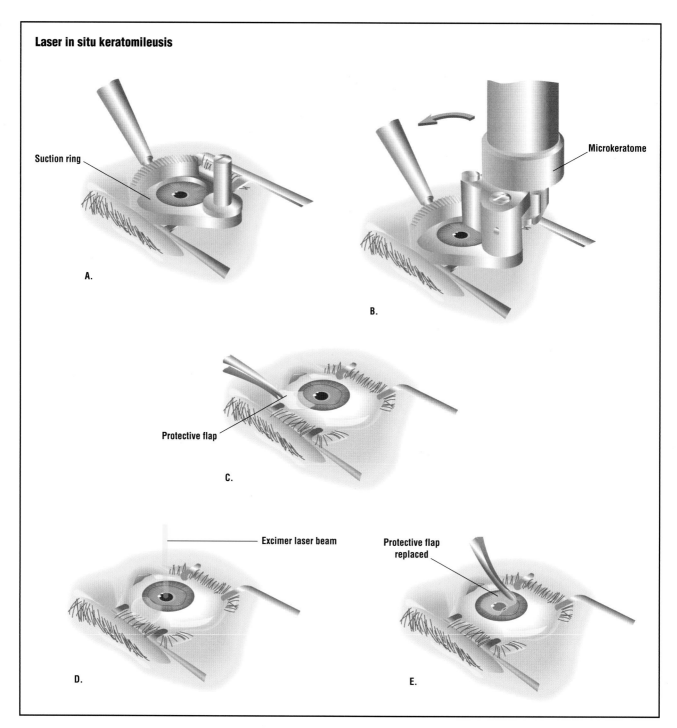

Suction ring

Microkeratome

A.

B.

Protective flap

C.

Excimer laser beam

Protective flap
replaced

D.

E.

In LASIK surgery, the eye is held open with a speculum, and a suction ring is attached to the eyeball (A). A microkeratome is used to shave the protective flap off the top of the eye (B), which is then pulled back (C). A computer-controlled laser is used to reshape the cornea (D), and the protective flap is replaced (E). *(Illustration by GGS Information Services. Cengage Learning, Gale.)*

use the hinged flap technique. Dr. Stephen Brint, as part of a clinical trial in 1991, performed the first LASIK procedure in the United States.

As of 2003, there are two types of LASIK. The standard LASIK procedure and custom LASIK, which relatively few surgeons have the technology to perform.

Ablation—During LASIK, the vaporization of eye tissue.

Astigmatism—Asymmetric vision defects due to irregularities in the cornea.

Cornea—The clear, curved tissue layer in front of the eye. It lies in front of the colored part of the eye (iris) and the black hole in the center of the iris (pupil).

Corneal topography—Mapping the cornea's surface with a specialized computer that illustrates corneal elevations.

Dry eye—Corneal dryness due to insufficient tear production.

Enhancement—A secondary refractive procedure performed in an attempt to achieve better visual acuity.

Excimer laser—An instrument that is used to vaporize tissue with a cold, coherent beam of light with a single wavelength in the ultraviolet range.

Hyperopia—The inability to see near objects as clearly as distant objects, and the need for accommodation to see objects clearly.

Intraocular lens (IOL) implant—A small, plastic device (IOL) that is usually implanted in the lens capsule of the eye to correct vision after the lens of the eye is removed. This is the implant used in cataract surgery.

Macular degeneration—A condition usually associated with age in which the area of the retina called the macula is impaired due to hardening of the arteries (arteriosclerosis). This condition interferes with vision.

Microkeratome—A precision surgical instrument that can slice an extremely thin layer of tissue from the surface of the cornea.

Myopia—A vision problem in which distant objects appear blurry. Myopia results when the cornea is too steep or the eye is too long and the light doesn't focus properly on the retina. People who are myopic or nearsighted can usually see near objects clearly, but not far objects.

Nomogram—A surgeon's adjustment of the excimer laser to fine-tune results.

Presbyopia—A condition affecting people over the age of 40 where the system of accommodation that allows focusing of near objects fails to work because of age-related hardening of the lens of the eye.

Retina—The sensory tissue in the back of the eye that is responsible for collecting visual images and sending them to the brain.

Stroma—The thickest part of the cornea between Bowman's membrane and Decemet's membrane.

Standard LASIK

Standard LASIK takes from 10 to 20 minutes to perform and the results are immediate. It's standard practice in LASIK operating rooms to have a clock on the wall so patients immediately can note they are able to read a clock face or other items that previously were blurry.

Immediately before the procedure, the ophthalmologist may request corneal topography (a corneal map) to compare with previous maps to ensure the treatment plan is still correct. The surgeon may also measure the cornea's thickness if he didn't previously. After these tests, a technician or co-managing optometrist will perform a refraction to make sure the refractive correction the surgeon will program into the laser is correct.

Three sets of eye drops will be administered twice before surgery. The first drop anesthetizes the cornea, the second drop prevents infection and the third drop controls inflammation after LASIK. Patients may be given a sedative, such as Valium. This is administered to calm nervous patients or to help patients sleep after the procedure.

After the prep work is completed, the patient reclines on a laser bed and the surgeon is seated directly behind the patient. If the procedure is being done on both eyes on the same day, the surgeon will patch the second eye. An eyelid speculum is inserted in the eye to be treated first to hold the eyelids apart. The patient stares at the blinking light of a laser microscope and must fixate his or her gaze on that light. The patient must remain still throughout the procedure.

The surgeon checks the refractive numbers on the laser. Because each patient's cornea is shaped differently, the surgeon may have to adjust the level of correction. Laser companies provide an algorithm to determine the correction level, and the surgeon may alter the level because of a patient's special needs. The adjustments are called nomograms. After the adjustments, the surgeon checks the microkeratome blade for defects.

The surgeon then indents the cornea to mark the flap location. The surgeon places a suction ring in the center of the sclera. A technician will activate the microkeratome's suction. The patient's vision dims at this point. The surgeon tests pressure by touching the cornea with a tonometer. Before using the microkeratome, sterile saline solution is squirted into the suction ring to lubricate the cornea. The microkeratome head is placed in the gear tracks of the suction ring, and the surgeon guides the microkeratome across the suction ring to create a flap. The microkeratome stops just short of traveling completely across the cornea. It leaves a hinge of tissue, commonly called a flap. After the flap is created, the surgeon removes the suction ring and slips a spatula under it and moves it to the side, exposing the stroma (inner cornea).

Once the stroma is exposed, the laser ablation begins, ranging from 30 to 60 seconds. The ablation flattens the cornea of myopic patients; steepens the cornea of hyperopic patients; and reshapes the cornea of astigmatic patients. After the ablation, the surgeon replaces the flap. More saline solution is squirted to remove any debris and enable the flap to move back into place without interruption. The surgeon ensures the flap is in place and removes any wrinkles. The surgeon places a shield over the eye to keep the flap in place. No **stitches** are used.

If bilateral LASIK is being performed, the patient must remain still while he is prepared for treatment on the remaining eye.

Custom LASIK

About half of all LASIK procedures are deemed "custom" LASIK. The difference between standard LASIK and custom LASIK lies in the diagnosis and who can be treated. With custom LASIK, surgeons use a wavefront analyzer (aberrometer) that beams light through the eye and finds irregularities based on how the light travels through the eye. It creates a three-dimensional corneal map to create a customized pattern for each patient. For standard LASIK, each patient with the same refractive error is treated with the same setting on the excimer laser, barring a few adjustments. The new technology individualizes treatment not only for refractive errors, but also for visual disorders that previous corneal mapping technology could not detect. As of early 2003, there was only one FDA-approved laser capable of the customized ablations, but others were awaiting approval.

Besides the customized excimer laser, the surgical procedure is the same. Surgeons now can treat patients who have higher-order aberrations, such as contrast sensitivity. Therefore, custom LASIK can successfully treat glare, night vision and other contrast problems.

Diagnosis/Preparation

Before LASIK, patients need to have a complete eye evaluation and comprehensive medical history taken. Soft contact lens wearers should stop wearing their lenses at least one week before the initial exam. Gas permeable lens wearers should not wear their lenses from three weeks to a month before the exam. Contact lens wear can alter the cornea's shape, which should be allowed to return to its natural shape before the initial exam.

The initial exam

During the first exam, the surgeon's staff will take a comprehensive medical history to determine if there are underlying medical problems that will prevent a successful surgery. This screening process will determine patients who should not have the procedure including:

- pregnant women or women who are breastfeeding
- patients with very small or very large refractive errors
- patients with low contrast sensitivity
- patients with scarred corneas or macular disease
- people with autoimmune diseases
- diabetics
- glaucoma patients
- patients with persistent blepharitis

The physician will also ask about medication. Some prescription medicines have been known to cause postsurgical scarring or cause flecks under the corneal flap. It is important for the patient to disclose any prescriptions or over-the-counter medicines taken regularly. Allergies to prescription medicine must also be discussed.

A complete eye exam will be performed to determine refractive error, uncorrected visual acuity and best corrected visual acuity. A cycloplegic refraction using eye drops to dilate the pupils also will be performed. Other examination procedures include corneal mapping, a keratometer reading to determine the curvature of the central part of the cornea, a slit lamp exam to determine any damage to the cornea and evidence of glaucoma and cataracts. A fundus exam also will be performed to check for retinal holes and macular degeneration and macular disease. Other tests are done to rule out glaucoma.

While those tests check general eye health, others more closely relate to the outcome of LASIK surgery. A corneal pachymeter measures the cornea's thickness. This is important because surgeons remove tissue during surgery. A pupilometer measures the pupil when it is naturally dilated in a dark room without drops. Patients with large pupils have been known to have complications after LASIK, such as glare and halos.

Treatment options/Informed consent

After the exam, the patient and physician discuss treatment options and expectations. Patients who expect to see perfectly after LASIK are usually not considered good candidates because they usually are dissatisfied with the results. Surgeons also discuss how patients will handle presbyopia, which occurs during the patient's 40s. LASIK does not correct for presbyopia, and patients will need reading glasses to accommodate for reading when presbyopia occurs. Sometimes patients 40 and older opt for monovision to treat presbyopia, where one eye is left untreated or one eye is only partially corrected. Monovision means one eye is for short-term vision and the other is for distance vision.

The doctor will advise the patient of any possible LASIK complications, explain the procedure and answer questions. After deciding on a treatment option, the patient is required to sign an **informed consent** form.

At this time, payment will also be discussed. Insurance usually does not cover LASIK, although some offer a limited benefit for the procedure. Some laser centers offer payment plans and some physicians have begun using credit companies to handle payments. LASIK can cost anywhere from $999 to $3,000 per eye. The cost varies greatly from surgeon to surgeon. Most of the fees are global, and cover all the pre-operative and postoperative exams as well as the procedure. Patients should be advised of what the fee covers, and if retreatments to the original surgery are included in that price.

Presurgery preparations

The patient is advised to discontinue contact lens wear immediately and refrain from using creams, lotions, make-up or perfume for at least two days before surgery. Patients may also be asked to scrub their eyelashes for a period of time to remove any debris. Patients also must find transportation to and from the surgery, and also to and from the first postoperative visit. Medication and distorted vision make it unsafe for the patients to drive after LASIK.

Aftercare

After LASIK, patients may experience burning, itching or a foreign body sensation. They should be advised not to touch the eye as that could damage the flap. Many physicians recommend sleeping after the surgery. Patients may also experience glare, starbursts, or halos that should improve after the first few days. Patients are advised to seek help immediately if they feel severe eye pain, or if symptoms worsen.

The first follow-up visit is 24–48 hours after surgery. The physician will remove the eye shield, check the patient's vision, and may prescribe more antibiotic drops or artificial tears. Patients must refrain from strenuous activity, such as contact sports, for at least a month. The use of creams, lotions, and make-up must also be avoided for at least two weeks. Hot tubs and swimming pools should be avoided for at least two months. Patients are advised that refraining from these activities and products will help stem infection and aid healing of the cornea.

Patients will have regularly scheduled visits post-LASIK for at least six months. Vision gradually improves the first few months after surgery. In some cases, if the vision does not meet expectations and the surgeon believes it can be further corrected, he will perform an enhancement. Enhancements are usually done for undercorrection. Overcorrected patients usually need eyeglasses or contact lenses.

Risks

Surgeons separate LASIK complications into two categories.

Intraoperative risks

- Cornea perforation. This complication has almost disappeared because of advances in microkeratome design.
- Flap complications. Newer microkeratomes also have reduced the likelihood of "free caps," where the cap becomes unhinged. An experienced surgeon replaces the cap after ablation. In some cases, the procedure must be aborted while the eye heals.
- Laser hot spots. Higher energy surrounding the laser beam can cause irregular astigmatism. Proper laser testing before the procedure eliminates this risk.
- Central islands. This refers to a raised area in the central part of the treated zone that receives insufficient laser treatment. Any raised area can decrease the laser's effectiveness. The island either shrinks by itself or can be remedied with retreatment.
- Decentered ablation. This occurs when the laser beam is aimed incorrectly. This can result in permanent halos and ghost images.

Postoperative complications

- Undercorrection or overcorrection. Undercorrection can usually be treated with an enhancement, but overcorrection will require the use of eyeglasses or contact lenses.

- Debilitating symptoms. These can be permanent or transient, and include glare, halos, double vision and poor nighttime vision. Some patients may also lose contrast sensitivity.
- Dry eye. This also can be permanent or transient. Most patients experience some dry eye immediately after surgery. Some patients continue to experience dry eye and are treated with artificial tears or punctal plugs.
- Displaced flap. Occurs after the eye is hit or rubbed. If immediate attention is given by the surgeon, who must lift the flap and clean under it, no long-term effects occur.
- Nonspecific diffuse intralamellar keratitis. Commonly known as Sands of the Sahara, this complication can range from corneal haze to eye clouding that resembles swirling sand. It is treated with topical steroids, although severe cases may require eye irrigation.
- Epithelial ingrowth. The cells of the lower cornea migrate under the corneal cap. The surgeon must lift the cap and remove the cells. If untreated, vision is impaired.
- Striae. These are wrinkles in the flap that can reduce visual acuity. The surgeon must lift the corneal flap and smooth the wrinkles.
- Photophobia. Extreme sensitivity to light can last a few days or a week after surgery.
- Infection. This rarely occurs after LASIK. It is treated with antibiotics.

Normal results

After LASIK, most patients are able to see well enough to pass a driver's license exam without glasses or contact lenses. Some patients will still need corrective lenses, but the lenses won't need to be as powerful.

Because LASIK is a relatively new procedure, there is limited information on long-term regression. If patients are being treated for myopia, they should be aware they will have to rely on spectacles with the onset of presbyopia.

Morbidity and mortality rates

Information about mortality rates following LASIK is limited because the procedure is elective. Complications that can lead to more serious conditions, such as infection, are treated with **topical antibiotics** after LASIK. The most serious possible complication from LASIK is blindness from an untreated complication. As of 2000, there had been no reports of blindness-induced LASIK. One incidence

of legal blindness was reported after a severely myopic patient had retinal hemorrhages. However, it was inconclusive whether or not LASIK was the causative agent.

Alternatives

Nonsurgical alternatives

Nonsurgical alternatives to LASIK are contact lenses and eyeglasses, which can also correct refractive errors. Continuous-wear contact lenses, which a patient can sleep in for as long as 30 days, can provide the same effect as LASIK if the patient wants good vision upon waking. Orthokeratology involves a rigid gas permeable contact lens the patient wears for a predetermined amount of time to reshape the cornea. After removing the lens, it takes weeks for the cornea to return to its normal shape. At that time, the patient repeats the process.

Corneal rings and implants are another alternative for myopes. These require surgery without lasers and involve a corrective lens surgically implanted in the eye. One of the biggest benefits to these procedures is that they are reversible. However, they may not provide the crisp vision of a successful LASIK. There also are several different types of intraocular lenses being tested to treat myopia and hyperopia.

Surgical alternatives

There also are surgical alternatives to LASIK. They include:

- Conductive keratoplasty. This uses radio frequency waves to shrink corneal collagen. It is used to treat mild to moderate hyperopia.
- Photorefractive keratectomy (PRK). PRK also uses an excimer laser and is similar to LASIK. However, in PRK, the surface of the cornea is removed by the laser. PRK patients have a longer recovery time and may need steroidal eye drops for months after surgery. Its success rate is similar to that of LASIK.
- Radial keratotomy (RK). RK was the first widely used surgical correction for mild to moderate myopia. The surgeon alters the shape of the cornea without a laser. This is one of the oldest refractive procedures, and has proved successful on lower and moderate corrections.
- Astigmatic keratotomy (AK). AK is a variation of RK used to treat mild to moderate astigmatism. AK has proved successful if the errors are mild to moderate.
- Laser thermal keratoplasty (LTK). LTK was approved as to treat hyperopia in 2000. An LTK patient's vision

WHO PERFORMS THE PROCEDURE AND WHERE IS IT PERFORMED?

An ophthalmologist performs LASIK, but because it is a relatively new technology, the surgeon may not have received training as part of his residency. It is more likely the surgeon has completed continuing medical education courses or may have had training provided by the laser companies. He may also have received training as part of membership in an organization such as the American Society of Refractive Surgeons.

Before and aftercare probably will be provided by a co-managing optometrist. The optometrist usually performs the pre- and postoperative exams, and also discusses the patient's suitability for LASIK and any potential problems.

Ophthalmic technicians may perform preliminary testing, including corneal topography and corneal measuring. Laser technicians are required to have special training provided by the laser manufacturer.

Surgeons may perform LASIK in a hospital where they rely on the hospital staff for support. Because lasers are expensive, some surgeons pool their resources and purchase a laser that they share at a freestanding surgery center. LASIK is also provided by surgeons at surgery centers owned by refractive surgery companies. These businesses hire support staff, optometrists and surgeons to perform LASIK.

is overcorrected for one to three months, and the effect of improved near vision may diminish over time as distance vision improves. Some regression has been noted.

Resources

BOOKS

Yanoff, M et al. Ophthalmology. 2nd ed. St. Louis: Mosby, 2004.

ORGANIZATIONS

American Academy of Ophthalmology. PO Box 7424, San Francisco, CA 94120-7424 (415) 561-8500. http://www.aao.org

American Society of Cataract and Refractive Surgery. 4000 Legato Road, Suite 850, Fairfax, VA 22033-4055. (703) 591-2220. <ascrs@ascrs.org>. http://www.ascrs.org.

QUESTIONS TO ASK THE DOCTOR

- How many LASIK procedures have you performed and how long have you been performing them?
- Who will handle the aftercare, the ophthalmologist or co-managing optometrist?
- What is the experience of the laser support team?
- How many of your patients achieve 20/20 or better?
- What percentage of your patients have serious complications? Minor complications?
- Who will treat complications, if any, after the procedure?
- If the patient needs an enhancement, is that an extra expense, or is it covered in the original fee?

OTHER

"Basik Lasik: Tips on LASIK Eye Surgery." Federal Trade Commission. August 2000 [cited February 22, 2003]. http://www.ftc.gov/bcp/conline/pubs/health/lasik.htm.

Croes, Keith. "Custom LASIK: The Next Generation in Laser Eye Surgery." All About Vision. [cited February 22, 2003]. http://www.allaboutvision.com/visionsurgery/custom_lasik.htm.

Gonzalez, Jeanne Michelle. "To Increase LASIK Volume, Know Your Market." Ocular Surgery News. September 1, 2002 [cited February 23, 2003]. http://www.osnsupersite.com/view.asp?ID=3473.

Gottlieb, Howard O.D. "The Changing LASIK Patient." Ophthalmology Management. February 2001 [cited February 22, 2003]. http://www.ophmanagement.com/archive_results.asp?loc=archive/2001/february/0201038.htm.

"LASIK Eye Surgery." U.S. Food and Drug Administration Center for Devices and Radiological Health. October 1, 2002 [cited February 20, 2003]. http://www.fda.gov/cdrh/lasik.

"Refractive Errors and Refractive Surgery." American Academy of Ophthalmology. [cited February 23, 2003]. http://www.aao.org/aao/newsroom/facts/errors.cfm.

Mary Bekker

Laser iridotomy

Definition

Laser iridotomy is a surgical procedure that is performed on the eye to treat angle closure glaucoma, a condition of increased pressure in the front chamber

Laser iridotomy

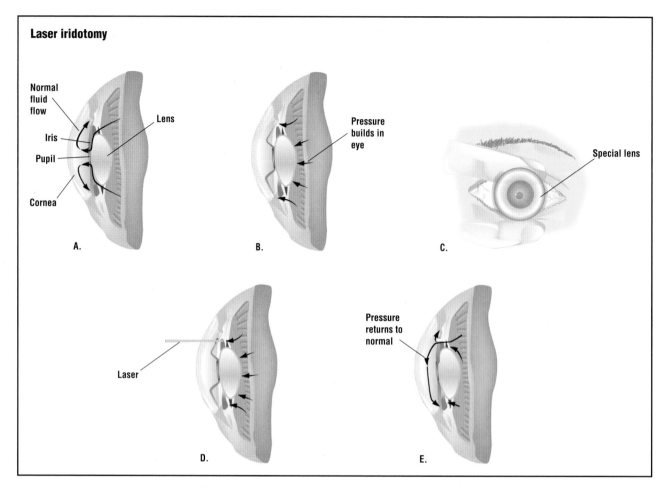

Normally intraocular fluid flows freely between the anterior and posterior sections of the eye (A). As pressure builds in the eye, this circulation is cut off (B). In a laser iridotomy, a special lens is placed on the eye (C). A laser is used to create a hole in part of the iris (D), allowing fluid to flow more normally and intraocular pressure to return to normal (E). *(Illustration by GGS Information Services. Cengage Learning, Gale.)*

(anterior chamber) that is caused by sudden (acute) or slowly progressive (chronic) blockage of the normal circulation of fluid within the eye. The block occurs at the angle of the anterior chamber that is formed by the junction of the cornea with the iris. All one needs to do to see this angle is to look at a person's eye from the side. Angle closure of the eye occurs when the trabecular meshwork, the drainage site for ocular fluid, is blocked by the iris. Laser iridotomy was first used to treat angle closures in 1956. During this procedure, a hole is made in the iris of the eye, changing its configuration. When this occurs, the iris moves away from the trabecular meshwork, and proper drainage of the intraocular fluid is enabled.

The angle of the eye refers to a channel in which the trabecular meshwork is located. To maintain the integrity of the eye, fluid must always be present in the anterior (front) and posterior (back) chambers of the eye. The fluid, known as aqueous fluid, is made in the ciliary processes, which are located behind the iris. Released continuously into the posterior chamber of the eye, aqueous fluid circulates throughout the eye. Eventually the fluid returns to the general circulation of the body, first passing through a space between the iris and the lens, then flowing into the anterior chamber of the eye and down the angle, where the trabecular meshwork is located. Finally, the fluid leaves the eye. An angle closure occurs when drainage of the aqueous fluid through the trabecular meshwork is blocked and the intraocular pressure builds up as a result.

For most types of angle closure, or narrow angle glaucoma, laser iridotomy is the procedure of choice. Changes in intraocular pressure (IOP) can alter the name of the condition when the IOP in the eye becomes elevated above 22 mm/Hg as a result of an angle closure. Then, angle closure becomes angle closure glaucoma. Lowering of the IOP is important because extreme elevations in IOP can damage the retina and the optic nerve permanently. The lasers used to perform this surgery are either the Nd:Yag laser or, if a patient has a bleeding disorder, the argon laser. The majority of patients with glaucoma do not have angle closure glaucoma, but rather have an open angle glaucoma, a type of glaucoma in which the angle of the eye is open.

An angle closure occurs when ocular anomalies (abnormalities) temporarily or permanently block the trabecular meshwork, restricting drainage of the ocular fluid. The anatomical anomalies that make an individual susceptible to an angle closure are, for example, an iris that is bent forward in the anterior chamber (front) of the eye, a small anterior chamber of the eye, and a narrow entrance to the angle of the eye. Some conditions that cause an angle closure are a pupillary block, a plateau iris, phacolytic glaucoma, and malignant glaucoma. The end result of all of these situations is an elevation of the IOP due to a build-up of aqueous fluid in the back part of the eye. The IOP rises quickly when an acute angle attack occurs and within an hour the pressure can be dangerously elevated. The sclera or white of the affected eye becomes red or injected. The patient will usually experience decreased vision and ocular pain with an acute angle closure. In severe cases of acute angle glaucoma, the patient may experience nausea and vomiting. Individuals with neurovascular glaucoma caused by uncontrolled diabetes or hypertension may have similar symptoms, but treatment for this type of glaucoma is very different.

Within a normal eye, the iris is in partial contact with the lens of the eye behind it. Individuals with narrow angles are at greater risk of angle closure by pupillary block because their anterior chamber is shallow; thus, the iris is closer to the lens and more likely to adhere completely to the lens, creating a pupillary block. Patients who experience a pupillary block may have had occasionally temporary blocks prior to a complete angle closure. Pupillary block can be started by prolonged exposure to dim light. Therefore, it not uncommon for an acute angle closure to occur as an individual with a narrow angle emerges from a dark environment such as a theater into bright light. It can also be brought on by neurotransmitter release during emotional stress or by medications taken for other medical conditions. Pupil dilation may be a side effect of one or more of those medications. However, pupillary block is the most common cause of angle closure, and laser iridotomy effectively treats this condition.

The irises of individuals with plateau iris is bunched up in the anterior chamber, and it is malpositioned

KEY TERMS

Angle—A channel in the anterior part of the eye in which the trabecular meshwork is located.

Angle closure—A blockage of the angle of the eye, causing an increase in pressure in the eye and possible glaucoma.

Aphakic—Having no lens in the eye.

Cataract—Condition that causes the lens to become opaque.

Glaucoma—A group of diseases of the eye, often caused by increased pressure (IOP), which can cause blindness if not treated.

Gonioscopy—Examination of the anterior chamber of the eye using a special instrument called a gonioscope.

Hyperosmotic agents—Causing abnormally rapid osmosis.

Iridectomy—Removal of a portion of the iris.

Iridoplasty—Surgery to alter the iris.

Iris—The colored part of the eye that is located in the anterior chamber.

Malignant glaucoma—Glaucoma the gets worse even after iridectomy.

Mannitol—A type of diuretic.

Laser iridotomy—A procedure, using either the Nd:Yag laser or the argon laser, to penetrate the iris, such that a hole, through which the fluid in the eye can drain, is formed.

Osmosis—Passage of a solvent through a membrane from an area of greater concentration to an area of lesser concentration.

Phacolytic glaucoma—Type of glaucoma causing dissolution of the lens.

Photocoagulation—Condensation of material by laser.

Pilocarpine—Drug used to treat glaucoma.

Trabecular meshwork—Area of fibrous tissue that forms a canal between the iris and cornea, through which aqueous humor flows.

Uveitis—Inflammation of the iris and ciliary bodies.

along the trabecular meshwork. Plateau iris develops into glaucoma when the iris bunches up further; this occurs on dilation of the iris, which temporarily closes off the angle of the eye. Laser iridotomy is often performed as a preventive measure in these patients, but is not a guarantee against future angle closure. This is because changes within the eye, such as narrowing of the angle and increase in lens size can lead to iris plateau syndrome, where the iris closes the angle of the eye even if a laser iridotomy has already been performed. Peripheral laser iridoplasty and other surgical techniques can be performed if the angle still closes after iridotomy.

Other causes of narrow angle glaucoma are not as common. Phacolytic glaucoma results when a cataract becomes hypermature and the proteins of the lens with the cataract leak out to block the angle and the trabecular meshwork. Laser iridotomy is not effective for this type of angle closure. Malignant glaucoma exists secondary to prior ocular surgery, and is the result of the movement of anatomical structures within the eye such that the meshwork is blocked. Patients who have no intraocular lens (aphakic) are at increased risk for angle closure, as well.

Laser iridotomy is also performed prophylactically (preventively) on asymptomatic individuals with narrow angles and those with pigment dispersion. Individuals with a narrow angle are at higher risk of an acute angle closure, especially upon dilation of the eye. Pigment dispersion is a condition in which the iris pigment is shed and is dispersed throughout the anterior part of the eye. If the dispersion occurs because of bowing of the iris (the case in 60% of patients with pigment dispersion) a laser iridotomy will decrease the bowing or concavity of the iris and subsequent pigment dispersion. This decreases the risk of these individuals to develop pigmentary glaucoma, a condition in which the dispersed pigment may clog the trabecular meshwork. Laser iridotomy is also done on the fellow eye of a patient who has had an angle closure of one eye, as the probability of an angle closure in the second eye is 50%.

There are other indications for laser iridotomy. It is performed on patients with nanophthalmos, or small eyes. Laser iridotomy may be also be indicated for patients with malignant glaucoma to help identify the etiology of elevated IOP. Because laser iridotomy changes the configuration of the iris, it is sometimes used to open the angle of the eye prior to performing a laser argon laser trabeculoplasty, if the angle is narrow. Laser trabeculoplasty is another laser procedure used to treat pigmentary and pseudoexfoliation glaucoma.

Laser iridotomy cannot be performed if the cornea is edematous or opacified, nor if the angle is completely closed. If an inflammation (such as uveitis or neovascular glaucoma) has caused the angle to close, laser iridotomy cannot be performed.

Purpose

The purpose of a laser iridotomy is to allow an equalization of pressure between the anterior (front) and posterior (back) chambers of the eye by making a hole in the superior peripheral iris. Once the laser iridotomy is completed, the intraocular fluid flows freely from the posterior to the anterior part of the eye, where it is drained via the trabecular meshwork. The result of this surgery is a decrease in IOP.

When laser iridotomy is performed on patients with chronic angle closure, or on patients with narrow angles with no history of angle closure, the chances of future pupillary blocks are decreased.

Demographics

Acute angle glaucoma occurs in one in 1,000 individuals. Angle-closure glaucoma generally expresses itself in populations born with a narrow angle. Individuals of Asian and Eskimo ancestry appear to be at greater risk of developing it. Family history, as well as age, are risk factors. Older women are more often affected than are others. Laser iridotomy is performed on the same groups of individuals as those likely to experience angle closures due to pupillary block or plateau iris. They are performed more often on females (whose eyes are smaller than those of males), and more often performed on the smaller eyes of far-sighted people than on those of the nearsighted because angle closures occur more frequently in those who are far-sighted. Most laser iridotomies are performed on those over age 40 with a family history of plateau iris or narrow angles. However, preventative plateau iris laser iridotomies are performed on patients in their 30s. Individuals who are aphakic (have no intraocular lens) are at greater risk of angle closure and undergo laser iridotomy more frequently than phakic patients. Phakic patients are those who either have an intact lens or who are psuedophakic (have had a lens implant after the removal of a cataract removal).

Description

After the cornea swelling has subsided and the IOP has been lowered, which is usually 48 hours after an acute angle closure, laser iridotomy can be performed. Pilocarpine is applied topically to the eye to constrict the pupil prior to surgery. When the pupil is constricted, the iris is thinner and it is easier for the surgeon to form a penetrating hole. If the eye is still edematous (swollen)—often the situation when the

IOP is extremely high—glycerin is applied to the eye to enable the surgeon to visualize the iris. Apraclonidine, an IOP-lowering drop, is applied one hour before surgery. Immediately prior to surgery, an anesthetic is applied to the eye.

Next, an iridotomy contact lens, to which methylcellulose is added for patient comfort, is placed on the upper part of the front of the eye. This lens increases magnification and helps the surgeon to project the laser beam accurately. The patient is asked to look downwards as the surgeon applies laser pulses to the iris, until a hole is formed. Once the hole has penetrated the iris, iris material bursts through the opening, followed by aqueous fluid. At this point, the surgeon can also see the anterior part of the lens capsule through the opening. The hole, or iridotomy, is formed on the upper section of the iris at an 11:00 or 1:00 position, so that the hole is covered by the eyelid. In an aphakic eye, the hole may be made on the inferior iris. After performing the laser iridotomy, the surgeon may place a gonioscopy lens on the eye if the angle has been opened. There is no pain associated with this surgery, although heat may be felt at the site of the lasering.

If a patient has a tendency to bleed, the argon laser will be used to pre-treat the patient prior to completing the procedure with an Nd:Yag laser, or the argon laser alone may be used. The argon laser is capable of photocoagulation, and thus minimizes any bleeding that occurs as the iris is penetrated. Formation of a hole is more difficult with the argon laser because it operates with a decreased power density and the tissue response to the argon laser has greater variability. The argon laser can be used with more patients who have medium-brown irises, however, since the energy of this laser is readily absorbed by irises of this color.

Diagnosis/Preparation

To determine if laser iridotomy is indicated, the surgeon must first determine if and how the angle is occluded. The eye is anesthetized and the aonioscopic lens, which enables the surgeon to see the interior of the eye, is placed on the front of the eye. This is done at the slit lamp biomicroscope in a dark room. In cases of prophylactic surgery, an image of the eye is taken with a **ultrasound** biomicroscope in both dim and bright light; this shows the doctor how the patient's iris moves with dilation and constriction, and how this movement can close an angle if the patient has ocular features that predispose the eye to an angle closure.

When an angle is completely occluded (blocked), the elevated IOP usually causes corneal edema (swelling). Because this swelling can obscure the surgeon's view of the iris, prior to performing a laser iridotomy, the IOP must be lowered. One technique to lower the IOP is corneal indentation, in which the gentle pressure is applied several times to the cornea with a lens or hook to open the angle. This pressure on the cornea causes a shift in the internal structures of the eye, enhances aqueous drainage, and lowers the IOP.

The doctor can attempt to lower the IOP medically, as well. One drug that lowers the pressure is acetazolamide, which is given either orally or by intravenous (IV) to decrease aqueous production in the eye. This may be administered up to four times a day, until the adhesion is broken. Another method of lowering the IOP, if acetazolamide is not effective, is the use of hyperosmotic agents, which through osmosis causes drainage of the aqueous fluid from the eye into the rest of the body. Hyperosmotic agents are given orally; an example of such an agent is glycerine. Given by IV, mannitol can be used. As the fluid drains from the eye, the vitreous—the jellylike substance behind the lens in the posterior chamber—shrinks. As it shrinks, the lens in the eye pulls away from the vitreous, creating an opening to the anterior chamber such that aqueous fluid can flow to the anterior chamber. The success of this procedure is increased, due to gravity, if the patient is laying supine (on the back).

Once the IOP has begun to decrease, the pressure is further decreased using topical glaucoma medications, such as pilocarpine, or beta blockers. Any inflammation that occurs because of the iridotomy must be controlled with steroid eye drops.

If glaucomatous-like visual field is present prior to surgical intervention, the prognosis for the patient is not as good as if the visual field were completely intact. Thus, a visual field test may be done prior to surgery.

Aftercare

Immediately after the procedure, another drop of aproclonidine is applied to the eye. The IOP is checked every hour for a several hours postsurgery. If the IOP increases dramatically, then the increased IOP is treated until lowered. Because of inflammation is inherent in this procedure, **corticosteroids** are applied to the eye every five minutes for 30 minutes, then hourly for six hours. This therapy is then continued four times a day for a week. Thereafter, the patient is seen by the surgeon at one week postsurgery and again at two to six weeks postsurgery. If there are complications, the patient is seen more frequently.

After the pressure has been stabilized, a visual field test to determine the extent of damage to the optic nerve may be performed again.

Risks

The greatest risk of laser iridotomy is an increase in intraocular pressure. Usually, the IOP spike is transient and of concern to the surgeon only during the first 24 hours after surgery. However, if there is damage to the trabecular meshwork during **laser surgery**, the intraocular pressure may not be lowered enough and extended medical intervention or filtration surgery is required. Patients who undergo preventative laser iridotomy do not experience as great an elevation in IOP.

The second greatest risk of this procedure is anterior uvetis, or inflammation within the eye. Usually the inflammation subsides within several days, but can persist for up to 30 days. Thus, the follow-up care for laser iridotomy includes the application of topical corticosteroids. A posterior synechia, in which the iris may again adhere to the lens, may occur if intraocular inflammation is not properly managed.

Other risks of this procedure include the following: swelling of, abrasions to, or opacification of the cornea; damage to the corneal endothelium (the part of the cornea that pumps oxygen and nutrients into the iris); bleeding of the iris during surgery, which is controlled during surgery by using the iridotomy lens to increase pressure on the eye; and macular edema, which can be avoided by careful aim of the laser during surgery to avoid the macula. The macula is the part of the eye where the highest concentration of photoreceptors is found. Perforations of the retina are rare. Distortion of the pupil and rupture of the lens capsule are other possible complications. Opacification of the anterior part of the lens is common, but this does not increase the risk of cataract formation when compared with the general population.

When the iridotomy hole is large, or if the eyelid does not completely cover the opening, some patients report such side effects as glare and double vision. The argon laser produces larger holes. Patients may also complain of an intermittent horizontal line in their vision. This may occur when the eyelid is raised just enough such that a small section of the inferior part of the hole is exposed, and disappears when the eyelid is lowered. Blurred vision may occur as well, but usually disappears 30 minutes after surgery.

Normal results

In successful laser iridotomy, the IOP differential between the anterior and posterior chambers is relieved and IOP is decreased, and the pupil is able to constrict normally. These are the results of the flatter configuration of the iris after laser iridotomy. If an angle closure is treated promptly, the patient will have minimal or no loss of vision. This procedure is successful in up to 44% of patients treated.

WHO PERFORMS THE PROCEDURE AND WHERE IS IT PERFORMED?

A laser iridotomy is performed in an office setting by an ophthalmologist, a doctor or osteopathic doctor with residency training in the treatment of eye diseases. The doctor who performs a laser iridotomy may have advanced fellowship training in the treatment of glaucoma, after completing his or her three-year residency.

Morbidity and mortality rates

For up to 64% of patients, one to three years after laser iridotomy, the IOP will rise above 21 mmHg, and long-term medical treatment is required. One-third of argon laser iridotomies will close within six to 12 weeks after surgery and will require a repeat laser iridotomy. Approximately 9% of Nd:Yag laser iridotomies must be redone for this reason. Closure of the iridotomy site is more likely if a uveitis presented after surgery. Up to 45% of patients will have anterior lens opacities after laser iridotomy, but these opacifications do not put the patient at an increased risk of cataracts.

Alternatives

An alternative to laser iridotomy is surgical **iridectomy**, a procedure in which part of the iris is removed surgically. This was the procedure of choice prior to the development of laser iridotomy. The risks for iridectomy are greater than for the laser iridotomy, because it involves an incision through the sclera, the white tunic covering of the eye that surrounds the cornea. The most common complication of an iridectomy is cataract formation, occurring in more than 50% of patients who have had a surgical iridectomy. Since an incision in the eye is required for surgical iridectomy, other procedures, such as filtration surgery—if needed in the future—will be more difficult to perform. Studies comparing the visual outcomes and IOP control of laser iridotomy with surgical iridectomy show equivalent results.

In the case of acute angle closures that occur because of reasons other than, or in addition to pupillary block, argon laser peripheral iridoplasty is performed.

QUESTIONS TO ASK THE DOCTOR

Will this procedure successfully lower the pressure in my eye indefinitely, or will I need further surgery or medication?

What is the probability that my other eye will also need surgery?

What will my vision be like after surgery?

Which laser will you use for my surgery?

How many laser iridotomies have you performed?

During this procedure, several long burns of low power are placed in the periphery of the iris. The iris contracts and pulls away from the angle, opening it up and relieving the IOP.

Resources

BOOKS

Albert, Daniel M., M.D. Ophthalmic Surgery Principles and Techniques. Oxford, England: Blackwell Science, 1999.

Albert, Daniel M., M.D., and Frederick A. Jakobiec. Principles and Practice of Ophthalmology 2nd ed. Philadelphia, PA: W. B. Saunders Company, 2000.

Albert, Daniel, M. and Mark J. Lucarelli, MD. Clinical Atlas of Procedures in Ophthalmic Surgery1st ed. Chicago, IL: American Medical Association Press, 2003.

Azuara-Blanco, Augusto, M.D., Ph.D., et. al. Handbook of Glaucoma. 1st ed. London, England: Taylor & Francis, 2007.

Kanski, Jack J. M. D., et. al. Glaucoma A Colour Manual of Diagnosis and Treatment.Oxford, England: Butterworth-Heinemann, 2003.

Ritch, Robert, M. D., et. al. The Glaucomas.St. Louis, MO: 1996.

PERIODICALS

Breingan, Peter J. M. D., et. al. "Iridolenticular Contact Decreases Following Laser Iridotomy For Pigment Dispersion Syndrome." Archives of Ophthalmology117 (March 1999): 325-28.

Brown, Reay H.,M. D., et. al. "Glaucoma Laser Treatment Parameters and Practices of ASCRS Members–1999 Survey." Journal of Cataract and Refractive Surgery 26 (May 2000): 755-65.

Nolan, Winifred P., et. el. "YAG Laser Iridotomy Treatment for Primary Angle Closure in East Asian Eyes." British Journal of Ophthalmology84 (2000): 1255-59.

Wu, Shiu-Chen, M. D., et. al. "Corneal Endothelial Damage After Neodymium: YAG Laser Iridotomy." Ophthalmic Surgery and Lasers 31 (October 2000): 411-16.

ORGANIZATIONS

American Academy of Ophthalmology. P. O. Box 7424, San Francisco, CA 94120-7424. (415) 561-8500. http://www.aao.org.

Canadian Ophthalmological Society (COS). 610-1525 Carling Avenue, Ottawa ON K1Z 8R9 Canada. http://www.eyesite.ca>.

National Eye Institute. 2020 Vision Place, Bethesda, MD 20892-3655. (301) 496-5248. http://nei.nih.gov.

Prevent Blindness America. 500 East Remington Road, Schaumburg, IL 60173. (800) 331-2020. http://www.prevent-blindness.org.

Wills Eye Hospital. 840 Walnut Street, Philadelphia, PA 19107. (215) 928-3000. http://www.willseye.org.

OTHER

"Lasers in Eye Surgery."http://www.karger.ch/gazette/64/kohnen/art_5_2.htm

"Laser Iridotomy and Iridoplasty."http://cuth.cataegu.ac.kr/~jwkim/glaucoma/doctor/LI.htm

"Narrow Angle Glaucoma and Acute Angle Closure Glaucoma." http://www.M.D.eyedocs.com/edacuteglaucoma.htm

National Cancer Institute (NCI) Physician Data Query (PDQ). Intraocular (Eye) Melanoma: Treatment, January 2, 2003 [cited April 2, 2003]. http://www.nci.nih.gov/cancerinfo/pdq/treatment/intraocularmelanoma/healthprofessional.

National Eye Institute (NEI).Facts About Glaucoma. 2008. NIH Publication No. 99–651.http://www.nei.nih.gov/health/glaucoma/glaucoma_facts.asp.

Tanasescu, I., and F. Grehn. "Advantage of Surgical Iridectomy Over Nd:YAG Laser Iridotomy in Acute Primary Angle Closure Glaucoma." Presentation on September 29, 2001, at the 99th annual meeting of the Deutsche Ophthalmologische Gesellschaft. http://www.dog.org/2001/mo_13.htm.

Waheed, Nadia K., and C. Stephen Foster. "Melanoma, Iris." eMedicine, July, 2005 [cited April 2, 2003]. http://www.emedicine.com/oph/topic405.htm.

Martha Reilly, OD
Laura Jean Cataldo, RN, EdD

Laser posterior capsulotomy

Definition

Laser posterior capsulotomy, or YAG laser capsulotomy, is a noninvasive procedure performed on the eye to remove the opacification (cloudiness) that develops on the posterior capsule of the lens of the eye after extraction of a cataract. This differs from the anterior capsulotomy that the surgeon makes during cataract extraction to remove a cataract and implant an intraocular lens (IOL). Laser posterior capsulotomy is performed with Nd:YAG laser, which uses a wavelength to disrupt the opacification on the posterior lens capsule. The energy emitted from the laser forms a hole in the lens capsule, removing a central area of the opacification. This posterior capsule opacification (PCO) is also referred to as a secondary cataract.

PCO formation is an attempt by the eye to make a new lens from remaining lens material. One form of PCO is a fibrosis that forms inside the capsule by lens epithelial (outer lining) cells that migrate from the anterior capsule to the posterior capsule when the anterior lens capsule is opened to remove the primary cataract and insert the IOL. Opacification is also be formed by residual lens cortex cells. The epithelial cells can transform into myofibroblasts and proliferate; myofibroblasts are precursors to muscle cells and capable of contraction. The deposit of collagen on these cells leaves the posterior lens capsule with a white, fibrous appearance. This type of opacification can appear within days of cataract surgery. The greatest capsule opacification is found around the edges of the IOL, where the anterior and posterior lens capsules adhere and form a seam, called Soemmering's ring.

Elschnig's pearls are a proliferation of cells on the outside of the capsule. This type of PCO can be several layers thick and develops months to years after cataract surgery. Elschnig's pearls can also appear along the margins of a previously performed laser capsulotomy.

A secondary cataract will also form from wrinkling of the lens capsule, either secondary to contraction of the myofibroblasts on the capsule or because of stretching of the capsule by haptics, or hooks, used to hold the IOL in place.

Posterior capsule opacification is the most common complication of cataract removal or extraction. It does not occur when an anterior chamber lens is implanted, because in this procedure the capsule is usually extracted along with the cataract, and a lens is attached to the iris in the front part of the eye, called the anterior chamber. This technique for cataract removal is not often performed.

Purpose

The purpose of a laser capsulotomy is to remove a PCO. This procedure dramatically improves visual acuity and contrast sensitivity and decreases glare. The visual acuity before capsulotomy can be as poor as 20/400, but barring any other visual or ophthalmologic conditions, the patient will see as well after a laser posterior capsulotomy as after removal of the original

---

KEY TERMS

Anterior chamber—The part of the eye located behind the cornea and in front of the iris and lens; it is filled with aqueous fluid.

Cataract—An opacification of the lens in the eye. There are three types of cataracts: subcapsular, which forms inside the capsule in which the lens is located; nuclear, which is a natural yellowing of the lens nucleus; cortical, which refers to spoke-type opacities within the cortex layer of the lens.

Lens capsule—The "bag" is a membrane that holds the lens in place and holds a posterior lens implant when a cataract is removed.

Macula—This is the part of the retina in which the highest concentration of photoreceptors are found.

Posterior capsule opacification (PCO)—This refers to the opacities that form on the back of the lens capsule after cataract removal or extraction. It is synonymous with a secondary cataract.

Posterior chamber—This is the part of the eye located behind the lens of the eye and includes the retina, where the photoreceptors are located.

Vitreous—This is the jelly-like substance that fills the space between the lens capsule and the retina.

---

cataract. Laser capsulotomies are usually performed once a patient's vision is 20/30.

Demographics

Approximately 20% of patients who undergo cataract extraction with placement of an intraocular lens into the posterior lens capsule will eventually undergo a laser capsulotomy, although a PCO may appear in up to 50% of patients who have undergone cataract surgery. The average time after cataract extraction for this procedure to be performed is two years, but it may be performed as early as three months after cataract removal, or as late as five years afterward.

Patients who fall into groups with an increased incidence of a secondary cataract formation have an increased rate of YAG capsulotomy. Patients who are younger when undergoing cataract removal are more likely to develop a PCO than are geriatric patients. This is particularly true of pediatric patients who are experiencing ocular growth. The incidence of PCO is higher in women than in men. Fifty percent of patients who experience papillary, or iris capture, of the IOL, which occurs if the IOL moves through the pupil (a hole in the iris) from its position in the posterior chamber of the eye to the anterior chamber, will form a PCO and benefit from laser capsulotomy.

The degree and incidence of capsule opacification also varies with the type of implant used in the initial cataract operation. Larger implants are associated with decreased opacification, and round-edged silicone implants are associated with a greater incidence of opacification than are acrylic implants, which have a square-edged design. These two types of IOLs are called foldable implants because they unfold after being placed in the eye, allowing for a smaller incision on the front of the eye during cataract surgery. Also, the incidence of PCO is less with a silicone IOL than with a rigid IOL. The greater the amount of remaining lens material after extraction, especially in the area of Soemmering's ring, the greater the probability of PCO formation and laser capsulotomy. Also, diabetic patients are more likely to require a YAG capsulotomy than are non-diabetic patients. This is especially true for YAG capsulotomies performed on diabetics 18 months or later after cataract removal. The extent of diabetic retinopathy does not correlate with incidence of PCO or laser capsulotomy. Finally, insufficient dilation of the pupil during cataract surgery and inexperience of the surgeon doing cataract removal contribute to an increased risk of secondary cataract formation.

Description

Laser capsulotomy is usually performed in an ophthalmologist's office as an outpatient procedure. Before beginning the capsulotomy, the patient is given an **informed consent** for the procedure. An hour before the laser capsulotomy, a drop of a pressure-lowering drug such as timoptic or apraclonidine is administered. A weak dilating drop to enlarge the pupil is applied to the eye. The eye may be anesthetized locally if the doctor uses a special contact lens for the procedure.

The patient then puts the head in the chinrest of a slit lamp microscope, to which a laser is attached. The doctor then may place a special lens on the front of the eye. It is important that the patient remain still as the doctor focuses on the posterior capsule. A head strap to help keep the patient's head in place may be used. While focusing on the posterior capsule, the doctor, with repeated bursts from the Nd:Yag laser in a circular manner, disrupts the PCO. An opening forms on the posterior part of the lens capsule as part of the PCO falls off of the posterior capsule and into the vitreous. Another drop of apraclonidine, or other pressure-lowering eyedrop, is applied to the eye as a preventative measure for increased pressure in the eye, which is experienced by most patients after the procedure. This is a brief procedure lasting only a few minutes and is not associated with pain.

Diagnosis/Preparation

Prior to performing a posterior capsulotomy, the doctor will perform a thorough ophthalmic examination and review any systemic medical problems. The ophthalmologic includes evaluation of visual acuity, slit-lamp biomicroscope examination of the eye to assess the extent and type of opacification and rule out inflammation or swelling in the front of the eye, measurement of intraocular pressure, and a thorough evaluation of the fundus or back of the eye to check for retinal detachments and macular problems, which would limit the extent to which the YAG capsulotomy could improve vision. A potential acuity meter (PAM) may be used to ascertain best expected visual acuity after YAG capsulotomy, and brightness acuity testing will determine the extent of glare experienced by the patient. Contrast sensitivity testing is employed by some doctors.

This procedure cannot be performed in the presence of certain preexisting ophthalmologic conditions. For example, irregularities of the cornea would interfere with the ability of the doctor to see the posterior capsule. Also, a laser capsulotomy could not be performed if there is ongoing inflammation in the eye, or if swelling of the macula (a part of the retina) is present. A laser capsulotomy would be contraindicated with glass IOLs. If macular edema is suspected, which can occur in up to 30% of patients who have undergone cataract surgery, a test called a fluoroscein **angiography** may also be performed.

Aftercare

After a laser capsulotomy, the patient will remain in the office for one to four hours so that the pressure in the eye can be evaluated. The patient can then resume normal everyday activities. After surgery, pressure-lowering eyedrops may be used for a week if the intraocular pressure is raised significantly. Cycloplegic agents to keep the pupil dilated and to prevent spasm of the muscles in the iris, and steroids to reduce inflammation may also be prescribed for up to a week. Follow-up visits are scheduled at one day, one week, one month, three months, and six months after capsulotomy.

Risks

One risk of laser capsulotomy is damage to the intraocular implant. Factors that determine the extent of damage to the IOL include the inherent resistance of a particular IOL to damage by the laser, the amount of energy used in the procedure, the position of the IOL within the lens capsule, and the focusing accuracy of the surgeon. The thicker the opacification of the lens capsule, the greater the amount of energy needed to remove it. The accuracy of the surgeon is improved when there is less opacification on the lens capsule.

In addition, during laser capsulotomy, the IOL can be displaced into the eye's vitreous. This happens more often in eyes with a rigid implant, rather than with acrylic or silicone IOLs, and also if a larger implant is used. If the posterior capsule ruptures during extraction of the primary cataract, risk of lens displacement is also increased. Displacement risk is also increased if the area over which the laser capsulotomy is done is large. The most serious complication of a capsulotomy is IOL damage so extensive that extraction would be required. This is a rare complication.

Another risk of this surgery is the re-formation of Elschnig's pearls over the opening created by the capsulotomy. This occurs in up to 80% of patients within two years of laser capsulotomy. Most of time, these PCOs will resolve over time without treatment, but 20% of patients will require a second laser capsulotomy. This secondary opacification by Elschnig pearls represents a spatial progression of the opacification that caused the initial secondary cataract.

Other risks to take into account when considering a posterior capsulotomy are macular edema, macular holes, corneal edema, inflammation of the iris, retinal detachment, and increased pressure in the eye, as well as glaucoma. These risks escalate with increased laser energy and with increased size of the capsulotomy area. Retinal detachments are usually treated with removal of the vitreous behind the lens capsule. Macular edema is treated by application of topical anti-inflammatory drops or intraocular steroid injections. Steroids control iritis (inflammation of the iris), either topically or intraocularly. Macular holes are also treated by removal of the vitreous (the substance that fills the main area of the eyeball), followed by one to three weeks of facedown positioning. Elevated intraocular pressure and glaucoma are treated with anti-glaucoma drops or glaucoma surgery, if necessary.

Finally, increased glare at night may result when the size of the capsulotomy is smaller than the diameter of the pupil during dark conditions.

Normal results

Within one to two days after surgery, maximum visual acuity will be attained by almost 99% of patients.

WHO PERFORMS THE PROCEDURE AND WHERE IS IT PERFORMED?

The procedure is usually performed in the office of an ophthalmologist or an osteopathic physician. The training of an ophthalmologist includes a year of internship and at least three years of residency training in the treatment of eye diseases and in eye surgery after graduation from medical school. In states where doctors of optometry are permitted by law to use lasers, and if trained in laser surgery, an optometrist may do the laser capsulotomy. A co-managing optometrist may perform some of the preoperative testing and postoperative follow-up.

Once the opacification is removed, most patients will not need a change in spectacle prescription. However, patients who have undergone implantation of a rigid IOL may experience an increase in hyperopia, or far-sightedness, after a capsulotomy. For a few weeks after surgery, the presence of visual floaters, which are pieces of the excised capsule, is normal. But, the presence of floaters months after this timeframe, especially if accompanied by flashes of light, may signal a retinal tear or detachment and require immediate attention. Also, if vision suddenly or gradually worsens after an initial improvement, further follow-up to determine the cause of a decrease in visual function is imperative.

Morbidity and mortality rates

The probability of a retinal detachment after capsulotomy is 1.6–1.9%. This represents a two-fold increase of retinal detachment over the rate for all patients undergoing cataract surgery, regardless if a posterior capsulotomy was done or not. Macular edema occurs in up to 2.5% of patients who undergo a laser capsulotomy and is more likely to occur when the capsulotomy is performed soon after cataract extraction, or in younger individuals. Rarely does glaucoma develop after laser capsulotomy, although as many as two-thirds of patients will experience transient increased intraocular pressure.

Alternatives

The alternative to laser capsulotomy is surgical capsulotomy of the PCO and the adjacent anterior vitreous. There is an increased risk of retinal detachment when this invasive intraocular surgery is employed. The other alternative is to leave the PCO in place. This leaves the patient with permanent decreased visual acuity.

QUESTIONS TO ASK THE DOCTOR

- What are the alternatives to laser capsulotomy?
- Am I a good candidate for this procedure?
- What will my vision be like after the procedure?
- How many of these procedures have you performed?

Resources

BOOKS

Albert, Daniel M., M.D. Ophthalmic Surgery Principles and Techniques. Oxford, England: Blackwell Science, 1999.

Albert, Daniel M., M.D., and Frederick A. Jakobiec. Principles and Practice of Ophthalmology 2nd ed. Philadelphia, PA: W. B. Saunders Company, 2000.

Albert, Daniel, M. and Mark J. Lucarelli, MD. Clinical Atlas of Procedures in Ophthalmic Surgery 1st ed. Chicago, IL: American Medical Association Press, 2003.

Azuara-Blanco, Augusto, M.D, Ph.D., et. al. Handbook of Glaucoma. 1st ed. London, England: Taylor & Francis, 2007.

Ritch, Robert, M. D., et. al. The Glaucomas. St. Louis, MO: 1996.

Gills, James P. Cataract Surgery: The State of the Art. Thorofare, NJ: Slack Inc., 1997.

Jaffe, Norman. Atlas of Ophthalmic Surgery. London: Mosby-Wolfe, 1996.

Steinert, Roger F. Cataract Surgery: Technique, Complications, & Management. 2nd ed. Philadelphia, PA: W. B. Saunders, 2003.

PERIODICALS

Baratz, K. H., et al. "Probability of Nd:YAG Laser Capsulotomy After Cataract Surgery in Olmsted County, Minnesota." American Journal of Ophthalmology 131 (February 2001): 161–166.

Charles, Steve. "Vitreoretinal Complications of YAG Laser Capsulotomy." Ophthalmology Clinics of North America 14 (December 2001): 705–9.

Chua, C. N, et al. "Refractive Changes following Nd:YAG Capsulotomy." Eye 15 (June 2001): 303–5.

Hayashi, Ken. "Posterior Capsule Opacification After Surgery In Patients With Diabetes Mellitus." American Journal of Ophthalmology 134 (July 2002): 10–16.

Hu, Chao-Yu., et al. "Change in the Area of Laser Posterior Capsulotomy: 3 Month Follow-Up." Journal of Cataract and Refractive Surgery 27 (April 2001): 537–42.

Kurosaka, Daijiro, et al. "Elschnig Pearl Formation Along the Neodymium:YAG Laser Posterior Capsulotomy Margin." Journal of Cataract and Refractive Surgery 28 (October 2002): 1809–1813.

O'Keefe, Michael, et al. "Visual Outcomes and Complications of Posterior Chamber Intraocular Lens Implantation in the First Year of Life." Journal of Cataract and Refractive Surgery 27 (December 2001): 2006–11.

Sundelin, Karin, and Johan Sjostrand. "Posterior Capsule Opacification 5 Years After Extracapsular Cataract Extraction." Journal of Cataract and Refractive Surgery 25 (February 1999): 246–50.

Trinavarant, A., et al. "Neodymium: YAG laser Damage Threshold of Foldable Intraocular Lenses." Journal of Cataract and Refractive Surgery 27 (May 2001): 775–880.

ORGANIZATIONS

American Academy of Ophthalmology. P. O. Box 7424, San Francisco, CA 94120-7424. (415) 561-8500. http://www.aao.org.

Canadian Ophthalmological Society (COS). 610-1525 Carling Avenue, Ottawa ON K1Z 8R9 Canada. http://www.eyesite.ca>.

National Eye Institute. 2020 Vision Place, Bethesda, MD 20892-3655. (301) 496-5248. http://nei.nih.gov.

Prevent Blindness America. 500 East Remington Road, Schaumburg, IL 60173. (800) 331-2020. http://www.prevent-blindness.org.

Wills Eye Hospital. 840 Walnut Street, Philadelphia, PA 19107. (215) 928-3000. http://www.willseye.org.

OTHER

"Lasers in Eye Surgery."http://www.karger.ch/gazette/64/kohnen/art_5_2.htm

"Narrow Angle Glaucoma and Acute Angle Closure Glaucoma." http://www.M.D.eyedocs.com/edacuteglaucoma.htm

National Cancer Institute (NCI) Physician Data Query (PDQ). Intraocular (Eye) Melanoma: Treatment, January 2, 2003 [cited April 2, 2003]. http://www.nci.nih.gov/cancerinfo/pdq/treatment/intraocularmelanoma/healthprofessional.

National Eye Institute (NEI).Facts About Glaucoma. 2008. NIH Publication No. 99–651.http://www.nei.nih.gov/health/glaucoma/glaucoma_facts.asp.

Waheed, Nadia K., and C. Stephen Foster. "Melanoma, Iris." eMedicine, July, 2005 [cited April 2, 2003]. http://www.emedicine.com/oph/topic405.htm.

Martha Reilly, OD
Laura Jean Cataldo, RN, EdD

Laser skin resurfacing

Definition

Laser skin resurfacing involves the application of laser light to the skin in order to remove fine wrinkles and tighten the skin surface. It is most often used on the skin of the face.

Purpose

The purpose of laser skin resurfacing is to use the heat generated by extremely focused light to remove the upper to middle layers of the skin. This procedure eliminates superficial signs of aging and softens the appearance of other lesions such as scars. Upon healing, the surface of the skin has a younger appearance. Microscopic analysis of skin after laser resurfacing shows that the healed surface more closely resembles younger, healthier skin in many aspects.

Demographics

According to the American Society for Aesthetic **Plastic Surgery**, there were more than 72,000 laser skin resurfacing procedures performed in the United States in 2002. Almost all persons of sufficient age have one or more symptoms of aging or damaged skin that can be treated by this procedure, including fine lines in the skin, known as rhytides; discoloration of the skin; acne scarring; and surgical or other types of scars.

Description

A central component of the laser skin resurfacing technique is the laser device. Laser is an acronym for light amplification by stimulated emission of radiation. This device produces an intense beam of light of a specific, known wavelength. Laser light is produced by high-energy stimulation of different substances such as crystals, liquid dyes, and gases. For skin resurfacing, two types of lasers produce light that is well absorbed by the upper to middle layers of the skin: light produced from carbon dioxide gas (CO_2) and light produced from a crystal made of eribium, yttrium, aluminum, and garnet (Er:YAG). Combination lasers are also commercially available.

There are as yet no standard parameters for laser use in all skin resurfacing procedures. Settings are determined on a case-by-case basis by the laser surgeon who relies on his or her own experience.

Before the procedure begins, medication is often given to relax the patient and reduce pain. For small areas, local topical (surface-applied) anesthetics are often used to numb the area to be treated. Alternatively, for large areas, nerve block-type anesthesia is used. Some laser surgeons use **conscious sedation** (twilight anesthesia) alone or in combination with other techniques.

During the procedure, the patient lies on his or her back on the surgical table, eyes covered to protect them from the laser light. Laser passes are performed over the area being treated, utilizing computer control

KEY TERMS

Acetic acid—Vinegar; very dilute washes of the treated areas with a vinegar solution are suggested by some surgeons after laser skin resurfacing.

Carbon dioxide—Abbreviated CO_2; a gas that produces light that is well absorbed by the skin, so is commonly used for skin resurfacing treatments.

Erbium:YAG—A crystal made of erbium, yttrium, aluminum, and garnet that produces light that is well absorbed by the skin, so it is used for skin resurfacing treatments.

Hydrogel—A gel that contains water, used as a dressing after laser skin resurfacing.

Milia—Small bumps on the skin that are occur when sweat glands are clogged.

Rhytides—Very fine wrinkles, often of the face.

Topical—Applied to the skin surface.

of the laser for precise results. In general, more passes are needed with Er:YAG lasers than carbon dioxide laser treatment.

Because areas of the body other than the face have relatively low numbers of the cells central to the healing process, laser skin resurfacing is not generally used anywhere but on the face, as elsewhere the healing process may be so slow as to result in scarring.

Diagnosis/Preparation

An initial consideration is to determine which laser would be best for any particular skin resurfacing procedure. Carbon dioxide lasers have been in use longer and have been shown to produce very good results. However, the healing times tend to be long and redness can persist for several months. In contrast, because the light produced by the Er:YAG laser is more efficiently absorbed by the skin, less light energy and shorter pass times can be used, which significantly shortens the healing time. Unfortunately, the results obtained with this laser have not been as consistently good as with a carbon dioxide laser. Patients should therefore discuss the two laser types and the condition of their skin with their doctor to determine which would be better for their particular situation.

Although controversial, some studies have reported abnormal scarring in patients previously treated with 13 cis-retinoic acid (Accutane), so many surgeons will

WHO PERFORMS THE PROCEDURE AND WHERE IS IT PERFORMED?

The procedure is performed by an experienced laser surgeon or a dermatological surgeon with special training in the use of the laser. It is performed in a special suite adapted for laser use, often located at the surgeon's offices.

require a six-month break from the medication before performing laser skin resurfacing.

Laser skin resurfacing does increase the chance of recurrent or initial herpes simplex virus infection (cold sores) during the healing process. Even with no patient history of the problem, it is important that anti-viral medicine is administered before, the morning of, and following laser skin resurfacing.

Aftercare

After the procedure, any treated areas are dressed for healing. Surgeons are divided on whether the wound should remain open or closed (covered) during the healing process. For example, surgeons that adopt a closed procedure can use a dressing that is primarily hydrogel held on a mesh support to cover the wound. This kind of dressing is changed daily while the epithelium (outer layer of skin) is restored. Open **wound care** involves frequent soaks in salt water or dilute acetic acid, followed by application of ointment. Whatever wound treatment is used, it is important to keep the healing skin hydrated.

Full restoration of the epithelial layer occurs in seven to 10 days after treatment with a carbon dioxide laser and three to five days after treatment with a Er:YAG laser, although redness can persist for many weeks afterward.

Risks

Risks of this procedure include skin redness that persists beyond the initial healing period, swelling, burning sensations, or itching. These risks tend to be short term and lessen over time. More long-term problems can include scarring, increased or decreased pigmentation of the skin, and infection during healing. Finally, the formation of milia, bumps that form due to obstruction of the sweat glands, can occur, although this can be treated after healing with retinoic acid.

QUESTIONS TO ASK THE DOCTOR

- What characteristics of my skin abnormality suggest using laser skin resurfacing to treat it?
- Which laser would be best to treat my skin condition?
- Would dermabrasion or chemical treatments be a better option?
- What is the expected cosmetic outcome for the laser resurfacing treatment in my case?

Normal results

Normal results of this procedure include reduction in the fine lines found in aging skin, improving skin texture, making skin coloration more consistent, and softening the appearance of scars. In a recent study, more than 93% of patients subjectively rated their results from the procedure either very good or excellent.

Morbidity and mortality rates

The morbidity and mortality rates for this cosmetic procedure are close to zero.

Alternatives

Surgical techniques such as facelifts or **blepharoplasty** (eyelid surgery) are often recommended when facial aging is beyond the restorative powers of a laser treatment and the most common alternative technique. Patients should also consider other skin resurfacing techniques such as **dermabrasion** or chemical peels, as these are more effective than laser resurfacing for certain skin conditions and certain skin types.

Resources

BOOKS
Habif TP. Clinical Dermatology. 4th ed. St. Louis: Mosby, 2004.
Roberts, Thomas L. III, and Jason N. Pozner. "Aesthetic Laser Surgery." In Plastic Surgery: Indications, Operations, and Outcomes, Volume 5, edited by Craig A. Vander Kolk, et al. St. Louis, MO: Mosby, 2000.

PERIODICALS
Roy D. "Ablative facial resurfacing." Dermatol Clin 23 (2005): 549–559.

ORGANIZATIONS
American Society for Aesthetic Plastic Surgery. 11081 Winners Circle, Los Alamitos, CA 90720. (800) 364-2147 or (562) 799-2356. www.surgery.org.

American Society of Plastic Surgeons. 444 E. Algonquin Rd., Arlington Heights, IL 60005. (800) 475-2784. www.plasticsurgery.org.

OTHER

Tanzi, Elizabeth L. "Cutaneous Laser Resurfacing: Erbuim: YAG." eMedicine, January 10, 2002.

Michelle Johnson, MS, JD

Laser surgery

Definition

The term "laser" means light amplification by stimulated emission of radiation. Laser surgery uses a laser light source to remove tissues that are diseased or unwanted, to treat blood vessels that are bleeding, or to terminate tumors or lesions. Laser beams are strong beams of light produced by electrically stimulating a particular material, in the case of laser surgery, most often carbon dioxide, argon, or neodymium.

The special light beam is focused to treat tissues by heating the cells until they burst. There are a number of different laser types. Each has a different use and color. Three types of laser that are commonly used are: the carbon dioxide (CO_2) laser; the YAG laser (yttrium aluminum garnet); and the argon laser.

Purpose

Laser surgery is used to:

- cut or destroy tissue that is abnormal or diseased without harming healthy, normal tissue
- shrink or destroy tumors and lesions
- close off nerve endings to reduce postoperative pain
- cauterize (seal) blood vessels to reduce blood loss
- seal lymph vessels to minimize swelling and decrease spread of tumor cells
- remove moles, warts, and tattoos
- decrease the appearance of skin wrinkles

Precautions

Anyone who is thinking about having laser surgery should ask the surgeon to:

- explain why laser surgery is likely to be of greater benefit than traditional surgery
- describe the surgeon's experience in performing the laser procedure the patient is considering

Because some lasers can temporarily or permanently discolor the skin of blacks, Asians, and Hispanics, a dark-skinned patient should make sure that the surgeon has successfully performed laser procedures on people of color. Potential problems include infection, pain, scarring, and changes in skin color.

Some types of laser surgery should not be performed on pregnant women or on patients with severe cardiopulmonary disease or other serious health problems.

Additionally, because some laser surgical procedures are performed under **general anesthesia**, its risks should be fully discussed with the anesthesiologist. The patient should fully disclose all over-the-counter and prescription medications that are being taken, as well as the foods and beverages that are generally consumed; some can interact with agents used in anesthesia.

Description

Lasers are used to perform many surgical procedures. Lasers of various wavelengths are used remove tissue, cut, coagulate, and vaporize. Often times, lasers can take the place of conventional surgical tools—scalpels, cryosugery probes, electrosurgical units, or microwave devices—to carry out standard procedures such as **mastectomy** (breast surgery). By using lasers, surgeons can accomplish more complex tasks and reduce blood loss, decrease postoperative patient discomfort, decrease the chances of infection to the wound, reduce the spread of some cancers, minimize the extent of surgery (in some cases), and achieve better outcomes in wound healing. Also, because lasers are more precise, the laser can penetrate tissue by adjusting the intensity of the light.

Lasers are also extremely useful in both open and laparoscopic procedures. Breast surgery, hernia repair, **bowel resection**, **hemorrhoidectomy**, gallbladder removal, and solid organ surgery are among the common types of laser surgery.

The first working laser was introduced in 1960. Initially used to treat diseases and disorders of the eye, the device was first used to treat diseases and disorders of the eye, whose transparent tissues gave ophthalmic surgeons a clear view of how the narrow, concentrated beam was being directed. Dermatologic surgeons also helped to pioneer laser surgery, and developed and improved upon many early techniques and more refined surgical procedures.

Types of lasers

The three types of lasers most often used in medical treatment are the:

KEY TERMS

Argon—A colorless, odorless gas.

Astigmatism—A condition in which one or both eyes cannot filter light properly and images appear blurred and indistinct.

Canker sore—A blister-like sore on the inside of the mouth that can be painful but is not serious.

Carbon dioxide—A heavy, colorless gas that dissolves in water.

Cardiopulmonary disease—Illness of the heart and lungs.

Cardiopulmonary resuscitation (CPR)—An emergency procedure used to restore circulation and prevent brain death to a person who has collapsed, is unconscious, is not breathing, and has no pulse.

Cauterize—To use heat or chemicals to stop bleeding, prevent the spread of infection, or destroy tissue.

Cornea—The outer, transparent lens that covers the pupil of the eye and admits light.

Endometriosis—An often painful gynecologic condition in which endometrial tissue migrates from the inside of the uterus to other organs inside and beyond the abdominal cavity.

Glaucoma—A disease of the eye in which increased pressure within the eyeball can cause gradual loss of vision.

Invasive surgery—A form of surgery that involves making an incision in the patient's body and inserting instruments or other medical devices into it.

Laparoscopic procedures—Surgical procedures during which surgeons rely on a laparoscope—a pencil-thin instrument that has its own lighting system and miniature video camera. To perform surgeries, only small incisions are needed to insert the instruments and the miniature camera.

Nearsightedness—A condition in which one or both eyes cannot focus normally, causing objects at a distance to appear blurred and indistinct. Also called myopia.

Ovarian cyst—A benign or malignant growth on an ovary. An ovarian cyst can disappear without treatment or become extremely painful and have to be surgically removed.

Pilonidal cyst—A special kind of abscess that occurs in the cleft between the buttocks. Forms frequently in adolescence after long trips that involve sitting.

Vaporize—To dissolve solid material or convert it into smoke or gas.

Varicose veins—Swollen, twisted veins, usually occurring in the legs, that occur more often in women than in men.

• Carbon dioxide (CO_2) laser. Primarily a surgical tool, this device converts light energy to heat strong enough to minimize bleeding, while cutting through or vaporizes tissue.

• Neodymium:yttrium-aluminum-garnet (Nd:YAG) laser. Capable of penetrating tissue more deeply than other lasers, the Nd:YAG laser enables blood to clot quickly, allowing surgeons to see and can enable surgeons to see and touch body parts that could otherwise be reached only through open (invasive) surgery.

• Argon laser. This laser provides the limited penetration needed for eye surgery and superficial skin disorders. In a special procedure known as photodynamic therapy (PDT), this laser uses light-sensitive dyes to shrink or dissolve tumors.

Laser applications

Sometimes described as "scalpels of light," lasers are used alone or with conventional **surgical instruments** in a array of procedures that:

• improve appearance

• relieve pain

• restore function

• save lives

Laser surgery is often standard operating procedure for specialists in:

• cardiology (branch of medicine which deals with the heart and its diseases)

• dentistry (branch of medicine which deals with the anatomy and development and diseases of the teeth)

• dermatology (science which treats the skin, its structure, functions, and its diseases)

• gastroenterology (science which treats disorders of the stomach and intestines)

• gynecology (science which treats of the structure and diseases of women)

• neurosurgery (surgery of the nervous system)

• oncology (cancer treatment)

• ophthalmology (treatment of disorders of the eye)

- orthopedics (treatment of disorders of bones, joints, muscles, ligaments, and tendons)

- otolaryngology (treatment of disorders of the ears, nose, and throat)

- pulmonology (treatment of disorders of the respiratory system)

- urology (treatment of disorders of the urinary tract and of the male reproductive system)

Routine uses of lasers, include eliminating birthmarks, skin discoloration, and skin changes due to aging, and removing benign, precancerous, or cancerous tissues or tumors. Lasers are used to stop a patient's snoring, remove tonsils, remove or transplant hair, and relieve pain and restore function in patients who are too weak to undergo major surgery. Lasers are also used to treat:

- angina (chest pain)

- cancerous or noncancerous tumors that cannot be removed or destroyed

- cold and canker sores, gum disease, and tooth sensitivity or decay

- ectopic pregnancy (development of a fertilized egg outside the uterus)

- endometriosis

- fibroid tumors

- gallstones

- glaucoma, mild-to-moderate nearsightedness and astigmatism, and other conditions that impair sight

- migraine headaches

- noncancerous enlargement of the prostate gland

- nosebleeds

- ovarian cysts

- ulcers

- varicose veins

- warts

- numerous other conditions, diseases, and disorders

Advantages of laser surgery

Often referred to as "bloodless surgery," laser procedures usually involve less bleeding than conventional surgery. The heat generated by the laser keeps the surgical site free of germs and reduces the risk of infection. Because a smaller incision is required, laser procedures often take less time (and cost less money) than traditional surgery. Sealing off blood vessels and nerves reduces bleeding, swelling, scarring, pain, and the length of the recovery period.

Disadvantages of laser surgery

Although many laser surgeries can be performed in a doctor's office, rather than in a hospital, the person guiding the laser must be at least as thoroughly trained and highly skilled as someone performing the same procedure in a hospital setting. The American Society for Laser Medicine and Surgery urges that:

- All operative areas be equipped with oxygen and other drugs and equipment required for cardiopulmonary resuscitation (CPR).

- Nonphysicians performing laser procedures be properly trained, licensed, and insured.

- A qualified and experienced supervising physician be able to respond to and manage unanticipated events or other emergencies within five minutes of the time they occur.

- Emergency transportation to a hospital or other acute care facility (ACF) be available whenever laser surgery is performed in a non-hospital setting.

Diagnosis/Preparation

Because laser surgery is used to treat so many diverse conditions, the patient should ask the physician for detailed instructions about how to prepare for a specific procedure. Diet, activities, and medications may not have to be limited prior to surgery, but some procedures require a **physical examination**, a medical history, and conversation with the patient that:

- enables the doctor to evaluate the patient's general health and current medical status

- provides the doctor with information about how the patient has responded to other illnesses, hospital stays, and diagnostic or therapeutic procedures

- clarifies what the patient expects the outcome of the procedure to be

Aftercare

Most laser surgeries can be performed on an outpatient basis, and patients are usually permitted to leave the hospital or medical office when their **vital signs** have stabilized. A patient who has been sedated should not be discharged until recovery from the anesthesia is complete, unless a responsible adult is available to accompany the patient home.

The doctor may prescribe analgesic (pain-relieving) medication, and should provide easy-to-understand, written instructions on how to take the medication. The doctor should also be able to give the patient a good estimate of how the patient's recovery should progress, the recovery time, and what to do in case complications or emergency arise. The amount of time it takes for the patient to recover from surgery depends on the surgery and on the individual. Recovery time for laser surgery is, for the most part, faster than for traditional surgery.

Risks

Like traditional surgery, laser surgery can be complicated by:

- hemorrhage
- infection
- perforation (piercing) of an organ or tissue

Laser surgery can also involve risks that are not associated with traditional surgical procedures. Being careless or not practicing safe surgical techniques can severely burn the patient's lungs. Patients must wear protective eye shields while undergoing laser surgery on any part of the face near the eyes or eyelids, and the United States Food and Drug Administration has said that both doctors and patients must use special wavelength-specific, protective eyewear whenever a CO_2 laser is used.

There are other kinds of dangers that laser surgery can impose of which the patient should be aware. Laser beams have the capacity to do a great deal of damage when coupled with high enough energy and absorption. They can ignite clothing, paper, and hair. Further, the risk of fire from lasers increases in the presence of oxygen. Hair should be protected and clothing should be tied back, or removed, within the treatment areas. It is important to guard against electric shock, as lasers require the use of high voltage. Critically, installation must ensure proper wiring.

Laser beams can burn or destroy healthy tissue, cause injuries that are painful and sometimes permanent, and actually compound problems they are supposed to solve. Errors or inaccuracies in laser surgery can worsen a patient's vision, for example, and lasers can scar and even change the skin color of some patients.

All of the above risks, precautions, and potential complications should be discussed by the doctor with the patient.

Normal results

The nature and severity of the problem, the skill of the surgeon performing the procedure, and the patient's general health and realistic expectations are among the factors that influence the outcome of laser surgery. Successful procedures can enable patients to feel better, look younger, and enjoy longer, fuller, more active lives.

A patient who is considering any kind of laser surgery should ask the doctor to provide detailed information about what the outcome of the surgery is expected to be, what the recovery process will involve, and how long it will probably be before a normal appearance is regained and the patient can resume normal activities.

A person who is considering any type of laser surgery should ask the doctor to provide specific and detailed information about what could go wrong during the procedure and what the negative impact on the patient's health or appearance might be.

Lighter or darker skin may appear, for example, when a laser is used to remove sun damage or age spots from an olive- or dark-skinned individual. This abnormal pigmentation may or may not disappear over time.

Scarring or rupturing of the cornea is uncommon, but laser surgery on one or both eyes can:

- increase sensitivity to light or glare
- reduce night vision
- permanently cloud vision, or cause sharpness of vision to decline throughout the day

Signs of infection following laser surgery include:

- burning
- crusting of the skin
- itching
- pain
- scarring
- severe redness
- swelling

Resources

BOOKS

Goldberg, David J. *Laser Dermatology: Pearls and Problems.* Malden, MA: Blackwell Pub., 2008.

Vij, D.F. and K. Mahesh, eds. *Medical Applications of Lasers.* Boston: Kluwer Academic, 2002.

Waynant, Ronald W., ed. *Lasers in Medicine.* Boca Raton: CRC Press, 2002.

PERIODICALS

"Laser Dermatology; Pearls and Problems." *SciTech Book News* (March 2008).

Parlette, Eric C., Michael S. Kaminer and Kenneth A. Arndt. "The Art of Tattoo Removal: Of the Multiple Removal Approaches, Laser Therapy is the Gold Standard." *Plastic Surgery Products* 18.1 (Jan 2008): 18-20.

ORGANIZATIONS

American Society for Dermatologic Surgery. 930 N. Meacham Road, P.O. Box 4014, Schaumburg, IL 60168-4014. (847) 330-9830. http://www.asds-net.org.

American Society for Laser Medicine and Surgery. 2404 Stewart Square, Wausau, WI 54401.(715) 845-9283. http://www.aslms.org.

Cancer Information Service. 9000 Rockville Pike, Building 31, Suite 10A18, Bethesda, MD 20892. 1-800-4-CANCER. <http://wwwicic.nci.nih.gov>.

Mayo Clinic. Division of Colon and Rectal Surgery. 200 First Street. SW, Rochester, MN 55905. (507) 284-2511. http://www.mayoclinic.org/colorectalsurgery-rst/laparoscopicsurgery.html.

Mayo Clinic. Mayo Foundation for Medical Education and Research, 200 First Street. SW, Rochester, MN 55905. (507) 284-2511. <http://http://www.mayoclinic.com.

National Cancer Institute. Building 31, Room 10A31, 31 Center Drive, MSC 2580, Bethesda, MD 20892-2580. (800) 422-6237. http://www.nci.nih.gov.

Laith Farid Gulli, MD, MS
Randi B. Jenkins, BA
Bilal Nasser, MD, MS
Robert Ramirez, BS
Robert Bockstiegel

LASIK *see* **Laser in-situ keratomileusis (LASIK)**

Lateral release *see* **Knee arthroscopic surgery**

Laxatives

Definition

Laxatives are medicines that promote bowel movements.

Purpose

Laxatives are used to treat constipation—the passage of small amounts of hard, dry stools, usually fewer than three times a week. Before recommending the use of laxatives, a physician should perform differential diagnosis. Prolonged constipation may be evidence of a significant problem, such as localized peritonitis or **diverticulitis**. Complaints of constipation may be associated with obsessive-compulsive disorder. Use of laxatives should be avoided in these cases. Patients should be aware that patterns of defecation are highly variable, and may vary from two to three times daily to two to three times weekly.

Laxatives may also be used prophylacticly for patients such as those recovering from a myocardial infarction (heart attack) or those who have had recent surgery and should not strain during defecation.

Description

Laxatives may be grouped by mechanism of action.

Saline cathartics include dibasic sodium phosphate (Phospo-Soda), magnesium citrate, magnesium hydroxide (milk of magnesia), magnesium sulfate (Epsom salts), sodium biphosphate, and others. They act by attracting and holding water in the intestinal tissues, and may produce a watery stool. Magnesium sulfate is the most potent of the laxatives in this group.

Stimulant and irritant laxatives increase the peristaltic movement of the intestine. Product examples include cascara and bisadocyl (Dulcolax). Castor oil works in a similar fashion.

Bulk-producing laxatives increase the volume of the stool, and will both soften the stool and stimulate intestinal motility. Psyllium (Metamucil, Konsil) and methylcellulose (Citrucel) are examples of this type. The overall effect is similar to that of eating high-fiber foods, and this class of laxative is most suitable for regular use.

Docusate (Colace) is the only representative example of the stool softener class. It holds water within the fecal mass, providing a larger, softer stool. Docusate has no effect on acute constipation, since it must be present before the fecal mass forms to have any effect, but may be useful for prevention of constipation in patients with recurrent problems, or those who are about to take a constipating drug such as narcotic **analgesics**.

Mineral oil is an emollient laxative. It acts by retarding intestinal absorption of fecal water, thereby softening the stool.

The hyperosmotic laxatives are glycerin and lactulose (Chronulac, Duphalac), both of which act by holding water within the intestine. Lactulose may also increase peristaltic action of the intestine.

Precautions

Short-term use of laxatives is generally safe except in cases of appendicitis, fecal impaction, or intestinal obstruction. Lactulose is composed of two sugar molecules, galactose and fructose, and should not be administered to patients who require a low-galactose diet.

KEY TERMS

Carbohydrates—Compounds such as cellulose, sugar, and starch that contain only carbon, hydrogen, and oxygen, and are a major part of the diets of people and other animals.

Cathartic colon—A poorly functioning colon, resulting from the chronic abuse of stimulant cathartics.

Colon—The large intestine.

Diverticulitis—Inflammation of the part of the intestine known as the diverticulum.

Fiber—Carbohydrate material in food that cannot be digested.

Hyperosmetic—Hypertonic, containing a higher concentration of salts or other dissolved materials than normal tissues.

Osteomalacia—A disease of adults, characterized by softening of the bone; similar to rickets, which is seen in children.

Pregnancy category— A system of classifying drugs according to their established risks for use during pregnancy: category A: controlled human studies have demonstrated no fetal risk; category B: animal studies indicate no fetal risk, and there are no adequate and well-controlled studies in pregnant women; category C: no adequate human or animal studies, or adverse fetal effects in animal studies, but no available human data; category D: evidence of fetal risk, but benefits outweigh risks; category X: evidence of fetal risk, which outweigh any benefits.

Steatorrhea—An excess of fat in the stool.

Stool—The solid waste that is left after food is digested. Stool forms in the intestines and passes out of the body through the anus.

Chronic use of laxatives may result in fluid and electrolyte imbalances, steatorrhea, osteomalacia, diarrhea, cathartic colon, and liver disease. Excessive intake of mineral oil may cause impaired absorption of oil soluble vitamins, particularly A and D. Excessive use of magnesium salts may cause hypermanesemia.

Lactulose and magnesium sulfate are pregnancy category B. Casanthranol, cascara sagrada, danthron, docusate sodium, docusate calcium, docusate potassium, mineral oil, and senna are category C. Casanthranol, cascara sagrada, and danthron are excreted in breast milk, resulting in a potential increased incidence of diarrhea in the nursing infant.

Interactions

Mineral oil and docusate should not be used in combination. Docusate is an emulsifying agent that will increase the absorption of mineral oil.

Bisacodyl tablets are enteric coated, and so should not be used in combination with antacids. The antacids will cause premature rupture of the enteric coating.

Recommended dosage

The patient should consult specialized drug references, or ask a physician or pharmacist about a specific medication.

Resources

PERIODICALS

"Constipation, Laxatives and Dietary Fiber." *HealthTips* (April 1993): 9.

"Overuse Hazardous: Laxatives Rarely Needed." *FDA Consumer* (April 1991): 33.

ORGANIZATIONS

National Digestive Diseases Information Clearinghouse. 2 Information Way, Bethesda, MD 20892-3570. <nddic @aerie.com>. http://www.niddk.nih.gov/Brochures/ NDDIC.htm.

OTHER

"Effectiveness of Laxatives in Adults." Centre for Reviews and Dissemination, University of York. [cited June 2003] http://www.york.ac.uk/inst/crd/ehc71.htm.

"Laxatives (Oral)." Medline Plus Drug Information. [cited June 2003] http://www.nlm.nih.gov/medlineplus/druginfo/ uspdi/202319.html.

Samuel D. Uretsky, PharmD

LDL cholesterol test

Definition

An LDL test measures the low density lipoprotein fraction of a person's total cholesterol.

Purpose

The purpose of an LDL test is to evaluate an individual's risk of cardiovascular (heart) disease.

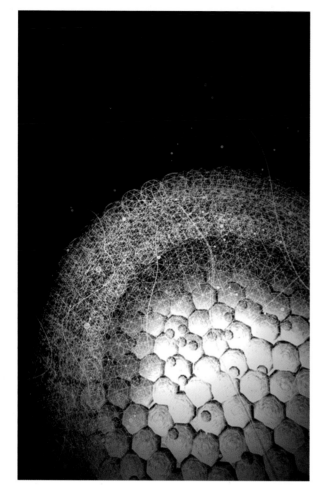

Microscopic view of lipoproteins. *(MedicalRF.com / Alamy)*

Description

The LDL test is a component of a **lipid profile**. A lipid profile includes four blood tests: total cholesterol, HDL cholesterol, LDL cholesterol and triglycerides.

LDL stands for low density lipoproteins. It is also known as the so-called bad cholesterol. It slowly accumulates on the inner walls of arteries. This buildup is known as plaque. Over time, it creates a condition known as atherosclerosis.

Dietary fats, including cholesterol, are absorbed from the small intestines. They are converted into triglycerides, which are then packaged into lipoproteins. All of these products are transported into the liver by chylomicrons. After a fast (not eating) lasting at least 12 hours, chylomicrons are absent from the bloodstream. This is the reason why persons that are having an LDL test must fast overnight.

A healthy LDL level is 129 mg/dL or less (in the optimal or near optimal ranges).

WHO PERFORMS THE PROCEDURE AND WHERE IS IT PERFORMED?

- LDL cholesterol tests are typically ordered by a family doctor, internist or geriatrician.
- A blood sample is usually obtained by a nurse, phlebotomist or medical technologist.
- The blood sample is tested or processed by a medical technologist.
- Results are usually reviewed, returned to the person being tested and interpreted by the physician initially ordering the LDL test.

- Optimal: Less than 100 mg/dL
- Near optimal: 100–129 mg/dL
- Borderline high: 130–159 mg/dL
- High: 160–189 mg/dL
- Very high: 190 mg/dL and higher

Pharmaceutical interventions are based, in part, on LDL test values.

An optimal range is defined as less than 70mg/dL for persons with a history of heart disease or those at very high risk for atherosclerotic disease.

Ranges for laboratory values may vary slightly among different laboratories.

Recommended dosage

LDL cholesterol testing is a component of a lipid profile. A lipid profile can be ordered at any time. Routine lipid profiles that are used to monitor the effectiveness of drugs intended to reduce serum cholesterol are usually performed every three months.

Precautions

A fast (not eating) for a minimum of 12 hours before drawing blood contributes to a more accurate measurement of lipids in the blood. No other precautions are needed.

At the time of drawing blood, the only precaution needed is to clean the venipuncture site with alcohol.

Side effects

The most common side effects of an LDL test are minor bleeding (hematoma) or bruising at the site of venipuncture.

QUESTIONS TO ASK YOUR DOCTOR

- Why are LDL cholesterol tests needed?
- What do the results indicate for my health?
- What treatment options do I have?

Interactions

There are no interactions for an LDL test.

Resources

BOOKS

Fischbach, F. T. and M. B. Dunning. *A Manual of Laboratory and Diagnostic Tests.* 8th ed. Philadelphia: Lippincott Williams & Wilkins, 2008.

McGhee, M. *A Guide to Laboratory Investigations.* 5th ed. Oxford, UK: Radcliffe Publishing Ltd, 2008.

Price, C. P. *Evidence-Based Laboratory Medicine: Principles, Practice, and Outcomes.* 2nd ed. Washington, DC: AACC Press, 2007.

Scott, M.G., A. M. Gronowski, and C. S. Eby. *Tietz's Applied Laboratory Medicine.* 2nd ed. New York: Wiley-Liss, 2007.

Springhouse, A. M.. *Diagnostic Tests Made Incredibly Easy!.* 2nd ed. Philadelphia: Lippincott Williams & Wilkins, 2008.

PERIODICALS

Amati, L., M. Chilorio, E. Jirillo, and V. Covelli. "Early pathogenesis of atherosclerosis: the childhood obesity." *Current Pharmaceutical Design* 13, no. 36 (2007): 3696–3700.

Leigh-Hunt, N., and M. Rudolf. "A review of local practice regarding investigations in children attending obesity clinics and a comparison of the results with other studies." *Child Care Health and Delivery* 34, no. 1 (2008): 55–58.

Shephard, M. D., B. C. Mazzachi, and A. K. Shephard. "Comparative performance of two point-of-care analysers for lipid testing." *Clinical Laboratory* 53, no. 9-12 (2007): 561–566.

Wright, J. T., S. Harris-Haywood, S. Pressel, et al. "Clinical outcomes by race in hypertensive patients with and without the metabolic syndrome: Antihypertensive and Lipid-Lowering Treatment to Prevent Heart Attack Trial." *Archives of Internal Medicine* 168, no. 2 (2008): 207–217.

ORGANIZATIONS

American Association for Clinical Chemistry. http://www.aacc.org/AACC/.

American Society for Clinical Laboratory Science. http://www.ascls.org/.

American Society of Clinical Pathologists. http://www.ascp.org/.

College of American Pathologists. http://www.cap.org/apps/cap.portal.

OTHER

American Clinical Laboratory Association. "Information about clinical chemistry." 2008 [cited February 24, 2008]. http://www.clinical-labs.org/.

Clinical Laboratory Management Association. "Information about clinical chemistry." 2008 [cited February 22, 2008]. http://www.clma.org/.

Lab Tests On Line. "Information about lab tests." 2008 [cited February 24, 2008]. http://www.labtestsonline.org/.

National Accreditation Agency for Clinical Laboratory Sciences. "Information about laboratory tests." 2008 [cited February 25, 2008]. http://www.naacls.org/.

L. Fleming Fallon, Jr, MD, DrPH

KEY TERMS

Hematoma—A collection of blood that has entered a closed space.

Phlebotomist—Health care professional trained to obtain samples of blood.

Leg lengthening or shortening

Definition

Leg lengthening or shortening involves a variety of surgical procedures used to correct legs of unequal lengths, a condition referred to as limb length discrepancy (LLD). LLD occurs because a leg bone grows more slowly on one leg than on the other leg. Surgical treatment is indicated for discrepancies exceeding 1 in (2.5 cm).

Purpose

Leg lengthening or shortening surgery, also known as bone lengthening, bone shortening, correction of unequal bone length, femoral lengthening, or femoral shortening, has the goal of correcting LLD and associated deformities while preserving function of muscles and joints. It is performed to:

- Lengthen an abnormally short leg (bone lengthening or femoral lengthening). Leg lengthening is usually recommended for children whose bones are skeletally immature, meaning that they are still growing. The surgery can add up to 6 in (15.2 cm) in length.

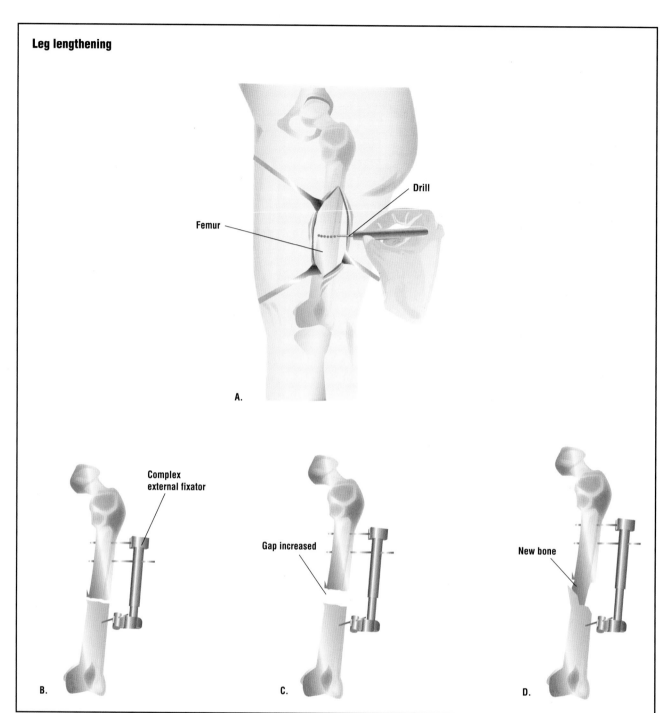

Leg lengthening

To lengthen a leg surgically, an incision is made in the leg to access the femur (A). A surgical drill is used to weaken the femur so the surgeon can break it. During the operation, screws are drilled into the bone on both sides of the break, and an external fixator is applied (B). The gap between the two pieces of bone is increased gradually (C), so new bone growth results in a longer leg (D). *(Illustration by GGS Information Services. Cengage Learning, Gale.)*

The leg lengthening and deformity correction process is based on the principle of distraction osteogenesis, meaning that a bone that has been cut during surgery can be gradually distracted (pulled apart), stimulating new bone formation (osteogenesis) at the site of the lengthening. The procedure basically involves breaking a bone of the leg and attaching pins through the leg into the bone. The pins pull the bones apart by

KEY TERMS

Arthrodesis—The surgical immobilization of a joint, also called joint fusion.

Cerebral palsy—Group of disorders characterized by loss of movement or loss of other nerve functions. These disorders are caused by injuries to the brain that occur during fetal development or near the time of birth.

Diaphysis—The shaft of a long bone.

Epiphysiodesis—An surgical procedure that partially or totally destroys an epiphysis and may incorporate a bone graft to produce fusion of the epiphysis or premature cessation of its growth; usually performed to equalize leg length.

Epiphysis—A part of a long bone where bone growth occurs from.

Fibula—The long bone in the lower leg that is next to the tibia. It supports approximately one-sixth of the body weight and produces the outer prominence of the ankle.

Femur—The thighbone. The large bone in the thigh that connects with the pelvis above and the knee below.

Fixator—A device providing rigid immobilization through external skeletal fixation by means of rods

(attached to pins which are placed in or through the bone.

Ilizarov method—A bone fixation technique using an external fixator for lengthening limbs, correcting deformities, and assisting the healing of fractures and infections. The method was designed by the Russian orthopedic surgeon Gavriil Abramovich Ilizarov (1921-1992).

Medullary cavity—The marrow cavity in the shaft of a long bone.

Non-union—Bone fracture or defect induced by disease, trauma, or surgery that fails to heal within a reasonable time span.

Osteotomy—The surgical cutting of a bone.

Poliomyelitis—Disorder caused by a viral infection (poliovirus) that can affect the whole body, including muscles and nerves.

Septic arthritis—A pus-forming bacterial infection of a joint.

Tibia—The large bone between the knee and foot that supports five-sixths of the body weight.

---

about 0.4 in (1 mm) each day and the bone grows new bone to try to mend the gap. It takes about a month to grow an inch (2.5 cm).

- Shorten an abnormally long leg (bone shortening or femoral shortening). Shortening a longer leg is usually indicated for patients who have achieved skeletal maturity, meaning that their bones are no longer growing. This surgery can produce a very precise degree of correction.

- Limit the growth of a normal leg to allow a short leg to grow to a matching length (epiphysiodesis). During childhood and adolescence, the long bones—femur (thighbone) or tibia and fibula (lower leg bones)—each consist of a shaft (diaphysis) and end parts (epiphyses). The epiphyses are separated from the shaft by a layer of cartilage called the epiphyseal or growth plate. As the limbs grow during childhood and adolescence, the epiphyseal plates absorb calcium and develop into bone. By adulthood, the plates have been replaced by bone. Epiphysiodesis is an operation performed on the epiphyseal plate in one of the patient's legs that slows down the growth of a specific bone.

Leg lengthening or shortening surgery is usually recommended for severe unequal leg lengths resulting from:

- poliomyelitis, cerebral palsy, or septic arthritis
- small, weak (atrophied) muscles
- short, tight (spastic) muscles
- hip diseases, such as Legg-Perthes disease
- previous injuries or bone fractures that may have stimulated excessive bone growth
- scoliosis (abnormal spine curvature)
- birth defects of bones, joints, muscles, tendons, or ligaments

Guidelines for treatment are tailored to patient needs and are usually as follows:

- LLD < 0.79 in (2 cm): orthotics (lift in shoe)
- LLD = 0.79-3.2 in (2-6 cm): epiphysiodesis or shortening procedure
- LLD > 3.2 in (6 cm): lengthening procedure
- LLD > 5.9-7.9 in (15-20 cm): lengthening procedure, staged or combined with epiphysiodesis (Amputation if performed if the procedure fails.)

Demographics

According to the Maryland Center for Limb Lengthening and Reconstruction, the rate of increase of the leg length difference is progressive in the United States with one-fourth of the LLD present at birth, one-third by age one year, and one-half by age three in girls and age four in boys.

LLD is common in the general population, with 23% of the population having a discrepancy of 0.4 in (1 cm) or more. One person out of 1,000 requires a corrective device such as a shoe lift.

Description

Leg lengthening

Leg lengthening is performed under **general anesthesia**, so that the patient is deep asleep and can't feel pain. Of the several surgical techniques developed, the Ilizarov method, or variation thereof, is the one most often used. An osteotomy is performed, meaning that the bone to be lengthened is cut, usually the lower leg bone (tibia) or upper leg bone (femur). Metal pins or screws are inserted through the skin and into the bone. Pins are placed above and below the cut in the bone and the skin incision is stitched closed. An external fixator is attached to the pins in the bone. The fixator is used after surgery to gradually pull the cut bone apart, creating a gap between the ends of the cut bone in which new bone growth can occur. The fixator functions much like a bone scaffold and will be used very gradually, so that the bone lengthens in extremely small steps. The original Ilizarov external fixator consists of stainless steel rings connected by threaded rods. Each ring is attached to the underlying bone segment by two or more wires, placed under tension to increase stability, yet maintain axial motion. Titanium pins are also used for supporting the bone segments. Several fixators are available and the choice depends on the desired goal and on specific patient requirements.

Other surgical techniques, such as the Wagner method, or acute lengthening, are used much less commonly. The Wagner technique features more rapid lengthening followed by **bone grafting** and plating. The advantage of the Ilizarov technique is that it does not require an additional procedure for grafting and plating. However, there are reports indicative of higher pain scores associated with the Ilizarov method and conflicting reports concerning the level of complications associated with each technique.

Leg shortening

Leg shortening surgery is also performed under general anesthesia. Generally, femoral shortening is preferred to tibial shortening, as larger resections are possible. Femoral shortening can be performed by open or closed methods at various femur locations. The bone to be shortened is cut, and a section is removed. The ends of the cut bone are joined together, and a metal plate with screws or an intermedullary rod down the center of the bone is placed across the bone incision to hold it in place during healing.

Epiphysiodesis

Epiphysiodesis is also performed under general anesthesia. The surgeon makes an incision over the epiphyseal plate at the end of the bone in the longer leg. He then proceeds to destroy the epiphyseal plate by scraping or drilling it to restrict further growth.

Diagnosis/Preparation

LLD is a common problem that is frequently discovered during the growing years. A medical history specific to the problem of limb length discrepancy is taken by the treating physician to provide information as to the cause of discrepancy, previous treatment, and neuromuscular status of the limb. The patient is first evaluated standing on both legs to assess pelvic obliquity, relative height of the knees, presence of angular deformity, foot size, and heel pad thickness. Overall discrepancy is assessed by having the patient stand with the shorter leg on graduated blocks until the pelvis is level. Examination is then performed with the patient prone, hips extended and knees flexed to 90 degrees. In this position, the respective lengths of the femur and tibia segments of the two legs can be compared, and the relative contribution of the difference within each segment to the overall LLD can be roughly assessed.

Imaging studies, such as x rays, are the diagnostic tool of choice to fully evaluate the patient. A leg series of x rays shows the overall picture of the affected leg. The extent of LLD and required alignment can be measured with precision, and bone abnormalities involving specific parts of the leg can also be seen. The x rays are usually repeated at six to 12 month intervals to establish the growth pattern of the limbs. When several determinations of limb length have been compiled, the remaining growth and the ultimate discrepancy between the legs can be calculated, and a treatment plan selected based on predicting future growth and discrepancy, which is in turn dependent on an accurate record of past and present growth. Treatment is rarely started solely on the basis of a single determination of the existing discrepancy in a skeletally immature child. **CT scans** are not performed routinely but may be helpful in confirming the diagnosis or more accurately measure the amount of discrepancy.

For LLD patients with a nonfunctional foot, most physicians recommend **amputation**. In patients with a functional foot, the surgical procedure recommendations generally fall into one of the following three groups:

- The first group involves patients with a leg discrepancy less than 10%. There is little disagreement that these patients can benefit from lengthening procedures.

- The second group involves patients with a leg discrepancy exceeding 30%. Amputation is usually recommended for these patients.

- The third group involves patients a discrepancy ranging between 10 and 30%. Lengthening more than 4 in (10 cm) in a leg with associated knee, ankle, and foot abnormalities is very complex. At skeletal maturity, an average lower-extremity length is often 31.5–39.4 in (80–110 cm) and a 10% discrepancy represents 3.1–4.3 in (8–11 cm).

In the case of leg lengthening, the patient is also seen and evaluated for the design of the external fixator before surgery.

One week before surgery, patients are usually scheduled for a blood and urine test. They are asked to have nothing at all to eat or drink after midnight on the night before surgery.

Aftercare

After the operation, nursing staff teach patients how to clean and care for the skin around the pins that attach the external fixator to the limb (pinsite care). Patients are also shown how to recognize and treat early signs of infection and not to neglect pinsite care, which takes about 30 minutes every day until the apparatus is removed. It is very important in preventing infection from developing.

After an epiphysiodesis procedure, hospitalization is required for about a week. Occasionally, a cast is placed on the operated leg for three to four weeks. Healing usually requires from eight to 12 weeks, at which time full activities can be resumed.

In the case of leg shortening surgery, two to three weeks of hospitalization is common. Occasionally, a cast is placed on the leg for three to four weeks. Muscle weakness is common, and muscle-strengthening therapy is started as soon as tolerated after surgery. Crutches are required for six to eight weeks. Some patients may require from six to 12 months to regain normal knee control and function. The intramedullary rod is usually removed after a year.

In the case of leg lengthening surgery, hospitalization may require a week or longer. Intensive physical therapy is required to maintain a normal range of leg motion. Frequent visits to the treating physician are also required to adjust the external fixator and

> ### WHO PERFORMS THE PROCEDURE AND WHERE IS IT PERFORMED?
>
> Leg lengthening/shortening surgery is performed in a hospital, by a treatment team usually consisting of an experienced orthopedic surgeon and residents specialized in extremity lengthening and deformity correction, physiotherapists, nurses, and other qualified orthopedic staff. Orthopedics is a medical specialty that focuses on the diagnosis, care and treatment of patients with disorders of the bones, joints, muscles, ligaments, tendons, nerves and skin. Orthopedic surgery is a specialty of immense variety, and includes LLD repair.

attentive care of the pins holding the device is essential to prevent infection. Healing time depends on the extent of lengthening. A rule of thumb is that each 0.4 in (1 cm) of lengthening requires some 36 days of healing. A large variety of external fixators are now available for use. Today's fixators are very durable, and are generally capable of holding full weight. Most patients can continue many normal activities during the three to six months the device is worn.

Metal pins, screws, **staples**, rods, or plates are used in leg lengthening/shortening surgery to stabilize bone during healing. Most orthopedic surgeons prefer to plan to remove any large metal implants after several months to a year. Removal of implanted metal devices requires another surgical procedure under general anesthesia.

During the recovery period, physical therapy plays a very important role in keeping the patient's joints flexible and in maintaining muscle strength. Patients are advised to eat a nutritious diet and to take calcium supplements. To speed up the bone healing process, gradual weight-bearing is encouraged. Patients are usually provided with an external system that stimulates bone growth at the site, either an **ultrasound** device or one that creates a painless electromagnetic field.

Risks

All the risks associated with surgery and the administration of anesthesia exist, including adverse reactions to medications, bleeding and breathing problems.

Specific risks associated with LLD surgery include:

- osteomyelitis (bone infection)
- nerve injury that can cause loss of feeling in the operated leg

QUESTIONS TO ASK THE DOCTOR

- Is surgery the best solution?
- How long does bone lengthening take?
- What is an external fixator?
- What are the major risks of the procedure?
- What kind of pain is to be expected after surgery and for how long?
- What are the risks associated with the surgery?
- How long will it take to resume normal walking?
- When will I be fitted with the external fixator?

- injury to blood vessels
- poor bone healing (non-union)
- avascular necrosis (AVN) of the femoral head as a result of vascular damage during surgery
- chondrolysis (destruction of cartilage) following insertion of rods and pins
- hardware failure, failure of epiphysiodesis, failure of slip progression
- unequal limb lengths if one leg fails to heal properly (The physician may need to reverse the direction of the external fixator device to strengthen it, causing a slight discrepancy between the two legs.)
- joint stiffness (contractures) may occur during lengthening, especially significant lengthenings
- pin loosening in the anchor sites

Another serious specific risk associated with leg lengthening/shortening surgery is infection of the pins or wires going through the bone and/or resting on the skin that may result in further bone or skin infections (osteomyelitis, cellulitis, staph infections).

Normal results

Epiphysiodesis usually has good outcomes when performed at the correct time in the growth period, though it may result in an undesirable short stature. Bone shortening may achieve better correction than epiphysiodesis, but requires a much longer convalescence. Bone lengthening is completely successful only 40% of the time and has a much higher rate of complications. Recovery time from leg lengthening surgery varies among patients, with the consolidation phase sometimes lasting a long period, especially in adults. Generally speaking, children heal in half the time as it takes an adult patient. For example, when the desired goal is 1.5 in (3.8 cm) of new bone growth,

a child will wear the fixation device for three months, while an adult will need to wear it for six months.

Alternatives

A LLD of 0.8 in (2 cm) or less is usually not a functional problem and non-surgical treatment options are preferred. The simplest forms do not involve surgery:

- Orthotics. Often leg length can be equalized with a sole or heel lift attached to or inserted inside the shoe. This measure can effectively level a difference of 0.4–2.0 in (1.0–5.0 cm) and correct about two thirds of the LLD. Up to 0.4 in (1 cm) can be inserted in a shoe. Beyond this, the lift gets heavy, awkward, and can cause problems such as ankle sprains and falls. The shoes look unsightly and patients complain of gait instability with such a large lift. A foot-in-foot prosthesis can be used for larger LLDs but they tend to be bulky and used as a temporary measure.
- Physical therapy. LLD results in the pelvis tilting sideways since one side of the body is higher than the other side. In turn, this causes a "kink" in the spine known as a scoliosis. Thus, leg length discrepancies can alter the mechanics of the pelvis so that the normal stabilizing and controlling action of specific muscles is altered. A common approach is to use exercises designed to modify the mechanics through specific strengthening of muscles that are weak and stretching of muscles that are restricting movement.

Resources

BOOKS

Golyakhovsky, V. and V. H. Frankel. *Operative Manual of Ilizarov Techniques.* Chicago: Year Book Medical Publishers, 1993.

Maiocchi, A. B. *Operative Principles of Ilizarov: Fracture, Treatment, Nonunion, Osteomyelitis, Lengthening Deformity Correction.* Phildalephia: Lippincott, Williams & Wilkins, 1991.

Menelaus, M. B., ed. *The Management of Limb Inequality.* Edinburgh: Churchill Livingstone, Pub., 1997.

Watts, H., Williams, M. *Who Is Amelia?: Caring for Children With Limb Difference.* Rosemont, IL: American Academy of Orthopaedic Surgeons, 1998.

PERIODICALS

Aarnes, G. T., H. Steen, P. Ludvigsen, L. P. Kristiansen, and O. Reikeras. "High frequency distraction improves tissue adaptation during leg lengthening in humans." *Journal of Orthopaedic Research* 20 (July 2002): 789–792.

Barker, K. L., A. H. Simpson, and S. E. Lamb. "Loss of knee range of motion in leg lengthening." *Journal of Orthopaedics Sports and Physical Therapy* 31 (May 2001): 238–144.

Bidwell, J. P., G. C. Bennet, M. J. Bell, and P. J. Witherow. "Leg lengthening for short stature in Turner's syndrome." *Journal of Bone and Joint Surgery (British)* 82 (November 2000): 1174–1176.

Choi, I. H., J. K. Kim, C. Y. Chung, et al. "Deformity correction of knee and leg lengthening by Ilizarov method in hypophosphatemic rickets: outcomes and significance of serum phosphate level." *Journal of Pediatric Orthopaedics* 22 (September-October 2002): 626–631.

Kocaoglu, M., L. Eralp, A. C. Atalar, and F. E. Bilen. "Correction of complex foot deformities using the Ilizarov external fixator." *Journal of Foot and Ankle Surgery* 41 (January-February 2002): 30–39.

Lee, S. H., G. Szoke, and H. Simpson. "Response of the physis to leg lengthening." *Journal of Pediatric Orthopaedics* 10 (October 2001): 339–343.

Lindsey, C. A., M. R. Makarov, S. Shoemaker, et al. "The effect of the amount of limb lengthening on skeletal muscle." *Clinical Orthopaedics and Related Research* 402 (September 2002): 278–287.

Nanchahal, J. and M. F. Pearse. "Management of soft-tissue problems in leg trauma in conjunction with application of the Ilizarov fixator assembly." *Plastic and Reconstructive Surgery* 111 (March 2003): 1359–1360.

ORGANIZATIONS

American Academy of Orthopaedic Surgeons. 6300 North River Road, Rosemont, Illinois 60018-4262. (847) 823-7186. http://www.aaos.org

American College of Foot and Ankle Surgeons. 515 Busse Highway, Park Ridge, Illinois, 60068. (847) 292-2237. (800) 421-2237. http://www.acfas.org/.

OTHER

"Epiphysiodesis." Institute of Child Health. [cited April 2003]. http://www.ich.ucl.ac.uk/factsheets/test_procedure_operations/epiphysiodesis/index.html.

"Ilizarov Method." Northwestern orthopaedics. [cited April 2003]. http://www.orthopaedics.northwestern.edu/orthopaedics/nmff/ilizarov.htm.

"Leg lengthening/shortening." MedlinePlus. [cited April 2003]. http://www.nlm.nih.gov/medlineplus/ency/article/002965.htm.

Monique Laberge, Ph.D.

Leg veins x ray *see* **Phlebography**

Length of hospital stay

Definition

The length of time a patient is required to stay overnight in the hospital is determined by their medical condition.

Description

The length of time a patient needs to stay in the hospital depends upon what type of care they require, how sick they are, and whether they need medications that cannot be administered at home. According to the United States Centers for Disease Control and Prevention (CDC), the average length of hospital stay statistically increases with age.

Conditions that May Require a Length of Hospital Stay

- Very High Fever
- Significantly Altered Vital Signs – Pulse, Blood Pressure, Breathing Rate, Temperature
- Severe Alterations in the Heartbeat
- Major Trauma - Injuries including Burns, Lacerations, and other Trauma
- Organ Failure
- Need for Intravenous (IV) Medications
- Psychotic Episodes
- Being Homicidal or Suicidal
- Recovery from Surgery
- Complications from Surgery
- Severe Allergic Reactions
- Severe Adverse Effects of Medications
- Drug-induced Delirium
- Severe Infections – Bacterial, Fungal, or Viral
- Inability to Breathe
- Inability to Urinate
- Chemical Toxicity from Poison
- Radiation Sickness
- Debilitating Diseases

Length of Hospital Stay after Surgery

Whether or not a hospital stay is necessary after surgery depends on the type of surgical procedure and whether there are any medical complications. More invasive surgical procedures often require longer hospital stays than minimally invasive procedures. Patients may require a specific time period of hospital-based rest and recovery if their post-surgical medical condition is serious enough to warrant the supervision of a doctor. Post-surgical complications may require a length of hospital stay until they can be resolved, which may or may not include several overnight stays.

The presence of a fever after surgery may necessitate a length of time staying in the hospital. Fever may be a sign of surgically related systemic infection that could become life threatening. If the operative site is very swollen or showing other signs of local

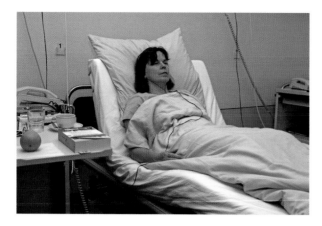

(Bildagenteur-online / Alamy)

infection, the patient may need to remain in the hospital. Operative sites that are still bleeding may also be cause to stay in the hospital. Generally speaking, a patient may be required to be able to think clearly, remain upright without fainting, drink fluids and consume light food without vomiting, breathe normally, urinate normally, be able to walk, and be free of severe pain before they are allowed to leave the hospital after a surgical procedure.

After a surgical procedure requiring **general anesthesia**, a patient is required to be awake and able to think clearly before they are discharged from the hospital. While many patients may experience some feelings of mental confusion after having general anesthesia, staying overnight is only necessary if the mental state has deteriorated beyond normal responses to anesthesia, such as seen with postoperative delirium. Delirium is a severe state of mental confusion, disorientation, agitation, and general incoherence. Delirium may also include hallucinations. Postoperative delirium is a temporary state of delirium that may be caused by multiple factors relating to the surgical procedure. A postoperative temporary state of delirium may occur if the patient experiences a lack of oxygen, hypotension, or sepsis as a result of the surgical procedure. With proper treatment, post-operative delirium usually only requires a hospital stay of about 72 hours.

If a patient is unable to keep down fluids or food, the length of hospital stay necessary after surgery is increased. The patient will need fluids through an IV route to remain hydrated until they may hydrate themselves by drinking fluids. Similarly, a patient who cannot keep down food after surgery may require a feeding tube for nourishment. Many patients may experience vomiting merely as an after effect of general anesthesia. In this case, problems with vomiting usually resolve themselves within hours and the length of hospital stay after surgery may be very short.

If there are complications with the patient's ability to breathe after a surgical procedure, a hospital stay will be necessary until the issue is resolved. In this case, a breathing tube and respirator is medically necessary and the length of stay is determined by whatever condition is causing the breathing problem. The ability to urinate after surgery can be affected by certain types of anesthesia used during the procedure. Anesthesia-based urinary retention may require a hospital stay that ranges from hours to several days before it is resolved. Additionally, some types of surgery may cause serious problems with the kidneys that first show up as urinary retention. Patients must be able to urinate before being allowed to go home.

Because patients must be generally well and on the road to recovery after surgical procedures, length of hospital stay is affected by a patient's ability to walk. Surgery is often associated with postoperative pain and some fatigue that greatly limits activity level. An activity level that is too high can also cause internal bleeding at surgical sites, and so bed rest is often encouraged. However, most patients should be able to walk short distances, such as to the bathroom, or they may require a hospital stay.

Severe pain is also associated with increased length of hospital stay after surgery. Often, if the pain is very severe, an IV form of morphine is used in the hospital. Additionally, severe pain after surgery may be an indication that something is wrong, or a surgical complication has occurred. Until severe pain is resolved and there are no apparent surgical complications, patients may be required to stay in the hospital.

Length of Hospital Stay after Childbirth

Childbirth can cause significant physical trauma to a woman's body. Even without medical complications, the act of birthing takes a significant physical toll that usually requires a length of hospital stay. Usually, a normal vaginal birth with no complications results in a hospital stay that ranges from one to four days. When childbirth causes tearing of the skin or muscle around the vagina and surrounding area, it may create the need for a longer hospital stay. The more severe the tearing, the more likely it will need a longer stay for treatment and healing. Very severe tearing involving the rectum or post-tear infections may require the longest hospital length of stay. Childbirth done by caesarean delivery is performed through a surgical incision in the abdominal wall as well as the wall of the uterus. This method of childbirth is associated with the greatest length of hospital stay, usually from four to nine days. Infection of the incision site increases length of stay.

KEY TERMS

Caesarean Delivery—Childbirth performed through a surgical incision in the abdominal wall as well as the wall of the uterus, as opposed to normal vaginal delivery.

Delirium—An altered state of consciousness that includes confusion, disorientation, incoherence, agitation, and defective perception (such as hallucinations).

Laceration—A ragged wound.

Malignant Neoplasm—Any malignant cancerous growth or tumor caused by uncontrolled cell division and capable of spreading to other parts of the body than where it formed.

Morphine—A very strong painkiller often used post-surgically.

Pneumonia—An inflammatory lung disease that affects the ability of the respiratory system to function.

Vital Signs—The physiological aspects of body function basic to life. They are temperature, pulse, breathing rate, and blood pressure.

Average Length of Hospital Stay

Research done by the CDC determined the average length of short-term hospital stay for various medical conditions in 2005. The categories studied were diverse, ranging from psychiatric disorders to heart disease and injuries. The length of hospital stay in the categories studied was longest for psychiatric disorders, which had an average of eight days. One of the shortest lengths of hospital stay was for childbirth, which averaged 2.6 days. In 2005, the following were some of the medical conditions that averaged between four and six days length of hospital stay: heart disease, bone fractures, diabetes, urinary tract infections, and pneumonia. Malignant neoplasms (cancer) had an average length of short-term hospital stay that ranged between seven and nine days. These specific categories of disease were chosen for the study because in 2005 they were responsible for millions of hospital discharges.

Resources

BOOKS

Beers, Mark H. "Surgery." In *The Merck Manual of Medical Information: 2nd Home Edition*. Whitehouse Station, NJ: Merck & Co., 2004. Also available online at http://www.merck.com/mmhe/sec25/ch301/ch301a.html [Accessed April 10, 2008].

OTHER

CDC Vital and Health Statistics. National Hospital Discharge Survey: Advance Data 2005. Number 385, July 2007. http://www.cdc.gov/nchs/data/ad/ad385.pdf

CDC Vital and Health Statistics. National Hospital Discharge Survey: 2005 Annual Summary with Detailed Diagnosis and Procedure Data. Series 13, Number 165, December 2007. http://www.cdc.gov/nchs/data/series/sr_13/sr13_165.pdf

"Episiotomy." Medicine Net. http://www.medicinenet.com/episiotomy/article.htm [Accessed April 10, 2008].

Sehdev, Harish M. "Cesarean Delivery." Emedicine. August 6, 2005. http://www.emedicine.com/MED/topic3283.htm [Accessed April 10, 2008].

Maria Basile, PhD

Ligation for varicose veins *see* **Vein ligation and stripping**

Limb salvage

Definition

Limb salvage surgery is a type of surgery primarily performed to remove bone and soft-tissue cancers occurring in limbs in order to avoid **amputation**.

Purpose

Limb salvage surgery is performed to remove cancer and avoid amputation, while preserving the patient's appearance and the greatest possible degree of function in the affected limb. The procedure is most commonly performed for bone tumors and bone sarcomas, but is also performed for soft tissue sarcomas affecting the extremities. This complex alternative to amputation is used to cure cancers that are slow to spread from the limb where they originate to other parts of the body, or that have not yet invaded soft tissue.

Twenty years ago, the standard of care for a patient with a cancer in a limb was to amputate the affected extremity. Limb salvage surgery was an exception to the rule. Today, it is the exception that a patient loses a limb as part of cancer treatment. This is due to improvements in surgical technique, both resection and reconstruction, imaging methods (computed tomography [CT scan] and **magnetic resonance imaging** [MRI]), and survival rates of patients treated with chemotherapy.

In recent years, limb salvage has been extended more and more to patients severely affected by chronic

KEY TERMS

Resection—Remove of a part of an organ.

Sarcoma—A form of cancer that arises in the supportive tissues such as bone, cartilage, fat, or muscle.

degenerative bone and joint diseases, such as rheumatoid arthritis, those facing diabetic limb amputation, and those with acute and chronic limb wounds.

Demographics

According to the National Cancer Institute, primary bone cancer is rare, with only 2,500 new cases diagnosed each year in the United States. More commonly, bones are the site of tumors that result from the spread of other primary cancers—that is, from cancers that spread other organs, such as the breasts, lungs, and prostate. Bone cancers occur more frequently in children and young adults.

Description

Also called limb-sparing surgery, limb salvage involves removing the cancer and about an inch of healthy tissue surrounding it. In addition, if had been removed, the removed bone is replaced. The replacement can be made with synthetic metal rods or plates (prostheses), pieces of bone (grafts) taken from the patient's own body (autologous transplant), or pieces of bone removed from a donor body (cadaver) and frozen until needed for transplant (allograft). In time, transplanted bone grows into the patient's remaining bone. Chemotherapy, radiation, or a combination of both treatments may be used to shrink the tumor before surgery is performed.

Limb salvage is performed in three stages. Surgeons remove the cancer and a margin of healthy tissue, implant a prosthesis or bone graft (when necessary), and close the wound by transferring soft tissue and muscle from other parts of the patient's body to the surgical site. This treatment cures some cancers as successfully as amputation.

Surgical techniques

BONE TUMORS. Surgeons remove the malignant lesion and a cuff of normal tissue (wide excision) to cure low-grade tumors of bone or its components. To cure high-grade tumors, they also remove muscle, bone, and other tissues affected by the tumor (radical resection).

SOFT TISSUE SARCOMAS. Surgeons use limb-sparing surgery to treat about 80% of soft tissue sarcomas affecting extremities. The surgery removes the tumor, lymph nodes, or tissues to which the cancer has spread, and at least 1 inch (2.5 cm) of healthy tissue on all sides of the tumor.

Radiation and/or chemotherapy may be administered before or after the operation. Radiation may also be administered during the operation by placing a special applicator against the surface from which the tumor has just been removed, and inserting tubes containing radioactive pellets at the site of the tumor. These tubes remain in place during the operation and are removed several days later.

To treat a soft tissue sarcoma that has spread to the patient's lung, the doctor may remove the original tumor, administer radiation or chemotherapy treatments to shrink the lung tumor, and surgically remove the lung tumor.

Diagnosis/Preparation

Before deciding that limb salvage is appropriate for a particular patient, the treating doctor considers what type of cancer the patient has, the size and location of the tumor, how the illness has progressed, and the patient's age and general health.

After determining that limb salvage is appropriate for a particular patient, the doctor makes sure that the patient understands what the outcome of surgery is likely to be, that the implant may fail, and that additional surgery—even amputation—may be necessary.

Physical and occupational therapists help prepare the patient for surgery by introducing the muscle-strengthening, ambulation (walking), and range of motion (ROM) exercises the patient will begin performing right after the operation.

Aftercare

During the five to 10 days the patient remains in the hospital following surgery, nurses monitor sensation and blood flow in the affected extremity and watch for signs that the patient may be developing pneumonia, pulmonary embolism, or deep-vein thrombosis.

The doctor prescribes broad-spectrum **antibiotics** for at least the first 48 hours after the operation and often prescribes medication (prophylactic anticoagulants) and antiembolism stockings to prevent blood clots. A drainage tube placed in the wound for the first 24–48 hours prevents blood (hematoma) and fluid (seroma) from accumulating at the surgical site. As postoperative pain becomes less intense, mild narcotics or anti-inflammatory medications replace the epidural catheter or patient-controlled analgesic pump used to relieve pain immediately after the operation.

Exercise intervention

Limb salvage requires extensive surgical incisions, and patients who have these operations need extensive rehabilitation. The amount of bone removed and the type of reconstruction performed dictate how soon and how much the patient can **exercise**, but most patients begin muscle-strengthening, continuous passive motion (CPM), and ROM exercises the day after the operation and continue them for the next 12 months.

A patient who has had upper-limb surgery can use the opposite side of the body to perform hand and shoulder exercises. Patients should not do active elbow or shoulder exercises for two to eight weeks after having surgery involving the bone between the shoulder and elbow (humerus). Rehabilitation following lower-extremity limb salvage focuses on strengthening the muscles that straighten the legs (quadriceps), maintaining muscle tone, and gradually increasing weight-bearing so that the patient is able to stand on the affected limb within three months of the operation. A patient who has had lower-extremity surgery may have to learn a new way of walking (gait retraining) or wear a lift in one shoe.

Goals of rehabilitation

Physical and occupational therapy regimens are designed to help the patient move freely, function independently, and accept changes in body image. Even patients who look the same after surgery as they did previously may feel that the operation has altered their appearance.

Before a patient goes home from the hospital or rehabilitation center, the doctor decides whether the patient needs a walker, brace, cane, or other device, and should make sure that the patient can climb stairs. Also, the doctor should emphasize the life-long importance of preventing infection and give the patient written instructions about how to prevent and recognize infection, as well as what steps to take if infection does develop.

Risks

The major risks associated with limb salvage are: superficial or deep infection at the site of the surgery; loosening, shifting, or breakage of implants; rapid loss of blood flow or sensation in the affected limb; and severe blood loss and anemia from the surgery.

WHO PERFORMS THE PROCEDURE AND WHERE IS IT PERFORMED?

Limb salvage surgery is performed in a hospital setting by experienced orthopedic surgeons with demonstrated expertise in limb salvage.

Postoperative infection is a serious problem. Chemotherapy or radiation can weaken the immune system, and extensive bone damage can occur before the infection is identified. Tissue may die (necrosis) if the surgeon used a large piece of tissue (flap) to close the wound. This is most likely to occur if the surgical site was treated with radiation before the operation. Treatment for postoperative infection involves removing the graft or implant, inserting drains at the infected site, and giving the patient oral or intravenous (IV) antibiotic therapy for as long as 12 months. Doctors may have to amputate the affected limb.

Normal results

A patient who has had limb salvage surgery will remain disease-free as long as a patient whose affected extremity has been amputated.

Salvaged limbs always function better than artificial ones. However, it takes a year for patients to learn to walk again following lower-extremity limb salvage, and patients who have undergone upper-extremity salvage must master new ways of using the affected arm or hand.

Successful surgery reduces the frequency and severity of patient falls and fractures that often result from disease-related changes in bone. Although successful surgery results in limbs that look and function very much like normal, healthy limbs, it is not unusual for patients to feel that their appearance has changed.

Some patients may also need additional surgery within five years of the first operation.

Morbidity and mortality rates

Orthopedic oncologists recognize that an operation to remove a tumor that spares the limb is associated with an incidence of tumor recurrence higher than that following an amputation. However, because there is no significant difference in overall survival rates, the increased rate of recurrence in patients who undergo limb salvage surgery is considered acceptable.

QUESTIONS TO ASK THE DOCTOR

- What are the possible complications involved in limb salvage surgery?
- How do I prepare for surgery?
- What type of anesthesia will be used?
- How is the surgery performed?
- How long will I be in the hospital?
- How much limb salvage surgery do you perform in a year?
- Why do you think limb salvage will be successful in my case?
- How will I look and feel after the operation?
- Will I be able to enjoy my favorite sports and other activities after the operation?

Alternatives

If the cancer's location makes it impossible to remove the malignancy without damaging or removing vital organs, essential nerves, or key blood vessels, or if it is impossible to reconstruct a limb that will function satisfactorily, salvage surgery may not be an appropriate treatment and amputation of the limb becomes the only alternative treatment.

Resources

BOOKS

Brown, K., ed. Complications of Limb Salvage: Prevention Management and Outcome UK: International Society of Limb Salvage, 1991.

Lerner, A., et al. Severe Injuries to the Limbs: Staged Treatment 1st ed. New York: Springer, 2007.

Malawer, Martin M., and Paul H. Sugarbaker. Musculoskeletal Cancer Surgery: Treatment of Sarcomas and Allied Diseases 1st ed. New York: Springer, 2001.

Sidawy, Anton N. Diabetic Foot: Lower Extremity Arterial Disease and Limb Salvage 2nd ed. New York: Lippincott Williams & Wilkins 2005.

Yarbro, Connie Henke, et al. Cancer Nursing 5th ed. Sudbury, MA: Jones and Bartlett, 2000.

PERIODICALS

Nehler, M. R., Hiatt, W. R., and L. M. Taylor Jr. "Is revascularization and limb salvage always the best treatment for critical limb ischemia?" Journal of Vascular Surgery 37 (March 2003): 704-708.

Neville, R. F. "Diabetic revascularization: Improving limb salvage in the absence of autogenous vein." Seminars in Vascular Surgery 16 (March 2003): 19-26.

Plotz, W., Rechl, H., Burgkart, R., Messmer, C., Schelter, R., Hipp, E., and R. Gradinger. "Limb salvage with tumor endoprostheses for malignant tumors of the knee." Clinical Orthopaedics 405 (December 2002): 207-215.

Tefera, G., Turnipseed, W., and T. Tanke. "Limb salvage angioplasty in poor surgical candidates." Vascular and Endovascular Surgery 37 (March-April 2003): 99-104.

Teodorescu, V. J., Chun, J. K., Morrisey, N. J., Faries, P. L., Hollier, L. H., and M. L. Marin. "Radial artery flow-through graft: A new conduit for limb salvage." Journal of Vascular Surgery 37 (April 2003): 816-820.

van Etten, B., van Geel, A. N., de Wilt, J. H., and A. M. Eggermont. "Fifty tumor necrosis factor-based isolated limb perfusions for limb salvage in patients older than 75 years with limb-threatening soft tissue sarcomas and other extremity tumors." Annals of Surgical Oncology 10 (January-February 2003): 32-37.

ORGANIZATIONS

American Academy of Orthopaedic Surgeons (AAOS). 6300 North River Road, Rosemont, Illinois 60018-4262. (847) 823-7186. www.aaos.org

American Diabetes Association (ADA). 1701 North Beauregard Street, Alexandria, VA 22311. (800) DIABETES. www.diabetes.org

International Society of Limb Salvage (ISOLS). E-mail: rjesusgarcia.dot@epm.br (UK). www.isols.org

OTHER

"Adult Soft Tissue Sarcoma." CancerNet 2000.[cited July 11, 2001]. www.cancernet.nci.nih.gov

"Bone Cancer."CancerNet 2000. [cited July 11, 2001]. www.cancernet.nci.nih.gov

"Bone Cancer." ACS Cancer Resource Center American Cancer Society. 2006. [cited February, 2008]. http://www.cancer.org/docroot/CRI/content/CRI_2_4_1X_What_Is_bone_cancer_ 2.asp?sitearea = CRI

"Limb salvage after osteosarcoma resection." AAOS On-Line Service April 1997 Bulletinhttp://www2.aaos.org/aaos/archives/bulletin/apr97/temple.htm.

Limb Salvage Center.www.limbsalvagecentre.com/.

Maureen Haggerty
Monique Laberge, PhD
Laura Jean Cataldo, RN, EdD

Lipid profile

Definition

A lipid profile includes data or results from four blood tests: total cholesterol, HDL cholesterol, LDL cholesterol and triglycerides.

WHO PERFORMS THE PROCEDURE AND WHERE IS IT PERFORMED?

- A lipid profile is typically ordered by a family doctor, internist, or geriatrician.
- A blood sample is usually obtained by a nurse, phlebotomist, or medical technologist.
- The blood sample is tested or processed by a medical technologist.
- Results are usually reviewed, returned to the person being tested and interpreted by the physician initially ordering the lipid profile.

Purpose

The purpose of a lipid profile is to help evaluate an individual's risk of cardiovascular disease.

Description

A lipid profile quantifies four different forms of lipids that are found in the blood: total cholesterol, HDL cholesterol, LDL cholesterol and triglycerides. Dietary fats, including cholesterol, are absorbed from the small intestines. They are converted into triglycerides, which are then packaged into lipoproteins. All of these products are transported into the liver by chylomicrons. After a fast (not eating) lasting at least 12 hours, chylomicrons are absent from the bloodstream. This is the reason why persons that are having a lipid profile must fast overnight.

Humans make 75 to 80% of the cholesterol that they need. The remainder comes from their diet. Because it is important, the body stores extra cholesterol. Total cholesterol is just that: a measure of cholesterol in the blood. It is a useful measure but it can be refined, usually into the other three components of a lipid profile.

HDL stands for high density lipoproteins. HDL cholesterol is a fraction of total cholesterol. It is also known as so-called good cholesterol because high levels of HDL cholesterol seem to provide protection against a heart attack. A majority of experts feel that HDL cholesterol returns cholesterol to the liver where it is eliminated from the body. On average, 25 to 33% of all cholesterol in the blood is the HDL variety.

LDL stands for low density lipoproteins. It is also known as the so-called bad cholesterol. It slowly accumulates on the inner walls of arteries. This buildup is

QUESTIONS TO ASK YOUR DOCTOR

- Why is a lipid profile needed?
- What do the results indicate for my health?
- What treatment options do I have?

known as plaque. Over time, it creates a condition known as atherosclerosis.

Triglycerides are made (synthesized) in the body. Synthesis can be increased by being overweight, living a sedentary lifestyle (minimal to no physical activity), smoking, eating a diet that is high in carbohydrates (more than 60% of total calories) or consuming excess alcohol. People with high triglyceride levels often develop diabetes or heart disease.

Physicians calculate the ratio of HDL to LDL values to assess disease risk related to blood lipid levels.

- Very low risk: 3.3 to 3.4
- Low risk: 3.8 to 4.0
- Average risk: 4.5 to 5.0
- Moderate risk: 7.0 to 9.5
- High risk: above 11

Pharmaceutical interventions are based on the HDL to LDL ratio.

Recommended dosage

Lipid profiles can be ordered at any time. Routine lipid profiles that are used to monitor the effectiveness of drugs intended to reduce serum cholesterol are usually performed every three months.

Precautions

A fast (not eating) for a minimum of 12 hours before drawing blood contributes to a more accurate measurement of lipid in the blood. No other precautions are needed.

At the time of drawing blood, the only precaution needed is to clean the venipuncture site with alcohol.

Side effects

The most common side effects of a lipid profile are minor bleeding (hematoma) or bruising at the site of venipuncture.

KEY TERMS

Hematoma—A collection of blood that has entered a closed space.

Phlebotomist—Health care professional trained to obtain samples of blood.

Interactions

There are no interactions for a lipid profile.

Resources

BOOKS

Fischbach, F. T. and M. B. Dunning. *A Manual of Laboratory and Diagnostic Tests*. 8th ed. Philadelphia: Lippincott Williams & Wilkins, 2008.

McGhee, M. *A Guide to Laboratory Investigations*. 5th ed. Oxford, UK: Radcliffe Publishing Ltd, 2008.

Price, C. P. *Evidence-Based Laboratory Medicine: Principles, Practice, and Outcomes*. 2nd ed. Washington, DC: AACC Press, 2007.

Scott, M.G., A. M. Gronowski, and C. S. Eby. *Tietz's Applied Laboratory Medicine*. 2nd ed. New York: Wiley-Liss, 2007.

Springhouse, A. M.. *Diagnostic Tests Made Incredibly Easy!*. 2nd ed. Philadelphia: Lippincott Williams & Wilkins, 2008.

PERIODICALS

Amati, L., M. Chilorio, E. Jirillo, and V. Covelli. "Early pathogenesis of atherosclerosis: the childhood obesity." *Current Pharmaceutical Design* 13, no. 36 (2007): 3696–3700.

Leigh-Hunt, N., and M. Rudolf. "A review of local practice regarding investigations in children attending obesity clinics and a comparison of the results with other studies." *Child Care Health and Delivery* 34, no. 1 (2008): 55–58.

SHephard, M. D., B. C. Mazzachi, and A. K. Shephard. "Comparative performance of two point-of-care analysers for lipid testing." *Clinical Laboratory* 53, no. 9-12 (2007): 561–566.

Wright, J. T., S. Harris-Haywood, S. Pressel, et al. "Clinical outcomes by race in hypertensive patients with and without the metabolic syndrome: Antihypertensive and Lipid-Lowering Treatment to Prevent Heart Attack Trial." *Archives of Internal Medicine* 168, no. 2 (2008): 207–217.

ORGANIZATIONS

American Association for Clinical Chemistry. http://www.aacc.org/AACC/.

American Society for Clinical Laboratory Science. http://www.ascls.org/.

American Society of Clinical Pathologists. http://www.ascp.org/.

College of American Pathologists. http://www.cap.org/apps/cap.portal.

OTHER

American Clinical Laboratory Association. "Information about clinical chemistry." 2008 [cited February 24, 2008]. http://www.clinical-labs.org/.

Clinical Laboratory Management Association. "Information about clinical chemistry." 2008 [cited February 22, 2008]. http://www.clma.org/.

Lab Tests On Line. "Information about lab tests." 2008 [cited February 24, 2008]. http://www.labtestsonline.org/.

National Accreditation Agency for Clinical Laboratory Sciences. "Information about laboratory tests." 2008 [cited February 25, 2008]. http://www.naacls.org/.

L. Fleming Fallon, Jr, MD, DrPH

Lipid tests

Definition

Lipid tests are routinely performed on plasma, which is the liquid part of blood without the blood cells. Lipids themselves are a group of organic compounds that are greasy and cannot be dissolved in water, although they can be dissolved in alcohol. Lipid tests include measurements of total cholesterol, triglycerides, high-density lipoprotein (HDL) cholesterol, and low-density lipoprotein (LDL) cholesterol. Lipid tests may also be performed on amniotic fluid, which is the fluid that surrounds the fetus during pregnancy. Prenatal lipid tests include tests for lecithin and other pulmonary (lung) surfactants that cover the air spaces in the lungs with a thin film.

Purpose

Blood tests

The purpose of blood lipid testing is to determine whether abnormally high or low concentrations of a specific lipid are present. Low levels of cholesterol are associated with liver failure and inherited disorders of cholesterol production. Cholesterol is a primary component of the plaques that form in atherosclerosis and is therefore the major risk factor for the rapid progression of coronary artery disease (CAD). High blood cholesterol may be inherited or result from such other conditions as biliary obstruction, diabetes mellitus, hypothyroidism, and nephrotic syndrome. In addition, cholesterol levels may be increased in persons who eat foods that are rich in saturated fats and cholesterol, and who lead a sedentary lifestyle.

Amniocentesis—A procedure for removing amniotic fluid from the womb using a fine needle.

Atherosclerosis—A disease of the coronary arteries in which cholesterol is deposited in plaques on the arterial walls. The plaque narrows or blocks blood flow to the heart. Atherosclerosis is sometimes called coronary artery disease, or CAD.

High-density lipoprotein (HDL)—A type of lipoprotein that protects against CAD by removing cholesterol deposits from arteries or preventing their formation.

Hypercholesterolemia—The presence of excessively high levels of cholesterol in the blood.

Hypertriglyceridemia—The presence of excessively high levels of TAG in the blood.

Lecithin—A phospholipid found in high concentrations in surfactant.

Lipid—Any organic compound that is greasy, insoluble in water, but soluble in alcohol. Fats, waxes, and oils are examples of lipids.

Lipoprotein—A complex molecule that consists of a protein membrane surrounding a core of lipids. Lipoproteins carry cholesterol and other lipids from the

digestive tract to the liver and other body tissues. There are five major types of lipoproteins.

Low-density lipoprotein (LDL)—A type of lipoprotein that consists of about 50% cholesterol and is associated with an increased risk of CAD.

Plaque—An abnormal deposit on the wall of an artery. Plaque is made of cholesterol, triglyceride, dead cells, lipoproteins and calcium.

Sedentary—Characterized by inactivity and lack of exercise. A sedentary lifestyle is a risk factor for high blood cholesterol levels.

Surfactant—A compound made of fats and proteins that is found in a thin film along the walls of the air sacs of the lungs. Surfactant keeps the surface pressure low so that the sacs can inflate easily and not collapse.

Tocolytic drug—A compound given to women to stop the progression of labor.

Triglyceride (TAG)—A chemical compound that forms about 95% of the fats and oils stored in animal and vegetable cells. TAG levels are sometimes measured as well as cholesterol levels when a patient is screened for heart disease.

Low levels of triglyceride are seen in persons with malnutrition or malabsorption. Increased levels are associated with diabetes mellitus, hypothyroidism, pancreatitis, glycogen storage diseases, and estrogens. Diets rich in either carbohydrates or fats may cause elevated triglyceride levels in some persons. Although triglycerides are not a component of the plaque associated with atherosclerosis, they increase the viscosity (thickness) of the blood and promote obesity, which can contribute to coronary disease. The majority of cholesterol and triglyceride testing is performed to screen persons at increased risk of coronary artery disease.

Amniotic fluid tests

Lipid tests are performed on amniotic fluid to determine the maturity of the fetal lungs. These tests are performed prior to delivery to ensure that there is sufficient pulmonary surfactant to prevent collapse of the lungs when the baby exhales (breathes out).

Description

Cholesterol screening can be performed with or without fasting, but it should include tests of total and

HDL cholesterol levels. The frequency of cholesterol testing depends on the patient's risk of developing CAD. Adults over 20 with total cholesterol levels below 200 mg/dL should be tested once every five years. People with higher levels should be tested for LDL cholesterol levels, and tested at least once per year thereafter if their LDL cholesterol is 130 mg/dL or higher. The National Cholesterol Education Program (NCEP) suggests further evaluation when the patient has any of the symptoms of CAD, or if she or he has two or more of the following risk factors for CAD:

- high blood pressure
- history of cigarette smoking
- diabetes
- low HDL levels
- family history of CAD
- age over 45 years (men) or 55 years (women)

Measurements of cholesterol and triglyceride levels are routinely performed in all patients.

Measurement of pulmonary surfactants

Lecithin is the principal pulmonary surfactant secreted by the alveolar cells of the lung. Lecithin and the other surfactants prevent collapse of the air sacs when the baby exhales. During the first half of gestation, the levels of lecithin and another lipid known as sphingomyelin in the amniotic fluid are approximately equal. During the second half of pregnancy, however, lecithin production increases while the sphingomyelin level remains constant. Infants born prematurely may suffer from respiratory distress syndrome (RDS) because the levels of pulmonary surfactant in their lungs are insufficient to prevent collapse of the air sacs. Tests for RDS are called fetal lung maturity (FLM) tests. The reference method for determining fetal lung maturity is the ratio between lecithin and sphingomyelin in the amniotic fluid, or the L/S ratio.

Precautions

Tests for triglycerides and LDL cholesterol must be performed following a 12-hour fast. Acute illness, high fever, starvation, or recent surgery lowers the blood cholesterol and triglyceride levels. If possible, patients should also stop taking any medications that may affect the accuracy of the test.

Amniotic fluid is collected by a process called **amniocentesis**. This procedure is usually performed after the 30th week of gestation to evaluate the maturity of the baby's lungs. A miscarriage (spontaneous abortion) may occur as a consequence of this procedure, although its overall incidence following amniocentesis is less than 1%. Possible complications of amniocentesis include premature labor and placental bleeding. The fluid that is withdrawn may be contaminated with blood or meconium (a dark-green material in the intestines of a fetus), which may interfere with some fetal lung maturity tests.

Preparation

Patients who are scheduled for a **lipid profile** test should fast (except for water) for 12–14 hours before the blood sample is drawn. If the patient's LDL cholesterol is to be measured, he or she should also avoid alcohol for 24 hours before the test. When possible, patients should also stop taking any medications that may affect the accuracy of the test results. These drugs include **corticosteroids**; estrogen or androgens; oral contraceptives; some **diuretics**; antipsychotic medications, including haloperidol; some **antibiotics**; and niacin. Antilipemics are drugs that lower the concentration of fatty substances in the blood. When these medications are taken by the patient, blood testing may be done frequently to evaluate liver function as well as lipid levels.

Aftercare

Aftercare following blood lipid tests includes routine care of the skin around the needle puncture. Most patients have no aftereffects, but some may have a small bruise or swelling. A washcloth soaked in warm water usually relieves any discomfort. In addition, the patient can resume taking any prescription medications that were discontinued before the test.

Care after amniocentesis requires that the clinician monitor the patient for any signs of infection or possible injury to the fetus. Some things to look for are fever, vaginal bleeding, or vaginal discharge. The patient may feel sick and there may be some cramping. She should be advised to rest and avoid strenuous activity. If the mother appears to be going into labor, she should be given supportive care. She may be given medications known as tocolytic agents to prevent the premature birth of the baby.

Risks

The primary risk to the patient from blood tests of lipid levels is a mild stinging or burning sensation during the venipuncture, with minor swelling or bruising afterward.

Although amniocentesis is much safer in the third trimester, and is less risky when it is performed with the guidance of **ultrasound** technology, does present a risk of miscarriage and fetal injury. The mother should be monitored for any signs of bleeding, infection, or impending labor.

Normal results

The normal values for serum lipids depend on the patient's age, sex, and race. Normal values for people in Western countries are usually given as 140-220 mg/dL for total cholesterol in adults, although as many as 5% of the population have a total cholesterol higher than 300 mg/dL. Among Asians, the figures are about 20% lower. As a rule, both total and LDL cholesterol levels rise as people get older. Normal values for HDL cholesterol are also age- and sex-dependent. The range for males 20–29 years is approximately 30–63 mg/dL; for females of the same age group it is 33–83 mg/dL. Normal values for fasting triglycerides are also age- and sex-dependent. The reference range for adult males 20–29 years is 45–200 mg/dL; for females of the same age group it is 37–144 mg/dL. As with cholesterol, the normal range rises with age.

Since a person's diet and lifestyle affect normal values, which are determined by the interval between the 5th and 95th percentile of the group, it is more helpful to evaluate cholesterol and triglycerides from the perspective of desirable plasma levels. The desirable values defined by the Nation Cholesterol Education Program (NCEP) in 2001 are as follows:

- Total cholesterol: Less than 200 mg/dL; 200–239 mg/dL is considered borderline high; and greater than 240 mg/dL is high.
- HDL cholesterol: Less than 40mg/dL is low.
- LDL cholesterol: Less than 100 mg/dL is optimal; near-optimal is 100–129 mg/dL; borderline high is 130-159 mg/dL; high is 160–189 mg/dL; and very high is any value over 190 mg/dL.
- Total cholesterol: HDL ratio: Under 4.0 in males; 3.8 in females.

Fetal lung maturity tests

Low levels of surfactant in amniotic fluid are denoted by an L/S ratio lower than 2.0 or a lecithin level lower than or equal to 0.10 mg/dL. Lung development can be delayed in premature births and in babies whose mothers have diabetes.

Patient education

Nurses should explain the results of abnormal blood lipid tests to patients and advise them on lifestyle changes. Patient education is important in fetal lung maturity testing. The situation faced by the expectant parents may be very critical; the more information they are given, the better choices they can make.

Resources

BOOKS

Henry, J. B. Clinical Diagnosis and Management by Laboratory Methods, 20th ed. Philadelphia, PA: W. B. Saunders Company, 2001.

"Hyperlipidemia." Section 2, Chapter 15 in The Merck Manual of Diagnosis and Therapy, edited by Mark H. Beers, MD, and Robert Berkow, MD. Whitehouse Station, NJ: Merck Research Laboratories, 1999.

McPherson, Richard A., and Matthew R. Pinncus.Henry's Clinical Diagnosis and Management by Laboratory Methods, 21st ed. Philadelphia, PA: W. B. Saunders Company, 2006.

"Prenatal Diagnostic Techniques: Amniocentesis." Section 18, Chapter 247 in The Merck Manual of Diagnosis and Therapy, edited by Mark H. Beers, MD, and Robert Berkow, MD. Whitehouse Station, NJ: Merck Research Laboratories, 1999.

Wallach, Jacques. Interpretation of Diagnostic Tests, 8th ed. Philadelphia, PA: Lippincott Williams & Wilkins, 2006.

ORGANIZATIONS

American Dietetic Association. (800) 877-1600. www.eatright.org..

National Cholesterol Education Program: National Heart, Lung, and Blood Institute (NHLBI), National Institutes of Health. PO Box 30105, Bethesda, MD, 20824-0105. (301) 251-1222. http://www.nhlbi.nih.gov/about/ncep/.

OTHER

MedLine Plus. "High blood cholesterol and triglycerides". October, 2006.http://www.nlm.nih.gov/medlineplus/ency/article/000403.htm&gt

Jane E. Philips
Mark A. Best
Laura Jean Cataldo, RN, EdD

Liposuction

Definition

Liposuction, also known as lipoplasty or suction-assisted lipectomy, is **cosmetic surgery** performed to remove unwanted deposits of fat from under the skin. The surgeon sculpts and re-contours a person's body by removing excess fat deposits that have been resistant to reduction by diet or **exercise**. Removal of fat cells is permanent.

Purpose

Liposuction is intended to reduce and smooth the contours of the body and improve a person's appearance. Its goal is cosmetic improvement. Liposuction does not remove large quantities of fat and is not intended as a weight-reduction technique. The average amount of fat removed is about 1 quart (1 liter). Although liposuction is not intended to remove cellulite (lumpy fat), some doctors believe that it improves the appearance of areas that contain cellulite, including thighs, hips, buttocks, abdomen, and chin. A technique called liposhaving shows more promise at reducing cellulite. Liposhaving can be done under **local anesthesia** and is reported to be less traumatic to the skin than liposuction. Liposuction is most often performed by board-certified plastic surgeons.

Demographics

Liposuction is the most commonly performed cosmetic procedure for men in the United States and the second most common cosmetic procedure (after breast augmentation) for women. In 2006, about 403,680

KEY TERMS

Cellulite—Dimpled skin that is caused by uneven fat deposits beneath the surface.

Epinephrine—Epinephrine, also called adrenalin, occurs naturally in the body and causes blood vessels to constrict or narrow. As a drug, it is used to reduce bleeding.

Hemoglobin—The component of blood that carries oxygen to the tissues.

Liposhaving—Involves removing fat that lies closer to the surface of the skin by using a needle-like instrument that contains a sharp-edged shaving device.

liposuction procedures were performed in the United States. This is more than double the amount performed ten years earlier.

Description

Most liposuction procedures are performed under local anesthesia. Local anesthesia produces loss of sensation without loss of consciousness. The tumescent, or wet, technique is used most often. In this technique, a large volume of very dilute anesthetic is injected under the person's skin, making the tissue swollen (tumescent) and firm. Epinephrine is added to the solution to reduce bleeding, which allows the removal of larger amounts of fat.

The physician first numbs the skin with an injection of local anesthetic. After the skin is desensitized, the doctor makes a series of tiny incisions no larger than 0.12–0.25 in (3–6 mm) in length. Flooding the area with more dilute anesthetic, fat is then extracted with suction through a long, blunt hollow tube called a cannula. The doctor repeatedly pushes the cannula through the fat layers in a radiating pattern creating tunnels, thus removing fat and re-contouring the area.

Some newer modifications to the procedure include the use of a cutting cannula called a liposhaver. Formerly some surgeons used **ultrasound** to help break up the fat deposits, but this technique has largely been abandoned because it created greater safety risks than the tumescent technique. Larger incisions may be closed with a suture or staple, while micro incisions are covered with **bandages** but do not need sutures. Incisions usually heal completely within two weeks and should leave few or no scars

The length of time required to perform the procedure varies with the amount of fat that is to be removed and the number of areas to be treated. Most operations take from 30 minutes up to two hours, but extensive procedures can take longer. Risk of complications increases the more extensive the procedure. The length of time required also varies with the manner in which the anesthetic is injected.

The cost of liposuction varies depending upon the fees commonly charged in the region of the country where it is performed, the extent of the area being treated, and the person performing the procedure. In the mid-2000s, an increasing trend was for Americans to go overseas to have cosmetic procedures performed in countries where they cost substantially less than in the United States. These procedures are cosmetic and are not covered by most insurance policies.

Diagnosis/Preparation

Liposuction is most successful when performed on persons who have firm, elastic skin and concentrated pockets of fat in areas that are characterized by cellulite. To get good results after fat removal, the skin must contract to conform to the new contours without sagging. Older persons have less elastic skin and, consequently, may not be good candidates for this procedure. People with generalized fat distribution, rather than localized pockets, are not good candidates. Candidates should be in good general health and free of heart or lung disease. People who have poor circulation or who have had recent surgery at the intended site of fat reduction are not good candidates.

The doctor will conduct a **physical examination** and may order blood work to determine clotting time and hemoglobin level for transfusions, in case the need should arise. The person may be placed on **antibiotics** before surgery to ward off potential infection.

Aftercare

Liposuction is normally an outpatient procedure. Patients should plan to have someone available to drive them home and stay with them for the next 12–24 hours. If the tumescent technique is used, the patient will feel little or no pain for 24 hours following the procedure but after that may have soreness and swelling for several weeks. After some liposuction surgery, the patient may need to wear a support garment continuously for 2–3 weeks. If ankles or calves were treated, support hose should be worn for up to 6 weeks. The support garments can be removed during bathing. A drainage tube placed under the skin in the

WHO PERFORMS THE PROCEDURE AND WHERE IS IT PERFORMED?

Many liposuction surgeries are performed by plastic surgeons or by dermatologists. Any licensed physician may legally perform liposuction. Liposuction may be performed in a private professional office, an outpatient center, or in a hospital.

QUESTIONS TO ASK THE DOCTOR

Candidates for liposuction surgery should consider asking the following questions:

- What will be the resulting appearance?
- Is the surgeon board certified in plastic and reconstructive surgery?
- How many liposuction procedures has the surgeon performed?
- What is the surgeon's complication rate?
- How much will the procedure cost and is any of it covered by insurance?

area of the procedure may be needed to prevent fluid build-up.

The incisions involved in this procedure are tiny, but the surgeon may close them with metal sutures or **staples**. These will be removed a few days surgery. Some micro-incisions are small enough that the doctor may not need to close them with sutures. Minor bleeding or seepage through the incision site(s) is common after this procedure. Wearing the elastic bandage or support garment helps reduce fluid loss.

The patient usually can return to normal activity within a week. Any postoperative bruising is expected to go away within 10–14 days. Postoperative swelling begins to go down after a week. It may take 3–6 months for the final contour to be reached depending on the extent of the surgery.

Risks

Liposuction under local anesthesia using the tumescent technique is exceptionally safe so long as the patient is in good health. The main hazards associated with this surgery involve migration of a blood clot or fat globule to the heart, brain, or lungs. Such an event can cause a heart attack or stroke. Ultrasound assisted liposuction has largely been abandoned because of safety concerns such as burns and complications such as scarring.

Staying in bed increases the risk of clot formation, but too much activity can result in increased swelling of the surgical area. Such swelling is a result of excess fluid and blood accumulation, and generally comes from not wearing the compression garments. If necessary, this excess fluid can be drained with a needle in the doctor's office.

Infection is another complication, but this rarely occurs. If the physician is skilled and works in a sterile environment, infection should not be much of a concern.

The greatest risk of complications arises when too much fat is removed or too many parts of the body are

worked on at one time. If too much fat is removed, the skin may peel in that area. Smokers are at increased risk for shedding skin because their circulation is impaired. Removing too much fat may also cause the patient to go into shock.

Normal results

The loss of fat cells is permanent, and the patient should have smoother, more pleasing body contours without excessive bulges. Nevertheless, if the patient overeats, the remaining fat cells will grow in size. Although the patient may gain weight, the body should retain the new proportions and the suctioned area should remain proportionally smaller.

Tiny scars at the site of incision are normal. The doctor usually makes the incisions in places where the scars are not likely to show.

In some instances, the skin may appear rippled, wavy, or baggy after surgery. Pigmentation spots may develop. The re-contoured area may be uneven. This unevenness can be corrected with a second procedure that is less extensive than the first.

Morbidity and mortality rates

The morbidity rate from liposuction is less than 1%. Mortality is exceedingly rare.

Alternatives

Some of the alternatives to liposuction include modifying diet to lose excess body fat, exercise, accepting one's body and appearance as it is, or using clothing or makeup to downplay or emphasize body or facial features.

Resources

BOOKS

Loftus, Jean M. The Smart Woman's Guide to Plastic Surgery., 2nd. ed. New York: McGraw-Hill, 2008.

Olesen, R, Merrell. Cosmetic Surgery for Dummies. Hoboken, NJ: Wiley, 2005

Perry, Arthur W. Straight Talk About Cosmetic Surgery. New Haven, CT: Yale University Press, c2007.

Shelton, Ron M. and Terry Malloy. Liposuction: A Question and Answer Guide to Today's Popular Cosmetic Procedure. New York: Berkley Books, 2004.

ORGANIZATIONS

American Board of Plastic Surgery. Seven Penn Center, Suite 400, 1635 Market Street, Philadelphia, PA 19103-2204. (215) 587-9322. http://www.abplsurg.org.

American College of Surgeons. 633 North Saint Claire Street, Chicago, IL 60611. (312) 202-5000. http://www.facs.org.

American Society for Aesthetic Plastic Surgery. 11081 Winners Circle, Los Alamitos, CA 90720.(888) 272-7711. http://www.surgery.org.

American Society for Dermatologic Surgery. 5550 Meadowbrook Drive, Suite 120, Rolling Meadows, IL 60006 (847) 956-0900. http://www.asds-net.org.

American Society of Plastic and Reconstructive Surgeons. 444 E. Algonquin Rd., Arlington Heights, IL 60005. (847) 228-9900. http://www.plasticsurgery.org.

OTHER

"Liposuction." United States Food and Drug Administration. 2005. [cited January 24, 2008]. http://www.fda.gov/womens/getthefacts/liposuction.html.

L. Fleming Fallon, Jr., M.D., Ph. D.
Tish Davidson, A. M.

Lithotripsy

Definition

Lithotripsy is the use of high-energy shock waves to fragment and disintegrate kidney stones. The shock wave, created by using a high-voltage spark or an electromagnetic impulse outside of the body, is focused on the stone. The shock wave shatters the stone, allowing the fragments to pass through the urinary system. Since the shock wave is generated outside the body, the procedure is termed extracorporeal shock wave lithotripsy (ESWL). The name is derived from the roots of two Greek words, *litho*, meaning stone, and *trip*, meaning to break.

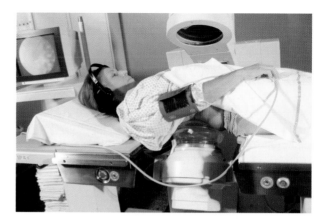

A woman undergoing lithotripsy. *(Phanie / Photo Researchers, Inc.)*

Purpose

ESWL is used when a kidney stone is too large to pass on its own, or when a stone becomes stuck in a ureter (a tube that carries urine from the kidney to the bladder) and will not pass. Kidney stones are extremely painful and can cause serious medical complications if not removed.

Demographics

For an unknown reason, the number of persons in the United States developing kidney stones has been increasing over the past 20 years. White people are more prone to develop kidney stones than are persons of color. Although stones occur more frequently in men, the number of women who develop them has been increasing over the past 10 years, causing the ratio to change. Kidney stones strike most people between the ages of 20 and 40. Once persons develop more than one stone, they are more likely to develop others. Lithotripsy is not required for treatment in all cases of kidney stones.

Description

Lithotripsy uses the technique of focused shock waves to fragment a stone in the kidney or the ureter. The affected person is placed in contact with a water-filled cushion (older machines require that the individual is actually seated in a tub of water). A sophisticated machine called Lithotripter produces the focused shock waves. A high-voltage electrical discharge is passed through a spark gap under water. The shock waves thus produced are focused on the stone inside the person's body. The shock waves are created and focused on the stone with the help of a machine called a C-Arm Image Intensifier. The wave shatters and

KEY TERMS

Aneurysm—A dilation of the wall of an artery that causes a weak area prone to rupture.

Bladder—Organ in which urine is stored prior to urination.

Bleeding disorder—A problem related to the clotting mechanism of the blood.

Cardiologist—A physician who specializes in problems of the heart.

EKG—A graphical tracing of the electrical activity of the heart.

Extracorporeal shock wave lithotripsy (ESWL)—The use of focused shock waves, generated outside the body, to fragment kidney stones.

Gravel—The debris that is formed from a fragmented kidney stone.

Intravenous pyelogram (IVP)—A type of x ray. After obtaining an x ray of the lower abdomen, a radio-opaque dye is injected into the veins. X rays are then obtained every 15 minutes for the next hour. The dye pinpoints the location of kidney stones. It is also used to determine the anatomy of the urinary system.

Kidney stone—A hard mass that forms in the urinary tract that can cause pain, bleeding, obstruction, and/or infection. Stones are primarily composed of calcium.

Stent—A plastic tube placed in the ureter prior to the ESWL procedure, which facilitates the passage of gravel and urine.

Ultrasound—A diagnostic imaging modality that uses sound waves to determine internal structures of the body.

Ureter—A tube that carries urine from the kidney to the bladder.

Urethra—A tube that carries urine from the bladder to the outside of the body.

Urologist—A physician who specializes in problems of the urinary system.

---

fragments the stone. The resulting debris, called gravel, can then pass through the remainder of the ureter, through the bladder, and through the urethra during urination. There is minimal chance of damage to skin or internal organs because biologic tissues are resilient, not brittle, and because the shock waves are not focused on them.

WHO PERFORMS THE PROCEDURE AND WHERE IS IT PERFORMED?

Lithotripsy is performed by a technician or other individual with specialized training under the supervision of a physician. The physician in charge usually has specialized training in urology. Lithotripsy is most often performed as an outpatient procedure in a facility affiliated with a hospital.

The shock wave is characterized by a very rapid pressure increase in the transmission medium and is quite different from **ultrasound**. The shock waves are transmitted through a person's skin and pass harmlessly through soft tissues. The shock wave passes through the kidney and strikes the stone. At the edge of the stone, energy is transferred into the stone, causing small cracks to form on the edge of the stone. The same effect occurs when the shock wave exits the stone. With successive shock waves, the cracks open up. As more cracks form, the size of the stone is reduced. Eventually, the stone is reduced to small particles, which are then flushed out of the kidneys or ureter naturally during urination.

Diagnosis/Preparation

ESWL should not be considered for persons with severe skeletal deformities, people weighing more than 300 lb (136 kg), individuals with abdominal aortic aneurysms, or persons with uncontrollable bleeding disorders. Women who are pregnant should not be treated with ESWL. Individuals with cardiac **pacemakers** should be evaluated by a cardiologist familiar with ESWL. The cardiologist should be present during the ESWL procedure in the event the pacemaker needs to be overridden.

Prior to the lithotripsy procedure, a complete **physical examination** is performed, followed by tests to determine the number, location, and size of the stone or stones. A test called an intravenous pyelogram (IVP) is used to locate the stones, which involves injecting a dye into a vein in the arm. This dye, which shows up on x ray, travels through the bloodstream and is excreted by the kidneys. The dye then flows down the ureters and into the bladder. The dye surrounds the stones. In this manner, x rays are used to evaluate the stones and the anatomy of the urinary system. Blood tests are performed to determine if any potential bleeding problems exist. For women of childbearing age, a pregnancy

QUESTIONS TO ASK THE DOCTOR

Individuals contemplating a lithotripsy procedure should consider asking the following questions:

- Is the doctor board certified in urology?
- How many lithotripsy procedures has the doctor performed?
- What is the doctor's complication rate?

test is done to make sure they are not pregnant. Older persons have an EKG test to make sure that no potential heart problems exist. Some individuals may have a stent placed prior to the lithotripsy procedure. A stent is a plastic tube placed in the ureter that allows the passage of gravel and urine after the ESWL procedure is completed.

The process of lithotripsy generally takes about one hour. During that time, up to 8,000 individual shock waves are administered. Depending on a person's pain tolerance, there may be some discomfort during the treatment. **Analgesics** may be administered to relieve this pain.

Aftercare

Most persons pass blood in their urine after the ESWL procedure. This is normal and should clear after several days to a week. Lots of fluids should be taken to encourage the flushing of any gravel remaining in the urinary system. Treated persons should follow up with a urologist in about two weeks to make sure that everything is progressing as planned. If a stent has been inserted, it is normally removed at this time.

Risks

Abdominal pain is fairly common after ESWL, but it is usually not a cause for worry. However, persistent or severe abdominal pain may imply an unexpected internal injury. Occasionally, stones may not be completely fragmented during the first ESWL treatment and further lithotripsy procedures may be required.

Some people are allergic to the dye material used during an IVP, so it cannot be used. For these people, focused sound waves, called ultrasound, can be used to identify where the stones are located.

Normal results

In most cases, stones are reduced to gravel and passed within a few days. Individuals may return to work whenever they feel able.

Morbidity and mortality rates

Colicky renal pain is very common when gravel is being passed. Other problems may include perirenal hematomas (blood clots near the kidneys) in 66% of the cases; nerve palsies; pancreatitis (inflammation of the pancreas); and obstruction by stone fragments. **Death** is extremely rare and usually due to an undiagnosed associated or underlying condition that is aggravated by the lithotripsy procedure.

Alternatives

Before the advent of lithotripsy, surgery was used to remove kidney stones. This approach is uncommon today, but occasionally used when other conditions prevent the use of lithotripsy. Attempts are occasionally made to change the pH of urine so as to dissolve kidney stones. This treatment has limited success.

Resources

BOOKS

Brenner, BM et al Brenner & Rector's The Kidney. 7th ed. Philadelphia: Saunders, 2004.

Wein, AJ et al. Campbell-Walsh Urology. 9th ed. Philadelphia: Saunders, 2007.

PERIODICALS

Ather, M. H., and M. A. Noor. "Does Size and Site Matter for Renal Stones Up to 30 mm in Size in Children Treated by Extracorporeal Lithotripsy?" Urology 61, no.1 (2003): 212–215.

Downey, P., and D. Tolley. "Contemporary Management of Renal Calculus Disease." Journal of the Royal College of Surgery (Edinburgh) 47, no.5 (2002): 668–675.

Hochreiter, W. W., H. Danuser, M. Perrig, and U. E. Studer. "Extracorporeal Shock Wave Lithotripsy for Distal Ureteral Calculi." Journal of Urology 169, no.3 (2003): 878–880.

Rajkumar, P., and G. F. Schmitgen. "Shock Waves Do More Than Just Crush Stones: Extracorporeal Shock Wave Therapy in Plantar Fasciitis." International Journal of Clinical Practice 56, no.10 (2002): 735–737.

ORGANIZATIONS

American Foundation for Urologic Disease. 1128 North Charles Street, Baltimore, MD 21201. (800) 242-2383 or (410) 468-1800. E-mail: admin@afud.org. www.afud.org.

American Lithotripsy Society. 305 Second Avenue, Suite 200, Waltham, MA 02451.

American Medical Association. 515 N. State Street, Chicago, IL 60610. (312) 464-5000. http://www.ama-assn.org.

American Urological Association. 1120 North Charles Street, Baltimore, MD 21201-5559. (410) 727-1100. http://www.auanet.org/index_hi.cfm.

National Kidney Foundation. 30 East 33rd Street, New York, NY 10016. (800) 622-9010, (781) 895-9098. Fax: (781) 895-9088. E-mail: als@lithotripsy.org. http://www.kidney.org.

OTHER

Case Western Reserve University. [cited March 17, 2003] http://www.cwru.edu/artsci/dittrick/artifactspages/b-2lithotripsy.htm.

Global Lithotripsy Services. [cited March 17, 2003] http://www.gls-lithotripsy.com/Howdoes.html.

Lifespan. [cited March 17, 2003] http://www.lifespan.org/mininvasive/revised/patient/gallstones/lithotripsy.htm.

National Institute of Diabetes and Digestive and Kidney Diseases. [cited March 17, 2003] http://www.niddk.nih.gov/health/urolog/pubs/stonadul/stonadul.htm#whogets.

National Library of Medicine. [cited March 17, 2003] http://www.nlm.nih.gov/medlineplus/ency/article/007113.htm.

L. Fleming Fallon, Jr, MD, DrPH

Liver biopsy

Definition

A liver biopsy is a medical procedure performed to obtain a small piece of liver tissue for diagnostic testing. The sample is examined under a microscope by a pathologist, a doctor who specializes in the effects of disease on body tissues; in this case, to detect abnormalities of the liver. Liver biopsies are sometimes called percutaneous liver biopsies, because the tissue sample is obtained by going through the patient's skin. This is a useful diagnostic procedure with very low risk and little discomfort to the patient.

Purpose

A liver biopsy is usually done to evaluate the extent of damage that has occurred to the liver because of chronic and acute disease processes or toxic injury. Biopsies are often performed to identify abnormalities in liver tissues after other techniques have failed to yield clear results. In patients with chronic hepatitis C, liver biopsy may be used to assess the patient's prognosis and the likelihood of responding to antiviral treatment.

A liver biopsy may be ordered to diagnose or stage any of the following conditions or disorders:

- jaundice
- cirrhosis
- repeated abnormal results from liver function tests
- alcoholic liver disease
- unexplained swelling or enlargement of the liver (hepatomegaly)
- suspected drug-related liver damage such as acetaminophen poisoning
- hemochromatosis, a condition of excess iron in the liver
- intrahepatic cholestasis, the build up of bile in the liver
- hepatitis
- primary cancers of the liver such as hepatomas, cholangiocarcinomas, and angiosarcomas
- metastatic cancers of the liver (more than 20 times as common in the United States as primary cancers)
- post-liver transplant to measure graft rejection
- fever of unknown origin
- suspected tuberculosis, sarcoidosis, or amyloidosis
- genetic disorders such as Wilson's disease (a disorder in which copper accumulates in the liver, brain, kidneys, and corneas)

Demographics

According to the American Liver Foundation, liver disease affects approximately 25 million (one in 10) Americans annually. Cirrhosis accounts for over 27,000 deaths each year. Liver disease is the third most common cause of **death** among individuals between the ages of 25 and 59, and the seventh most common cause of all disease-related deaths.

Description

Percutaneous liver biopsy is sometimes called aspiration biopsy or fine-needle aspiration (FNA) because it is done with a hollow needle attached to a suction syringe. The special needles used to perform a liver biopsy are called Menghini or Jamshedi needles. The amount of specimen collected should be about 0.03–0.7 fl oz (1–2 cc). In many cases, the biopsy is done by a radiologist, doctor who specializes in x rays and imaging studies. The radiologist will use computed tomography (CT) scan or **ultrasound** to guide the needle to the target site for the biopsy. Some ultrasound-guided biopsies are performed using a biopsy gun that has a spring mechanism that contains a cutting sheath. This type of procedure gives a greater yield of tissue.

An hour or so before the biopsy, the patient will be given a sedative to aid in relaxation. The patient is then asked to lie on the back with the right elbow to

Liver Biopsy

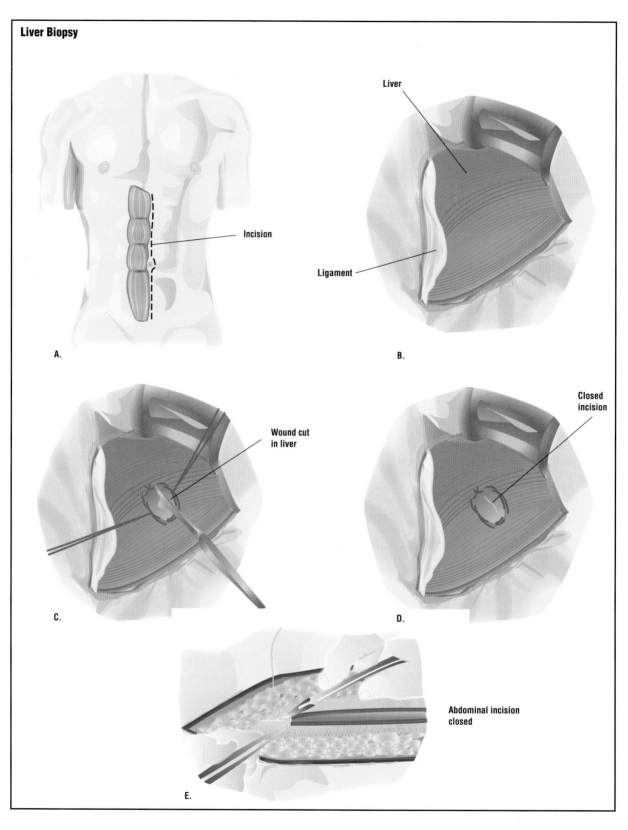

A.

B.

C.

D.

E.

In a traditional liver biopsy, access to the liver is gained through an incision in the abdomen (A). A wedge-shaped section is cut into the liver and removed (C). The liver incision is (D). The abdominal incision is then repaired (E). *(Illustration by GGS Information Services. Cengage Learning, Gale.)*

KEY TERMS

Aspiration—The technique of removing a tissue sample for biopsy through a hollow needle attached to a suction syringe.

Bile—Liquid produced by the liver that is excreted into the intestine to aid in the digestion of fats.

Biliary—Relating to bile.

Biopsy—The surgical removal and microscopic examination of living tissue for diagnostic purposes.

Cholestasis—A blockage in the flow of bile.

Cirrhosis—A progressive disease of the liver characterized by the death of liver cells and their replacement with fibrous tissue.

Formalin—A clear solution of diluted formaldehyde that is used to preserve liver biopsy specimens until they can be examined in the laboratory.

Hepatitis—Inflammation of the liver, caused by infection or toxic injury.

Jaundice—Also termed icterus; an increase in blood bile pigments that are deposited in the skin, eyes, deeper tissue, and excretions. The skin and whites of the eye will appear yellow.

Menghini needle/Jamshedi needle—Special needles used to obtain a sample of liver tissue by aspiration.

Metastatic cancer—A cancer that has been transmitted through the body from a primary cancer site.

Percutaneous biopsy—A biopsy in which the needle is inserted and the sample removed through the skin.

Prothrombin test—A common test to measure the amount of time it takes for a patient's blood to clot; measurements are in seconds.

Vital signs—A person's essential body functions, usually defined as the pulse, body temperature, and breathing rate.

The doctor prepares the needle by drawing sterile saline solution into a syringe. The syringe is then attached to the biopsy needle, which is inserted into the patient's chest wall. The doctor then draws the plunger of the syringe back to create a vacuum. At this point, the patient is asked to take a deep breath and hold it. The needle is inserted into the liver and withdrawn quickly, usually within two seconds or less. The negative pressure in the syringe draws or pulls a sample of liver tissue into the biopsy needle. As soon as the needle is withdrawn, the patient can breathe normally. This step takes only a few seconds. Pressure is applied at the biopsy site to stop any bleeding and a bandage is placed over it. The liver tissue sample is placed in a cup with a 10% formalin solution and sent to the laboratory immediately. The entire procedure takes 10–15 minutes. Test results are usually available within a day.

Most patients experience minor discomfort during the procedure (up to 50% of patients), but not severe pain. According to a medical study of adult patients undergoing percutaneous liver biopsy, pain was most often described as mild to moderate (i.e., a rating of three on a scale of one to 10). Mild medications of a non-aspirin type can be given after the biopsy if the pain persists for several hours.

Diagnosis/Preparation

Liver biopsies require some preparation by the patient. Since **aspirin** and ibuprofen (Advil, Motrin) are known to cause excessive bleeding by inhibiting platelets and lessening clotting function, the patient should avoid taking any of these medications for at least a week before the biopsy. The doctor should check the patient's records to see whether he or she is taking any other medications that may affect blood clotting. Both a platelet count (or **complete blood count**) and a **prothrombin time** (to assess how well the patient's blood clots) are performed prior to the biopsy. These tests determine whether there is an abnormally high risk of uncontrolled bleeding from the biopsy site, which may contraindicate the procedure. The patient should limit food or drink for a period of four to eight hours before the biopsy.

Patients should be told what to expect in the way of discomfort pre- and post-procedure. In addition, they should be advised about what medications they should not take before or after the biopsy. It is important for the clinician to reassure the patient concerning the safety of the procedure.

Before the procedure, the patient or family member must sign a consent form. The patient will be questioned about any history of allergy to the local

the side and the right hand under the head. The patient is instructed to lie as still as possible during the procedure. He or she is warned to expect a sensation resembling a pinch in the right shoulder when the needle passes a certain nerve (the phrenic nerve), but to remain motionless in spite of the momentary pain.

The doctor will then mark a spot on the skin of the abdomen where the needle will be inserted. The right side of the upper abdomen is thoroughly cleansed with an antiseptic solution, generally iodine. The patient is then given a local anesthetic at the biopsy site.

anesthetic, and then will be asked to empty the bladder so that he or she will be more comfortable during the procedure. **Vital signs**, including pulse rate, temperature, and breathing rate will be noted so that the doctor can tell during the procedure if the patient is having any physical problems.

When performing the liver biopsy and blood collection that precedes it, the physician and other health care providers will follow universal precautions to maintain sterility for the prevention of transmission of blood-borne pathogens.

Some patients should not have percutaneous liver biopsies. They include those with any of the following conditions:

- a platelet count below 50,000
- a prothrombin test time greater than three seconds over the reference interval, indicating a possible clotting abnormality
- a liver tumor with a large number of veins
- a large amount of abdominal fluid (ascites)
- infection anywhere in the lungs, the lining of the chest or abdominal wall, the biliary tract, or the liver
- benign tumors (angiomas) of the liver, which consist mostly of enlarged or newly formed blood vessels and may bleed heavily
- biliary obstruction (bile may leak from the biopsy site and cause an infection of the abdominal cavity)

Aftercare

Liver biopsies are now performed as outpatient procedures in most hospitals. Patients are asked to lie on their right sides for one hour and then to rest quietly for three more hours. At regular intervals, a nurse checks the patient's vital signs. If there are no complications, the patient is discharged, but will be asked to stay in an area that is within an hour from the hospital in case delayed bleeding occurs.

Patients should arrange to have a friend or relative take them home after discharge. Bed rest for a day is recommended, followed by a week of avoiding heavy work or strenuous **exercise**. The patient can immediately resume eating a normal diet.

Some mild soreness in the area of the biopsy is expected after the anesthetic wears off. Irritation of the muscle that lies over the liver can also cause mild discomfort in the shoulder for some patients. **Acetaminophen** can be taken for minor soreness, but aspirin and ibuprofen products are best avoided. The patient should, however, call the doctor if there is severe pain in the abdomen, chest, or shoulder; difficulty breathing; or persistent bleeding. These signs

> # WHO PERFORMS THE PROCEDURE AND WHERE IS IT PERFORMED?
>
> The liver biopsy requires the skill of many clinicians, including the radiologist, hepatologist, and pathologist, to make the diagnosis. Nurses will assist the physician during the biopsy procedure and in caring for the patient after the procedure. Tissues are prepared for microscopic evaluation by a histologic technician in the pathology lab. The procedure is generally performed on an outpatient basis in a hospital.

may indicate that there has been leakage of bile into the abdominal cavity, or that air has been introduced into the cavity around the lungs.

Risks

The complications associated with a liver biopsy are usually minor; most will occur in the first two hours following the procedure, and greater than 95% in the first 24 hours. The most significant risk is prolonged internal bleeding. Other complications from percutaneous liver biopsies include the leakage of bile or the introduction of air into the chest cavity (pneumothorax). There is also a small chance that an infection may occur. The risk that an internal organ such as the lung, gallbladder, or kidney might be punctured is decreased when using the ultrasound- or CT-guided procedure.

Normal results

After the biopsy, the liver sample is sent to the pathology laboratory and examined. A normal (negative) result would find no evidence of pathology in the tissue sample. It should be noted that many diseases of the liver are focal and not diffuse; an abnormality may not be detected if the sample was taken from an unaffected site. If symptoms persist, the patient may need to undergo another biopsy.

The pathologist will perform a visual inspection of the sample to note any abnormalities in appearance. In cirrhosis, the sample will be fragmented and hard. Fatty liver, seen in heavy drinkers, will float in the formalin solution and will be yellow. Carcinomas are white. The pathologist will also look for deposition of bile pigments (green), indicating cholestasis (obstruction of bile flow). In preparation for microscopic examination, the tissue will be frozen and cut into

QUESTIONS TO ASK THE DOCTOR

- Why is a biopsy indicated in my case?
- How many biopsies do you perform each year? What is your rate of complications?
- What will happen when I get the results?
- What alternatives are available to me?

thin sections, which will be mounted on glass slides and stained with various dyes to aid in identifying microscopic structures. Using the microscope, the pathologist will examine the tissue samples, and identify abnormal cells and any deposited substances such as iron or copper. In liver cancer, small dark malignant cells will be visible within the liver tissue. An infiltration of white blood cells may signal infection. The pathologist also checks for the number of bile ducts, and determines whether they are dilated. He or she also looks at the health of the small arteries and portal veins. Fibrosis will appear as scar tissue, and fatty changes are diagnosed by the presence of lipid droplets. Many different findings may be noted and a differential diagnosis (one out of many possibilities) can often be made. In difficult cases, other laboratory tests such as those assessing liver function enzymes will aid the clinician in determining the final diagnosis.

Morbidity and mortality rates

Post-biopsy complications that require hospitalization occur in approximately 1–3% of cases. Moderate pain is reported by 20% of patients, and 3% report pain severe enough to warrant intravenous pain relief. The mortality rate is approximately one in 10,000. In about 0.4% of cases, a patient with liver cancer will develop a fatal hemorrhage from a percutaneous biopsy. These fatalities result because some liver tumors are supplied with a large number of blood vessels and thus may bleed excessively.

Alternatives

Liver biopsy is an invasive and sometimes painful procedure that is also expensive (in 2002, direct costs associated with liver biopsy were $1,500–2,000). In some instances, blood tests may provide enough information to health care providers to make an accurate diagnosis and therefore avoid a biopsy. Occasionally, a biopsy may be obtained using a laparoscope (an instrument inserted through the abdominal wall that allows the doctor to visualize the liver and obtain a

sample) or during surgery if the patient is undergoing an operation on the abdomen. Imaging techniques (such as ultrasound) may also be employed during a liver biopsy, in order to allow more accurate placement of the biopsy needle.

Resources

BOOKS

Feldman, M, et al.. Sleisenger & Fordtran's Gastrointestinal and Liver Disease. 8th ed. St. Louis: Mosby, 2005.

Khatri, VP and JA Asensio. Operative Surgery Manual. 1st ed. Philadelphia: Saunders, 2003.

Townsend, CM et al. Sabiston Textbook of Surgery. 17th ed. Philadelphia: Saunders, 2004.

PERIODICALS

Dienstag, Jules L. "The Role of Liver Biopsy in Chronic Hepatitis C." Hepatology 36, no. 5 (November 2002): 152–60.

ORGANIZATIONS

American Liver Foundation. 1425 Pompton Avenue, Cedar Grove, NJ 07009. (800) 465-4837. http://www.liver foundation.org.

Jane E. Phillips, PhD
Stephanie Dionne Sherk
Rosalyn Carson-DeWitt, MD

Liver function tests

Definition

Liver function tests, or LFTs, include tests that are routinely measured in all clinical laboratories. LFTs include bilirubin, a compound formed by the breakdown of hemoglobin; ammonia, a breakdown product of protein that is normally converted into urea by the liver before being excreted by the kidneys; proteins that are made by the liver, including total protein, albumin, prothrombin, and fibrinogen; cholesterol and triglycerides, which are made and excreted via the liver; and the enzymes alanine aminotransferase (ALT), aspartate aminotransferase (AST), alkaline phosphatase (ALP), gamma-glutamyl transferase (GGT), and lactate dehydrogenase (LDH). Other liver function tests include serological tests (to demonstrate antibodies); DNA tests for hepatitis and other viruses; and tests for antimitochondrial and smooth muscle antibodies, transthyretin (prealbumin), protein electrophoresis, bile acids, alpha-fetoprotein, and a constellation of other enzymes that help differentiate

KEY TERMS

Bile acid—A detergent that is made in the liver and excreted into the intestine to aid in the absorption of fats.

Biliary—Relating to bile.

Cirrhosis—A liver disease where there is a loss of normal liver tissues, replaced by scar tissue. This is usually caused by chronic alcohol abuse, but also can be caused by blockage of the bile ducts.

Detoxification—A process of altering the chemical structure of a compound to make it less toxic.

Hepatitis—Inflammation of the liver.

Hepatocyte—Liver cell.

Isoenzyme—One of a group of enzymes that brings about the same reactions on the same chemicals, but are different in their physical properties.

Jaundice—Hyperbilirubinemia, or too much bilirubin in the blood. Bilirubin will be deposited in the skin and the mucosal membranes. The whites of the eyes and the skin appear yellow.

Lipoprotein—A chemical combination of a protein and a lipid (fats).

Neonatal jaundice—A disorder in newborns where the liver is too premature to conjugate bilirubin, which builds up in the blood.

necrotic (characterized by the **death** of tissue) versus obstructive liver disease.

Purpose

Liver function tests done individually do not give the physician much information, but used in combination with a careful history, **physical examination**, and imaging studies, they contribute to making an accurate diagnosis of the specific liver disorder. Different tests will show abnormalities in response to liver inflammation; liver injury due to drugs, alcohol, toxins, or viruses; liver malfunction due to blockage of the flow of bile; and liver cancers.

Precautions

Blood for LFTs is collected by sticking a needle into a vein. The nurse or phlebotomist (person trained to draw blood) performing the procedure must be careful to clean the skin before sticking in the needle.

Bilirubin: Drugs that may cause increased blood levels of total bilirubin include anabolic steroids, **antibiotics**, antimalarials, ascorbic acid, Diabinese, codeine, **diuretics**, epinephrine, oral contraceptives, and vitamin A.

Ammonia: Muscular exertion can increase ammonia levels, while cigarette smoking produces significant increases within one hour of inhalation. Drugs that may cause increased levels include alcohol, **barbiturates**, narcotics, and diuretics. Drugs that may decrease levels include antibiotics, levodopa, lactobacillus, and potassium salts.

ALT: Drugs that may increase ALT levels include **acetaminophen**, ampicillin, codeine, dicumarol, indomethacin, methotrexate, oral contraceptives, **tetracyclines**, and verapamil. Previous intramuscular injections may cause elevated levels.

GGT: Drugs that may cause increased GGT levels include alcohol, phenytoin, and phenobarbital. Drugs that may cause decreased levels include oral contraceptives.

LDH: Strenuous activity may raise levels of LDH. Alcohol, anesthetics, **aspirin**, narcotics, procainamide, and fluoride may also raise levels. Ascorbic acid (vitamin C) can lower levels of LDH.

Description

The liver is the largest and one of the most important organs in the body. As the body's "chemical factory," it regulates the levels of most of the biomolecules found in the blood, and acts with the kidneys to clear the blood of drugs and toxic substances. The liver metabolizes these products, alters their chemical structure, makes them water soluble, and excretes them in bile. Laboratory tests for total protein, albumin, ammonia, transthyretin, and cholesterol are markers for the synthetic (chemical-producing) function of the liver. Tests for cholesterol, bilirubin, ALP, and bile salts are measures of the secretory (excretory) function of the liver. The enzymes ALT, AST, GGT, LDH, and tests for viruses are markers for liver injury.

Some liver function tests are used to determine if the liver has been damaged or its function impaired. Elevations of these markers for liver injury or disease tell the physician that something is wrong with the liver. ALT and bilirubin are the two primary tests used largely for this purpose. Bilirubin is measured by two tests, called total and direct bilirubin. While total bilirubin is elevated in various liver diseases, it is also increased in certain (hemolytic) anemias caused by increased red blood cell turnover. Neonatal hyperbilirubinemia (jaundice) is a condition caused by an immature liver than cannot conjugate (process) the bilirubin. The level of total bilirubin in the blood becomes elevated and must be monitored closely in order to prevent damage to the brain caused by unconjugated bilirubin, which has a high affinity for brain tissue. Bilirubin levels can be decreased by exposing the baby to UV light. Direct bilirubin is formed only by the liver, and therefore, it is specific for hepatic or biliary disease. Its concentration in the blood is very low (0–0.2 mg/dL) and therefore, even slight increases are significant. Highest levels of direct bilirubin are seen in obstructive liver diseases. However, direct bilirubin is not sensitive to all forms of liver disease and is not always elevated in the earliest stages of disease. Therefore, ALT is needed to exclude a diagnosis.

Although ALT is present in other tissues, its concentration in the liver is far greater than any other tissue. The enzyme is very sensitive to liver injury. Consequently, if ALT or direct bilirubin is increased, then some form of liver disease is likely. If both are normal, then liver disease is unlikely.

These two tests, along with others, are used to help make a diagnosis. The most useful tests for this purpose are the liver function enzymes and the ratio of direct to total bilirubin. These tests are used to differentiate diseases characterized primarily by hepatocellular damage (necrosis, or cell death) from those characterized by obstructive damage (cholestasis or blockage of bile flow). Liver cell damage may be caused by viral hepatitis, hepatitis induced by drugs or poisons (toxic hepatitis), alcoholic hepatitis, hypoxic necrosis (a consequence of congestive heart failure), chronic hepatitis, and cirrhosis of the liver. Obstructive liver diseases include intrahepatic (within the liver) obstructive disease or extrahepatic (outside the liver) obstruction. In both cases, the direct bilirubin is often greatly elevated because the liver can conjugate the bilirubin, but this direct bilirubin cannot be excreted via the bile. In such cases the ratio of direct to total bilirubin is greater than 0.4.

Aspartate aminotransferase (AST) is not as specific for liver disease as ALT is. However, differentiation of acute and chronic forms of liver disease is aided by examining the ratio of ALT to AST, called the DeRitis ratio. In acute hepatitis, Reye's syndrome, and infectious mononucleosis, the ALT predominates. However, in alcoholic liver disease, chronic hepatitis, and cirrhosis, the AST predominates.

Alkaline phosphatase (ALP)is increased in obstructive liver diseases, but it is not specific for the liver. Increases are commonly seen in bone diseases, late pregnancy, leukemia, and some other malignancies. The enzyme gamma-glutamyl transferase (GGT) is used to help differentiate the source of an elevated ALP. GGT is greatly increased in obstructive jaundice, alcoholic liver disease, and hepatic cancer. When

the increase in GGT is two or more times greater than the increase in ALP, the source of the ALP is considered to be from the liver. When the increase in GGT is five or more times the increase in ALP, this points to a diagnosis of alcoholic hepatitis. GGT, but not AST and ALT, is elevated in the first stages of liver inflammation due to alcohol consumption, and GGT is useful as a marker for excessive drinking. GGT has been shown to rise after acute persistent alcohol ingestion and then fall when alcohol is avoided.

Lactate dehydrogenase (LDH) is found in almost all cells in the body. LDH is increased in megaloblastic and hemolytic anemias, leukemias and lymphomas, myocardial infarction, infectious mononucleosis, muscle wasting diseases, and both necrotic and obstructive jaundice. LDH is markedly increased in most cases of liver cancer. An enzyme pattern showing a marked increase in LDH and to a lesser degree ALP with only slightly increased transaminases (AST and ALT) is seen in cancer of the liver.

Some liver function tests are not sensitive enough to be used for diagnostic purposes, but are elevated in severe or chronic liver diseases. These tests are used primarily to indicate the extent of damage to the liver. Tests falling into this category are ammonia, total protein, albumin, cholesterol, transthyretin, fibrinogen, and the **prothrombin time**.

Analysis of blood ammonia aids in the diagnosis of severe liver diseases and helps to monitor the course of these diseases. Together with the AST and the ALT, ammonia levels are used to confirm a diagnosis of Reye's syndrome, a rare disorder usually seen in children and associated with infection and aspirin intake. Reye's syndrome is characterized by brain and liver damage following an upper respiratory tract infection, chickenpox, or influenza. Ammonia levels are also helpful in the diagnosis and treatment of hepatic encephalopathy, a serious brain condition caused by the accumulated toxins that result from liver disease and liver failure. Ammonia levels in the blood are normally very low. Increasing ammonia signals end-stage liver disease and a high risk of hepatic coma.

Albumin is the protein found in the highest concentration in blood, making up over half of the protein mass. A persistently low albumin in liver disease is a sign of progressive liver failure. In the acute stages of liver disease, proteins such as transthyretin (prealbumin) may be measured to give an indication of the severity of the disease.

Cholesterol is synthesized by the liver. Its balance is maintained by the liver's ability to remove cholesterol from lipoproteins, and use it to produce bile acids and salts that it excretes into the bile ducts. In obstructive jaundice caused by stones, biliary tract scarring, or cancer, the bile cannot be eliminated. Cholesterol and triglycerides may accumulate in the blood as low-density lipoprotein (LDL) cholesterol. In acute necrotic liver diseases, triglycerides may be elevated. In liver failure caused by necrosis, the liver's ability to synthesize cholesterol is reduced, and blood levels may be low.

The liver is responsible for production of the vitamin K clotting factors. In obstructive liver diseases a deficiency of vitamin K-derived clotting factors results from failure to absorb vitamin K. In obstructive jaundice, an intramuscular injection of vitamin K will be given. In severe necrotic disease, the liver cannot synthesize clotting factors from vitamin K.

The most prevalent liver disease is viral hepatitis. Tests for this condition include a variety of antigen and antibody markers and nucleic acid tests. In addition to hepatitis A-E, viral hepatitis may be caused by Epstein-Barr virus (EBV) and cytomegalovirus (CMV) infections of the liver. Tests for these viruses such as the infectious mononucleosis antibody test, anti-viral capsid antigen test (anti-VCA), and anti-CMV test are useful in diagnosing these infections.

Liver disease may be caused by autoimmune mechanisms in which autoantibodies destroy liver cells. Autoimmune necrosis is associated with systemic lupus erythematosus and chronic viral hepatitis, usually caused by hepatitis B and hepatitis C virus infections. These conditions give rise to anti-smooth muscle antibodies and anti-nuclear antibodies, and tests for these are useful markers for chronic hepatitis. Antibodies to mitochondrial antigens (antimitochondrial antibodies) are found in the blood of more than 90% of persons with primary biliary cirrhosis.

Preparation

Patients are asked to fast and to inform clinicians of all drugs, even over-the-counter drugs, that they are taking. Many times liver function tests are done on an emergency basis. Thus fasting and obtaining a medical history may not be possible.

Aftercare

Patients will have blood drawn into a vacuum tube and may experience some pain and burning at the site of injection. A gauze bandage may be placed over the site to prevent further bleeding. If the patient is suffering from severe liver disease, he or she may lack clotting factors. The nurse or caregiver should be careful to monitor bleeding in these patients after obtaining blood.

Normal results

Reference ranges vary from laboratory to laboratory and also depend upon the method used. However, normal values are generally framed by the ranges shown below.

- ALT: 5–35 IU/L. (Values for the elderly may be slightly higher, and values also may be higher in men and in African-Americans.)
- AST: 0–35 IU/L.
- ALP: 30–120 IU/LALP is higher in children, older adults and pregnant females.
- GGT: males 2–30 U/L; females 1–24 U/L.
- LDH: 0–4 days old: 290–775 U/L; 4–10 days: 545–2000 U/L; 10 days–24 months: 180–430 U/L; 24 months–12 years: 110–295 U/L; 12–60 years: 100–190 U/L; 60 years: >110–210 U/L.
- Bilirubin: (Adult, elderly, and child) Total bilirubin: 0.1–1.0 mg/dL; indirect bilirubin: 0.2–0.8 mg/dL; direct bilirubin: 0.0–0.3 mg/dL. (Newborn) Total bilirubin: 1–12 mg/dL. Note: critical values for adult: greater than 1.2 mg/dL. Critical values for newborn (requiring immediate treatment): greater than 15 mg/dL.
- Ammonia: 10–70 micrograms per dL (heparinized plasma). Normal values for this test vary widely, depending upon the age of the patient and the type of specimen.
- Albumin: 3.2–5.4 g/L.

Abnormal results

ALT: Values are significantly increased in cases of hepatitis, and moderately increased in cirrhosis, liver tumor, obstructive jaundice, and severe burns. Values are mildly increased in pancreatitis, heart attack, infectious mononucleosis, and shock. Most useful when compared with ALP levels.

AST: High levels may indicate liver cell damage, hepatitis, heart attack, heart failure, or gall stones.

ALP: Elevated levels occur in diseases that impair bile formation (cholestasis). ALP may also be elevated in many other liver disorders, as well as some lung cancers (bronchogenic carcinoma) and Hodgkin's lymphoma. However, elevated ALP levels may also occur in otherwise healthy people, especially among older people.

GGT: Increased levels are diagnostic of hepatitis, cirrhosis, liver tumor or metastasis, as well as injury from drugs toxic to the liver. GGT levels may increase with alcohol ingestion, heart attack, pancreatitis, infectious mononucleosis, and Reye's syndrome.

LDH: Elevated LDH is seen with heart attack, kidney disease, hemolysis, viral hepatitis, infectious mononucleosis, Hodgkin's disease, abdominal and lung cancers, germ cell tumors, progressive muscular dystrophy, and pulmonary embolism. LD is not normally elevated in cirrhosis.

Bilirubin: Increased indirect or total bilirubin levels can indicate various serious anemias, including hemolytic disease of the newborn and **transfusion** reaction. Increased direct bilirubin levels can be diagnostic of bile duct obstruction, gallstones, cirrhosis, or hepatitis. It is important to note that if total bilirubin levels in the newborn reach or exceed critical levels, exchange transfusion is necessary to avoid kernicterus, a condition that causes brain damage from bilirubin in the brain.

Ammonia: Increased levels are seen in primary liver cell disease, Reye's syndrome, severe heart failure, hemolytic disease of the newborn, and hepatic encephalopathy.

Albumin: Albumin levels are increased due to dehydration. They are decreased due to a decrease in synthesis of the protein which is seen in severe liver failure and in conditions such as burns or renal disease that cause loss of albumin from the blood.

Patient education

Health-care providers should inform the patient of any abnormal results and explain how these values reflect the status of their liver disease. It is important to guide the patient in ways to stop behaviors such as taking drugs or drinking alcohol, if these are the causes of the illness.

Resources

BOOKS

Feldman, M, et al.. Sleisenger & Fordtran's Gastrointestinal and Liver Disease. 8th ed. St. Louis: Mosby, 2005.
McPherson RA et al.Henry's Clinical Diagnosis and Management By Laboratory Methods. 21st ed. Philadelphia: Saunders, 2007.

OTHER

Jensen, J. E. Liver Function Tests. [cited April 4, 2003]. http://www.gastromd.com/lft.html.
National Institutes of Health. [cited April 4, 2003]. http://www.nlm.nih.gov/medlineplus/encyclopedia.html.
Worman, Howard J. Common Laboratory Tests in Liver Disease. [cited April 4, 2003]. http://www.cpmcnet.columbia.edu/dept/gi/labtests.html.

Jane E. Phillips, Ph.D.
Mark A. Best, M.D.
Rosalyn Carson-DeWitt, MD

Liver removal *see* **Hepatectomy**

Liver transplantation

Definition

Liver transplantation is a surgery that removes a diseased liver and replaces it with a healthy donor liver.

Purpose

A liver transplant is needed when the liver's function is reduced to the point that the life of the patient is threatened.

Demographics

Compared to whites, those with African-American, Asian, Pacific Islander, or Hispanic descent are three times more likely to suffer from end-stage renal disease (ESRD). Both children and adults can suffer from liver failure and require a transplant.

Patients with advanced heart and lung disease, who are human immunodeficiency virus (HIV) positive, and who abuse drugs and alcohol are poor candidates for liver transplantation. Their ability to survive the surgery and the difficult recovery period, as well as their long-term prognosis, is hindered by their conditions.

Description

The liver is the body's principle chemical factory. It receives all nutrients, drugs, and toxins, which are absorbed from the intestines, and performs the final stages of digestion, converting food into energy and replacement parts for the body. The liver also filters the blood of all waste products, removes and detoxifies poisons, and excretes many of these into the bile. It further processes other chemicals for excretion by the kidneys. The liver is also an energy storage organ, converting food energy to a chemical called glycogen that can be rapidly converted to fuel.

When other medical treatment interferes with the functioning of a damaged liver, a transplant is necessary. Since 1963, when the first human liver transplant was performed, thousands more have been performed each year. Cirrhosis, a disease that kills healthy liver cells, replacing them with scar tissue, is the most common reason for liver transplantation in adults. The most frequent reason for transplantation in children is biliary atresia—a disease in which the ducts that carry bile out of the liver, are missing or damaged.

Included among the many causes of liver failure that bring patients to **transplant surgery** are:

KEY TERMS

Acetaminophen—A common pain reliever (e.g., Tylenol).

Anesthesia—A safe and effective means of alleviating pain during a medical procedure.

Antibody—An antibody is a protein complex used by the immune system to identify and neutralize foreign objects, such as like bacteria and viruses. Each antibody recognizes a specific antigen unique to its target

Antigen—Any chemical that provokes an immune response.

Ascites—A buildup of fluid in the stomach as a result of liver failure.

Bile ducts—Tubes carrying bile from the liver to the intestines.

Biliary atresia—A disease in which the ducts that carry bile out of the liver are missing or damaged is the most frequent reason for transplantation in children. Biliary atresia of the major bile ducts causes cholestasis and jaundice, which does not become apparent until several days after birth; periportal fibrosis develops and leads to cirrhosis, with proliferation

of small bile ducts unless these are also atretic; giant cell transformation of hepatic cells also occurs.

Biliary system—The tree of tubes that carries bile.

Cirrhosis—A disease in which healthy liver cells are killed and replaced with scar tissue. Cirrhosis is the most common reason for liver transplantation in adults and is often a result of alcoholism.

Computed tomography (CT or CAT) scan—A radiologic imaging modality that uses computer processing to generate an image of the tissue density in a "slice" as thin as 1–10 mm in thickness through the patient's body. These images are spaced at intervals of 0.5 cm–1 cm. Cross-sectional anatomy can be reconstructed in several planes without exposing the patient to additional radiation. Called also computerized axial tomography (CAT) and computerized transaxial tomography (CTAT).

Electrocardiogram (EKG)—A graphic record showing the electrical activity of the heart.

Endoscopy—An instrument (endoscope) used to visualize a hollow organ's interior.

- Progressive hepatitis, mostly due to virus infection, accounts for more than one-third of all liver transplants.

- Alcohol damage accounts for approximately 20% of transplants.

- Scarring, or abnormality of the biliary system, accounts for roughly another 20% of liver transplants.

- The remainder of transplants come from various cancers, uncommon diseases, and a disease known as fulminant liver failure.

Fulminant liver failure most commonly happens during acute viral hepatitis, but is also the result of mushroom poisoning by *Amanita phalloides* and toxic reactions to overdose of some medicines, such as acetaminophen—a medicine commonly used to relieve pain and reduce fever. The person who is the victim of mushroom poisoning is a special category of candidate for a liver transplant because of the speed of the disease and the immediate need for treatment.

As the liver fails, all of its functions diminish. Nutrition suffers, toxins build, and waste products accumulate. Scar tissue accumulates on the liver as the disease progresses. Blood flow is increasingly restricted in the portal vein, which carries blood from

the stomach and abdominal organs to the liver. The resulting high blood pressure (hypertension) causes swelling of and bleeding from the blood vessels of the esophagus. Toxins build in the blood (liver encephalopathy), resulting in severe jaundice (yellowing of the skin and eyes), fluid accumulation in the abdomen (ascites), and deterioration of mental function. Eventually, **death** occurs.

There are three types of liver transplantation methods. They include:

- Orthotopic transplantation, the replacement of a whole diseased liver with a healthy donor liver.

- Heterotrophic transplantation, the addition of a donor liver at another site, while the diseased liver is left intact.

- Reduced-size liver transplantation, the replacement of a whole diseased liver with a portion of a healthy donor liver. Reduced-size liver transplants are most often performed on children.

When an orthotropic transplantation is performed, a segment of the inferior vena cava (the body's main vein to the heart) attached to the liver is taken from the donor, as well. The same parts are removed from the recipient and replaced by connecting the inferior vena

Hepatic artery—The blood vessel supplying arterial blood to the liver.

Heterotrophic transplantation—The addition of a donor liver at another site, while the diseased liver is left intact.

Interleukin-2 (IL-2)—A cytokine derived from T helper lymphocytes that causes proliferation of T-lymphocytes and activated B lymphocytes.

Immunosuppression—A disorder or condition where the immune response is reduced or absent.

Inferior vena cava—The biggest vein in the body, returning blood to the heart from the lower half of the body.

Jaundice—Yellowing of the skin and eyes caused by a buildup of bile or excessive breakdown of red blood cells.

Leukemia—A cancer of the white blood cells (WBCs).

Lymphoma—A cancer of lymphatic tissue.

Lymphoproliferative—An increase in the number of lymphocytes. Lymphocytes are a white blood cell (WBC) formed in lymphatic tissue throughout the body—in the lymph nodes, spleen, thymus, tonsils, Peyer patches, and sometimes in bone marrow), and in normal adults, comprising approximately 22–28% of the total number of leukocytes in the circulating blood.

Magnetic resonance imaging (MRI)—A test that provides pictures of organs and structures inside the body by using a magnetic field and pulses of radio wave energy to detect tumors, infection, and other types of tissue disease or damage, and helps to diagnose conditions that affect blood flow. The area of the body being studied is positioned inside a strong magnetic field.

Nephrotoxicity—The quality or state of being toxic to kidney cells.

Orthotopic transplantation—The replacement of a whole diseased liver with a healthy donor liver.

Portal vein—The blood vessel carrying venous blood from the abdominal organs to the liver.

Receptor—A structural protein molecule on the cell surface or within the cytoplasm that binds to a specific factor, such as a drug, hormone, antigen, or neurotransmitter.

cava, the hepatic artery, the portal vein, and the bile ducts.

When there is a possibility that the afflicted liver may recover, a heterotypic transplantation is performed. The donor liver is placed in a different site, but it still has to have the same connections. It is usually attached very close to the patient's original liver; if the original liver recovers, the donor liver will wither away. If the patient's original liver does not recover, that liver will dry up, leaving the donor in place.

Reduced-size liver transplantation puts part of a donor liver into a patient. A liver can actually be divided into eight pieces—each supplied by a different set of blood vessels. In the past, just two of these sections have been enough to save a patient suffering from liver failure, especially if it is a child. It is possible, therefore, to transplant one liver into at least two patients and to transplant part of a liver from a living donor—and for both the donor and recipients to survive. Liver tissue grows to accommodate its job provided that the organ is large enough initially. Patients have survived with only 15–20% of their original liver intact, assuming that that portion was healthy from the beginning.

As of 2003, the availability of organs for transplant was in crisis. In October 1997, a national distribution system was established that gives priority to patients who are most ill and in closest proximity to the donor livers. Livers, however, are available nationally. It is now possible to preserve a liver out of the body for 10–20 hours by flushing it with cooled solutions of special chemicals and nutrients, if necessary. This enables transport cross-country.

Description

Once a donor liver has been located and the patient is in the **operating room** and under **general anesthesia**, the patient's heart and blood pressure are monitored. A long cut is made alongside of the ribs; sometimes, an upwards cut may also be made. When the liver is removed, four blood vessels that connect the liver to the rest of the body are cut and clamped shut. After getting the donor liver ready, the transplant surgeon connects these vessels to the donor vessels. A connection is made from the bile duct (a tube that drains the bile from the liver) of the donor liver to the bile duct of the liver of the patient's bile duct. In some cases, a small piece of the intestine is connected to the new donor bile duct. This connection is called

Roux-en-Y. The operation usually takes between six and eight hours; another two hours is spent preparing the patient for surgery. Therefore, a patient will likely be in the operating room for eight to 10 hours.

Split-liver techniques means that a single, perfect donor liver from a larger cadaver may be split for transplantation into more than one patient. Usually, the left lobe (comprising about 40% of the entire liver) will go to a small adult, adolescent, or child, while the larger right lobe (comprising about 60% of the entire liver) will go to an adult. When an infant requires a liver transplant, 20% of a normal-sized liver may be utilized, and the other 80% can go to another individual awaiting transplant. The success rate of this split-liver technique is somewhat lower than with whole organs (about 80% success rate versus about 90% success rate), but the obvious advantage is that more patients awaiting transplant can be served.

The United Network for Organ Sharing (UNOS) data indicates that patients in need of organ transplants outnumber available organs three to one.

Diagnosis/Preparation

The liver starts to fail only when more than half of it is damaged. Thus, once a person demonstrates symptoms of liver failure, there is not much liver function left. Signs and symptoms of liver failure include:

- jaundice
- muscle wasting (loss of muscle)
- forgetfulness, confusion, or coma
- fatigue
- itching
- poor blood clotting
- build-up of fluid in the stomach (ascites)
- infections
- bleeding in the stomach

A doctor will diagnose liver disease; a liver specialist, a transplant surgeon, and other doctors will have to be consulted, as well, before a patient can be considered for a liver transplant. Before transplantation takes place, the patient is first determined to be a good candidate for transplantation by going through a rigorous medical examination. Blood tests, consultations, and x rays will be needed to determine if the patient is a good candidate. Other tests that may be conducted are: computed tomography (CAT or CT) scan, magnetic resonance image (MRI), **ultrasound**, routine **chest x ray**, endoscopy, sclerotherapy and rubber-band ligation, transjugular intrahepatic portosystemic shunt (TIPS), creatinine clearance, cardiac testing (echocardiogram [ECHO]) and/or **electrocardiogram** [EKG or ECG]), and pulmonary function test [PFTs]), **liver biopsy**, and nutritional evaluation. A dietitian will evaluate the patient's nutritional needs and design an eating plan. Since a patient's emotional state is as important as their physical state, a psychosocial evaluation will be administered.

Once test results are reviewed and given to the liver transplant selection committee, the patient will be assessed for whether he or she is an appropriate candidate. Some patients are deemed too healthy for a transplant and will be followed and retested at a later date if their liver gets worse. Other patients are determined to be too sick to survive a transplant. The committee will not approve a transplant for these patients. Once a patient is approved, they will be placed on a waiting list for a donor liver. When placed on the waiting list, a patient will be given a score based on the results of the blood tests. The higher a patient's score, the sicker the patient is. This results in the patient earning a higher place on the waiting list.

Suitable candidates boost their nutritional intakes to ensure that they are as healthy as possible before surgery. Drugs are administered that will decrease organ rejection after surgery. The medical committee consults with the patient and family, if available, to explain the surgery and any potential complications. Many problems can arise during the waiting period. Medicines should be changed as needed, and blood tests should be done to ensure a patient is in the best possible health for the transplant surgery. Psychological counseling during this period is recommended, as well.

When a donor is found, it is important that the transplant team be able to contact the patient. The patient awaiting the organ must not eat or drink anything from the moment the hospital calls. On the other hand, the liver may not be good enough for transplantation. Then, the operation will be cancelled, although this does not happen often.

Aftercare

Following surgery, the patient will wake up in the surgical **intensive care unit** (SICU). During this time, a tube will be inserted into the windpipe to facilitate breathing. It is removed when the patient is fully awake and strong enough to breathe on his or her own. There may be other tubes that are removed as the patient recovers. When safe to leave the SICU, the patient is moved to the transplant floor. Walking and eating will become the primary focus. Physical therapy may be started to help the patient become active, as it is an important part of recovery. When the patient begins to feel hungry and the bowels are working, regular food that is low in salt will be given.

A patient should expect to spend about 10–14 days in the hospital, although some stays may be shorter or longer. Before leaving the hospital, a patient will be advised of: signs of infection or rejection, how to take medications and change **dressings**, and how to understand general health problems. Infection can be a real danger, because the medications taken compromise the body's defense systems. The doctors will conduct blood tests, ultrasounds, and x rays to ensure that the patient is doing well.

The first three months after transplant are the most risky for getting infections, such as the flu, so patients should follow these precautions:

- Avoid from people who are ill.
- Wash hands frequently.
- Tell the doctor if you are exposed to any disease.
- Tell the doctor if a cold sore, rash, or water blister appears on the body or spots appear in the throat or on the tongue.
- Stay out of crowds and rooms with poor circulation.
- Do not swim in lakes or community pools during the three months following transplant.
- Eat meats that are well-cooked.
- Stay away from soil, including those in which houseplants are grown, and gardens, during the three months following transplant.
- Take all medications as directed.
- Learn to report the early symptoms of infection.

To ensure that the transplant is successful and that the patient has a long and healthy life, a patient must get good medical care, prevent and treat complications, keep in touch with doctors and nurses, and follow their advice. Nutrition plays a big part in the success of a liver transplant, so what a patient eats after the transplant is very important.

Medications needed following liver transplantation

Successfully receiving a transplanted liver is only the beginning of a lifelong process. Patients with transplanted livers have to stay on **immunosuppressant drugs** for the rest of their lives to prevent organ rejection. Although many patients can reduce the dosage after the initial few months, virtually none can discontinue drugs altogether. For adolescent transplant recipients, post transplantation is a particularly difficult time, as they must learn to take responsibility for their own behavior and medication, as well as balance their developing sexuality in a body that has been transformed by the adverse effects of immunosuppression. Long-term outcome and tailoring of immunosuppression is of great importance.

Cyclosporine has long been the drug of experimentation in the immunosuppression regimen, and has been well-tolerated and effective. Hypertension, nephrotoxicity, and posttransplant lymphoproliferative disease (PTLD) are some of the long-term adverse effects. Tacrolimus has been developed more recently, and has improved the cosmetic adverse effects of cyclosporine, but has similar rates of hypertension and nephrotoxicity, and possibly a higher rate of PTLD. Prednisone, azathioprine, and tacrolimus are often combined with cyclosporine for better results. Newer immunosuppressive agents promise even better results.

There has been a recent, welcome development in renal sparing drugs, such as mycophenolate mofetil, which has no cosmetic adverse effects, does not require drug level monitoring, and is thus particularly attractive to teenagers. If started prior to irreversible renal dysfunction, recent research demonstrates recovery of renal function with mycophenolate mofetil. There is little published data on the use of sirolimus (rapamycin) in the pediatric population, but preliminary studies suggest that the future use of interleukin-2 receptor antibodies may be beneficial for immediate post-transplant induction of immunosuppression. When planning immunosuppression for adolescents, it is important to consider the effects of drug therapy on both males and females in order to maintain fertility and to ensure safety in pregnancy. Adequate practical measures and support should reduce noncompliance in this age group, and allow good, long-term function of the transplanted liver.

Risks

Early failure of the transplant occurs once in four surgeries and has to be repeated. Some transplants never work, some patients succumb to infection, and some suffer immune rejection. Primary failure is apparent within one or two days. Rejection usually starts at the end of the first week. There may be problems like bleeding of the bile duct after surgery, or blood vessels of the liver may become too narrow. The surgery itself may need revision because of narrowing, leaking, or blood clots at the connections. These issues may be solved with or without more surgery depending on the severity.

Infections are a constant risk while on immunosuppressive agents, because the immune system is supposed to prevent them. A method has not yet been devised to control rejection without hampering immune

WHO PERFORMS THE PROCEDURE AND WHERE IS IT PERFORMED?

A transplant surgeon will perform the surgery in a hospital that has a special unit called a transplant center.

QUESTIONS TO ASK THE DOCTOR

- What should I do to prepare for this operation?
- Who will tell me about the transplant process?
- Can I tour the transplant center?
- Who are the members of the transplant team and what are their jobs?
- Is there a special nursing unit for transplant patients?
- How many attending surgeons are available to do my type of transplant?
- Does the hospital do living donor transplants?
- Is a living donor transplant a choice in my case? If so, where will the living donor evaluation be done?
- What is the organ recovery cost if I have a living donor?
- Will I also need to change my lifestyle?
- How long will I have to stay in the hospital?
- Why is recovery such a slow process?

defenses against infections. Not only do ordinary infections pose a threat, but because of the impaired immunity, transplant patients are susceptible to the same opportunistic infections (OIs) that threaten acquired immune deficiency syndrome (AIDS) patients–pneumocystis pneumonia, herpes and cytomegalovirus (CMV) infections, fungi, and a host of bacteria.

Drug reactions are also a continuing threat. Every drug used to suppress the immune system has potential problems. As previously stated, hypertension, nephrotoxicity, and PTLD are some of the long-term adverse effects with immunosupressive drugs like cyclosporine. Immunosuppressants also hinder the body's ability to resist cancer. All drugs used to prevent rejection increase the risk of leukemias and lymphomas.

There is also a risk of the original disease returning. In the case of hepatitis C, reoccurrence is a risk factor for orthotropic liver transplants. Newer antiviral drugs hold out promise for dealing with hepatitis. In alcoholics, the urge to drink alcohol will still be a problem. Alcoholics Anonymous (AA) is the most effective treatment known for alcoholism.

Transplant recipients can get high blood pressure, diabetes, high cholesterol, thinning of the bones, and can become obese. Close medical care is needed to prevent these conditions.

Normal results

For a successful transplant, good medical care is important. Patients and families must stay in touch with their medical teams and drugs must be taken as advised to prevent infection and rejection of the new organ. However, sometimes because of the way it is preserved, the new liver doesn't function as it should, and a patient may have to go back on to the waiting list to receive a new liver.

Morbidity and mortality

Twenty-five million or one in 10 Americans are or have been afflicted with liver or biliary diseases. As of July 1, 2006, there were 17,298 patients on the UNOS National Transplant Waiting List who were waiting for a liver transplantation. During the year running from July 2006 to July 2007, 6,532 liver transplants were performed. Of these, 6,274 were deceased donor transplants, and 258 were living donor transplants. For liver transplants performed from July 1, 1999 through June 30, 2001, the one-year survival rate was 86% for adults; 1,861 patients died while on the UNOS waiting list for the year ending June 30, 2002. More than 80% of children survive transplantation to adolescence and adulthood.

Since the introduction of cyclosporine and tacrolimus (drugs that suppress the immune response and keep it from attacking and damaging the new liver), success rates for liver transplantation have reached 80–90%.

Infections occur in about half of transplant patients and often appear during the first week. Biliary complications are apparent in about 22% of recipient patients (and 6% of donors), and vascular complications occur in 9.8% of recipient patients. Other complications in donors include re-operation (4.5%) and death (0.2%).

There are potential social, economic, and psychological problems, and a vast array of possible medical and surgical complications. Close medical surveillance must continue for the rest of the patient's life.

Alternatives

There is no treatment that can help the liver with all of its functions; thus, when a person reaches a certain stage of liver disease, a liver transplant may be the only way to save the patient's life.

Resources

BOOKS

Abhinav, Humar, M.D., I. Hertz Marshall, M.D., Laura J., Blakemore, M.D., eds. Manual of Liver Transplant Medical Care. Minneapolis, MN: Fairview Press, 2002.

Feldman, M, et al.. Sleisenger & Fordtran's Gastrointestinal and Liver Disease. 8th ed. St. Louis: Mosby, 2005.

Khatri, VP and JA Asensio. Operative Surgery Manual. 1st ed. Philadelphia: Saunders, 2003.

Townsend, CM et al. Sabiston Textbook of Surgery. 17th ed. Philadelphia: Saunders, 2004.

PERIODICALS

Brown, R.S., Jr., M. W. Russo, M. Lai, M. L. Shiffman, M. C. Richardson, J. E. Everhart, et al. "A survey of liver transplantation from living adult donors in the United States." New England Journal of Medicine 348, no. 9 (February, 2003):818-25.

Goldstein, M. J., E. Salame, S. Kapur, M. Kinkhabwala, D. LaPointe-Rudow, N. P. P. Harren, et al. "Analysis of failure in living donor liver transplantation: differential outcomes in children and adults." World Journal of Surgery 27, no. 3 (2003):356-64.

Kelly, D. A. "Strategies for optimizing immunosuppression in adolescent transplant recipients: a focus on liver transplantation." Paediatric Drugs 5, no. 3 (2003): 177-83.

Longheval, G., P. Vereerstraeten, P. Thiry, M. Delhaye, O. Le Moine, J. Deviere, et al. "Predictive models of short- and long-term survival in patients with nonbiliary cirrhosis." Liver Transplantation: Official Publication of the American Association for the Study of Liver Diseases and the International Liver Transplantation Society 9, no. 3 (March, 2003):260-7.

Neff, G. W., A. Bonham, A. G. Tzakis, M. Ragni, D. Jayaweera, E. R. Schiff, et al. "Orthotopic liver transplantation in patients with human immunodeficiency virus and end-stage liver disease." Liver Transplantation: official publication of the American Association for the Study of Liver Diseases and the International Liver Transplantation Society 9, no. 3 (March, 2003): 239-47.

Papatheodoridis, G. V., V. Sevastianos, and A. K. Burrouhs. "Prevention of and treatment for hepatitis B virus infection after liver transplantation in the nucleoside analogues era." American Journal of Transplantation 3, no. 3 (March, 2003):250-8.

ORGANIZATIONS

American Liver Foundation. 75 Maiden Lane, Suite 603, New York, NY. 10038. (800) 465-4837 or (888) 443-7872. Fax: (212) 483.8179. E-mail: info@liverfoundation. org.http://www.liverfoundation.org.

Hepatitis Foundation International (HFI). 504 Blick Drive, Silver Spring, MD. 20904-2901. (800) 891-0707 or (301) 622-4200. Fax: (301) 622-4702. Email: hfi@comcast. net.http://www.hepfi.org

National Digestive Diseases, Information Clearinghouse. 2 Information Way, Bethesda, MD. 20892-3570. Email: nddic@info.niddk.nih.gov.

National Institutes of Health, 9000 Rockville Pike, Bethesda, Maryland. 20892. (301) 496-4000. Email: NIHInfo@OD.NIH.GOV. http://www.nih.gov.

United Network for Organ Sharing. 500-1100 Boulders Parkway, P.O. Box 13770. Richmond, VA. 23225. (888) 894-6361 or (804) 330-8500. http://www.unos.org

OTHER

U.S. National Library of Medicine and the National Institutes of Health. Liver Transplantation. 2003. [cited March 13, 2003]. www.nlm.nih.gov/medlineplus/ livertransplantation.html.

J. Ricker Polsdorfer, M.D.
Crystal H. Kaczkowski, M.Sc.
Rosalyn Carson-DeWitt, MD

▌Living will

Definition

A living will is a legal document with which patients instruct healthcare providers about their wishes with respect to medical procedures, in case they become incapacitated. The living will and the durable medical **power of attorney** are two federally mandated parts of what is known as advance medical directives.

Purpose

Advance medical directives are legal mechanisms to assure that patients' wishes about medical procedures are carried out in their final days or when they are incapacitated. The documents reflect patients' rights of consent and medical choice under conditions in which patients can no longer choose for themselves what medical interventions they wish to undergo.

In 1990, recognizing the importance of patient treatment wishes at the end of life, Congress enacted the Patient Self-Determination Act (PSDA). This federal law requires that patients admitted to hospitals, **nursing homes**, home health agencies, HMOs, and hospices be informed of their right under state law to prepare advance healthcare directives and to have the

KEY TERMS

Durable medical power of attorney—A legal document that empowers a person to make medical decisions for the patient should the patient be unable to make the decisions.

Medical directives—Legal documents that include a declaration of wishes pertaining to medical treatment (living will) and the stipulation of a proxy decision maker (power of attorney).

Patient Self-Determination Act (PSDA)—Federal law that ensures that medical providers offer the option of medical directives to patients and include the documents in their medical records.

Surrogate—A person who represents the wishes of the patient, chosen by the patient and stipulated by a legal document as power of attorney.

documents entered into their medical record. Each state has different requirements for the living will and the power of attorney. It is important to research and create advance medical directives before an accident or illness. Living wills have become customary in many parts of the country and are broadly respected by health care providers. However, most Americans do not have a living will or a medical power of attorney to ensure its compliance.

Description

The living will can be a very broad or a very focused document, according to the wishes of the patient. It is the patient's declaration, a written statement of what he or she wants to occur in the event of a serious accident or illness. It is primarily directed to medical personnel about the type of care the patient wishes to receive or not receive, in situations of terminal illness or incapacitation.

The document commonly includes medical procedures that are usually administered to patients who are seriously ill, such as:

- blood or plasma transfusion
- cardiopulmonary resuscitation (CPR)
- dialysis
- administration of drugs
- use of a respirator
- surgery
- tissue and organ donation

The living will declaration can also include issues of pain medication, food, and water. Most states recognize that relief from pain and discomfort are procedures that most people wish to have and these are not considered life-prolonging treatments. In some states, however, food and water may be considered life prolonging, and the consideration to forego them may fall within the rights of the patient to refuse. What may be included in the living will depends upon the state.

The living will—in some states called instructions, directive to physicians, or declaration—does not require a surrogate (an appointed person) to make decisions for the patient. Most states include these types of instructions in their medical durable power of attorney forms. Not all states, however, recognize separate living wills as legally binding; California, for instance, does not.

Preparation

The living will should be given careful thought, and be talked about with patient's family, physician, and care providers. It is highly recommended that discussion of patient wishes occur before medical treatment is necessary, because the living will involves the patient's family and loved ones, who are expected to assist in its implementation. It should be researched for the state in which the patient is most likely to receive medical care, and be dated and signed before two witnesses.

The living will may be drafted on standardized forms, with or without the assistance of an attorney. The document may be revoked in writing, or orally, by either the patient (the person making the advance directive) or by a designated proxy (a surrogate) at any time. If the patient does not specify in the living will a particular element of treatment or treatment withdrawal, then it is not included. It is important that living wills be as specific and detailed as possible.

Most hospitals offer advance medical directive resources, commonly in the religious office attached to the hospital. Coupled with a durable medical power of attorney, the living will ensures in advance that patient wishes about the quality of **death** are respected.

Normal results

The living will, whether prepared prior to hospitalization or prepared once the patient is admitted, is placed in the patient's medical chart along with other documents such as the medical power of attorney declaration. Providers are required by federal law to honor this declaration of the patient's wishes. The document serves as a statement of intentions on the part of the patient and can be very important to family members, healthcare providers, and patient proxy during a very distressful and uncertain time.

Resources

BOOKS

Burnell, George M. *Freedom to Choose: How to Make End-of-Life Decisions on Your Own Terms.* Amityville, NY: Baywood Publishing, 2007.

Mirarchi, Ferdinando. *Understanding Your Living Will: What You Need to Know Before a Medical Emergency.* Omaha, NE: Addicus Books, 2006.

Schneiderman, L. J. *Embracing Our Mortality: Medical Choices in an Age of Miracles* New York: Oxford University Press, 2008.

ORGANIZATIONS

Caring Connections. 1700 Diagonal Road, Suite 625, Alexandria, Virginia 22314. (703) 837-1500. Fax: (703) 837-1233. Toll-free hotline: (800) 658-8898. http://www.caringinfo.org/ (accessed April 1, 2008).

U.S. Living Will Registry. 523 Westfield Ave., P.O. Box 2789, Westfield, NJ 07091-2789. Toll-free: (800) LIV-WILL or (800) 548-9455. http://www.uslivingwillregistry.com/ (accessed April 1, 2008).

OTHER

Advance Directives, Living Wills, Powers of Attorney: What's the Difference?. Nolo Law for All. http://www.nolo.com/resource.cfm/catID/EDC82D5A-7723-4A77-9E10DDB947D1F801/309/292/295/ (accessed April 1, 2008).

Living Wills and Other Advance Directives. http://www.intelihealth.com/IH/ihtIH?d = dmtContent&c = 227472&p = ~br,IHW|~st,24479|~r,WSIHW000|~b,*| (accessed April 1, 2008).

Nancy McKenzie, PhD
Robert Bockstiegel

Lobectomy, hepatic *see* **Hepatectomy**

▌Lobectomy, pulmonary

Definition

A lobectomy is the removal of a lobe, or section, of the lung.

Purpose

Lobectomies are performed to prevent the spread of cancer to other parts of the lung or other parts of the body, as well as to treat patients with such noncancerous diseases as chronic obstructive pulmonary disease

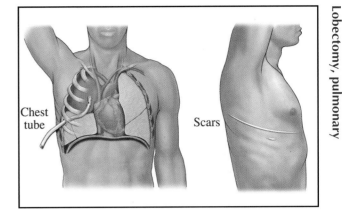

A post-operative lobectomy. *(Nucleus Medical Art, Inc. / Alamy)*

(COPD). COPD includes emphysema and chronic bronchitis, which cause airway obstruction.

Demographics

Lung cancer

Lung cancer is the leading cause of cancer-related deaths in the United States. About 213,380 patients were newly diagnosed with lung cancer in 2007 (about 114,760 in men and 98,620 in women). It is expected to claim nearly 160,390 lives in 2007 (89,510 in men and 70,880 in women). Lung cancer kills more people than cancers of the breast, prostate, colon, and pancreas combined. Cigarette smoking accounts for nearly 90% of cases of lung cancer in the United States.

Lung cancer is the second most common cancer among both men and women and is the leading cause of **death** from cancer in both sexes. In addition to the use of tobacco as a major cause of lung cancer among smokers, second-hand smoke contributes to the development of lung cancer among nonsmokers. Exposure to asbestos and other hazardous substances is also known to cause lung cancer. Air pollution is also a probable cause, but makes a relatively small contribution to incidence and mortality rates. Indoor exposure to radon may also make a small contribution to the total incidence of lung cancer in certain geographic areas of the United States.

In each of the major racial/ethnic groups in the United States, the rates of lung cancer among men are about two to three times greater than the rates among women. Among men, age-adjusted lung cancer incidence rates (per 100,000) range from a low of about 14 among Native Americans to a high of 117 among African Americans, an eight-fold difference. For women, the rates range from approximately 15

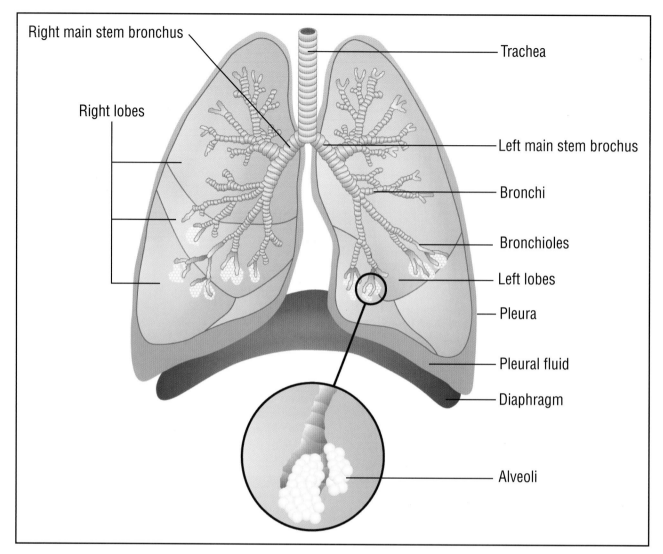

Right main stem bronchus

Right lobes

Trachea

Left main stem brochus

Bronchi

Bronchioles

Left lobes

Pleura

Pleural fluid

Diaphragm

Alveoli

(Cengage Learning, Gale.)

per 100,000 among Japanese Americans to nearly 51 among Native Alaskans, only a three-fold difference.

Chronic obstructive pulmonary disease

The following are risk factors for COPD:

- current smoking or a long-term history of heavy smoking

- employment that requires working around dust and irritating fumes

- long-term exposure to second-hand smoke at home or in the workplace

- a productive cough (with phlegm or sputum) most of the time

- shortness of breath during vigorous activity

- shortness of breath that grows worse even at lower levels of activity

- a family history of early COPD (before age 45)

Description

Lobectomies of the lung are also called pulmonary lobectomies. The lungs are a pair of cone-shaped breathing organs within the chest. The function of the lungs is to draw oxygen into the body and release carbon dioxide, which is a waste product of the body's cells. The right lung has three lobes: a superior lobe, a middle lobe, and an inferior lobe. The left lung has only two, a superior and an inferior lobe. Some lobes exchange more oxygen than others. The lungs are covered by a thin membrane called the pleura. The bronchi are two tubes which lead from the trachea

KEY TERMS

Bronchodilator—A drug that relaxes the bronchial muscles, resulting in expansion of the bronchial air passages.

Corticosteroids—Any of various adrenal-cortex steroids used as anti-inflammatory agents.

Emphysema—A chronic disease characterized by loss of elasticity and abnormal accumulation of air in lung tissue.

Mycobacterium—Any of a genus of nonmotile, aerobic, acid-fast bacteria that include numerous saprophytes and the pathogens causing tuberculosis and leprosy.

Perfusion scan—A lung scan in which a tracer is injected into a vein in the arm. It travels through the bloodstream and into the lungs to show areas of the lungs that are not receiving enough air or that retain too much air.

Pulmonary rehabilitation—A program to treat COPD, which generally includes education and counseling, exercise, nutritional guidance, techniques to improve breathing, and emotional support.

Ventilation scan—A lung scan in which a tracer gas is inhaled into the lungs to show the quantity of air that different areas of the lungs are receiving.

V/Q scan—A test in which both a perfusion scan and ventilation scan are done (separately or together) to show the quantity of air that different areas of the lungs are receiving.

(windpipe) to the right and left lungs. Inside the lungs are tiny air sacs called alveoli and small tubes called bronchioles. Lung cancer sometimes involves the bronchi.

To perform a lobectomy, the surgeon makes an incision (**thoracotomy**) between the ribs to expose the lung while the patient is under **general anesthesia**. The chest cavity is examined and the diseased lung tissue is removed. A drainage tube (chest tube) is then inserted to drain air, fluid, and blood out of the chest cavity. The ribs and chest incision are then closed.

A newer, minimally invasive lobectomy technique is called video-assisted thorascopic surgery (or VATS). This technique involves the use of three tiny incisions and micro-surgery tools, along with a scope. Thus far, research suggests that this technique offers many of the advantages of the classic technique, with fewer complications and a quicker recovery time. VATS, however, is

still only practiced at certain select centers, where surgeons have been specially trained in the relatively new method.

Lung surgery may be recommended for the following reasons:

- presence of tumors
- small areas of long-term infection (such as highly localized pulmonary tuberculosis or mycobacterial infection)
- lung cancer
- abscesses
- permanently enlarged (dilated) airways (bronchiectasis)
- permanently dilated section of lung (lobar emphysema)
- injuries associated with lung collapse (atelectasis, pneumothorax, or hemothorax)
- a permanently collapsed lung (atelectasis)

Diagnosis/Preparation

Diagnosis

In some cases, the diagnosis of a lung disorder is made when the patient consults a physician about chest pains or other symptoms. The symptoms of lung cancer vary somewhat according to the location of the tumor; they may include persistent coughing, coughing up blood, wheezing, fever, and weight loss. Patients with a lung abscess often have symptoms resembling those of pneumonia, including a high fever, loss of appetite, general weakness, and putrid sputum. The doctor will first take a careful history and listen to the patient's breathing with a **stethoscope**. Imaging studies include x-ray studies of the chest and **CT scans**. If lung cancer is suspected, the doctor will obtain a tissue sample for a biopsy. If a lung abscess is suspected, the doctor will send a sample of the sputum to a laboratory for culture and analysis.

For patients with lungs that have been damaged by emphysema or chronic bronchitis, pulmonary function tests are conducted prior to surgery to determine whether the patient will have enough healthy lung tissue remaining after surgery. A test may be used before surgery to help determine how much of the lung can safely be removed. This test is called a quantitative ventilation/perfusion scan, or a quantitative V/Q scan.

Preparation

Patients should not take **aspirin** or ibuprofen for seven to 10 days before surgery. Patients should also consult their physician about discontinuing any blood-thinning medications such as Coumadin (warfarin).

The night before surgery, patients should not eat or drink anything after midnight.

Aftercare

If no complications arise, the patient is transferred from the surgical **intensive care unit** (ICU) to a regular hospital room within one to two days. Patients may need to be hospitalized for seven to 10 days after a lobectomy. A tube in the chest to drain fluid will probably be required, as well as a mechanical ventilator to help the patient breathe. The chest tube normally remains in place until the lung has fully re-expanded. Oxygen may also be required, either on a temporary or permanent basis. A respiratory therapist will visit the patient to teach him or her deep breathing exercises. It is important for the patient to perform these exercises in order to re-expand the lung and lower the risk of pneumonia or other infections. The patient will be given medications to control postoperative pain. The typical recovery period for a lobectomy is one to three months following surgery.

Risks

The specific risks of a lobectomy vary depending on the specific reason for the procedure and the general state of the patient's health; they should be discussed with the surgeon. In general, the risks for any surgery requiring a general anesthetic include reactions to medications and breathing problems. As previously mentioned, patients having part of a lung removed may have difficulty breathing and may require the use of oxygen. Excessive bleeding, wound infections, and pneumonia are possible complications of a lobectomy. The chest will hurt for some time after surgery, as the surgeon must cut through the patient's ribs to expose the lung. Patients with COPD may experience shortness of breath after surgery.

Normal results

The outcome of lobectomies depends on the general condition of the patient's lung. This variability is related to the fact that lung tissue does not regenerate after it is removed. Therefore, removal of a large portion of the lung may require a person to need oxygen or ventilator support for the rest of his or her life. On the other hand, removal of only a small portion of the lung may result in very little change to the patient's quality of life.

QUESTIONS TO ASK THE DOCTOR

Lobectomies are performed in a hospital by a thoracic surgeon, who is a physician who specializes in chest, heart, and lung surgery. Thoracic surgeons may further specialize in one area, such as heart surgery or lung surgery. They are board-certified through the Board of Thoracic Surgery, which is recognized by the American Board of Medical Specialties. A doctor becomes board certified by completing training in a specialty area and passing a rigorous examination.

Morbidity and mortality rates

A small percentage of patients undergoing lung lobectomy die during or soon after the surgery. This percentage varies from about 3–6% depending on the amount of lung tissue removed. Of cancer patients with completely removable stage-1 non-small cell cancer of the lung (a disease in which malignant cancer cells form in the tissues of the lung), 50% survive five years after the procedure.

Alternatives

Lung cancer

The treatment options for lung cancer are surgery, radiation therapy, and chemotherapy, either alone or in combination, depending on the stage of the cancer.

After the cancer is found and staged, the cancer care team discusses the treatment options with the patient. In choosing a treatment plan, the most significant factors to consider are the type of lung cancer (small cell or non-small cell) and the stage of the cancer. It is very important that the doctor order all the tests needed to determine the stage of the cancer. Other factors to consider include the patient's overall physical health; the likely side effects of the treatment; and the probability of curing the disease, extending the patient's life, or relieving his or her symptoms.

Chronic obstructive pulmonary disease

Although surgery is rarely used to treat COPD, it may be considered for people who have severe symptoms that have not improved with medication therapy. A significant number of patients with advanced COPD face a miserable existence and are at high risk of death, despite advances in medical technology. This

QUESTIONS TO ASK THE DOCTOR

- What benefits can I expect from a lobectomy?
- What are the risks of this operation?
- What are the normal results?
- How long will my recovery take?
- Are there any alternatives to this surgery?

group includes patients who remain symptomatic despite the following:

- smoking cessation
- use of inhaled bronchodilators
- treatment with antibiotics for acute bacterial infections, and inhaled or oral corticosteroids
- use of supplemental oxygen with rest or exertion
- pulmonary rehabilitation

After the severity of the patient's airflow obstruction has been evaluated, and the foregoing interventions implemented, a pulmonary disease specialist should examine him or her, with consideration given to surgical treatment.

Surgical options for treating COPD include laser therapy or the following procedures:

- Bullectomy. This procedure removes the part of the lung that has been damaged by the formation of large air-filled sacs called bullae.

- Lung volume reduction surgery. In this procedure, the surgeon removes a portion of one or both lungs, making room for the remaining lung tissue to work more efficiently. Its use is considered experimental, although it has been used in selected patients with severe emphysema.

- Lung transplant. In this procedure a healthy lung from a donor who has recently died is given to a person with COPD.

Resources

BOOKS

Abeloff, MD et al. Clinical Oncology. 3rd ed. Philadelphia: Elsevier, 2004.

Mason, RJ et al. Murray & Nadel's Textbook of Respiratory Medicine. 4th ed. Philadelphia: Saunders, 2007.

Tierney, Lawrence M., Stephen J. McPhee, and Maxine A. Papadakis, eds. Current Medical Diagnosis & Treatment 2003, 42nd ed. New York, NY: McGraw-Hill/Appleton & Lange, 2002.

PERIODICALS

Grann, Victor R., and Alfred I. Neugut. "Lung Cancer Screening at Any Price?" Journal of the American Medical Association289 (2003): 357-358.

Mahadevia, Parthiv J., Lee A. Fleisher, Kevin D. Frick, et al. "Lung Cancer Screening with Helical Computed Tomography in Older Adult Smokers: A Decision and Cost-Effectiveness Analysis." Journal of the American Medical Association 289 (2003): 313-322.

Pope III, C. Arden, Richard T. Burnett, Michael J. Thun, et al. "Lung Cancer, Cardiopulmonary Mortality, and Long-Term Exposure to Fine Particulate Air pollution." Journal of the American Medical Association 287 (2002): 1132-1141.

ORGANIZATIONS

American Cancer Society. 1599 Clifton Road, N.E., Atlanta, GA 30329-4251. (800) 227-2345. www.cancer.org.

American Lung Association, National Office. 1740 Broadway, New York, NY 10019. (800) LUNG-USA. www.lungusa.org.

National Cancer Institute (NCI), Building 31, Room 10A03, 31 Center Drive, Bethesda, MD 20892-2580. Phone: (800) 4-CANCER. (301) 435-3848. www.nci.nih.gov.

National Comprehensive Cancer Network. 50 Huntingdon Pike, Suite 200, Rockledge, PA 19046. (215) 728-4788. Fax: (215) 728-3877. www.nccn.org/.

National Heart, Lung and Blood Institute (NHLBI). 6701 Rockledge Drive, P.O. Box 30105, Bethesda, MD 20824-0105. (301) 592-8573. www.nhlhi.nih.gov/.

OTHER

Aetna InteliHealth Inc. Lung Cancer. [cited May 17, 2003]. www.intelihealth.com..

American Cancer Society (ACS). Cancer Reference Information. [cited March 31, 2008]. http://www.cancer.org/docroot/cri/cri_0.asp.

Michael Zuck, Ph.D.
Crystal H. Kaczkowski, M.Sc.
Rosalyn Carson-DeWitt, MD

Local anesthesia *see* **Anesthesia, local**

Long-term care insurance

Definition

Long-term care (LTC) insurance provides for a person's care in cases of chronic illness or disability. Policies for LTC provide insurance coverage for times when an individual cannot independently manage the essential activities of daily living (ADLs). These are universally known as feeding, dressing, bathing, toileting, and walking, as well as moving oneself from a bed to a chair (transferring). However, disabilities are not confined to these physical situations; they can be mental as well. The key element is that they limit the individual's ability to perform any of these functions.

Purpose

The purpose of LTC insurance is to provide coverage for a succession of caregiving services for the elderly, the chronically ill, the disabled, or the seriously injured. This care may be provided in a skilled nursing facility (SNF); a nursing home; a mental hospital; in a person's home with a registered nurse (RN); a licensed practical nurse (LPN) or nurse's aide; or even in an assisted living facility (ALF). It is important to note the societal changes responsible for the increased need for professional services to care for our loved ones. Although today's families are smaller and a number of women are working outside the home, the majority of LTC continues to be provided by unpaid, informal caregivers—family members and friends.

In 2003, more than 24 million households in the United States included a caregiver who was 50 years of age or older. Approximately three in four unpaid caregivers were women—and one-third of them are more than 65 years old. Many caregivers, especially women, balance multiple roles by providing care for both their parents and their children. Caring for a loved one full-time can overwhelm even the most devoted family member. As a result, more caregivers than ever are turning to outside resources to help with the care of a family member.

Demographics

In 2030, it is anticipated that people aged 65 and over will comprise 20% of the population. The United States Census Bureau is projecting that the population aged 65 and over will be 39.7 million in 2010, 53.7 million in 2020, and 70.3 million in 2030. As of 2003, at least 6.4 million people aged 65 and over require LTC; one in two people over the age of 85 require this kind of care now, and at least half of the population who are over the age of 85 will need help with ADLs.

Although the elderly rely on LTC most frequently, younger persons who have chronic illnesses, severe disabilities, or have experienced a serious injury may also benefit from having LTC insurance.

Advantages to purchasing LTC insurance

The financial risks of illness and injury are rarely considered when one is healthy and able, but that is also when the greatest choice of products with the best flexibility in cost is available for those considering LTC insurance. Having a LTC insurance policy

KEY TERMS

Chronic illness—A condition that lasts a year or longer, limits activity, and may require ongoing care.

Estate planning—Preparation of a plan of administration and disposition of one's property before or after death, including will, trusts, gifts, and power of attorney.

Indemnity—Protection, as by insurance, against damage or loss.

Long-term care (LTC)—The type of care one may need if one can no longer perform activities of daily living (ADLs) alone, such as eating, bathing or getting dressed. It also includes the kind of care one would need with a severe cognitive impairment, such as Alzheimer's disease. Care can be received in a variety of settings, including the home, assisted living facilities, adult day care centers, or hospice facilities.

Medicaid—Public assistance funded through the state to individuals unable to pay for health care. Medicaid can be accessed only when all prior assets and funds are depleted.

Medicare—A government program, administered by the Social Security Administration, which provides financial assistance to individuals over the age of 65 for hospital and medical expenses. Medicare does not cover long-term care expenses.

Skilled nursing facility (SNF)—A facility equipped to handle individuals with 24-hour nursing needs, postoperative recuperation, or complex medical care demands, as well as chronically-ill individuals who can no longer live independently. These facilities must be licensed by the state in which they operate to meet standards of safety, staffing, and care procedures.

enables access to quality care and choice of care provider when the need is greatest. Purchasing a policy when a person does not need it gives them the opportunity to investigate the company's financial stability (whether it is solid and how it is rated), operating performance, insurance industry rating, and its claims ratio. Rates should be guaranteed renewable; and coverage should not be canceled because of age or a change in a person's health; nor should premiums be increased on a class-wide basis.

There are several government organizations that can be of assistance in the purchase, evaluation, and monitoring of LTC insurance. One is the state health insurance assistance program—SHIP—that can review the policy before the actual purchase. Another excellent organization is the Health Insurance Association of America (HIAA), which protects consumers from the financial risks of injury and illness by providing affordable and flexible services that represent a choice. In the United States, HIAA focuses on managed care, and, specifically, advocates on issues such as disability income and LTC insurance.

The mission of the Health Insurance Association of America is to preserve financial security, freedom of choice, and dignity in LTC insurance. Because of its mission, HIAA seeks to:

- provide access to quality care and let a person choose where care is obtained
- eliminate out-of-pocket costs and avoid reliance on government programs for the poor
- ensure quality of life for a patient's caregivers

Description

Advantages

Having a LTC insurance policy cuts out-of-pocket costs and keeps the patient from having to rely on government assistance programs. Studies from the United States Department of Health and Human Services estimate that people with LTC insurance save between $60,000 and $75,000 in nursing home costs, more than $100,000 for assisted living, and actually ensure a higher quality of life for their caregiver. By having LTC at home, spouses and other family members are able to continue working or run errands while their loved one is being care for.

People of all ages usually prefer to receive LTC in their own homes, or in homelike assisted-living facilities. More than three-quarters of older Americans in need of LTC live in their communities. Most receive no paid services. The majority of LTC is provided by unpaid, informal caregivers, such as family members and friends.

Government assistance

Long-term care options can be uncoordinated and expensive for individuals, their families, and public programs. According to AARP (formerly known as American Association of Retired Persons) millions of Americans have no access to LTC services. They are caught in the trap of having too much money to qualify for government assistance, but not enough money to afford the types of services they need.

Recent changes in the United States federal tax law allow for a portion of a long-term insurance premium to be tax-deductible. The amount of the deduction increases with the insured person's age.

Medicare may cover a month or two of home health care after a stay in the hospital, but benefits are then usually capped. This government program, administered by the Social Security Administration, is well known for providing financial assistance to seniors 65 years of age and older and to the disabled—for medical and hospital expenses—but it does not cover LTC expenses. Medicare Supplement Insurance does not cover LTC either.

The federal/state **Medicaid** program is available, but the criteria to qualify for assistance is strict. Those who meet the guidelines for Medicaid must demonstrate financial need to receive assistance; most individuals must deplete most or all of their savings and assets before becoming eligible for any benefits. In 2006, approximately two-thirds of nursing home residents were dependent on Medicaid to finance at least some of their care. For the majority of residents, LTC insurance is cost-prohibitive. To make matters worse, preexisting conditions often prevent them from obtaining coverage for which they might qualify.

Personal policies

Long-term care insurance policies are often complex. People who purchase them may not read the fine print and are later forced to cancel their policies because they do not fit their needs. Increasing rates factored into some long-term policies, known as climbing premiums, may also become prohibitively expensive. However, long-term care insurance can benefit consumers, provided that such items as affordability, coverage gaps, and timing of purchase are carefully considered.

It is advisable to check the financial stability and the claims ratio of an insurance company. Long-term insurance is a serious financial investment and should be considered a part of estate planning. A qualified, independent professional should be consulted to review the policy before purchase. The state health insurance assistance program (SHIP) is also available to answer questions.

The type of care that an individual seeks or requires is an important consideration before purchasing a policy. Currently, there is no universal standard for defining long-term care facilities. A placement that is covered under one company's policy may not be covered by another. Physicians can also play a part in denial of a placement by stating that the facility of choice is either not adequate or too advanced for an individual's needs.

When to purchase a policy is another important consideration. Individuals with a preexisting diagnosis for a debilitating condition or illness may not be eligible for coverage. This clause is common in most insurance policies of any type. However, purchasing a policy too far in advance of an anticipated need can work against a buyer. The health care industry is currently in a state of flux, and technological advances are rapid. The benefits provided in a policy that is purchased at one point in time may not match the care available in the distant future, giving the company reason to deny benefits.

Generally, LTC insurance operates as an indemnity program for potential nursing home and home health care costs. Additionally, many policies provide coverage for adult daycare, for care delivered in an assisted living facility, and for **hospice** care. Rarely are all costs covered. Some LTC policies are pure indemnity programs, which pay the insured a daily benefit contracted for by the insured. The pure indemnity program pays the full daily benefit regardless of the amount of care that the insured receives each day.

Other LTC policies pay for covered losses, or the cost of care actually received each day, up to the selected daily benefit level. This type of policy is referred to as a pool-of-money contract.

Insurance for LTC is available either as part of a group or as individual coverage, although most policies are currently purchased by individuals. Most policies cover skilled, custodial, and intermediate LTC services. A purchaser would be wise to consider a contract that covers all of these levels.

Benefits under a LTC contract are triggered in a tax-qualified policy when an insured person becomes unable to perform a number of activities associated with normal daily living or develops a cognitive impairment that requires supervision. Non–tax-qualified policies usually offer more liberal eligibility criteria. This includes long-term benefits required due to medical necessity.

Risks

Long-term care insurance policies can be expensive and may be restrictive in what they provide. Before purchasing the policy, persons should be certain that the cost is within their means and that the plan will meet their anticipated needs. Some policies allow policy holders to use survivor **death** benefits for health care needs. It is advisable for several different policies to be compared in detail. Policies that seem

---

QUESTIONS TO ASK BEFORE PURCHASING LTC INSURANCE

- Will the policy meet my needs?
- Is the policy affordable?
- What restrictions or exemptions exist?
- Under what conditions, if any, can this plan be canceled?
- Are there any laws to protect me from insurance companies or LTC facilities that provide substandard conditions and/or services?

---

too inexpensive when compared against the competition should be carefully evaluated. There may be hidden clauses in the contracts that limit coverage.

Organizations that can help consumers

The Health Insurance Association of America (HIAA) protects consumers from the financial risks of illness and injury by providing flexible and affordable products and services that embody freedom of choice, and advocates on a number of issues—including LTC insurance.

The United States Department of Health and Human Services oversees the Administration on Aging's Ombudsmen Program. Established in 1972 by the Older Americans Act, the Program operates throughout the country on behalf of aging residents. Its purpose is to investigate over 260,000 complaints annually regarding various topics, including selection and payment of LTC insurance policies. The ombudsmen advocate for residents of **nursing homes**, LTC homes, assisted living facilities, and similar adult care facilities; they have made dramatic differences in the lives of LTC residents. On behalf of individuals and groups of residents, they provide information to residents and their families about the LTC system and work to improve local, state and national level programs. Ombudsmen also provide an ongoing presence in LTC facilities, monitoring care and conditions and providing a voice for those who are unable to speak for themselves.

Resources

BOOKS

Matthews, J. *Long-Term Care: How to Plan and Pay for It.* 6th ed. Berkeley CA: NOLO, 2006.

Shelton, P. *Long-Term Care: Your Financial Planning Guide.* 4th ed. Richmond, VA: LTCi Publishing, 2007.

Truesdell, C. *Dignity for Life: Five Things You should Know Before Considering Long Term Care Insurance.* 4th ed. Kirkland, WA: LTC Financial Partners, 2007.

PERIODICALS

Kapp, M. B. "Medicaid planning, estate recovery, and alternatives for long-term care financing: identifying the ethical issues." *Care Management Journal* 7, no. 2 (2007): 73–78.

Prazich, M. N. "Long-term care insurance 101." *Northwest Dentistry* 86, no. 4 (2007): 31–34.

Quinn, J. B. "Insuring your future care." *Newsweek* 149, no. 25 (2007): 66–67.

Thomalla, K. C. "Should I purchase long-term care insurance?" *CDS Review* 100, no. 5 (2007): 16–20.

ORGANIZATIONS

AARP. 601 E. Street NW, Washington, DC 20049. (888) 687-2277. http://www.aarp.org.

American College of Healthcare Executives. One North Franklin, Suite 1700, Chicago, IL 60606-4425. (312) 424-2800. http://www.ache.org.

American Medical Association. 515 N. State Street, Chicago, IL 60610. (312) 464-5000. http://www.ama-assn.org.

Health Insurance Association of America. 601 Pennsylvania Avenue, NW, South Building, Washington, DC 20004-1204. (202) 778-3200. http://www.hiaa.org.

U.S. Administration on Aging (AOA), United States Department of Health and Human Services. 330 Independence Avenue, SW, Washington, DC 20201. (202) 619-0724. http://www.aoa.gov.

United States Department of Health and Human Services, 200 Independence Avenue, SW, Washington, DC 20201. (877) 696-6775. http://www.hhs.gov.

OTHER

American Health Care Association, National Center for Assisted Living. *Information about Long-term Care Insurance.* 2007 [cited December 26, 2007]. http://www.longtermcareliving.com.

The Federal Long Term Care Insurance Program. *Information about Long-term Care Insurance.* 2007 [cited December 26, 2007]. http://www.ltcfeds.com.

United Seniors Health. *Information about Long-term Care Insurance.* 2007 [cited December 26, 2007]. http://www.unitedseniorshealth.org.

American Association for Long-Term Care Insurance. *Information about Long-term Care Insurance.* 2007 [cited December 26, 2007]. http://www.aaltci.org/.

L. Fleming Fallon, Jr., MD, DrPH

Lower GI exam *see* **Barium enema**

LTC insurance *see* **Long-term care insurance**

Lumbar laminectomy *see* **Laminectomy**

Lumbar puncture *see* **Cerebrospinal fluid (CSF) analysis**

Lumpectomy

Definition

Lumpectomy is a type of surgery for breast cancer. It is considered "breast-conserving" surgery because only the malignant tumor and a surrounding margin of normal breast tissue are removed. Lymph nodes in the armpit (axilla) may also be removed. This procedure is also called lymph node dissection.

Purpose

Lumpectomy is a surgical treatment for newly diagnosed breast cancer. It is estimated that at least 50% of women with breast cancer are good candidates for this procedure. The location, size, and type of tumor are of primary importance when considering breast cancer surgery options. The size of the breast is another factor the surgeon considers when recommending surgery. The patient's psychological outlook, as well as her lifestyle and preferences, should also be taken into account when treatment decisions are being made.

The extent and severity of a cancer is evaluated, or "staged," according to a fairly complex system. Staging considers the size of the tumor and whether the cancer has spread (metastasized) to adjacent tissues, such as the chest wall, the lymph nodes, and/or to distant parts of the body. Women with early stage breast cancers are usually better candidates for lumpectomy. In most cases, a course of radiation therapy after surgery is part of the treatment. Chemotherapy or hormone treatment may also be prescribed.

In some instances, women with later stage breast cancer may be able to have lumpectomies. Chemotherapy may be administered before surgery to decrease tumor size and the chance of metastasis in selected cases.

Contraindications to lumpectomy

There are a number of factors that may prevent or prohibit a breast cancer patient from having a lumpectomy. The tumor itself may be too large or located in an area where it would be difficult to remove with good cosmetic results. Sometimes several areas of cancer are found in one breast, so the tumor cannot be removed as a single lump. A cancer that has already attached itself to nearby structures, such as the skin or the chest wall, needs more extensive surgery.

Certain medical or physical circumstances may also eliminate lumpectomy as a treatment option. Sometimes lumpectomy may be attempted, but the surgeon is unable to remove the tumor with a sufficient amount of surrounding normal tissue. This may

Lumpectomy

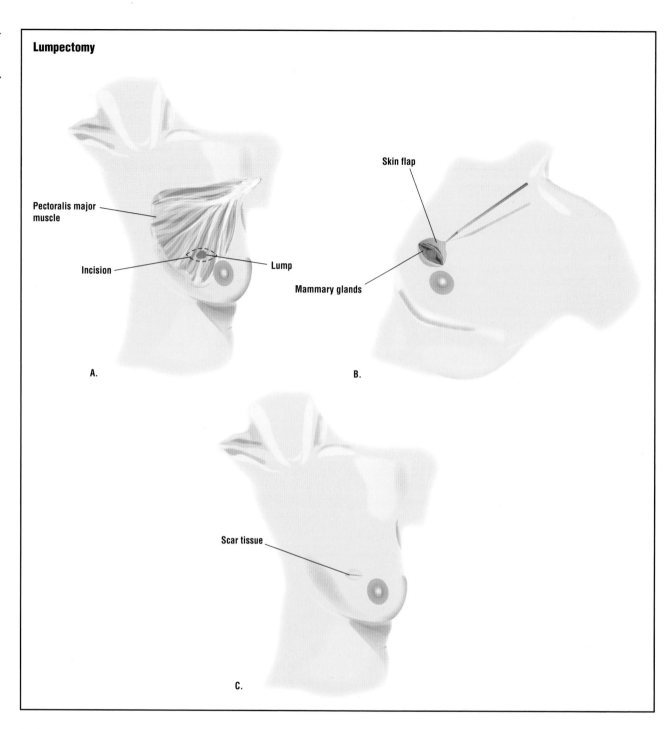

During a lumpectomy, a small incision is made around the area of the lump (A). The skin is pulled back, and the tumor removed (B). The incision is closed (C). *(Illustration by GGS Information Services. Cengage Learning, Gale.)*

be termed "persistently positive margins," or "lack of clear margins." Lumpectomy is suitable for women who have had previous lumpectomies and have a recurrence of breast cancer.

Because of the need for radiation therapy after lumpectomy, this surgery may be medically unacceptable. A breast cancer discovered during pregnancy is not amenable to lumpectomy because radiation therapy is part of the treatment. Radiation therapy cannot be administered to pregnant women because it may injure the fetus. If, however, delivery would be completed prior to the need for radiation, pregnant women may undergo lumpectomy. A woman who has already had therapeutic

KEY TERMS

Axillary lymph node—Lymph nodes under the arm.

Lymph node—A small mass of tissue in the form of a knot or protuberance. They are the primary source of lymph fluid, which serves in the body's defense by removing toxic fluids and bacteria.

Quadrantectomy—Removal of a quadrant, or about a quarter of the breast.

radiation to the chest area for other reasons cannot undergo additional exposure for breast cancer therapy.

The need for radiation therapy may also be a barrier due to nonmedical concerns. Some women simply fear this type of treatment and choose more extensive surgery so that radiation will not be required. The commitment of time, usually five days a week for six weeks, may not be acceptable for others. This may be due to financial, personal, or job-related constraints. Finally, in geographically isolated areas, a course of radiation therapy may require lengthy travel and perhaps unacceptable amounts of time away from family and other responsibilities.

Demographics

The American Cancer Society estimated that in 2007, 240,510 new cases of breast cancer would be diagnosed in the United States and 40,460 women would die as a result of the disease. Approximately one in eight women will develop breast cancer at some point in her life. The risk of developing breast cancer increases with age: women aged 30 to 40 have a one in 252 chance of developing breast cancer; women aged 40 to 50 have a one in 68 chance; women aged 50 to 60 have a one in 35 chance; and women aged 60 to 70 have a one in 27 chance—and these statistics do not even account for genetic and environmental factors.

Description

Any amount of tissue, from 1–50% of the breast, may be removed and called a lumpectomy. Breast conservation surgery is a frequently used synonym for lumpectomy. Partial **mastectomy**, **quadrantectomy**, segmental excision, wide excision, and tylectomy are other, less commonly used names for this procedure.

The surgery is usually done while the patient is under general anesthetic. Local anesthetic with additional sedation may be used for some patients. The

tumor and surrounding margin of tissue is removed and sent to a pathologist for examination. The surgical site is then closed. Newer techniques may use **magnetic resonance imaging** guidance to more accurately identify the breast tissue to be removed. Additionally, laser instruments may be used to perform the actual lumpectomy.

If axillary lymph nodes were not removed before, a second incision may be made in the armpit. The fat pad that contains lymph nodes is removed from this area and is also sent to the pathologist for analysis. This portion of the procedure is called an axillary lymph node dissection; it is critical for determining the stage of the cancer. Typically, 10 to 15 nodes are removed, but the number may vary. A newer alternative to axillary lymph node dissection involves removal of only one lymph node. This technique, called sentinel node biopsy, samples just the first lymph node to which the breast tissue drains. If the sentinel node is negative, it is likely that no cancer has spread to more distant lymph nodes. If the sentinel node is positive, then the surgeon may have to proceed with an axillary lymph node dissection. Surgical drains may be left in place in either location to prevent fluid accumulation. The surgery may last from one to three hours.

Diagnosis/Preparation

Routine preoperative preparations, such as having nothing to eat or drink the night before surgery, are typically ordered for a lumpectomy. Information about expected outcomes and potential complications is also part of preparation for lumpectomy, as it is for any surgical procedure. It is especially important that women know about sensations they might experience after the operation, so the they are not misinterpreted as signs of further cancer or poor healing.

If the tumor is not able to be felt (not palpable), a pre-operative localization procedure is needed. A fine wire, or other device, is placed at the tumor site, using x ray or **ultrasound** for guidance. This is usually done in the radiology department of a hospital. The woman is most often sitting up and awake, although some sedation may be administered.

Aftercare

The patient may stay in the hospital one or two days, or return home the same day. This generally depends on the extent of the surgery, the medical condition of the patient, and physician and patient preferences. A woman usually goes home with a small bandage. The inner part of the surgical site usually

WHO PERFORMS THE
PROCEDURE AND WHERE IS IT
PERFORMED?

Lumpectomy is usually performed by a general surgeon or surgical oncologist. Radiation therapy is administered by a radiation oncologist, and chemotherapy by a medical oncologist. The procedure is frequently done in a hospital setting (especially if lymph nodes are to be removed at the same time), but specialized outpatient facilities are sometimes preferred.

has dissolvable **stitches**. The skin may be sutured or stitched; or the skin edges may be held together with steristrips, which are special thin, clear pieces of tape.

After a lumpectomy, patients are usually cautioned against lifting anything that weighs over five pounds for several days. Other activities may be restricted (especially if the axillary lymph nodes were removed) according to individual needs. Pain is often enough to limit inappropriate motion. Women are often instructed to wear a well-fitting support bra both day and night for approximately one week after surgery.

Pain is usually well controlled with prescribed medication. If it is not, the patient should contact the surgeon, as severe pain may be a sign of a complication, which needs medical attention. A return visit to the surgeon is normally scheduled approximately ten days to two weeks after the operation.

Radiation therapy is usually started as soon as possible after lumpectomy. Other additional treatments, such as chemotherapy or hormone therapy, may also be prescribed. The timing of these is specific to each individual patient.

Risks

The risks are similar to those associated with any surgical procedure. Risks include bleeding, infection, breast asymmetry, anesthesia reaction, or unexpected scarring. A lumpectomy may also cause loss of sensation in the breast. The size and shape of the breast will be affected by the operation. Fluid can accumulate in the area where tissue was removed, requiring drainage.

If lymph node dissection is performed, there are several potential complications. A woman may experience decreased feeling in the back of her armpit. She may also experience other sensations, including numbness, tingling, or increased skin sensitivity. An

QUESTIONS TO ASK THE
DOCTOR

- Why is a lumpectomy recommended?
- What method of anesthesia/pain relief will be used?
- Will radiation or chemotherapy be administered?
- Will a lymph node dissection be performed?
- Am I a candidate for sentinel node biopsy?

inflammation of the arm vein, called phlebitis, can occur. There may be injury to the nerves controlling arm motion.

There is a risk of developing lymphedema (swelling of the arm) after axillary lymph node dissection. This swelling can range from mild to very severe. It can be treated with elastic **bandages** and specialized physical therapy, but it is a chronic condition, requiring continuing care. Lymphedema can arise at any time, even years after surgery.

Normal results

When lumpectomy is performed, it is anticipated that it will be the definitive surgical treatment for breast cancer. Other forms of therapy, especially radiation, are often prescribed as part of the total treatment plan. The expected outcome is no recurrence of the breast cancer.

Morbidity and mortality rates

The outcome of breast cancer is very dependent of the stage at the time of diagnosis. For stage 0 disease, the five-year survival is almost 100%. For stage I (early/lymph node negative), the five-year survival is alsom almost 100%. For stage II (early/lymph node positive), the five-year survival decreases to 81-92%. For stage III disease (locally advanced), the five-year survival is 54-67%. For women with stage IV (metastatic) breast cancer, the five-year survival is about 20%.

Approximately 17% of patients develop lymphedema after axillary lymph node dissection, while only 3% of patients develop lymphedema after sentinel node biopsy. Five percent of women are unhappy with the cosmetic effects of the surgery.

Alternatives

A procedure in which the entire affected breast is removed, called a mastectomy, has been shown to be equally effective in treating breast cancer as lumpectomy, in terms of rates of recurrence and survival. Some women may choose to have a mastectomy because they strongly fear a recurrence of breast cancer, and may consider a lumpectomy too risky. Others may feel uncomfortable with a breast that has had a cancer, and would experience more peace of mind with the entire breast removed.

Resources

BOOKS

Abeloff, MD et al.Clinical Oncology. 3rd ed. Philadelphia: Elsevier, 2004.

Khatri, VP and JA Asensio. Operative Surgery Manual. 1st ed. Philadelphia: Saunders, 2003.

Townsend, CM et al. Sabiston Textbook of Surgery. 17th ed. Philadelphia: Saunders, 2004.

PERIODICALS

Apantaku, Leila. "Breast-Conserving Surgery for Breast Cancer." American Family Physician 66, no. 12 (December 15, 2002): 2271-8.

Dershaw, D. David. "Breast imaging and the conservative treatment of breast cancer." Radiologic Clinics of North America 40, no. 3 (May 2002): 501-16.

ORGANIZATIONS

American Cancer Society. 1599 Clifton Rd. NE, Atlanta, GA 30329-4251. (800) 227-2345. http://www.cancer.org.

National Cancer Institute (NCI). (800) 4-CANCER. <http://cancertrials.nci.nih.gov/types/breast/treatment/sentnode>.

National Lymphedema Network. 2211 Post St., Suite 404, San Francisco, CA 94115-3427. (800) 541-3259 or (415) 921-1306. http://www.wenet.net/~lymphnet.

Ellen S. Weber, MSN
Stephanie Dionne Sherk

Lung biopsy

Definition

Lung biopsy is a procedure for obtaining a small sample of lung tissue for examination. The tissue is usually examined under a microscope, and may be sent to a microbiological laboratory for culture. Microscopic examination is performed by a pathologist.

Purpose

A lung biopsy is usually performed to determine the cause of abnormalities, such as nodules that appear on chest x rays. It can confirm a diagnosis of cancer, especially if malignant cells are detected in the patient's sputum or bronchial washing. In addition to evaluating lung tumors and their associated symptoms, lung biopsies may be used to diagnose lung infections, especially tuberculosis and Pneumocystis pneumonia, drug reactions, and chronic diseases of the lungs such as sarcoidosis and pulmonary fibrosis.

A lung biopsy can be used for treatment as well as diagnosis. **Bronchoscopy**, a type of lung biopsy performed with a long, flexible slender instrument called a bronchoscope, can be used to clear a patient's air passages of secretions and to remove airway blockages.

Demographics

Lung cancer is the leading cause of cancer-related deaths in the United States. About 213,380 patients were newly diagnosed with lung cancer in 2007 (about 114,760 in men and 98,620 in women). It is expected to claim nearly 160,390 lives in 2007 (89,510 in men and 70,880 in women). Lung cancer kills more people than cancers of the breast, prostate, colon, and pancreas combined. Cigarette smoking accounts for nearly 90% of cases of lung cancer in the United States.

Description

Overview

The right and left lungs are separated by the mediastinum, which contains the heart, trachea, lymph nodes, and esophagus. Lung biopsies sometimes involve **mediastinoscopy**.

Types of lung biopsies

Lung biopsies are performed using a variety of techniques, depending on where the abnormal tissue is located in the lung, the health and age of the patient, and the presence of lung disease. A bronchoscopy is ordered if a lesion identified on the x ray seems to be located on the wall (periphery) of the chest. If the suspicious area lies close to the chest wall, a needle biopsy can be done. If both methods fail to diagnose the problem, an open lung biopsy may be performed. When there is a question about whether the lung cancer or suspicious mass has spread to the lymph nodes in the mediastinum, a mediastinoscopy is performed.

BRONCHOSCOPIC BIOPSY. During the bronchoscopy, a thin, lighted tube (bronchoscope) is passed from the nose or mouth, down the windpipe (trachea) to the air passages (bronchi) leading to the lungs. Through the bronchoscope, the physician views the airways, and is able to clear mucus from blocked airways, and collect cells or tissue samples for laboratory analysis.

KEY TERMS

Bronchoscopy—A medical test that enables the physician to see the breathing passages and the lungs through a hollow, lighted tube.

Chest x ray—Brief exposure of the chest to radiation to produce an image of the chest and its internal structures.

Endotracheal tube—A hollow tube that is inserted into the windpipe to administer anesthesia.

Lung nodule—See pulmonary nodule.

Lymph nodes—Small, bean-shaped structures that serve as filters, scattered along the lymphatic vessels. Lymph nodes trap bacteria or cancer cells that are traveling through the lymphatic system.

Malignant—Cancerous.

Mediastinoscopy—A procedure that allows the physician to see the organs in the mediastinal space using a thin, lighted, hollow tube (a mediastinoscope).

Mediastinum—The area between the lungs, bounded by the spine, breastbone, and diaphragm.

Pleural cavity—The space between the lungs and the chest wall.

Pneumothorax—A condition in which air or gas enters the pleura (area around the lungs) and causes a collapse of the lung.

Pulmonary nodule—A lesion surrounded by normal lung tissue. Nodules may be caused by bacteria, fungi, or a tumor (benign or cancerous).

Sputum—A mucus-rich secretion that is coughed up from the passageways (bronchial tubes) and the lungs.

Sputum cytology—A lab test in which a microscope is used to check for cancer cells in the sputum.

Thoracentesis—Removal of fluid from the pleural cavity.

NEEDLE BIOPSY. The patient is mildly sedated, but awake during the needle biopsy procedure. He or she sits in a chair with arms folded in front on a table. An x-ray technician uses a computerized axial tomography (CAT) scanner or a fluoroscope to identify the precise location of the suspicious areas. Markers are placed on the overlying skin to identify the biopsy site. The skin is thoroughly cleansed with an antiseptic solution, and a local anesthetic is injected to numb the area. The patient will feel a brief stinging sensation when the anesthetic is injected.

The physician makes a small incision, about half an inch (1.25 cm) in length. The patient is asked to take a deep breath and hold it while the physician inserts the biopsy needle through the incision into the lung tissue to be biopsied. The patient may feel pressure, and a brief sharp pain when the needle touches the lung tissue. Most patients do not experience severe pain. The patient should refrain from coughing during the procedure. The needle is withdrawn when enough tissue has been obtained. Pressure is applied at the biopsy site and a sterile bandage is placed over the incision. A **chest x ray** is performed immediately after the procedure to check for potential complications. The entire procedure takes 30–60 minutes.

OPEN BIOPSY. Open biopsies are performed in a hospital **operating room** under **general anesthesia**. Once the anesthesia has taken effect, the surgeon makes an incision over the lung area, a procedure called a **thoracotomy**. Some lung tissue is removed and the incision is closed with sutures. Chest tubes are placed with one end inside the lung and the other end protruding through the closed incision. Chest tubes are used to drain fluid and blood, and re-expand the lungs. They are usually removed the day after the procedure. The entire procedure normally takes about an hour. A chest x ray is performed immediately after the procedure to check for potential complications.

VIDEO-ASSISTED THORACOSCOPIC SURGERY. A minimally-invasive technique, video-assisted thoracoscopic surgery (VATS) can be used to biopsy lung and mediastinal lesions. VATS may be performed on selected patients in place of open lung biopsy. While the patient is under general anesthetia, the surgeon makes several small incisions in the his or her chest wall. A thorascope, a thin, hollow, lighted tube with a tiny video camera mounted on it, is inserted through one of the small incisions. The other incisions allow the surgeon to insert special instruments to retrieve tissue for biopsy.

MEDIASTINOSCOPY. This procedure is performed under general anesthesia. A 2–3 inch (5–8 cm) incision is made at the base of the neck. A thin, hollow, lighted tube, called a mediastinoscope, is inserted through the incision into the space between the right and the left lungs. The surgeon removes any lymph nodes or tissues that look abnormal. The mediastinoscope is then removed, and the incision is sutured and bandaged. A mediastinoscopy takes about an hour.

Diagnosis/Preparation

Diagnosis

Before scheduling a lung biopsy, the physician performs a careful evaluation of the patient's medical history and symptoms, and performs a **physical examination**. Chest x rays and sputum cytology (examination of cells obtained from a deep-cough mucus sample) are other diagnostic tests that may be performed. An **electrocardiogram** (EKG) and laboratory tests may be performed before the procedure to check for blood clotting problems, anemia, and blood type, should a **transfusion** become necessary.

Preparation

During a preoperative appointment, usually scheduled within one to two weeks before the procedure, the patient receives information about what to expect during the procedure and the recovery period. During this appointment or just before the procedure, the patient usually meets with the physician (or physicians) performing the procedure (the pulmonologist, interventional radiologist, or thoracic surgeon).

A chest x ray or CAT scan of the chest is used to identify the area to be biopsied.

About an hour before the biopsy procedure, the patient receives a sedative. Medication may also be given to dry up airway secretions. General anesthesia is not used for this procedure.

For at least 12 hours before the open biopsy, VATS, or mediastinoscopy procedures, the patient should not eat or drink anything. Prior to these procedures, an intravenous line is placed in a vein in the patient's arm to deliver medications or fluids as necessary. A hollow tube, called an endotracheal tube, is passed through the patient's mouth into the airway leading to the lungs. Its purpose is to deliver the general anesthetic. The chest area is cleansed with an antiseptic solution. In the mediastinoscopy procedure, the neck is also cleansed to prepare for the incision.

Smoking cessation

Patients who will undergo surgical diagnostic and treatment procedures should be encouraged to stop smoking and stop using tobacco products. The patient needs to make the commitment to be a nonsmoker after the procedure. Patients able to stop smoking several weeks before surgical procedures have fewer postoperative complications. **Smoking cessation** programs are available in many communities. The patient should ask a health care provider for more information if he or she needs help with smoking cessation.

Informed consent

Informed consent is an educational process between health care providers and patients. Before any procedure is performed, the patient is asked to sign a consent form. Prior to signing the form, the patient should understand the nature and purpose of the diagnostic procedure or treatment, its risks and benefits, and alternatives, including the option of not proceeding with the test or treatment. During the discussions, the health care providers are available to answer the patient's questions about the consent form or procedure.

Aftercare

Needle biopsy

Following a needle biopsy, the patient is allowed to rest comfortably. He or she may be required to lie flat for two hours following the procedure to prevent the risk of bleeding. The nurse checks the patient's status at two-hour intervals. If there are no complications after four hours, the patient can go home once he or she has received instructions about resuming normal activities. The patient should rest at home for a day or two before returning to regular activities, and should avoid strenuous activities for one week after the biopsy.

Open biopsy, VATS, or mediastinoscopy

After an open biopsy, VATS, or mediastinoscopy, the patient is taken to the **recovery room** for observation. The patient receives oxygen via a face mask or nasal cannula. If no complications develop, the patient is taken to a hospital room. Temperature, blood oxygen level, pulse, blood pressure, and respiration are monitored. Chest tubes remain in place after surgery to prevent the lungs from collapsing, and to remove blood and fluids. The tubes are usually removed the day after the procedure.

The patient may experience some grogginess for a few hours after the procedure. He or she may have a sore throat from the endotracheal tube. The patient may also have some pain or discomfort at the incision site, which can be relieved by pain medication. It is common for patients to require some pain medication for up to two weeks following the procedure.

After receiving instructions about resuming normal activities and caring for the incision, the patient usually goes home the day after surgery. The patient should not drive while taking narcotic pain medication.

Patients may experience fatigue and muscle aches for a day or two because of the general anesthesia. The patient can gradually increase activities, as tolerated. Walking is recommended. Sutures are usually removed after one to two weeks.

The physician should be notified immediately if the patient experiences extreme pain, light-headedness, or difficulty breathing after the procedure. Sputum may be slightly bloody for a day or two after the procedure. Heavy or persistent bleeding requires evaluation by the physician.

Risks

Lung biopsies should not be performed on patients who have a bleeding disorder or abnormal blood clotting because of low platelet counts, or prolonged **prothrombin time** (PT) or **partial thromboplastin time** (PTT). Platelets are small blood cells that play a role in the blood clotting process. PT and PTT measure how well blood is clotting. If clotting times are prolonged, it may be unsafe to perform a biopsy because of the risk of bleeding. If the platelet count is lower than 50,000/cubic mm, the patient may be given a platelet transfusion as a temporary relief measure, and a biopsy can then be performed.

In addition, lung biopsies should not be performed if other tests indicate the patient has enlarged alveoli associated with emphysema, pulmonary hypertension, or enlargement of the right ventricle of the heart (cor pulmonale).

The normal risks of any surgical procedure include bleeding, infection, or pneumonia. The risk of these complications is higher in patients undergoing open biopsy procedures, as is the risk of pneumothorax (lung collapse). In rare cases, the lung collapses because of air that leaks in through the hole made by the biopsy needle. A chest x ray is done immediately after the biopsy to detect the development of this potential complication. If a pneumothorax occurs, a chest tube is inserted into the pleural cavity to re-expand the lung. Signs of pneumothorax include shortness of breath, rapid heart rate, or blueness of the skin (a late sign). If the patient has any of these symptoms after being discharged from the hospital, it is important to call the health care provider or emergency services immediately.

Bronchoscopic biopsy

Bronchoscopy is generally safe, and complications are rare. If they do occur, complications may include spasms of the bronchial tubes that can impair breathing, irregular heart rhythms, or infections such as pneumonia.

Needle biopsy

Needle biopsy is associated with fewer risks than open biopsy because it does not involve general anesthesia. Some hemoptysis (coughing up blood) occurs in 5% of needle biopsies. Prolonged bleeding or infection may also occur, although these are very rare complications.

Open biopsy

Possible complications of an open biopsy include infection or pneumothorax. If the patient has very severe breathing problems before the biopsy, breathing may be further impaired following the operation. Patients with normal lung function prior to the biopsy have a very small risk of respiratory problems resulting from or following the procedure.

Mediastinoscopy

Complications due to mediastinoscopy are rare. Possible complications include pneumothorax or bleeding caused by damage to the blood vessels near the heart. Mediastinitis, infection of the mediastinum, may develop. Injury to the esophagus or larynx may occur. If the nerves leading to the larynx are injured, the patient may be left with a permanently hoarse voice. All of these complications are rare.

Normal results

Normal results indicate no evidence of infection in the lungs, no detection of lumps or nodules, and cells that are free from cancerous abnormalities.

Abnormal results of needle biopsy, VATS, and open biopsy may be associated with diseases other than cancer. Nodules in the lungs may be due to active infections such as tuberculosis, or may be scars from a previous infection. In 33% of biopsies using a mediastinoscope, the biopsied lymph nodes prove to be cancerous. Abnormal results should always be considered in the context of the patient's medical history, physical examination, and other tests such as sputum examination, and chest x rays before a final diagnosis is made.

Morbidity and mortality rates

The risk of **death** from needle biopsy is rare. The risk of death from open biopsy is one in 3,000 cases. In mediastinoscopy, death occurs in fewer than one in 3,000 cases.

Alternatives

The type of alternative diagnostic procedures available depend upon each patient's diagnosis.

Some people may be eligible to participate in clinical trials, research programs conducted with patients

WHO PERFORMS THIS PROCEDURE AND WHERE IS IT PERFORMED?

Fiberoptic bronchoscopy is performed by pulmonologists, physician specialists in pulmonary medicine. CAT guided needle biopsy is done by interventional radiologists, physician specialists in radiological procedures. Thoracic surgeons perform open biopsies and VATS. Specially trained nurses, x-ray, and laboratory technicians assist during the procedures and provide pre- and postoperative education and supportive care.

The procedures are performed in an operating or procedure room in a hospital.

QUESTIONS TO ASK THE DOCTOR

- Why is this procedure being performed?
- Are there any alternative options to having this procedure?
- What type of lung biopsy procedure is recommended?
- Is minimally invasive surgery an option?
- Will the patient be awake during the procedure?
- Who will be performing the procedure? How many years of experience does this physician have? How many other lung biopsies has the physician performed?
- Can medications be taken the day of the procedure?
- Can the patient have food or drink before the procedure? If not, how long before the procedure should these activities be stopped?
- How long is the hospitalization?
- After discharge, how long will it take to recover from the procedure?
- How is pain or discomfort relieved after the procedure?
- What types of symptoms should be reported to the physician?
- When can normal activities be resumed?
- When cam driving be resumed?
- When can the patient return to work?
- When will the results of the procedure be given to the patient?
- How often are follow-up physician visits needed after the procedure?

to evaluate a new medical treatment, drug, or device. The purpose of clinical trials is to find new and improved methods of treating different diseases and special conditions. For more information on current clinical trials, visit the National Institutes of Health's ClinicalTrials.gov at http://www.clinicaltrials.gov or call (888) FIND-NLM [(888) 346-3656] or (301) 594-5983.

The National Cancer Institute (NCI) has conducted a clinical trial to evaluate a technology—low-dose helical computed tomography—for its effectiveness in screening for lung cancer. One study concluded that this test is more sensitive in detecting specific conditions related to lung cancer than other screening tests.

Resources

BOOKS

Abeloff, MD et al. Clinical Oncology. 3rd ed. Philadelphia: Elsevier, 2004.

Mason, RJ et al. Murray & Nadel's Textbook of Respiratory Medicine. 4th ed. Philadelphia: Saunders, 2007.

ORGANIZATIONS

American Association for Respiratory Care (AARC). 11030 Ables Lane, Dallas, TX 75229. E-mail: info@aarc.org. http://www.aarc.org.

American Cancer Society. 1599 Clifton Road, N.E., Atlanta, GA 30329. (800) 227-2345 or (404) 320-3333. http://www.cancer.org.

American College of Chest Physicians. 3300 Dundee Road, Northbrook, IL 60062-2348. (847) 498-1400. http://www.chestnet.org.

American Lung Association and American Thoracic Society. 1740 Broadway, New York, NY 10019-4374. (800)

586-4872 or (212) 315-8700. http://www.lungusa.org and http://www.thoracic.org.

Cancer Research Institute. 681 Fifth Avenue, New York, NY 10022. (800) 992-2623. http://www.cancerresearch.org.

Lung Line National Jewish Medical and Research Center. 14090 Jackson Street, Denver, CO 80206. (800) 222-5864. E-mail: lungline@njc.org. http://www.nationaljewish.org.

National Cancer Institute (National Institutes of Health). 9000 Rockville Pike, Bethesda, MD 20892. (800) 422-6237. http://www.nci.nih.gov.

National Heart, Lung and Blood Institute. Information Center. P.O. Box 30105, Bethesda, MD 20824-0105. (301) 251-2222. http://www.nhlbi.nih.gov.

OTHER

Dailylung.com. http://www.dailylung.com.
Chest Medicine On-Line. http://www.priory.com/chest.htm.
National Lung Health Education Program. http://www.nlhep.com.
Pulmonary Forum. http://www.pulmonarychannel.com.
Pulmonarypaper.org. P.O. Box 877, Ormond Beach, FL 32175. (800) 950- 3698. http://www.pulmonarypaper.org.

Barbara Wexler
Angela M. Costello
Rosalyn Carson-DeWitt, MD

Lung surgery *see* **Lobectomy, pulmonary**

Lung transplantation

Definition

Lung transplantation involves removal of one or both diseased lungs from a patient and the replacement of the lungs with healthy organs from a donor. Lung transplantation may refer to single, double, or even **heart-lung transplantation**.

Purpose

The purpose of lung transplantation is to replace a lung that no longer functions with a healthy lung. To perform a lung transplantation, there should be potential for rehabilitated breathing function. Other medical treatments should be attempted before transplantion is considered. Many candidates for this procedure have end-stage fibrotic lung disease, are dependent on **oxygen therapy**, and are likely to die of their disease in 12–18 months.

Demographics

In order to qualify for lung transplantation, a patient must suffer from severe lung disease such as:

- emphysema
- cystic fibrosis
- pulmonary fibrosis
- pulmonary hypertension
- bronchiectasis
- sarcoidosis
- silicosis

Patients with emphysema or chronic obstructive pulmonary disease (COPD) should be under 60 years of age, have a life expectancy without transplantation of two years or less, progressive deterioration, and emotional stability in order to be considered for lung transplantation. Young patients with end-stage silicosis may be candidates for lung or heart-lung transplantation. Patients with stage III or stage IV sarcoidosis with cor pulmonale (right-sided heart failure) should be considered as early as possible for lung transplantation.

Description

Once a patient has been selected as a possible organ recipient, the process of waiting for a donor organ match begins. The donor organ must meet specific requirements for tissue match in order to reduce the chance of organ rejection. It is estimated that it takes an average of one to two years to receive a suitable donor lung, and the wait is made less predictable by the necessity for tissue match. Patients on a recipient list must be available and ready to come to the hospital immediately when a donor match is found, since the life of the lungs outside the body is brief.

Single lung transplantation is performed via a standard **thoracotomy** (incision in the chest wall) with the patient under **general anesthesia**. Cardiopulmonary bypass (diversion of blood flow from the heart) is not always necessary for a single lung transplant. If bypass is necessary, it involves re-routing of the blood through tubes to a heart-lung bypass machine. Double lung transplantation involves implanting the lungs as two separate lungs, and cardiopulmonary bypass is usually required. The patient's lung or lungs are removed and the donor lungs are stitched into place. Drainage tubes are inserted into the chest area to help drain fluid, blood, and air out of the chest.

Heart-lung transplants always require the use of cardiopulmonary bypass. An incision is made through the middle of the sternum. The heart, lung, and supporting structures are transplanted into the recipient at the same time.

Diagnosis/Preparation

Patients who have diseases or conditions that may make them more susceptible to organ rejection are not selected for lung transplant. This includes patients who are acutely ill and unstable; have uncontrolled or untreatable pulmonary infection; significant dysfunction of other organs, particularly the liver, kidney, or central nervous system; and those with significant coronary disease or left ventricular dysfunction. Patients who actively smoke cigarettes or are dependent on drugs or alcohol may not be selected. There are a variety of protocols that are used to determine if a

Lung transplantation

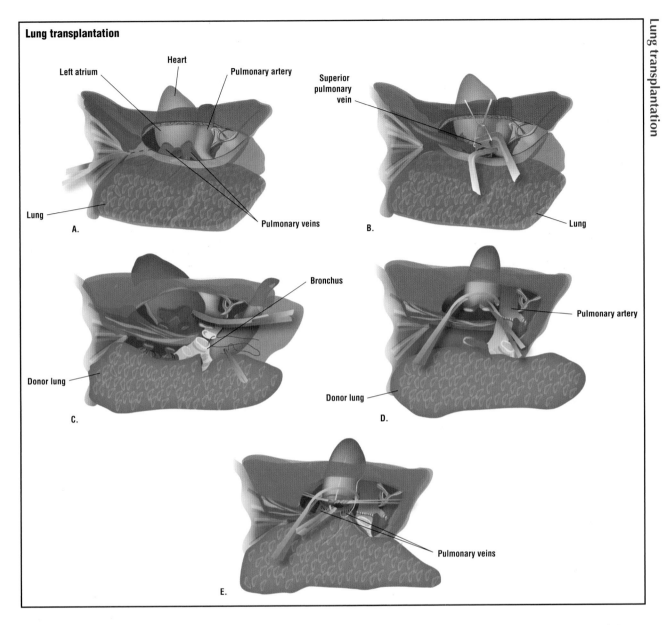

During a lung transplant, the chest is opened to reveal the heart, lungs, and major blood vessels (A). 2. Inferior and superior pulmonary veins and pulmonary artery are separated, and lung is removed (B). The bronchus of the donor lung is connected to the patient's existing bronchus (C). The pulmonary artery is attached (D), and the pulmonary vein and other blood vessels are also connected (E). *(Illustration by GGS Information Services. Cengage Learning, Gale.)*

patient will be placed on a transplant recipient list, and criteria may vary depending on location.

The following diagnostic tests are usually performed to evaluate a patient for lung transplantation:

- Arterial blood gases (ABG) test, which measures the amount of oxygen that the blood is able to carry to body tissues.
- Pulmonary function tests (PFTs), which measure lung volume and the rate of air flow through the lungs; the results measure the progress of the lung disease.

- Radiographic studies (x rays). The most common is the chest x ray (CXR), which takes an internal picture of the chest including the lungs, ribs, heart, and the contours of the major vessels of the chest.
- Computerized tomography (CT) scan. A chest CT scan is taken of horizontal slices of the chest to provide detailed images of the structure of the chest.
- Ventilation perfusion scan (lung scan, V/Q scan) is a test that compares right and left lung function.
- Electrocardiogram (EKG) is performed by placing electrodes on the chest and one electrode on each of

KEY TERMS

Anesthesia—The loss of feeling or sensation induced by use of drugs called anesthetics.

Bronchi—Any of the larger air passages of the lungs.

Bronchiectasis—Persistent and progressive dilation of bronchi or bronchioles as a consequence of inflammatory disease such as lung infections, obstructions, tumors, or congenital abnormality.

Bronchioles—The tiny branches of air tubes within the lungs that are the continuation of bronchi and connect to the lung air sacs (alveoli).

Cor pulmonale—Enlargement of the right ventricle of the heart caused by pulmonary hypertension that may result from emphysema or bronchiectasis; eventually, the condition leads to congestive heart failure.

Cystic fibrosis—A generalized disorder of infants, children, and young adults characterized by widespread dysfunction of the exocrine glands, and chronic pulmonary disease due to excess mucus production in the respiratory tract.

Emphysema—A pathological accumulation of air in tissues or organs, especially in the lungs.

Immunosuppressive—Relating to the weakening or reducing of the immune system's responses to

foreign material; immunosuppressive drugs reduce the immune system's ability to reject a transplanted organ.

Pulmonary—Refers to the respiratory system, or breathing function and system.

Pulmonary fibrosis—Chronic inflammation and progressive formation of fibrous tissue in the pulmonary alveolar walls, with steadily progressive shortness of breath, resulting in death from lack of oxygen or heart failure.

Pulmonary hypertension—Abnormally high blood pressure within the pulmonary artery.

Rejection—Occurs when the body tries to attack a transplanted organ because it reacts to the organ or tissue as a foreign object and produces antibodies to destroy it. Anti-rejection (immunosuppressive) drugs help prevent rejection.

Sarcoidosis—A chronic disease with unknown cause that involves formation of nodules in bones, skin, lymph nodes, and lungs.

Silicosis—A progressive disease that results in impairment of lung function and is caused by inhalation of dust containing silica.

the four limbs. A recording of the electrical activity of the heart is obtained to provide information about the rate and rhythm of the heartbeat, and to assess any damage.

- Echocardiogram (ECHO) is an ultrasound of the heart, performed to evaluate the impact of lung disease on the heart. It examines the chambers, valves, aorta, and the wall motion of the heart. ECHO also provides information concerning the blood pressure in the pulmonary arteries. This information is required to plan the transplantation surgery.

- Blood tests. Blood samples are required for both routine and specialized testing.

In addition to tests and criteria for selection as a candidate for transplantation, patients are prepared by discussing at length the procedure, risks, and expected prognosis with the doctor. Patients should continue to follow all therapies and medications for treatment of the underlying disease, unless otherwise instructed by their physician. Since lung transplantation takes place under general anesthesia, patients are advised not to take food or drink from midnight before the surgery.

Aftercare

Transplantation requires a long hospital stay, and recovery can last up to six months. Careful monitoring will take place in a **recovery room** immediately following the surgery and in the patient's hospital room. Patients must take immunosuppressive, or anti-rejection, drugs to reduce the risk of rejection of the transplanted organ. The body considers the new organ an invader and will fight its presence. The anti-rejection drugs lower the body's immune function in order to improve acceptance of the new organs. This also makes the patient more susceptible to infection.

Frequent check-ups, including x-ray and blood tests, will be necessary following surgery, probably for a period of several years.

Risks

Lung transplantation is a complicated and risky procedure, partly because of the organs and systems involved, and also because of the risk of rejection by the recipient's body. Acute rejection most often occurs within the first four months following surgery, but

WHO PERFORMS THE PROCEDURE AND WHERE IS IT PERFORMED?

Lung transplantations are performed in a specialized organ transplantation hospital. Every transplant hospital in the United States is a member of the United Network for Organ Sharing (UNOS) and must meet specific requirements.

Lung transplantations involve specialized transplant teams usually consisting of an anesthesiologist, an infectious disease specialist, a thoracic surgeon, an ear, nose, and throat (ENT) specialist, a cardiologist, and a transplant dietician who all perform with a high level of coordination.

QUESTIONS TO ASK THE DOCTOR

- Are there organizations who can help me afford the cost of transplantation?
- How does the lung matching process work?
- How do I get on the lung waiting list?
- How will they find the right donor for me?
- How many lung transplantations do you perform each year?
- What happens during transplantation?

may occur years later. Infection is a substantial risk for organ recipients. An early complication of the surgery can be poor healing of the bronchial and tracheal openings created during the surgery. A late complication and risk is chronic rejection. This can result in inflammation of the bronchial tubes or in late infection from the prolonged use of immunosuppressive drugs to fight rejection.

Normal results

Demonstration of normal results for lung transplantation patients include adequate lung function and improved quality of life, as well as lack of infection and rejection.

Morbidity and mortality rates

According to the Scientific Registry of Transplant Recipients (SRTR), a total of 1,000 lung transplants were performed in the United States in 2005, although the waiting list was comprised of 3,500 people. The survival rate after single-lung transplant was more than 82% at one year, almost 60% at three years, and almost 48% at five years.

Resources

BOOKS

Khatri, VP and JA Asensio. Operative Surgery Manual. 1st ed. Philadelphia: Saunders, 2003.

Mason, RJ et al. Murray & Nadel's Textbook of Respiratory Medicine. 4th ed. Philadelphia: Saunders, 2007.

Townsend, CM et al. Sabiston Textbook of Surgery. 17th ed. Philadelphia: Saunders, 2004.

PERIODICALS

Algar, F. J., et al. "Lung Transplantation in Patients under Mechanical Ventilation." Transplantation Proceedings, 35 (March 2003): 737–738.

Burns, K. E., B. A. Johnson, and A. T. Iacono. "Diagnostic Properties of Transbronchial Biopsy in Lung Transplant Recipients Who Require Mechanical Ventilation." Journal of Heart and Lung Transplantation, 22 (March 2003): 267–275.

Chan, K. M., and S. A. Allen. "Infectious Pulmonary Complications in Lung Transplant Recipients." Seminars in Respiratory Infections, 17 (December 2002): 291–302.

Helmi, M., R. B. Love, D. Welter, R. D. Cornwell, and K. C. Meyer. "Aspergillus Infection in Lung Transplant Recipients with Cystic Fibrosis: Risk Factors and Outcomes Comparison to Other Types of Transplant Recipients." Chest, 123 (March 2003): 800–808.

Kyle, U. G., L. Nicod, J. A. Romand, D. O. Slosman, A. Spiliopoulos, and C. Pichard. "Four-year Follow-up of Body Composition in Lung Transplant Patients." Transplantation, 75 (March 2003): 821–828.

Van Der Woude, B. T., et al. "Peripheral Muscle Force and Exercise Capacity in Lung Transplant Candidates." International Journal of Rehabilitation Research, 25 (December 2002): 351–355.

ORGANIZATIONS

American Society of Transplantation (AST). 17000 Commerce Parkway, Suite C, Mount Laurel, NJ 08054. (856) 439-9986. http://www.a-s-t.org.

Children's Organ Transplant Association, Inc. 2501 COTA Drive, Bloomington, IN 47403. (800) 366-2682. http://www.cota.org.

The National Heart, Lung, and Blood Institute (NHLBI). P.O. Box 30105, Bethesda, MD 20824-0105. (301) 592-8573. http://www.nhlbi.nih.gov/index.htm.

Second Wind Lung Transplant Association, Inc. 9030 West Lakeview Court, Crystal River, FL 34428. (888) 222-2690. http://www.arthouse.com/secondwind.

OTHER

"Lung Transplantation." The Brigham Women's Hospital.http://www.cheshire-med.com.

"Lung Transplantation." Medline Plus.http://www.nlm.nih.gov/medlineplus/lungtransplantation.html.

Teresa Norris, RN
Monique Laberge, PhD

Luque rod *see* **Spinal instrumentation**

Lymph node biopsy *see* **Sentinel lymph node biopsy**

Lymph node removal *see* **Lymphadenectomy**

Lymphadenectomy

Definition

Lymphadenectomy, also called lymph node dissection, is a surgical procedure in which lymph glands are removed from the body and examined for the presence of cancerous cells. A limited or modified lymphadenectomy removes only some of the lymph nodes in the area around a tumor; a total or radical lymphadenectomy removes all of the lymph nodes in the area.

Purpose

The lymphatic system is responsible for returning excess fluid from body tissues to the circulatory system and for defending against foreign or harmful agents such as bacteria, viruses, or cancerous cells. The major components of the lymphatic system are lymph capillaries, lymph vessels, and lymph nodes. Lymph is a clear fluid found in tissues that originates from the circulatory system. Lymph capillaries are tiny vessels that carry excess lymph to larger lymph vessels; these in turn empty to the circulatory system. Lymph nodes are small, oval- or bean-shaped masses found throughout the lymphatic system that act as filters against foreign materials. They tend to group in clusters in such areas as the neck (cervical lymph nodes), under the arm (axillary lymph nodes), the pelvis (iliac lymph nodes), and the groin (inguinal lymph nodes).

The lymphatic system plays an important role in the spread of cancerous cells throughout the body. Cancer cells can break away from their primary site of growth and travel through the bloodstream or lymphatic system to other sites in body. They may then begin growing at these distant sites or in the lymph nodes themselves; this process is called metastasis. Removal of the lymph nodes, then, is a way that doctors can determine if a cancer has begun to metastasize. Lymphadenectomy may also be pursued as a cancer treatment to help prevent further spread of abnormal cells.

Demographics

The American Cancer Society estimates that approximately 1,444,920 new cases of cancer were diagnosed in 2007, excluding carcinoma-in-situ and basal and squamous cell skin cancers. In 2007, 559,650 Americans are expected to die of cancer. This is 25% of all deaths within any year.

Description

Although the specific surgical procedure may differ according to which lymph nodes are to be removed, some steps are common among all lymphadenectomies. **General anesthesia** is usually administered for the duration of surgery; this ensures that the patient remain unconscious and relaxed, and awaken with no memory of the procedure.

First, an incision is made into the skin and through the subcutaneous layers in the area where the lymph nodes are to be removed. The lymph nodes are identified and isolated. They are then carefully taken out from surrounding tissues (that is, muscles, blood vessels, and nerves). In the case of axillary node dissection, the pad of fat under the skin of the armpit is removed; generally, about 10 to 20 lymph nodes are embedded in the fat and separately removed. The incision is sutured (stitched) closed with a drain left in place to remove excess fluid from the surgical site.

Alternatively, **laparoscopy** may be used as a less invasive method of removing lymph nodes. The laparoscope is a thin, lighted tube that is inserted into the abdominal cavity through a small incision. Images taken by the laparoscope may be seen on a video monitor connected to the scope. Certain lymph nodes, such as the pelvic and aortic lymph nodes, may be removed using this technology.

Diagnosis/Preparation

Lymph nodes may become swollen or enlarged as result of invasion by cancer cells. Swollen lymph nodes may be palpated (felt) during a physical exam. Before lymph nodes are removed, a small amount of tissue is usually removed. A biopsy will be performed on it to check for the presence of abnormal cells.

The patient will be asked to stop taking **aspirin** or aspirin-containing drugs for a period of time prior to surgery, as these can interfere with the blood's ability to

WHO PERFORMS THE PROCEDURE AND WHERE IS IT PERFORMED?

Lymphadenectomy is usually performed in a hospital operating room by a surgical oncologist, a medical doctor who specializes in the surgical diagnosis and treatment of cancers.

clot. Such drugs may include prescription blood thinners (for example, Coumadin and Heparin—generically known as warfarin. However, patients should discuss their medications with regard to their upcoming surgery with their doctors, and not make any adjustments or prescription changes on their own. No food or drink after midnight the night before surgery will be allowed.

Aftercare

Directly following surgery, the patient will be taken to the **recovery room** for constant monitoring and to recover from the effects of anesthesia. The patient may then be transferred to a regular room. If axillary nodes have been removed, the patient's arm will be elevated to help prevent postsurgical swelling. Likewise, the legs will be elevated if an inguinal lymphadenectomy had been performed. A drain placed during surgery to remove excess fluids from the surgical site will remain until the amount of fluid collected in the drain decreases significantly. The patient will generally remain in the hospital for one day.

Specific steps should be taken to minimize the risk of developing lymphedema, a condition in which excess fluid is not properly drained from body tissues, resulting in swelling. This swelling can sometimes become severe enough to interfere with daily activity. Common sites where lymphedema can develop are the arm or leg. Prior to being discharged, the patient will receive the following instructions for care of areas of the body that may be affected by lymph node removal:

- All cuts to the area should be properly cleaned, treated with an antibiotic ointment, and covered with a bandage.
- Heavy lifting should be avoided; bags should be carried on the unaffected arm.
- Tight jewelry and clothing with tight elastic bands should be avoided.
- Injections, blood draws, and blood pressure measurements should be done on the unaffected arm.
- Sunblock should be worn on the affected area to minimize the risk of sunburn.

QUESTIONS TO ASK THE DOCTOR

- Why is lymphadenectomy recommended?
- How many lymph nodes will be removed?
- How long will the procedure take?
- When will I find out the results?
- Am I a candidate for sentinel node biopsy?
- What will happen if the results are positive for cancer?

- Steps should be taken to avoid cuts to the skin. For example, an electric razor should be used to shave the affected area; protective gloves should be worn when working with abrasive items.

Risks

Some of the risks associated with lymphadenectomy include excessive bleeding, infection, pain, excessive swelling, vein inflammation (phlebitis), and damage to nerves during surgery. Nerve damage may be temporary or permanent and may result in weakness, numbness, tingling, and/or drooping. Lymphedema is also a risk whenever lymph nodes have been removed; it may occur immediately following surgery or from months to years later.

Normal results

After removed lymph nodes have been examined microscopically for the presence of cancerous cells, they may be labeled node-negative (no presence of cancer cells) or node-positive (presence of cancer cells). These findings are the basis for deciding the next step in cancer treatment, if one is indicated.

Morbidity and mortality rates

The rate of complications following lymphadenectomy depends on the specific lymph nodes being removed. For example, following axillary lymphadenectomy, there is a 17% chance of chronic lymphedema and 20% chance of abnormal skin sensations. The overall rate of complications following inguinal lymphadenectomy is approximately 15%, and 5–7% following pelvic lymphadenectomy.

Alternatives

A technique designed to spare the unnecessary removal of normal lymph nodes is called sentinel node biopsy. When lymph fluid moves out of a region, the sentinel lymph node is the first node it reaches. The theory behind **sentinel lymph node biopsy** is that if cancer is not present in the sentinel node, it is unlikely to have spread to other nearby nodes. This procedure may allow individuals with early stage cancers to avoid the complications associated with partial or radical removal of lymph nodes if there is little or no chance that cancer has spread to them. For example, while 17% of women have lymphedema after axillary node diseection, only 3% of women have this unpleasant complication after sentinel node biopsy.

Resources

BOOKS

Abeloff, MD et al.Clinical Oncology. 3rd ed. Philadelphia: Elsevier, 2004.

Khatri, VP and JA Asensio. Operative Surgery Manual. 1st ed. Philadelphia: Saunders, 2003.

Townsend, CM et al. Sabiston Textbook of Surgery. 17th ed. Philadelphia: Saunders, 2004.

ORGANIZATIONS

American Cancer Society. 1599 Clifton Rd. NE, Atlanta, GA 30329-4251. (800) 227-2345. http://www.cancer.org.

Society of Surgical Oncology. 85 W. Algonquin Rd., Suite 550, Arlington Heights, IL 60005. (847) 427-1400. http://www.surgonc.org.

OTHER

"All About Cancer: Detailed Guide." American Cancer Society. 2003 [cited April 9, 2003]. http://www.cancer.org/docroot/CRI/CRI_2_3.asp.

Stephanie Dionne Sherk

Magnetic resonance angiogram

Definition

A magnetic resonance angiogram uses the equipment and technology of magnetic resonance imaging (MRI) to assess the arterial system in the body. Unlike other radiologic techniques (x rays, CT scans), magnetic resonance imaging does not involve radiation. Instead, MRI employs a combination of magnetic fields and radio waves to generate images. The magnets cause hydrogen atoms in the subject's body to line up in a particular way; the radio waves then bounce off of these aligned hydrogen atoms. This signal is captured and recorded by a computer, which uses the information to create a two- or three-dimensional image of the tissue being studied. In order to be able to adequately image the arteries during a magnetic resonance angiogram, radioactive contrast is injected in the patient. This circulates throughout the arterial system, and "lights up" the arterial system. In this way, the outline of the arteries can be visualized, and any blockages, bulges, leaks, or other abnormalities can be evaluated.

Purpose

A magnetic resonance angiogram can be performed to assess a variety of conditions involving the arterial system throughout the body, including to

- Diagnose and monitor aneurysms
- Evaluate the extent of atherosclerosis in the coronary arteries, the carotid arteries in the neck, or in the major leg veins; may be useful prior to surgery to remove atherosclerotic plaques or to place a bypass stent
- Evaluate and monitor arteriovenous malformations, such as in the brain
- Diagnose aortic dissection

- Evaluate the arterial system that supplies the kidneys prior to kidney transplantation
- Assess the coronary arteries prior to bypass surgery
- Map out the arteries that supply a tumor prior to surgery to remove that tumor
- Evaluate any area of narrowing (stenosis) throughout the arterial system

Description

Prior to starting the scanner for an MRA, radioactive contrast is injected through an IV in the patient's arm. The classic MRI unit consists of an examination

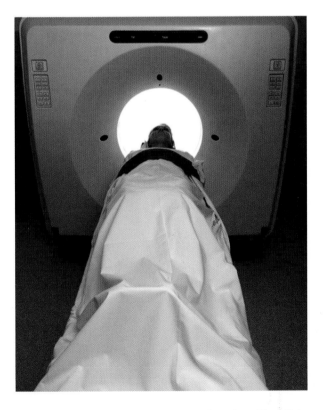

Patient undergoing magnetic resonance imaging. (PhotoSpin, Inc / Alamy)

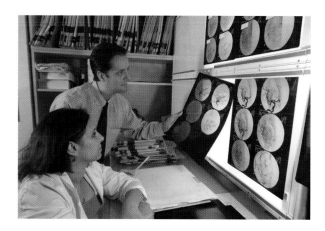

Doctors study MRA scans of the brain. *(Richard T. Nowitz / Phototake. Reproduced by permission.)*

table on which the patient lies, and a doughnut-shaped scanner into which the table slides. During the course of the MRA, which may take between thirty minutes and two hours, the patient must lie very still, and may at times be asked to hold his or her breath. Some people are bothered by the sounds that the MRI scanner makes, which include a variety of tapping, bumping, and fan sounds. Although no one is in the room with the patient, the patient can usually communicate with the MRI technician through a two-way sound system installed within the MRI unit.

Preparation

Because the strong magnetic field employed in MRA can interact with anything else that contains metal, it is crucial that the patient remove any jewelry, including from any piercings, prior to undergoing MRA. Other personal objects that should be removed include hearing aids, dentures, eyeglasses, hairpins. Pockets should be emptied of any metal-containing items, including coins, credit cards, Patients should inform the radiologist about any potentially metal-containing objects or medical devices that they have, such as tattoed eyeliner, a pacemaker, implanted defibrillator, aneurysm clips, cochlear implant, artificial limb, bone pin, medication patch, artificial heart valve, stent, infusion pump, or intrauterine device. People who have occupations in which they work frequently with metal should also inform the radiologist of this fact. In some cases, the MRA cannot be performed due to the presence of metal that cannot be removed and would be unsafe to expose to the magnetic fields of an MRI scanner. Sometimes, an x-ray will be ordered prior to an MRA in order to verify that there is not other metal in the body that would preclude performing the test.

KEY TERMS

Aneurysm—A weakness in the wall of an artery which can cause an area of outpouching or bulging. This weakness can break, resulting in massive bleeding.

Aortic dissection—A situation in which a tear in the interior lining of the wall of the aorta causes bleeding between the layers of that major artery.

Arteriovenous malformation—An anomaly present since birth in which the arteries and veins in a particular part of the body are caught up in a complex tangle, and in which there is an abnormal pattern of blood flowing from the arteries directly into the veins.

Atherosclerosis— A condition in which the major arteries throughout the body become obstructed by fatty plaques, causing narrowing, obstruction of blood flow, and ultimately hardening and stiffening of the arterial walls.

Some patients with a strong history of anxiety or claustrophobia find it difficult to be enclosed in the doughnut-shaped MRI machine. There are some open machines available that may cause less anxiety. Sometimes, a sedative can be used to help the patient relax during the MRA.

Women who are pregnant or who think they may be pregnant are advised against undergoing MRA. Women who are breastfeeding and who require MRA should feed their baby with formula for two days following the procedure, and should pump and discard their breast milk, since it will be contaminated with the radioactive dye.

Most MRI units have an upper limit of weight that they can hold. Patients over 300 pounds may not be able to undergo MRI, or may need to seek an open MRI unit for their study.

Aftercare

There is no aftercare necessary following an MRA. The patient can return to a normal diet and normal activities.

Risks

An MRA poses very little risk to the patient. Rarely, a patient may have an allergy to the radioactive contrast utilized.

Normal results

Normal results of an MRA would reveal normal arterial architecture, with fully patent arteries throughout the arterial tree. No narrowing, blockages, reduced blood flow, or outpouchings of the arterial walls are visualized in a normal MRA.

Abnormal results

An MRA is abnormal if there is reduced blood flow through any part of the arterial tree. This may result in being unable to visualize an area of an artery, due to an obstruction which prevents any blood flow (and therefore any dye) from reaching that part of the arterial system. Stenosis of an artery will cause the channel of dye to appear of smaller caliber than normal. An abnormal collection of dye may accumulate in an aneurysm pocket. An aortic dissection would reveal leakage of dye between the tissue planes of the aorta. Abnormal flow of dye into the venous system may indicate the presence of an arteriovenous malformation.

Morbidity and mortality rates

Under rare circumstances, patients may exhibit signs of allergy to the tracer.

Resources

BOOKS

Grainger, R. G., et al. *Grainger & Allison's Diagnostic Radiology: A Textbook of Medical Imaging.* 4th ed. Philadelphia: Saunders, 2001.

Mettler, F. A. *Essentials of Radiology,* 2nd ed. Philadelphia: Saunders, 2005.

Rosalyn Carson-DeWitt, MD

Magnetic resonance angiography
see **Magnetic resonance imaging**

▌Magnetic resonance imaging

Definition

Magnetic resonance imaging (MRI) is the newest, and perhaps most versatile, medical imaging technology available. Doctors can get highly refined images of the body's interior without surgery, using MRI. By using strong magnets and pulses of radio waves to manipulate the natural magnetic properties in the body, this technique makes better images of organs and soft tissues than those of other scanning technologies. MRI is particularly

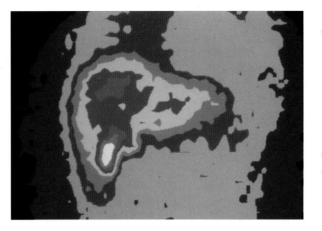

Nuclear scan of the liver and gallbladder. *(Collection CNRI / Phototake. Reproduced by permission.)*

useful for imaging the brain and spine, as well as the soft tissues of joints and the interior structure of bones. The entire body is visible to the technique, which poses few known health risks.

Purpose

MRI was developed in the 1980s. The latest additions to MRI technology are **angiography** (MRA) and spectroscopy (MRS). MRA was developed to study blood flow, while MRS can identify the chemical composition of diseased tissue and produce color images of brain function. The many advantages of MRI include:

• Detail. MRI creates precise images of the body based on the varying proportions of magnetic elements in different tissues. Very minor fluctuations in chemical composition can be determined. MRI images have greater natural contrast than standard x rays, computed tomography scan (CT scan), or ultrasound, all of which depend on the differing physical properties of tissues. This sensitivity lets MRI distinguish fine variations in tissues deep within the body. It also is particularly useful for spotting and distinguishing diseased tissues (tumors and other lesions) early in their development. Often, doctors prescribe an MRI scan to more fully investigate earlier findings of the other imaging techniques.

• Scope. The entire body can be scanned, from head to toe and from the skin to the deepest recesses of the brain. Moreover, MRI scans are not obstructed by bone, gas, or body waste, which can hinder other imaging techniques. (Although the scans can be degraded by motion such as breathing, heartbeat, and normal bowel activity.) The MRI process produces cross-sectional images of the body that are as sharp in the middle as on the edges, even of the brain through the skull. A close series of these two-dimensional images can provide a three-dimensional view of a targeted area.

- Safety. MRI does not depend on potentially harmful ionizing radiation, as do standard x-ray and CT scans. There are no known risks specific to the procedure, other than for people who might have metal objects in their bodies.

MRI is being used increasingly during operations, particularly those involving very small structures in the head and neck, as well as for preoperative assessment and planning. Intraoperative MRIs have shown themselves to be safe as well as feasible, and to improve the surgeon's ability to remove the entire tumor or other abnormality.

Given all the advantages, doctors would undoubtedly prescribe MRI as frequently as **ultrasound** scanning, but the MRI process is complex and costly. The process requires large, expensive, and complicated equipment; a highly trained operator; and a doctor specializing in radiology. Generally, MRI is prescribed only when serious symptoms and/or negative results from other tests indicate a need. Many times another test is appropriate for the type of diagnosis needed.

Doctors may prescribe an MRI scan of different areas of the body.

- Brain and head. MRI technology was developed because of the need for brain imaging. It is one of the few imaging tools that can see through bone (the skull) and deliver high quality pictures of the brain's delicate soft tissue structures. MRI may be needed for patients with symptoms of a brain tumor, stroke, or infection (like meningitis). MRI also may be needed when cognitive and/or psychological symptoms suggest brain disease (like Alzheimer's or Huntington's diseases, or multiple sclerosis), or when developmental retardation suggests a birth defect. MRI can also provide pictures of the sinuses and other areas of the head beneath the face. Recent refinements in MRI technology may make this form of diagnostic imaging even more useful in evaluating patients with brain cancer, stroke, schizophrenia, or epilepsy. In particular, a new 3-D approach to MRI imaging known as diffusion tensor imaging, or DTI, measures the flow of water within brain tissue, allowing the radiologist to tell where the normal flow of fluid is disrupted, and to distinguish more clearly between cancerous and normal brain tissue. The introduction of DTI has led to a technique known as fiber tracking, which allows the neurosurgeon to tell whether a space-occupying brain tumor has damaged or displaced the nerve pathways in the white matter of the brain. This information in turn improves the surgeon's accuracy during the actual operation.

- Spine. Spinal problems can create a host of seemingly unrelated symptoms. MRI is particularly useful for identifying and evaluating degenerated or herniated spinal discs. It can also be used to determine the condition of nerve tissue within the spinal cord.

- Joint. MRI scanning is most commonly used to diagnose and assess joint problems. MRI can provide clear images of the bone, cartilage, ligament, and tendon that comprise a joint. MRI can be used to diagnose joint injuries due to sports, advancing age, or arthritis. MRI can also be used to diagnose shoulder problems, like a torn rotator cuff. MRI can also detect the presence of an otherwise hidden tumor or infection in a joint, and can be used to diagnose the nature of developmental joint abnormalities in children.

- Skeleton. The properties of MRI that allow it to see through the skull also allow it to view the inside of bones. It can be used to detect bone cancer, inspect the marrow for leukemia and other diseases, assess bone loss (osteoporosis), and examine complex fractures.

- The rest of the body. While CT and ultrasound satisfy most chest, abdominal, and general body imaging needs, MRI may be needed in certain circumstances to provide better pictures or when repeated scanning is required. The progress of some therapies, like liver cancer therapy, needs to be monitored, and the effect of repeated x-ray exposure is a concern.

Precautions

MRI scanning should not be used when there is the potential for an interaction between the strong MRI magnet and metal objects that might be imbedded in a patient's body. The force of magnetic attraction on certain types of metal objects (including surgical steel) could move them within the body and cause serious injury. Metal may be imbedded in a person's body for several reasons.

- Medical. People with implanted cardiac pacemakers, metal aneurysm clips, or who have had broken bones repaired with metal pins, screws, rods, or plates must tell their radiologist prior to having an MRI scan. In some cases (like a metal rod in a reconstructed leg) the difficulty may be overcome.

- Injury. Patients must tell their doctors if they have bullet fragments or other metal pieces in their body from old wounds. The suspected presence of metal, whether from an old or recent wound, should be confirmed before scanning.

- Occupational. People with significant work exposure to metal particles (working with a metal grinder, for example) should discuss this with their doctor and radiologist. The patient may need pre-scan testing–usually a single, regular x ray of the eyes to see if any metal is present.

Chemical agents designed to improve the picture and/or allow for the imaging of blood or other fluid flow during MRA may be injected. In rare cases, patients may be allergic to or intolerant of these agents, and these patients should not receive them. If these chemical agents are to be used, patients should discuss any concerns they have with their doctor and radiologist.

The potential side effects of magnetic and electric fields on human health remain a source of debate. In particular, the possible effects on an unborn baby are not well known. Any woman who is, or may be, pregnant should carefully discuss this issue with her doctor and radiologist before undergoing a scan.

As with all medical imaging techniques, obesity greatly interferes with the quality of MRI.

Description

In essence, MRI produces a map of hydrogen distribution in the body. Hydrogen is the simplest element known, the most abundant in biological tissue, and one that can be magnetized. It will align itself within a strong magnetic field, like the needle of a compass. The earth's magnetic field is not strong enough to keep a person's hydrogen atoms pointing in the same direction, but the superconducting magnet of an MRI machine can. This comprises the "magnetic" part of MRI.

Once a patient's hydrogen atoms have been aligned in the magnet, pulses of very specific radio wave frequencies are used to knock them back out of alignment. The hydrogen atoms alternately absorb and emit radio wave energy, vibrating back and forth between their resting (magnetized) state and their agitated (radio pulse) state. This comprises the "resonance" part of MRI.

The MRI equipment records the duration, strength, and source location of the signals emitted by the atoms as they relax and translates the data into an image on a television monitor. The state of hydrogen in diseased tissue differs from healthy tissue of the same type, making MRI particularly good at identifying tumors and other lesions. In some cases, chemical agents such as gadolinium can be injected to improve the contrast between healthy and diseased tissue.

A single MRI exposure produces a two-dimensional image of a slice through the entire target area. A series of these image slices closely spaced (usually less than half an inch) makes a virtual three-dimensional view of the area.

Magnetic resonance spectroscopy (MRS) is different from MRI because MRS uses a continuous band of radio wave frequencies to excite hydrogen atoms in a variety of chemical compounds other than water. These compounds absorb and emit radio energy at characteristic frequencies, or spectra, which can be used to identify them. Generally, a color image is created by assigning a color to each distinctive spectral emission. This comprises the "spectroscopy" part of MRS. MRS is still experimental and is available in only a few research centers.

Doctors primarily use MRS to study the brain and disorders, like epilepsy, Alzheimer's disease, brain tumors, and the effects of drugs on brain growth and metabolism. The technique is also useful in evaluating metabolic disorders of the muscles and nervous system.

Magnetic resonance angiography (MRA) is another variation on standard MRI. MRA, like other types of angiography, looks specifically at fluid flow within the blood (vascular) system, but does so without the injection of dyes or radioactive tracers. Standard MRI cannot make a good picture of flowing blood, but MRA uses specific radio pulse sequences to capture usable signals. The technique is generally used in combination with MRI to obtain images that show both vascular structure and flow within the brain and head in cases of stroke, or when a blood clot or aneurysm is suspected.

Regardless of the exact type of MRI planned, or area of the body targeted, the procedure involved is basically the same and occurs in a special MRI suite. The patient lies back on a narrow table and is made as comfortable as possible. Transmitters are positioned on the body and the cushioned table that the patient is lying on moves into a long tube that houses the magnet. The tube is as long as an average adult lying down, and the tube is narrow and open at both ends. Once the area to be examined has been properly positioned, a radio pulse is applied. Then a two-dimensional image corresponding to one slice through the area is made. The table then moves a fraction of an inch and the next image is made. Each image exposure takes several seconds and the entire exam will last anywhere from 30-90 minutes. During this time, the patient is not allowed to move. If the patient moves during the scan, the picture will not be clear.

Depending on the area to be imaged, the radio-wave transmitters will be positioned in different locations.

- For the head and neck, a helmet-like hat is worn.
- For the spine, chest, and abdomen, the patient will be lying on the transmitters.
- For the knee, shoulder, or other joint, the transmitters will be applied directly to the joint.

Additional probes will monitor **vital signs** (like pulse, respiration, etc.).

The process is very noisy and confining. The patient hears a thumping sound for the duration of the procedure. Since the procedure is noisy, music supplied via earphones is often provided. Some patients get anxious or panic because they are in the small, enclosed tube. This is why vital signs are monitored and the patient and medical team can communicate between each other. If the chest or abdomen are to be imaged, the patient will be asked to hold his/her breath as each exposure is made. Other instructions may be given to the patient, as needed. In many cases, the entire examination will be performed by an MRI operator who is not a doctor. However, the supervising radiologist should be available to consult as necessary during the exam, and will view and interpret the results sometime later.

Preparation

In some cases (such as for MRI brain scanning or an MRA), a chemical designed to increase image contrast may be given by the radiologist immediately before the exam. If a patient suffers from anxiety or claustrophobia, drugs may be given to help the patient relax.

The patient must remove all metal objects (watches, jewelry, eye glasses, hair clips, etc). Any magnetized objects (like credit and bank machine cards, audio tapes, etc.) should be kept far away from the MRI equipment because they can be erased. Patients cannot bring their wallet or keys into the MRI machine. The patient may be asked to wear clothing without metal snaps, buckles, or zippers, unless a medical gown is worn during the procedure. The patient may be asked to remove any hair spray, hair gel, or cosmetics that may interfere with the scan.

Aftercare

No aftercare is necessary, unless the patient received medication or had a reaction to a contrast agent. Normally, patients can immediately return to their daily activities. If the exam reveals a serious condition that requires more testing and/or treatment, appropriate information and counseling will be needed.

Risks

MRI poses no known health risks to the patient and produces no physical side effects. Again, the potential effects of MRI on an unborn baby are not well known. Any woman who is, or may be, pregnant,

---

KEY TERMS

Angiography—Any of the different methods for investigating the condition of blood vessels, usually via a combination of radiological imaging and injections of chemical tracing and contrasting agents.

Diffusion tensor imaging (DTI)—A refinement of magnetic resonance imaging that allows the doctor to measure the flow of water and track the pathways of white matter in the brain. DTI is able to detect abnormalities in the brain that do not show up on standard MRI scans.

Gadolinium—A very rare metallic element useful for its sensitivity to electromagnetic resonance, among other things. Traces of it can be injected into the body to enhance the MRI pictures.

Hydrogen—The simplest, most common element known in the universe. It is composed of a single electron (negatively charged particle) circling a nucleus consisting of a single proton (positively charged particle). It is the nuclear proton of hydrogen that makes MRI possible by reacting resonantly to radio waves while aligned in a magnetic field.

Ionizing radiation—Electromagnetic radiation that can damage living tissue by disrupting and destroying individual cells. All types of nuclear decay radiation (including x rays) are potentially ionizing. Radio waves do not damage organic tissues they pass through.

Magnetic field—The three-dimensional area surrounding a magnet, in which its force is active. During MRI, the patient's body is permeated by the force field of a superconducting magnet.

Radio waves— Electromagnetic energy of the frequency range corresponding to that used in radio communications, usually 10,000 cycles per second to 300 billion cycles per second. Radio waves are the same as visible light, x rays, and all other types of electromagnetic radiation, but are of a higher frequency.

---

should carefully discuss this issue with her doctor and radiologist before undergoing a scan.

Normal results

A normal MRI, MRA, or MRS result is one that shows the patient's physical condition to fall within normal ranges for the target area scanned.

Abnormal results

Generally, MRI is prescribed only when serious symptoms and/or negative results from other tests indicate a need. There often exists strong evidence of a condition that the scan is designed to detect and assess. Thus, the results will often be abnormal, confirming the earlier diagnosis. At that point, further testing and appropriate medical treatment is needed. For example, if the MRI indicates the presence of a brain tumor, an MRS may be prescribed to determine the type of tumor so that aggressive treatment can begin immediately without the need for a surgical biopsy.

Morbidity and mortality rates

Morbidity rates are excessively miniscule. The most common problems are minor bleeding and bruising at the site of contrast injection. Since neither are reportable events, morbidity can only be estimated. Occasionally, an unknown allergy to seafood is discovered after injecting contrast. No deaths have been reported from MRI tests.

Alternatives Resources

Alternative resources include traditional x-rays and computed axial tomography (CT) scans.

Precautions

The main precaution needed is to clean the venipuncture site with alcohol before injecting contrast. Persons with claustrophobia should be given adequate medication to sedate them.

Side effects

The most common side effects of MRI are mild feelings of discomfort due to being enclosed during the test.

Resources

BOOKS

Culbreth, L. J., and C. Watson. Magnetic Resonance Imaging Technology. New York: Cambridge University Press, 2007.

Kastler, B. Understanding MRI. 2nd ed. Berlin: Springer-Verlag, 2008.

McRobbie, D. W., E. A. Moore, M. J. Graves, and M. R. Prince. MRI from Picture to Proton. 2nd ed. New York: Cambridge University Press, 2007.

Weishaupt, D., V. D. Koechli, and B. Marincek. How does MRI work?: An Introduction to the Physics and Function of Magnetic Resonance Imaging. 2nd ed. Berlin: Springer-Verlag, 2008.

PERIODICALS

Hara, H., T. Akisue, T. Fujimoto et al. "Magnetic resonance imaging of medullary bone infarction in the early stage." Clinical Imaging 32, no. 2 (2008): 147–151.

Rumboldt, Z. "Imaging of topographic viral CNS infections." Neuroimaging Clinics of North America 18, no. 1 (2002): 85–92.

Wada, R., and W. Kucharczyk. "Prion infections of the brain." Neuroimaging Clinics of North America 18, no. 1 (2008): 183–191.

Zhao, W., J. H. Choi, G. R. Hon, and M. A. Vannan. "Left ventricular relaxation." Heart Failure Clinics 4, no. 1 (2008): 37–46.

ORGANIZATIONS

American College of Radiology. 1891 Preston White Drive, Reston, VA 22091. (800) 227-5463. http://www.acr.org.

American Society of Radiologic Technologists. 15000 Central Ave. SE, Albuquerque, NM 87123-3917. (505) 298-4500. http://www.asrt.org.

Center for Devices and Radiological Health. United States Food and Drug Administration. 1901 Chapman Ave., Rockville, MD 20857. (301) 443-4109. http://www.fda.gov/cdrh.

OTHER

How Stuff Works. Information about MRI imaging. 2008 [cited February 24, 2008]. http://www.howstuffworks.com/mri.htm.

International Society for Magnetic Imaging in Medicine. Information about MRI tests. 2008 [cited February 25, 2008]. http://www.ismrm.org/.

National Library of Medicine. Information about MRI imaging. 2008 [cited February 24, 2008]. http://www.nlm.nih.gov/medlineplus/ency/article/003335.htm.

Radiology Info. Information about MRI imaging. 2008 [cited February 22, 2008]. http://www.radiologyinfo.org/en/info.cfm?pg = bodymr&bhcp = 1.

Kurt Richard Sternlof
L. Fleming Fallon, Jr, MD, DrPH
Rosalyn Carson-DeWitt, MD

Magnetic resonance spectroscopy
see Magnetic **resonance imaging**

Magnetic resonance venogram

Definition

A magnetic resonance venogram uses the equipment and technology of magnetic resonance imaging (MRI) to assess the body's venous system. Unlike other radiologic techniques (x-rays, CT scans), magnetic resonance imaging does not involve radiation.

Instead, MRI employs a combination of magnetic fields and radio waves to generate images. The magnets cause hydrogen atoms in the subject's body to line up in a particular way; the radio waves then bounce off of these aligned hydrogen atoms. This signal is captured and recorded by a computer, which uses the information to create a two- or three-dimensional image of the tissue being studied. In order to be able to adequately image the veins during a magnetic resonance venogram, radioactive contrast is injected in the patient. This circulates throughout the venous system, and "lights up" the venous system. In this way, the outline of the veins can be visualized, and any blockages, narrowing (stenosis), leaks, or other abnormalities can be evaluated.

Purpose

A magnetic resonance venogram can be performed to assess a variety of conditions involving the venous system throughout the body. MRV is particularly useful for the diagnosis of thrombosis (obstruction by blood clots) in the inferior vena cava (one of the very large major veins into which many of the veins in the body drain), renal (kidney) vein, and portal vein (a major vein in the liver). A thromboembolism (a blood clot that has traveled through the venous system to a point distant from its origination) in the pulmonary system can also be visualized. MRV can be used to demonstrate deep venous thrombosis anywhere in the body, such as the major leg veins or veins deep in the pelvis. Pelvic vein varicosities (enlarged, twisted, tortuous varicose veins) can also be assessed with MRV. MRV is an important method used to evaluate cerebral sinus venous thrombosis, a serious condition in which a clot blocks the drainage of blood from the brain. Lesions that occur in multiple sclerosis may also be visualized with MRV.

Description

Prior to beginning the MRV scan, radioactive contrast is injected through an IV. The classic MRI unit consists of an examination table on which the patient lies, and a doughnut-shaped scanner into which the table slides. During the course of the MRV, which may take between thirty minutes and two hours, the patient must lie very still, and may at times be asked to hold his or her breath. Some people are bothered by the sounds that the MRI scanner makes, which include a variety of tapping, bumping, and fan sounds. Although no one is in the room with the patient, the patient can usually communicate with the MRI technician through a two-way sound system installed within the MRI unit.

KEY TERMS

Multiple sclerosis—A chronic degenerative neurological disease in which demyelination of the nerves causes progressive weakness and loss of motor function.

Thromboembolism—A blood clot that originates in one area of the body, but travels through the venous system to another area, where it obstructs blood flow. This is particularly problematic when the thromboembolus lodges in the lung.

Thrombus— A blood clot that is blocking a blood vessel.

Varicose vein— A vein that is abnormally enlarged, swollen, and/or dilated, and may be twisted or tortuous.

Preparation

Because the strong magnetic field employed in MRV can interact with anything else that contains metal, it is crucial that the patient remove any jewelry, including from any piercings, prior to undergoing MRV. Other personal objects that should be removed include hearing aids, dentures, eyeglasses, hairpins. Pockets should be emptied of any metal-containing items, including coins, credit cards, Patients should inform the radiologist about any potentially metal-containing objects or medical devices that they have, such as tattoed eyeliner, a pacemaker, implanted defibrillator, aneurysm clips, cochlear implant, artificial limb, bone pin, medication patch, artificial heart valve, stent, infusion pump, or intrauterine device. People who have occupations in which they work frequently with metal should also inform the radiologist of this fact. In some cases, the MRV cannot be performed due to the presence of metal that cannot be removed and would be unsafe to expose to the magnetic fields of an MRI scanner. Sometimes, an x-ray will be ordered prior to an MRV in order to verify that there is not other metal in the body that would preclude performing the test.

Some patients with a strong history of anxiety or claustrophobia find it difficult to be enclosed in the doughnut-shaped MRI machine. There are some open machines available that may cause less anxiety. Sometimes, a sedative can be used to help the patient relax during the MRV.

Women who are pregnant or who think they may be pregnant are advised against undergoing MRV.

Women who are breastfeeding and who require MRV should feed their baby with formula for two days following the procedure, and should pump and discard their breast milk, since it will be contaminated with the radioactive dye.

Most MRI units have an upper limit of weight that they can hold. Patients over 300 pounds may not be able to undergo MRI, or may need to seek an open MRI unit for their study.

Aftercare

There is no aftercare necessary following an MRV. The patient can return to a normal diet and normal activities.

Risks

An MRV poses very little risk to the patient. Rarely, a patient may have an allergy to the radioactive contrast utilized.

Normal results

Normal results of an MRV would reveal normal venous architecture, with fully patent arteries throughout the venous tree. No narrowing, blockages, reduced blood flow, or outpouchings of the vein walls are visualized in a normal MRV.

Abnormal results

An MRV is abnormal if the veins appear to be dilated, enlarged, tortuous, or if there is reduced blood flow through any part of the venous tree. If a thrombus is completely obstructing a vein, the vein may not be visualized at all, since the obstruction will prevent any blood flow (and therefore any radioactive contract) from reaching that part of the venous system. When a thrombus is blocking a vein, the MRV may show the vein to be abnormally dilated, with a rim of increased radioactive intensity around the actual thrombus.

Resources

BOOKS

Grainger, R. G., et al. *Grainger & Allison's Diagnostic Radiology: A Textbook of Medical Imaging.* 4th ed. Philadelphia: Saunders, 2001.

Mettler, F. A. *Essentials of Radiology,* 2nd ed. Philadelphia: Saunders, 2005.

Rosalyn Carson-DeWitt, MD

Mallet toe surgery *see* **Hammer, claw, and mallet toe surgery**

Mammography

Definition

Mammography is the study of the breast using x rays. The actual test is called a mammogram. It is an x ray of the breast which shows the fatty, fibrous, and glandular tissues. There are two types of mammograms. A screening mammogram is ordered for women who have no problems with their breasts. It consists of two x-ray views of each breast: a craniocaudal (from above) and a mediolateral oblique (from the sides). A diagnostic mammogram is for evaluation of abnormalities in either men or women. Additional x rays from other angles, or special coned views of certain areas, are taken.

Purpose

The purpose of screening mammography is breast cancer detection. A screening test, by definition, is used for patients without any signs or symptoms, in order to detect disease as early as possible. Many studies have shown that having regular mammograms increases a woman's chances of finding breast cancer in an early stage, when it is more likely to be curable. It has been estimated that a mammogram may find a cancer as much as two or three years before it can be felt. The American Cancer Society (ACS) guidelines recommend an annual screening mammogram for every woman of average risk beginning at age 40. Radiologists look specifically for the presence of microcalcifications and other abnormalities that can be associated with malignancy. New digital mammography and computer-aided reporting can automatically enhance and magnify the mammograms for easier identification of these tiny calcifications.

The highest risk factor for developing cancer is age. Some women are at an increased risk for developing breast cancer, such as those with a positive family history of the disease. Beginning screening mammography at a younger age may be recommended for these women.

Diagnostic mammography is used to evaluate an existing problem, such as a lump, discharge from the nipple, or unusual tenderness in one area. It is also done to evaluate further abnormalities that have been seen on screening mammograms. The radiologist normally views the films immediately and may ask for additional views such as a magnification view of one specific area. Additional studies such as an **ultrasound** of the breast may be performed as well to determine if the lesion is cystic or solid. Breast-specific **positron emission**

KEY TERMS

Breast biopsy—A procedure where suspicious tissue is removed and examined by a pathologist for cancer or other disease. The breast tissue may be obtained by open surgery, or through a needle.

Craniocaudal—Head to tail, x-ray beam directly overhead the part being examined.

Radiographically dense—An abundance of glandular tissue that results in diminished anatomic detail on the mammogram.

tomography (PET) scans as well as an MRI (**magnetic resonance imaging**) may be ordered to further evaluate a tumor, but mammography is still the first choice in detecting small tumors on a screening basis.

Description

A mammogram may be offered in a variety of settings. Hospitals, outpatient clinics, physician's offices, or other facilities may have mammography equipment. In the United States only places certified by the Food and Drug Administration (FDA) are legally permitted to perform, interpret, or develop mammograms. Mammograms are taken with dedicated machines using high frequency generators, low kvp, molybdenum targets and specialized x-ray beam filtration. Sensitive high contrast film and screen combinations along with prolonged developing enable the visualization of minute breast detail.

In addition to the usual paperwork, a woman will be asked to fill out a questionnaire asking for information on her current medical history. Beyond her personal and family history of cancer, details about menstruation, previous breast surgeries, child bearing, birth control, and hormone replacement therapy are recorded. Information about breast self-examination (BSE) and other breast health issues are usually available at no charge.

At some centers, a technologist may perform a **physical examination** of the breasts before the mammogram. Whether or not this is done, it is essential for the technologist to record any lumps, nipple discharge, breast pain or other concerns of the patient. All visible scars, tattoos and nipple alterations must be carefully noted as well.

Clothing from the waist up is removed, along with necklaces and dangling earrings. A hospital gown or similar covering is put on. A small self-adhesive metal marker may be placed on each nipple by the x-ray technologist. This allows the nipple to be viewed as a reference point on the film for concise tumor location and easier centering for additional views.

Patients are positioned for mammograms differently, depending on the type of mammogram being performed:

- Craniocaudal position (CC): The woman stands or sits facing the mammogram machine. One breast is exposed and raised to a level position while the height of the cassette holder is adjusted to the same level. The breast is placed mid-film with the nipple in profile and the head turned away from the side being x rayed. The shoulder is relaxed and pulled slightly backward while the breast is pulled as far forward as possible. The technologist holds the breast in place and slowly lowers the compression with a foot pedal. The breast is compressed between the film holder and a rectangle of plastic (called a paddle). The breast is compressed until the skin is taut and the breast tissue firm when touched on the lateral side. The exposure is taken immediately and the compression released. Good compression can be uncomfortable, but it is very necessary. Compression reduces the thickness of the breast, creates a uniform density and separates overlying tissues. This allows for a detailed image with a lower exposure time and decreased radiation dose to the patient. The same view is repeated on the opposite breast.

- Mediolateral oblique position (MLO): The woman is positioned with her side towards the mammography unit. The film holder is angled parallel to the pectoral muscle, anywhere from 30 to 60 degrees depending on the size and height of the patient. The taller and thinner the patient the higher the angle. The height of the machine is level with the axilla (armpit). The arm is placed at the top of the cassette holder with a corner touching the armpit. The breast is lifted forward and upward and compression is applied until the breast is held firmly in place by the paddle. The nipple should be in profile and the opposite breast held away if necessary by the patient. This procedure is repeated for the other breast. A total of four x rays, two of each breast, are taken for a screening mammogram. Additional x rays, using special paddles, different breast positions, or other techniques may be taken for a diagnostic mammogram.

The mammogram may be seen and interpreted by a radiologist right away, or it may not be reviewed until later. If there is any questionable area or abnormality, extra x rays may be recommended. These may be taken during the same appointment. More commonly, especially for screening mammograms, the woman is called back on another day for these additional films.

A screening mammogram usually takes approximately 15 to 30 minutes. A woman having a diagnostic mammogram can expect to spend up to an hour for the procedure.

The cost of mammography varies widely. Many mammography facilities accept "self referral." This means women can schedule themselves without a physician's referral. However, some insurance policies do require a doctor's prescription to ensure payment. **Medicare** will pay for annual screening mammograms for all women over age 39.

Preparation

The compression or squeezing of the breast necessary for a mammogram is a concern of many women. Mammograms should be scheduled when a woman's breasts are least likely to be tender. One to two weeks after the first day of the menstrual period is usually best, as the breasts may be tender during a menstrual period. Some women with sensitive breasts also find that stopping or decreasing caffeine intake from coffee, tea, colas, and chocolate for a week or two before the examination decreases any discomfort. Women receiving hormone therapy may also have sensitive breasts. Over-the-counter pain relievers are recommended an hour before the mammogram appointment when pain is a significant problem.

Women should not put deodorant, powder, or lotion on their upper body on the day the mammogram is performed. Particles from these products can get on the breast or film holder and may show up as abnormalities on the mammogram. Most facilities will have special wipes available for those patients who need to wash before the mammogram.

Aftercare

No special aftercare is required.

Risks

The risk of radiation exposure from a mammogram is considered minimal and not significant. Experts are unanimous that any negligible risk is by far outweighed by the potential benefits of mammography. Patients who have **breast implants** must be x rayed with caution and compression is minimally applied so that the sac is not ruptured. Special techniques and positioning skills must be learned before a technologist can x ray a patient with breast implants.

Some breast cancers do not show up on mammograms, or "hide" in dense breast tissue. A normal (or negative) study is not a guarantee that a woman is cancer-free. The false-negative rate is estimated to be 15–20%, higher in younger women and women with dense breasts.

False positive readings are also possible. Breast biopsies may be recommended on the basis of a mammogram, and find no cancer. It is estimated that 75–80% of all breast biopsies resulted in benign (no cancer present) findings. This is considered an acceptable rate, because recommending fewer biopsies would result in too many missed cancers.

Normal results

A mammography report describes details about the x-ray appearance of the breasts. It also rates the mammogram according to standardized categories, as part of the Breast Imaging Reporting and Data System (BIRADS) created by the American College of Radiology (ACR). A normal mammogram may be rated as BIRADS 1 or negative, which means no abnormalities were seen. A normal mammogram may also be rated as BIRADS 2 or benign findings. This means there are one or more abnormalities but they are clearly benign (not cancerous), or variations of normal. Some kinds of calcifications, enlarged lymph nodes or obvious cysts might generate a BIRADS 2 rating.

Many mammograms are considered borderline or indeterminate in their findings. BIRADS 3 means either additional images are needed, or an abnormality is seen and is probably (but not definitely) benign. A follow-up mammogram within a short interval of six to 12 months is suggested. This helps to ensure that the abnormality is not changing, or is "stable." Only the affected side will be x rayed at this time. Some women are uncomfortable or anxious about waiting, and may want to consult with their doctor about having a biopsy. BIRADS 4 means suspicious for cancer. A biopsy is usually recommended in this case. BIRADS 5 means an abnormality is highly suggestive of cancer. A biopsy or other appropriate action should be taken.

Screening mammograms are not usually recommended for women under age 40 who have no special risk factors and a normal physical breast examination. A mammogram may be useful if a lump or other problem is discovered in a woman aged 30–40. Below age 30, breasts tend to be "radiographically dense," which means the breasts contain a large amount of glandular tissue which is difficult to image in fine detail. Mammograms for this age group are controversial. An ultrasound of the breasts is usually done instead.

Patient education

The mammography technologist must be empathetic to the patient's modesty and anxiety. He or she must explain that compression is necessary to improve the quality of the image but does not harm the breasts. Patients may be very anxious when additional films are requested. Explaining that an extra view gives the radiologist more information will help to ease the patient's tension. One in eight women in North America will develop breast cancer. Educating the public on monthly breast self-examinations and yearly mammograms will help in achieving an early diagnosis and therefore a better cure.

Resources

BOOKS

Grainger RG, et al. Grainger & Allison's Diagnostic Radiology: A Textbook of Medical Imaging. 4th ed. Philadelphia: Saunders, 2001.
Katz VL et al. Comprehensive Gynecology. 5th ed. St. Louis: Mosby, 2007.
Mettler, FA. Essentials of Radiology. 2nd ed. Philadelphia: Saunders, 2005.

ORGANIZATIONS

American Cancer Society (ACS), 1599 Clifton Rd., Atlanta, GA 30329. (800) ACS-2345. http://www.cancer.org.
Federal Drug Administration (FDA), 5600 Fishers Ln., Rockville, MD 20857. (800) 532-4440. http://www.fda.gov.
National Cancer Institute (NCI) and Cancer Information Service (CIS), Office of Cancer Communications, Bldg. 31, Room 10A16, Bethesda, MD 20892. (800) 4-CANCER (800) 422-6237. Fax: (800) 624-2511 or (301) 402-5874. <cancermail@cips.nci.nih.gov>. <http://cancernet.nci.nih.gov>.

Lorraine K. Ehresman
Lee A. Shratter, M.D.
Rosalyn Carson-DeWitt, MD

Managed care plans

Definition

Managed care plans are health-care delivery systems that integrate the financing and delivery of health care. Managed care organizations generally negotiate agreements with providers to offer packaged health care benefits to covered individuals.

Purpose

The purpose for managed care plans is to reduce the cost of health care services by stimulating competition and streamlining administration.

Description

A majority of insured Americans belongs to a managed care plan, a health care delivery system that applies corporate business practices to medical care in order to reduce costs and streamline care. The managed care era began in the late 1980s in response to skyrocketing health-care costs, which stemmed from a number of sources. Under the fee-for-service, or indemnity, model that preceded managed care, doctors and hospitals were financially rewarded for using a multitude of expensive tests and procedures to treat patients. Other contributors to the high cost of health care were the public health advances after World War II that lengthened the average lifespan of Americans. This put increased pressure on the health-care system. In response, providers have adopted state-of-the-art diagnostic and treatment technologies as they have become available.

Managed care companies attempted to reduce costs by negotiating lower fees with clinicians and hospitals in exchange for a steady flow of patients, developing standards of treatment for specific diseases, requiring clinicians to get plan approval before hospitalizing a patient (except in the case of an emergency), and encouraging clinicians to prescribe less expensive medicines. Many plans offer financial incentives to clinicians who minimize referrals and diagnostic tests, and some even apply financial penalties, or disincentives, on those considered to have ordered unnecessary care. The primary watchdog and accreditation agency for managed care organizations is the National Committee for Quality Assurance (NCQA), a non-profit organization that also collects and disseminates health plan performance data.

Three basic types of managed care plans exist: health maintenance organizations (HMOs), preferred provider organizations (PPOs), and point-of-service (POS) plans.

- HMOs, in existence for more than 50 years, are the best known and oldest form of managed care. Participants in HMO plans must first see a primary care provider, who may be a physician or an advanced practice registered nurse (APRN), in order to be referred to a specialist. Four types of HMOs exist: the Staff Model, Group Model, Network Model, and the Independent Practice Association (IPA). The Staff

KEY TERMS

Health maintenance organization (HMO)—Vertically integrated health-care provider employing many clinical professionals and usually owning or controlling a hospital.

Preferred provider organization (PPO)—Roster of professionals who have been approved to provide services to members of a particular managed care organization.

Model hires clinicians to work onsite. The Group Model contracts with group practice physicians on an exclusive basis. The Network Model resembles the group model except participating physicians can treat patients who are not plan members. The Independent Practice Association (IPA) contracts with physicians in private practice to see HMO patients at a prepaid rate per visit as a part of their practice.

• PPOs are more flexible than HMOs. Like HMOs, they negotiate with networks of physicians and hospitals to get discounted rates for plan members. But, unlike HMOs, PPOs allow plan members to seek care from specialists without being referred by a primary care practitioner. These plans use financial incentives to encourage members to seek medical care from providers inside the network.

• POS plans are a blend of the other types of managed care plans. They encourage plan members to seek care from providers inside the network by charging low fees for their services, but they add the option of choosing an out-of-plan provider at any time and for any reason. POS plans carry a high premium, a high deductible, or a higher co-payment for choosing an out-of-plan provider.

Several managed care theories such as those stressing continuity of care, prevention, and early intervention are applauded by health-care practitioners and patients alike. But managed care has come under fire by critics who feel patient care may be compromised by managed care cost-cutting strategies such as early hospital discharge and use of financial incentives to control referrals, which may make clinicians too cautious about sending patients to specialists. In general, the rise of managed care has shifted decision-making power away from plan members, who are limited in their choices of providers, and away from clinicians, who must concede to managed-care administrators regarding what is considered a medically necessary procedure. Many people would like to see managed care restructured to remedy this inequitable distribution of power. Such actions would maximize consumer choice and allow health-care practitioners the freedom to provide the best care possible. According to the American Medical Association, rejection of care resulting from managed care stipulations should be subjected to an independent appeals process.

The health-care industry today is dominated by corporate values of managed care and is subject to corporate principles such as cost cutting, mergers and acquisitions, and layoffs. To thrive in such an environment, and to provide health care in accordance with professional values, health-care practitioners must educate themselves on the business of health care, including hospital operations and administrative decision making, in order to influence institutional and regional health-care policies. A sampling of the roles available for registered nurses in a managed care environment include:

• Primary care provider. The individual responsible for determining a plan of care, including referrals to specialists.

• Case manager. The person who tracks patients through the health-care system to maintain continuity of care.

• Triage nurse. In a managed care organization, these individuals help direct patients through the system by determining the urgency and level of care necessary and advising incoming patients on self-care when appropriate.

• Utilization/Resource reviewer. This individual helps manage costs by assessing the appropriateness of specialized treatments.

Normal results

It is difficult to predict the effect of the managed care revolution on the health-care profession. All health-care providers will benefit from building broad coalitions at the state and federal levels to publicize their views on patient care issues. These coalitions will also be useful to monitor developing trends in the industry, including the impact of proposed mergers and acquisitions of health-care institutions on the provision of care.

See also Long-term insurance.

Resources

BOOKS

HCPro. *Managed Care and Ambulatory Surgery: Strategies for Contract Negotiation And Reimbursement.* Mission, KS: Opus Communications, 2004.

Kongstvedt, P. *Essentials of Managed Health Care.* 5th ed. Sudbury, MA: Jones and Bartlett, 2007.

Marcinko, D. E. *Dictionary of Health Insurance and Managed Care.* New York: Springer Publishing Company, 1999.

Mechanic, D. *Mental Health and Social Policy: Beyond Managed Care.* 5th ed. Boston, MA: Allyn and Bacon, 2007.

PERIODICALS

Landon, B. E., E. C. Schneider, S. L. Normand, S. H. Scholle, R. J., L. G. Pawlson, and A. M. Epstein. " Quality of care in Medicaid managed care and commercial health plans." *Journal of the American Medical Association* 298, no. 14 (2007): 1674–1681.

Lubell, J. " No advantage. Little quality progress at managed-care plans: report." *Modern Healthcare* 37, no. 39 (2007): 8–9.

Navarro, R., B. M. Mitrzyk and T. J. Bramley. "Chronic insomnia treatment and Medicare Part D: implications for managed care organizations." *American Journal of Managed Care* 13 (5 supp), (2007): S121–S124.

Reinke, T. " Better ways to pay providers. Paying for coordinating care and for packages of services–bundling and episodes of care–may be the best bet for a modification of the unfettered fee-for-service system." *Managed Care* 16, no. 7 (2007): 24–29.

ORGANIZATIONS

Alden March Bioethics Institute. 47 New Scotland Avenue, MC 153, Albany, NY 12208-3478. (518) 262-6082. <http://bioethics.org>.

American Association of Managed Care Nurses. 4435 Waterfront Drive, Suite 101, Glen Allen, VA 23060. (804) 747-9698. http://www.aamcn.org/ .

American College of Physicians. 190 N. Independence Mall West, Philadelphia, PA 19106-1572. 800) 523-1546, x2600, or (215) 351-2600. http://www.acponline.org.

American College of Surgeons. 633 North St. Clair Street, Chicago, IL 60611-32311. (312) 202-5000; Fax: (312) 202-5001. E-mail: postmaster@facs.org. http://www.facs.org.

American Hospital Association. One North Franklin, Chicago, IL 60606-3421. (312) 422-3000. http://www.aha.org/aha_app/index.jsp .

American Medical Association. 515 N. State Street, Chicago, IL 60610. (312) 464-5000. http://www.ama-assn.org.

American Nurses Association. 8515 Georgia Avenue, Suite 400, Silver Spring, MD 20910. (800) 274-4262. http://www.nursingworld.org.

National Committee for Quality Assurance. 1100 13th St., NW, Suite 1000, Washington, DC 20005. (202) 955-3500. http://www.ncqa.org.

OTHER

Centers for Medicare & Medicaid Services. Information about Long-Term Care Insurance. 2007 [cited December 26, 2007]. http://www.medicare.gov/choices/withdraws.asp .

Information about Long-Term Care Insurance. 2007 [cited December 26, 2007]. http://web.ncqa.org/.

Pennsylvania Health Law Project. Information about Long-Term Care Insurance. 2007 [cited December 26, 2007]. http://www.phlp.org/Website/Managed%20Care/Managed%20care.asp.

American Academy of Pediatrics. Information about Long-Term Care Insurance. 2007 [cited December 26, 2007]. http://www.aap.org/family/mancarbr.htm.

L. Fleming Fallon, Jr, MD, DrPH

Mantoux test

Definition

The Mantoux test is used to detect tuberculosis, an infectious disease caused by mycobacteria, usually *Mycobacterium tuberculosis*. Tuberculosis is a relatively common disease that usually affects the lungs, but it may also affect other organ systems and can be deadly.

Purpose

Many people infected with TB bacteria are asymptomatic and thus have a latent TB infection. Ten percent of latent TB infections will eventually become active TB, with a greater than 50% mortality rate. The Mantoux test is used to diagnose those with a latent TB infection. Once individuals are diagnosed with latent TB infection, treatment may begin which will substantially reduce the chance that a latent TB infection progresses to disease. The detection and treatment of latent TB infection is essential in controlling and potentially eliminating tuberculosis.

Precautions

Individuals who have been immunized for TB, have had a past cleared TB infection or are infected with a nontuberculous mycobacteria will respond to the Mantoux test similarly to those who have a latent infection, thus the Mantoux test must be interpreted with caution and if a positive result occurs, detailed history should be discussed. Recent scientific advances have led to the development of a more highly specific test for TB infection that may eventually replace the

Mantoux test as it is less likely to show a response in individuals who have been immunized for TB or infected with a nontuberculous mycobacteria.

Description

The Mantoux test is also known as the PPD test. PPD stands for Purified Protein Derivative. PPD is an antigen that is taken from dead tuberculosis bacteria. The test is administered by using .1 ml or 5 Tuberculin units of PPD. The solution is injected into the skin of the underside of the forearm with a small needle. A small raised bump forms where the solution is administered and the health care professional should mark two edges of the raised bump to mark the injection site. The bacteria that causes tuberculosis produces a delayed hypersensitivity reaction. Within 48-72 hours after the administration of the test, an individual who has been exposed to the bacteria usually reacts to the PPD antigen in the skin of the injection area. The reaction will cause a raised hardened area or induration, at the site of the injection. The size of this area is measured and the measurement of the induration together with the patient's risk factors will determine if the result is considered positive.

Preparation

In preparation for the test, it is important to remember that the results of the test need to be read by the healthcare provider 48-72 hours after the test is administered. The follow-up visit to have the test read should be planned before having the test administered. The healthcare provider should be notified if any surgeries or medical procedures are planned after the test or if a patient has allergies, is pregnant or breastfeeding. Lastly, the test should be postponed if the patient has a skin rash or sunburn on the underside of the forearms.

Aftercare

It is important not to scratch, rub or press on the injection site, nor should one use ointments, lotions or sunscreen on the site, until after the test results have been read by the healthcare provider.

Risks

Some people who are infected with tuberculosis may not have a reaction to the PPD test. This is called a false-negative result. Conversely, some people who are not infected with Mycobacterim Tuberculosis may have a positive PPD test result. This is called a false-positive result. For these reasons, the patient's medical history needs to be carefully taken into account for proper test result interpretation.

Results

Typically a negative reaction, where there is no induration present, or the induration measurement is below the cut-off for the particular patient's risk category, would indicate that the patient does not have a latent TB infection. There are different cut-offs for the measurement of an induration for different groups of people. If an induration is present and is greater than or equal to 5 mm, this result would be considered positive in individuals who are HIV positive or who are immunosuppressed for other reasons, have had recent contact with people who have TB, or those who have had a chest x-ray that shows changes consistent with TB. If an induration is present and is greater than or equal to 10mm, this result is considered positive in patients who are recent immigrants from areas where TB has a high incidence, IV drug users, individuals who live or work in high-risk settings, have medical conditions that place them at high risk or children under the age of four. If an induration is present and is greater than or equal to 15mm, this is considered positive for any individual, even those with no known risk factors.

Resources

BOOKS

Segen, J.C. and J. Wade. *Patient's Guide to Medical Tests: Everything You Need to Know About the Tests Your Doctor Orders.* New York, Checkmark Books, 2002.

PERIODICALS

Rothel, JS., P. Anderson. "Diagnosis of latent Mycobacterium tuberculosis infection: Is the demise of the Mantoux test imminent?" *Expert Review of Anti Infective Therapy* 3(6) (2005):981–983.

OTHER

"Mantoux Tuberculosis Skin Test Facilitator Guide." Centers for Disease Control and Prevention. National Center for HIV, STD and TB Prevention, Division of Tuberculosis Elimination. 1600 Clifton Road, MS E-10, Atlanta, GA 30333. (404)639-8140.www.cdc.gov/tb/pubs/Mantoux/guide.htm.

ORGANIZATIONS

Charles P. Felton National Tuberculosis Center, 2238 Fifth Avenue, First Floor, New York, NY 10037. (212)939-8254.http://www.harlemtbcenter.org/.

Renee Laux, M.S.

Marshall-Marchetti-Krantz procedure *see* Retropubic suspension

Mastectomy

Definition

Mastectomy is the surgical removal of the breast for the treatment or prevention of breast cancer.

Purpose

Mastectomy is performed as a surgical treatment for breast cancer. The severity of a breast cancer is evaluated according to a complex system called staging. This takes into account the size of the tumor and whether it has spread to the lymph nodes, adjacent tissues, and/or distant parts of the body. A mastectomy usually is the recommended surgery for more advanced breast cancers. Women with earlier stage breast cancers, who might also have breast-conserving surgery (**lumpectomy**), may choose to have a mastectomy. In the United States, approximately 50,000 women a year undergo mastectomy.

The size, location, and type of tumor are important considerations when choosing the best surgery to treat breast cancer. The size of the breast also is an important factor. A woman's psychological concerns and lifestyle choices also should be considered when making a decision.

There are many factors that may make a mastectomy the treatment of choice for a patient. Large tumors are difficult to remove with good cosmetic results. This is especially true if the woman has small breasts. Sometimes multiple areas of cancer are found in one breast, making removal of the whole breast necessary. The surgeon sometimes is unable to remove the tumor with a sufficient amount, or margin, of normal tissue surrounding it. In this situation, the entire breast needs to be removed. Recurrence of breast cancer after a lumpectomy is another indication for mastectomy.

Radiation therapy is almost always recommended following a lumpectomy. If a woman is unable to have radiation, a mastectomy is the treatment of choice. Pregnant women cannot have radiation therapy for fear of harming the fetus. A woman with certain collagen vascular diseases, such as systemic lupus erythematosus or scleroderma, would experience unacceptable scarring and damage to her connective tissue from radiation exposure. Any woman who has had therapeutic radiation to the chest area for other reasons cannot tolerate additional exposure for breast cancer therapy.

The need for radiation therapy after breast conserving surgery may make mastectomy more appealing for nonmedical reasons. Some women fear radiation and choose the more extensive surgery so radiation treatment will not be required. The commitment of time, usually five days a week for six weeks, may not be acceptable for other women. This may be due to financial, personal, or job-related factors. In geographically isolated areas, a course of radiation therapy may require lengthy travel and perhaps unacceptable amounts of time away from family or other responsibilities.

Some women choose mastectomy because they strongly fear recurrence of the breast cancer, and lumpectomy seems too risky. Keeping a breast that has contained cancer may feel uncomfortable for some patients. They prefer mastectomy, so the entire breast will be removed. However, studies have shown that survival rates for women choosing mastectomy and those undergoing breast-conserving surgery have been the same.

The issue of prophylactic or preventive mastectomy, or removal of the breast to prevent future breast cancer, is controversial. Women with a strong family history of breast cancer and/or who test positive for a known cancer-causing gene may choose to have both breasts removed. Patients who have had certain types of breast cancers that are more likely to recur may elect to have the unaffected breast removed. Although there is some evidence that this procedure can decrease the chances of developing breast cancer, it is not a guarantee. It is not possible to guarantee that all breast tissue has been removed. There have been cases of breast cancers occurring after both breasts have been removed.

Studies have shown that women who choose preventive mastectomy generally are satisfied with their choice, but also believe they lacked enough information before deciding, particularly about the surgery, genetic testing, and **breast reconstruction**. A recent study of women who underwent radical mastectomy of one breast and chose surgical removal of the other breast as a preventive measure reported that 83% were highly satisfied with their decision.

Precautions

The decision to have mastectomy or lumpectomy should be carefully considered. It is important that the woman be fully informed of all the potential risks and benefits of each surgical treatment before making a choice.

Description

There are several types of mastectomies. The radical mastectomy, also called the Halsted mastectomy, is rarely performed today. It was developed in the late 1800s, when it was thought that more extensive surgery was most likely to cure cancer. A radical mastectomy involves removal of the breast, all surrounding lymph nodes up to the collarbone, and the underlying chest muscle. Women often were left disfigured and disabled, with a large defect in the chest wall requiring **skin grafting**, and significantly decreased arm sensation and motion. Unfortunately, and inaccurately, it still is the operation many women picture when the word mastectomy is mentioned.

Surgery that removes breast tissue, nipple, an ellipse of skin, and some axillary or underarm lymph nodes, but leaves the chest muscle intact, usually is called a **modified radical mastectomy**. This is the most common type of mastectomy performed today. The surgery leaves a woman with a more normal chest shape than the older radical mastectomy procedure, and a scar that is not visible in most clothing. It also allows for immediate or delayed breast reconstruction.

In a **simple mastectomy**, only the breast tissue, nipple, and a small piece of overlying skin are removed. If a few of the axillary lymph nodes closest to the breast also are taken out, the surgery may be called an extended simple mastectomy.

There are other variations on the term mastectomy. A skin-sparing mastectomy uses special techniques that preserve the patient's breast skin for use in reconstruction, although the nipple still is removed. Total mastectomy is a confusing expression, as it may be used to refer to a modified radical mastectomy or a simple mastectomy. In 2003, surgeons reported on a new technique that spared the nipple in many women with early stage breast cancer.

Many women choose to have breast reconstruction performed in conjunction with the mastectomy. The reconstruction can be done using a woman's own abdominal tissue, or using saline-filled artificial expanders, which leave the breast relatively flat but partially reconstructed. Additionally, there are psychological benefits to coming out of the surgery with the first step to a reconstructed breast. Immediate reconstruction will add time and cost to the mastectomy procedure, but the patient can avoid the physical impact of a later surgery.

A mastectomy typically is performed in a hospital setting, but specialized outpatient facilities sometimes are used. The surgery is done under **general anesthesia**.

The type and location of the incision may vary according to plans for reconstruction or other factors, such as old scars. As much breast tissue as possible is removed. Approximately 10 to 20 axillary lymph nodes usually are removed. All tissue is sent to the pathology laboratory for analysis. If no immediate reconstruction is planned, surgical drains are left in place to prevent fluid accumulation. The skin is sutured and **bandages** are applied.

The surgery may take from two to five hours. Patients usually stay at least one night in the hospital, although outpatient mastectomy is increasingly performed for about 10% of all patients. Insurance usually covers the cost of mastectomy. If immediate reconstruction is performed, the length of stay, recovery period, insurance reimbursement, and fees will vary. In 1998, the Women's Health and Cancer Rights Act required insurance plans to cover the cost of breast reconstruction in conjunction with a mastectomy procedure.

Preparation

Routine preoperative preparations, such as not eating or drinking the night before surgery, typically are ordered for a mastectomy. On rare occasions, the patient also may be asked to donate blood in case a blood **transfusion** is required during surgery. The patient should advise the surgeon of any medications she is taking. Information regarding expected outcomes and potential complications also should be part of preparation for a mastectomy, as for any surgical procedure. It is especially important that women know about sensations they might experience after surgery, so they are not misinterpreted as a sign of poor wound healing or recurrent cancer.

Aftercare

In the past, women often stayed in the hospital at least several days. Now many patients go home the same day or within a day or two after their mastectomies. Visits from **home care** nurses can sometimes be arranged, but patients need to learn how to care for themselves before **discharge from the hospital**. Patients may need to learn to change bandages and/ or care for the incision. The surgical drains must be attended to properly; this includes emptying the drain, measuring fluid output, moving clots through the drain, and identifying problems that need attention from the doctor or nurse. If the drain becomes blocked, fluid or blood may collect at the surgical site. Left untreated, this accumulation may cause infection and/or delayed wound healing.

After a mastectomy, activities such as driving may be restricted according to individual needs. Pain is usually well controlled with prescribed medication. Severe pain may be a sign of complications, and should be reported to the physician. A return visit to the surgeon is usually scheduled 7 to 10 days after the procedure.

Exercises to maintain shoulder and arm mobility may be prescribed as early as 24 hours after surgery. These are very important in restoring strength and promoting good circulation. However, intense **exercise** should be avoided for a time after surgery in order to prevent injury. The specific exercises suggested by the physician will change as healing progresses. Physical therapy is an integral part of care after a mastectomy, aiding in the overall recovery process.

Emotional care is another important aspect of recovery from a mastectomy. A mastectomy patient may feel a range of emotions including depression, negative self-image, grief, fear and anxiety about possible recurrence of the cancer, anger, or guilt. Patients are advised to seek counseling and/or support groups and to express their emotions to others, whether family, friends, or therapists. Assistance in dealing with the psychological effects of the breast cancer diagnosis, as well as the surgery, can be invaluable for women.

Measures to prevent injury or infection to the affected arm should be taken, especially if axillary lymph nodes were removed. There are a number of specific instructions directed toward avoiding pressure or constriction of the arm. Extra care must be exercised to avoid injury, to treat it properly if it occurs, and to seek medical attention promptly when appropriate.

Additional treatment for breast cancer may be necessary after a mastectomy. Depending on the type of tumor, lymph node status, and other factors, chemotherapy, radiation therapy, and/or hormone therapy may be prescribed.

Risks

Risks that are common to any surgical procedure include bleeding, infection, anesthesia reaction, or unexpected scarring. After mastectomy and axillary lymph node dissection, a number of complications are possible. A woman may experience decreased feeling in the back of her armpit or other sensations including numbness, tingling, or increased skin sensitivity. Some women report phantom breast symptoms, experiencing itching, aching, or other sensations in the breast that has been removed. There may be scarring around where the lymph nodes were removed, resulting in

> ## KEY TERMS
>
> **Axillary**—Located in or near the armpit.
>
> **Lymphedema**—Swelling caused by an accumulation of fluid from faulty lymph drainage.
>
> **Mastectomy, modified radical**—Total mastectomy with axillary lymph node dissection, but with preservation of the pectoral muscles.
>
> **Mastectomy, radical**—Removal of the breast, pectoral muscles, axillary lymph nodes, and associated skin and subcutaneous tissue.
>
> **Mastectomy, simple**—Removal of only the breast tissue, nipple and a small portion of the overlying skin

decreased arm mobility and requiring more intense physical therapy.

Approximately 10% to 20% of patients develop lymphedema after axillary lymph node removal. This swelling of the arm, caused by faulty lymph drainage, can range from mild to severe. It can be treated with elevation, elastic bandages, and specialized physical therapy. Lymphedema is a chronic condition that requires continuing treatment. This complication can arise at any time, even years after surgery. A new technique called sentinel lymph node mapping and biopsy often eliminates the need for removing some or all lymph nodes by testing the first lymph node for cancer.

Normal results

A mastectomy is performed as the definitive surgical treatment for breast cancer. The goal of the procedure is that the breast cancer is completely removed and does not recur.

Abnormal results

An abnormal result of a mastectomy is the incomplete removal of the breast cancer or a recurrence of the cancer. Other abnormal results include long-lasting (chronic) pain or impairment that does not improve after several months of physical therapy.

Morbidity and mortality rates

Morbidity rates are modest. The most common problems include post-operative infections, unwanted scarring and issues related to emotional adjustment. A decade ago, exposure to silicone from a ruptured implant occasionally occurred. This has been eliminated with the use of saline-filled implants. Mortality is extremely uncommon, averaging fewer than ten deaths per year.

Alternatives Resources

There are no alternatives to mastectomy that is medically indicated. Options do exist for post-mastectomy **reconstructive surgery**. These include the use of pads and breast forms.

Resources

BOOKS

Disa, J. J., and M. C. Kuechel. 100 Questions and Answers About Breast Surgery. Sudbury, MA: Jones and Bartlett, 2005.

Dixon, J. M. Breast Surgery: A Companion to Specialist Surgical Practice. 3rd ed. Philadelphia: Saunders, 2006.

Freund, R. M., and A. VanDyne. Cosmetic Breast Surgery: A Complete Guide to Making the Right Decision–from A to Double D. New York: Marlowe & Company, 2004.

Mang, W., K. Lang, F. Niedel, N. S. Mackowski, N. Rossman, and M. Stock. Manual of Aesthetic Surgery 2. New York: SPringer, 2005.

Spear, S. L., S. C. Willey, G. L. Robb, D. C. Hammond, and N. Y. Nahabedian. Surgery of the Breast: Principles And Art. 2nd ed. Philadelphia: Lippincott Williams & Wilkins, 2005.

Steligo, K. The Breast Reconstruction Guidebook. 2nd ed. San Carlos, CA: Carlo Press, 2005.

PERIODICALS

Greenall, M. J." Is there any argument for delayed breast reconstruction after total mastectomy?" Annals of the royal College of Surgeons of England 89, no. 8 (2007): 754–756.

Guyomard, V., S. Leinster, and M. Wilkinson. " Systematic review of studies of patients' satisfaction with breast reconstruction after mastectomy." Breast 16, no. 6 (2007): 547–567.

Smith, B. " The case for immediate breast reconstruction." Annals of the royal College of Surgeons of England 89, no. 8 (2007): 757–759.

Yano, K., K. Hosokawa, T. Masuoka, K, Matsuda, A. Takada, T. Taguchi, Y. Tamaki, and S. Noguchi. "Options for immediate breast reconstruction following skin-sparing mastectomy." Breast Cancer 14, no. 4 (2007): 406–413.

ORGANIZATIONS

American Board of Plastic Surgery. Seven Penn Center, Suite 400, 1635 Market Street, Philadelphia, PA 19103-2204. (215) 587-9322. http://www.abplsurg.org.

American College of Surgeons. 633 North Saint Claire Street, Chicago, IL 60611. (312) 202-5000. http://www.facs.org/.

American Society for Aesthetic Plastic Surgery. 11081 Winners Circle, Los Alamitos, CA 90720. (888) 272-7711. http://www.surgery.org/.

American Society of Plastic Surgeons. 444 E. Algonquin Rd., Arlington Heights, IL 60005. (847) 228-9900. http://www.plasticsurgery.org.

OTHER

American Cancer Society. Information about Breast Reconstruction. [cited December 23, 2007]. http://www.cancer.org/docroot/CRI/content/CRI_2_6X_Breast_Reconstruction_After_Mastectomy_5. asp.

American Society of Plastic Surgeons. Information about Breast Reconstruction. [cited December 23, 2007]. http://www.plasticsurgery.org/patients_consumers/procedures/BreastReconstruction.cfm?CFID = 2081034&CFTOKEN = 88819197.

M. D. Anderson Cancer Center. Information about Breast Reconstruction. [cited December 23, 2007]. http://www.mdanderson.org/Diseases/BreastCancer/reconstruction/.

Mayo Clinic. Information about Breast Reconstruction. [cited December 23, 2007]. http://www.mayoclinic.com/health/breast-reconstruction/WO00083.

National Library of Medicine. Breast Implants. [cited December 23, 2007]. http://vsearch.nlm.nih.gov/vivisimo/cgi-bin/query-meta?v%3Aproject = medlineplus&query = breast + reconstruction .

Public Broadcasting System Breast Implants on Trial. [cited December 23, 2007]. http://www.pbs.org/search/search_ results.html?q = breast + reconstruction& neighborhood = none .

U.S. Food and Drug Administration. Breast Implants. [cited December 23, 2007]. http://google2.fda.gov/search?output = xml_no_dtd&lr = &proxystylesheet = FDA& client = FDA&site = FDA&getfields = *&q = breast + reconstruction.

L. Fleming Fallon, Jr, MD, DrPH

Mastoid tympanoplasty *see* **Mastoidectomy**

Mastoidectomy

Definition

A mastoidectomy is a surgical procedure that removes an infected portion of the mastoid bone when medicinal treatment is not effective.

Purpose

A mastoidectomy is performed to remove infected mastoid air cells resulting from ear infections, such as mastoiditis or chronic otitis, or by inflammatory disease of the middle ear (cholesteatoma). The mastoid air cells are open spaces containing air that are located throughout the mastoid bone, the prominent bone located behind the ear that projects from the temporal bone of the skull. The air cells are connected to a cavity

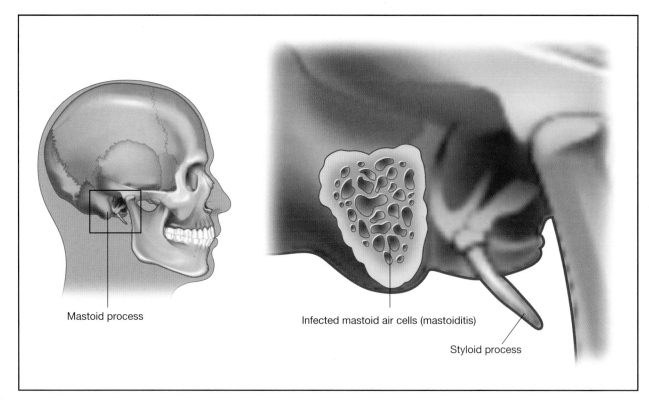

Mastoid process

Infected mastoid air cells (mastoiditis)

Styloid process

(Illustration by Electronic Illustrators Group.)

in the upper part of the bone, which is in turn connected to the middle ear. Aggressive infections in the middle ear can thus sometimes spread through the mastoid bone. When **antibiotics** can't clear this infection, it may be necessary to remove the infected area by surgery. The primary goal of the surgery is to completely remove infection so as to produce an infection-free ear. Mastoidectomies are also performed sometimes to repair paralyzed facial nerves.

Demographics

According to the American Society for Microbiology, middle ear infections increased in the United States from approximately 3 million cases in 1975 to over 9 million in 1997. Middle ear infections are now the second leading cause of office visits to physicians, and this diagnosis accounts for over 40% of all outpatient antibiotic use. Ear infections are also very common in children between the ages of six months and two years. Most children have at least one ear infection before their eighth birthday.

Description

A mastoidectomy is performed with the patient fully asleep under **general anesthesia**. There are several different types of mastoidectomy procedures, depending on the amount of infection present:

- Simple (or closed) mastoidectomy. The operation is performed through the ear or through a cut (incision) behind the ear. The surgeon opens the mastoid bone and removes the infected air cells. The eardrum is incised to drain the middle ear. Topical antibiotics are then placed in the ear.

- Radical mastoidectomy. The procedure removes the most bone and is usually performed for extensive spread of a cholesteatoma. The eardrum and middle ear structures may be completely removed. Usually the stapes, the "stirrup" shaped bone, is spared if possible to help preserve some hearing.

- Modified radical mastoidectomy. In this procedure, some middle ear bones are left in place and the eardrum is rebuilt by tympanoplasty.

After surgery, the wound is stitched up around a drainage tube and a dressing is applied.

Diagnosis/Preparation

The treating physician gives the patient a thorough ear, nose, and throat examination and uses detailed diagnostic tests, including an audiogram and

KEY TERMS

Audiogram—A test of hearing at a range of sound frequencies.

Mastoid air cells—Numerous small intercommunicating cavities in the mastoid process of the temporal bone that empty into the mastoid antrum.

Mastoid antrum—A cavity in the temporal bone of the skull, communicating with the mastoid cells and with the middle ear.

Mastoid bone—The prominent bone behind the ear that projects from the temporal bone of the skull.

Mastoiditis—An inflammation of the bone behind the ear (the mastoid bone) caused by an infection spreading from the middle ear to the cavity in the mastoid bone.

Otitis—Inflammation of the ear, which may be marked by pain, fever, abnormalities of hearing, hearing loss, tinnitus and vertigo.

Tympanoplasty—Procedure to reconstruct the tympanic membrane (eardrum) and/or middle ear bone as the result of infection or trauma.

imaging studies of the mastoid bone using x rays or **CT scans** to evaluate the patient for surgery.

The patient is prepared for surgery by shaving the hair behind the ear on the mastoid bone. Mild soap and a water solution are commonly used to cleanse the outer ear and surrounding skin.

Aftercare

The drainage tube inserted during surgery is typically removed a day or two later.

Painkillers are usually needed for the first day or two after the operation. The patient should drink fluids freely. After the **stitches** are removed, the bulky mastoid dressing can be replaced with a smaller dressing if the ear is still draining. The patient is given antibiotics for several days.

The patient should inform the physician if any of the following symptoms occur:

- bright red blood on the dressing

- stiff neck or disorientation (These may be signs of meningitis.)

- facial paralysis, drooping mouth, or problems swallowing

WHO PERFORMS THE PROCEDURE AND WHERE IS IT PERFORMED?

An mastoidectomy is performed in a hospital by surgeons specialized in otolaryngology, the branch of medicine concerned with the diagnosis and treatment of disorders and diseases of the ears, nose and throat. The procedure usually takes between two and three hours. It is occasionally performed on an outpatient basis in adults but usually involves hospitalization.

Risks

Complications do not often occur, but they may include:

- persistent ear discharge

- infections, including meningitis or brain abscesses

- hearing loss

- facial nerve injury (This is a rare complication.)

- temporary dizziness

- temporary loss of taste on the side of the tongue

Normal results

The outcome of a mastoidectomy is a clean, healthy ear without infection. However, both a modified radical and a radical mastoidectomy usually result in less than normal hearing. After surgery, a hearing aid may be considered if the patient so chooses.

Morbidity and mortality rates

In the United States, **death** from intracranial complications of cholesteatoma is uncommon due to earlier recognition, timely surgical intervention, and supportive antibiotic therapy. Cholesteatoma remains a relatively common cause of permanent, moderate, and conductive hearing loss.

Alternatives

Alternatives to mastoidectomy include the use of medications and delaying surgery. However, these alternative methods carry their own risk of complications and a varying degree of success. Thus, most physicians are of the opinion that patients for whom mastoidectomy is indicated should best undergo the operation, as it provides the patient with the best chance of successful treatment and the lowest risk of complications.

QUESTIONS TO ASK THE DOCTOR

- What are the alternatives to mastoidectomy?
- What are the risks associated with the surgery?
- How will the surgery affect hearing?
- What are the possible alternative treatments?
- How long will it take to recover from the surgery?
- How many mastoidectomies do you perform each year?

Resources

BOOKS

Fisch, H. and J. May. *Tympanoplasty, Mastoidectomy, and Stapes Surgery*. New York: Thieme Medical Pub., 1994.

PERIODICALS

Cristobal, F., Gomez-Ullate, R., Cristobal, I., Arcocha, A., and R. Arroyo. "Hearing results in the second stage of open mastoidectomy: A comparison of the different techniques." *Otolaryngology - Head and Neck Surgery* 122 (May 2000): 350-351.

Garap, J. P., and S. P. Dubey. "Canal-down mastoidectomy: experience in 81 cases." *Otology & Neurotology* 22 (July 2001): 451-456.

Jang, C. H. "Changes in external ear resonance after mastoidectomy: open cavity mastoid versus obliterated mastoid cavity." *Clinical Otolaryngology* 27 (December 2002): 509-511.

Kronenberg, J., and L. Migirov. "The role of mastoidectomy in cochlear implant surgery." *Acta Otolaryngologica* 123 (January 2003): 219-222.

ORGANIZATIONS

American Academy of Otolaryngology-Head and Neck Surgery, Inc. One Prince St., Alexandria VA 22314-3357. (703) 836-4444. http://www.entnet.org.

American Hearing Research Foundation. 55 E. Washington St., Suite 2022, Chicago, IL 60602. (312) 726-9670. http://www.american-hearing.org/.

Better Hearing Institute. 515 King Street, Suite 420, Alexandria, VA 22314. (703) 684-3391.

OTHER

"Mastoidectomy series." *MedlinePlus*. www.nlm.nih.gov/medlineplus/ency/presentations/100032_1.htm.

Carol A. Turkington
Monique Laberge, Ph.D.

Maze procedure for atrial fibrillation

Definition

The Maze procedure, also known as the Cox-Maze procedure, is a surgical treatment for chronic atrial fibrillation or atrial flutter. The procedure restores the heart's normal rhythm by surgically interrupting the conduction of abnormal impulses.

Purpose

When the heart beats too fast, blood no longer circulates effectively in the body. The Maze procedure is used to stop this abnormal beating so that the heart can begin its normal rhythm and pump more efficiently. The procedure is also intended to control heart rate and prevent blood clots and strokes.

Demographics

The Maze procedure has been performed since 1987 and was developed by Dr. James L. Cox. The average age of patients undergoing this procedure is about 52.

The Maze procedure is used to treat chronic or paroxysmal atrial fibrillation, a type of abnormal heart rhythm in which the upper chamber of the heart quivers instead of pumping in an organized way. In general, patients usually have atrial fibrillation for about eight years before undergoing the Maze procedure. The Maze procedure may be recommended for patients who need surgical treatment for coronary artery disease or valve disease. Therefore, the Maze procedure may be performed in combination with coronary artery bypass surgery (CABG), valve repair, valve replacement, or other cardiac surgery.

The Maze procedure may be recommended for patients whose atrial fibrillation has not been successfully treated with medications or other non-surgical interventional procedures. It may also be a treatment option for patients who have a history of stroke or cardiac thrombus.

Abnormal heart rhythms are slightly more common in men than in women, and the prevalence of abnormal heart rhythms, especially atrial fibrillation, increases with age. Atrial fibrillation is relatively uncommon in people under age 20.

Description

Elective Maze surgery is usually scheduled in advance. After arriving at the hospital, an intravenous (IV) catheter will be placed in the arm to deliver

Ablation—The removal or destruction of tissue.

Ablation therapy—A procedure used to treat arrhythmias, especially atrial fibrillation.

Ambulatory monitors—Small portable electrocardiograph machines that record the heart's rhythm, and include the Holter monitor, loop recorder, and trans-telephonic transmitter.

Anti-arrhythmic—Medication used to treat abnormal heart rhythms.

Anticoagulant—A medication, also called a blood thinner, that prevents blood from clotting.

Atria—The right and left upper chambers of the heart.

Cardiac catheterization—An invasive procedure used to create x rays of the coronary arteries, heart chambers and valves.

Cardioversion—A procedure used to restore the heart's normal rhythm by applying a controlled electric shock to the exterior of the chest.

Echocardiogram—An imaging procedure used to create a picture of the heart's movement, valves and chambers.

Electrocardiogram (ECG, EKG)—A test that records the electrical activity of the heart using small electrode patches attached to the skin on the chest.

Electrophysiology study (EPS)—A test that evaluates the electrical activity within the heart.

Head-upright tilt table test—A test used to determine the cause of fainting spells.

Implantable cardioverter-defibrillator (ICD)—An electronic device that is surgically placed to constantly monitor the patient's heart rate and rhythm. If a very fast, abnormal heart rate is detected, the device delivers electrical energy to the heart to resume beating in a normal rhythm.

Nuclear imaging—Method of producing images by detecting radiation from different parts of the body after a radioactive tracer material is administered.

Pacemaker—A small electronic device implanted under the skin that sends electrical impulses to the heart to maintain a suitable heart rate and prevent slow heart rates.

Pulmonary vein isolation—A surgical procedure used to treat atrial fibrillation.

Stress test—A test used to determine how the heart responds to stress.

Ventricles—The lower pumping chambers of the heart; the heart has two ventricles: the right and the left.

---

medications and fluids. **General anesthesia** is administered to put the patient to sleep.

In most cases, a traditional incision is made down the center of the patient's chest, cuts through the breastbone (sternum), and the rib cage is retracted open to expose the heart. The patient is connected to a heart-lung bypass machine, also called a cardiopulmonary bypass pump, which takes over for the heart and lungs during the surgery. The heart-lung machine removes carbon dioxide from the blood and replaces it with oxygen. A tube is inserted into the aorta to carry the oxygenated blood from the bypass machine to the aorta for circulation to the body. The heart-lung machine allows the heart's beating to be stopped so the surgeon can operate on a still heart.

Some patients may be candidates for off-pump surgery, in which the surgery is performed without the use of a heart-lung bypass machine. This is also called beating heart surgery.

The Maze surgery may be an option for some patients. The minimally invasive technique enables the surgeon to work on the heart through small chest holes called ports and other small incisions. Advantages of minimally invasive surgery over the traditional method include smaller incisions, a shorter hospital stay, a shorter recovery period, and lower costs.

During the procedure, precise incisions, also called lesions, are made in the right and left atria to isolate and stop the unusual electrical impulses from forming. The incisions form a maze through which the impulses can travel in one direction from the top of the heart to the bottom. When the heart heals, scar tissue forms and the abnormal electrical impulses can no longer travel through the heart.

These energy sources may be used during the procedure:

- Radiofrequency: A radiofrequency energy catheter is used to create the incisions or lesions in the heart.

- Microwave: A wand-like catheter is used to direct microwave energy to create the lesions in the heart.

- Cryothermy (also called cryoablation): Very cold temperatures are transmitted through a probe (cryoprobe) to create the lesions.

When these energy sources are used, the procedure is called surgical pulmonary vein isolation.

Diagnosis/Preparation

Diagnosis of abnormal heart rhythms

A doctor may be able to detect an irregular heartbeat during a physical exam by taking the patient's pulse. In addition, the diagnosis may be based upon the presence of certain symptoms, including:

- palpitations (feeling of skipped heartbeats or fluttering in the chest)
- pounding in the chest
- shortness of breath
- chest discomfort
- fainting
- dizziness or feeling light-headed
- weakness, fatigue, or feeling tired

Not everyone with abnormal heart rhythms will experience symptoms, so the condition may be discovered upon examination for another medical condition.

DIAGNOSTIC TESTS. Tests used to diagnose an abnormal heart rhythm or determine its cause include:

- blood tests
- chest x rays
- electrocardiogram
- ambulatory monitors such as the Holter monitor, loop recorder, and trans-telephonic transmitter
- stress test
- echocardiogram
- cardiac catheterization
- electrophysiology study (EPS)
- head-upright tilt table test
- nuclear medicine test such as a MUGA scan (multiple-gated acquisition scanning)

Preparation

During a preoperative appointment, usually scheduled within one to two weeks before surgery, the patient will receive information about what to expect during the surgery and the recovery period. The patient will usually meet the cardiologist, anesthesiologist, nurse clinicians, and surgeon during this appointment or just before the procedure.

Medication to thin the blood (blood thinner or anticoagulant) is usually given for at least three weeks before the procedure.

If the patient develops a cold, fever, or sore throat within a few days before the surgery, he or she should notify the surgeon's office.

From midnight before the surgery, the patient should not eat or drink anything.

The morning of the procedure, the patient should take all usual medications as prescribed, with a small sip of water, unless other instructions have been given. Patients who take diabetes medications or anticoagulants should ask their doctor for specific instructions.

The patient is usually admitted to the hospital the same day the surgery is scheduled. The patient should bring a list of current medications, allergies, and appropriate medical records upon **admission to the hospital**.

The morning of surgery, the chest area is shaved and heart monitoring begins. The patient is given general anesthesia before the procedure, so he or she will be asleep during the procedure.

The traditional Maze procedure takes about an hour to perform, while the surgical pulmonary vein isolation procedure generally takes only a few minutes to perform. However, the preparation and recovery time add a few hours to both procedures. The total time in the **operating room** for each of these procedures is about three to four hours.

Aftercare

Recovery in the hospital

The patient recovers in a surgical **intensive care unit** for one to two days after the surgery. The patient will be connected to chest and breathing tubes, a mechanical ventilator, a heart monitor, and other monitoring equipment. A urinary catheter will be in place to drain urine. The breathing tube and ventilator are usually removed about six hours after surgery, but the other tubes usually remain in place as long as the patient is in the intensive care unit.

Drugs are prescribed to control pain and to prevent unwanted blood clotting. Daily doses of **aspirin** are started within six to 24 hours after the procedure.

The patient is closely monitored during the recovery period. **Vital signs** and other parameters such as heart sounds and oxygen and carbon dioxide levels in arterial blood are checked frequently. The chest tube is checked to ensure that it is draining properly. The patient may be fed intravenously for the first day or two.

Chest physiotherapy is started after the ventilator and breathing tube are removed. The therapy includes coughing, turning frequently, and taking deep breaths. Sometimes oxygen is delivered via a mask to help loosen and clear secretions from the lungs. Other exercises will be encouraged to improve the patient's circulation and prevent complications from prolonged bed rest.

If there are no complications, the patient begins to resume a normal routine around the second day. This includes eating regular food, sitting up, and walking around a bit. Before being discharged from the hospital, the patient usually spends a few days under observation in a non-surgical unit. During this time, counseling is usually provided on eating right and starting a light **exercise** program to keep the heart healthy.

The average hospital stay after the Maze surgery is five to seven days, depending on the patient's rate of recovery.

Recovery at home

MEDICATIONS. The doctor may prescribe anti-arrhythmic medications (such as beta-blockers, digitalis, or calcium channel blockers) to prevent the abnormal heart rhythm from returning. Some patients may need to take a diuretic for four to eight weeks after surgery to reduce fluid retention that may occur after surgery. Potassium supplements may be prescribed along with the diuretic medications. Some patients may be prescribed anticoagulant medication such as warfarin and aspirin to reduce the risk of blood clots. The medications prescribed may be adjusted over time to determine the best dosage and type of medication so the abnormal heart rhythm is adequately controlled.

INCISION AND SKIN CARE. The incision should be kept clean and dry. When the skin is healed, the incision should be washed with soapy water. The scar should not be bumped, scratched, or otherwise disturbed. Ointments, lotions, and **dressings** should not be applied to the incision unless specific instructions have been given.

DISCOMFORT. While the incision scar heals, which takes one to two months, it may be sore. Itching, tightness, or numbness along the incision is common. Muscle or incision discomfort may occur in the chest during activity.

LIFESTYLE CHANGES. The patient needs to make several lifestyle changes after surgery, including:

- Quitting smoking. Smoking causes damage to blood vessels, increases the patient's blood pressure and heart rate, and decreases the amount of oxygen available in the blood.

- Managing weight. Maintaining a healthy weight, by watching portion sizes and exercising, is important. Being overweight increases the work of the heart.
- Participating in an exercise program. The cardiac rehabilitation exercise program is usually tailored for the patient, who will be supervised by fitness professionals.
- Making dietary changes. Patients should eat a lot of fruits, vegetables, grains, and non-fat or low-fat dairy products, and reduce fats to less than 30% of all calories.
- Taking medications as prescribed. Aspirin and other heart medications may be prescribed, and the patient may need to take these medications for life.
- Following up with health-care providers. An exercise test is often scheduled during one of the first follow-up visits to determine how effective the surgery was and to confirm that progressive exercise is safe. The patient needs to regularly see the physician for follow-up visits to monitor his or her recovery and control risk factors.

Risks

The Maze procedure is major surgery and patients may experience any of the normal complications associated with major surgery and anesthesia, such as the risk of bleeding, pneumonia, or infection. The risk of stroke is 1%. One common complication that has occurred early after surgery is fluid retention. However, **diuretics** are now prescribed to reduce the risk of this complication. To date, minimal long-term adverse effects have been reported in patients undergoing the Maze procedure.

Normal results

Full recovery from the Maze procedure takes six to eight weeks. Upon release from the hospital, the patient will feel weak because of the extended bed rest in the hospital. Within a few weeks, the patient should begin to feel stronger.

Most patients are able to drive in about three to four weeks, after receiving approval from their physician. Sexual activity can generally be resumed in three to four weeks, depending on the patient's rate of recovery.

It takes about six to eight weeks for the sternum to heal. During this time, the patient should not perform activities that cause pressure or put weight on the breastbone or tension on the arms and chest. Pushing and pulling heavy objects (such as mowing the lawn) should be avoided and lifting objects more than 20 lbs (9 kg) is not permitted. The patient should not hold his

WHO PERFORMS THE PROCEDURE AND WHERE IS IT PERFORMED?

Heart surgeons specially trained in the Maze procedure should perform this procedure. The Maze procedure takes place in an operating room in a hospital. When evaluating where to have the surgery performed, the patient should find out how many Maze procedures have been performed at that facility, how many Maze procedures are performed per month, when the surgeons at that facility started performing the procedure, and what the typical outcomes or results are for their patients.

or her arms above shoulder level for a long period of time. The patient should try not to stand in one place for longer than 15 minutes. Stair climbing is permitted unless other instructions have been given.

Within four to six weeks, people with sedentary office jobs can return to work; people with physical jobs (such as construction work or jobs requiring heavy lifting) must wait longer (up to 12 weeks).

In about 30% of all patients, atrial fibrillation will recur temporarily right after surgery. This is common. Medications are usually prescribed to control atrial fibrillation after surgery. About three months after the surgery, medications are often reduced and then stopped.

In about 7–10% of patients, a permanent pacemaker is needed as a result of the procedure or sometimes due to underlying sinus node dysfunction.

About 90–95% of patients have a return of normal heart rhythm within one year after the surgery. Among U.S. surgeons reporting their data in the January 2000 issue of Seminars in Thoracic and Cardiovascular Surgery, the overall success rate of the Maze procedure is from 90–98%. Some hospitals report a 98% success rate in lone atrial fibrillation patients (those who do not have any other underlying heart conditions) undergoing the traditional Maze procedure. An 80–90% success rate has been reported for the surgical pulmonary vein isolation procedure.

Morbidity and mortality rates

The overall operative mortality for patients undergoing the Maze procedure is 3%. The mortality rate increases among patients over age 65.

QUESTIONS TO ASK THE DOCTOR

- Am I a candidate for minimally invasive surgery?
- Am I a candidate for the "off-pump" surgery technique?
- Who will be performing the surgery? How many years of experience does this surgeon have? How many other Maze procedures has this surgeon performed?
- Can I take my medications the day of the surgery?
- Can I or drink the day of the surgery? If not, how long before the surgery should I stop eating or drinking?
- How long will I have to stay in the hospital after the surgery?
- After I go home from the hospital, how long will it take me to recover from surgery?
- What should I do if I experience symptoms similar to those I felt before surgery?
- What types of symptoms should I report to my doctor?
- What types of medications will I have to take after surgery?
- When will I be able I resume my normal activities, including work and driving?
- When will I find out if the surgery was successful?
- What if the surgery was not successful?
- If I have had the surgery once, can I have it again to correct future blockages?
- Will I have any pain or discomfort after the surgery? If so, how can I relieve this pain or discomfort?
- Are there any medications, foods, or activities I should avoid to prevent my symptoms from recurring?
- How often do I need to see my doctor for follow-up visits after the surgery?

Atrial fibrillation is not immediately life threatening, but it can lead to other heart rhythm problems. Follow-up data from the Framingham Heart Study and the Anti-arrhythmia Versus Implantable Defibrillators Trial have shown that atrial fibrillation is a predictor of increased mortality.

According to a 2002 study published in the *New England Journal of Medicine*, controlling a patient's heart rate is as important as controlling the patient's heart rhythm to prevent **death** and complications from cardiovascular causes. The study also concluded that anticoagulant therapy is important to reduce the risk of stroke and is appropriate therapy in patients who have recurring, persistent atrial fibrillation even after they received treatment.

Alternatives

Health care providers usually try to correct the heart rhythm with medication and recommend lifestyle changes and other interventional procedures such as **cardioversion** before recommending the Maze procedure.

Lifestyle changes often recommended to treat abnormal heart rhythms include:

- quitting smoking
- avoiding activities that prompt the symptoms of abnormal heart rhythms
- limiting alcohol intake
- limiting or not using caffeine, which may produce more symptoms in some people with abnormal heart rhythms
- avoiding stimulant-containing medications such as some cough and cold remedies

If the Maze procedure is not successful in restoring the normal heart rhythm, other treatments for abnormal heart rhythms include:

- permanent pacemakers
- implantable cardioverter-defibrillator
- ablation therapy

Resources

BOOKS

Khatri, VP and JA Asensio. Operative Surgery Manual. 1st ed. Philadelphia: Saunders, 2003.
Libby, P. et al. Braunwald's Heart Disease. 8th ed. Philadelphia: Saunders, 2007.
Townsend, CM et al. Sabiston Textbook of Surgery. 17th ed. Philadelphia: Saunders, 2004.

PERIODICALS

Gillinov AM. "Surgical approaches for atrial fibrillation." Medical Clinics of North America, 92 (2008): 203–215.
Khasnis A "Atrial fibrillation: A historical perspective." Medical Clinics of North America, 92 (2008): 1–15.

ORGANIZATIONS

American College of Cardiology. Heart House. 9111 Old Georgetown Rd., Bethesda, MD 20814-1699. (800) 253-4636 ext. 694 or (301) 897-5400. http://www.acc.org.
American Heart Association. 7272 Greenville Ave., Dallas, TX 75231. (800) 242-8721 or (214) 373-6300. http://www.americanheart.org.
The Cleveland Clinic Heart Center, The Cleveland Clinic Foundation. 9500 Euclid Avenue, F25, Cleveland, OH 44195. (800) 223-2273 ext. 46697 or (216) 444-6697. http://www.clevelandclinic.org/heartcenter.
National Heart, Lung and Blood Institute. National Institutes of Health. Building 1. 1 Center Dr., Bethesda, MD 20892. E-mail: <NHLBIinfo@rover.nhlbi.>. http://www.nhlbi.nih.gov.
Texas Heart Institute. Heart Information Service. P.O. Box 20345, Houston, TX 77225-0345. http://www.tmc.edu/thi.
North American Society of Pacing and Electrophysiology. 6 Strathmore Rd., Natick, MA 01760-2499. (508) 647-0100. http://www.naspe.org.

OTHER

About Atrial Fibrillation. http://www.aboutatrialfibrillation.com.
HeartCenterOnline. http://www.heartcenteronline.com.
The Heart: An Online Exploration. The Franklin Institute Science Museum. 222 North 20th Street, Philadelphia, PA, 19103. (215) 448-1200. <http://sln2.fi.edu/biosci/heart.html>.
Heart Information Network. http://www.heartinfo.org.
Heart Surgeon.com. http:www.heartsurgeon.com.

Angela M. Costello

Mean corpuscular hemoglobin *see* **Red blood cell indices**

Mean corpuscular volume *see* **Red blood cell indices**

▌ Mechanical circulation support

Definition

Mechanical circulatory support is used to treat patients with advanced heart failure. A mechanical pump is surgically implanted to provide pulsatile or non-pulsatile flow of blood to supplement or replace the blood flow generated by the native heart. Types of circulatory support pumps include pneumatic and electromagnetic pumps. Rotary pumps are also available.

Purpose

Heart failure causes low cardiac output, which results in inadequate blood pressure and reduced blood flow to the brain, kidneys, heart, and/or lungs. Pharmaceutical and surgical treatments (other than transplantation) are all typically exhausted before mechanical circulatory support is initiated. The extent of failure exhibited by one or both ventricles of the heart

KEY TERMS

Anticoagulant—Pharmaceutical to prevent clotting proteins and platelets in the blood to be activated to form a blood clot.

Cannulae—Tubes that provide access to the blood once inserted into the heart or blood vessels.

Cardiac—Of or relating to the heart.

Cardiac output—The liter per minute blood flow generated by contraction of the heart.

Cardiopulmonary bypass—Diversion of blood flow away from the right atrium and return of blood beyond the left ventricle to bypass the heart and lungs.

determines if univentricular or biventricular support is required. In either case, blood flow is supplemented or replaced by a mechanical circulatory support device. The device works by removing blood from the inlet of the ventricle(s) and reinjecting it at the outlet of the ventricle(s) in order to increase blood pressure and blood flow to the brain, kidneys, heart, and lungs.

Some devices, along with the intra-aortic balloon pump (IABP), centrifugal pump, and extracorporeal membrane oxygenation (ECMO), are systems that are meant to sustain the patient until the heart recovers. If recovery does not occur, or is not expected, then **heart transplantation** becomes the next desired course of treatment. In this case, intermediate- to long-term mechanical circulatory support devices are required.

Description

Short-, intermediate-, and long-term support requires bedside monitoring of the equipment and patient throughout treatment. The specialized nature of the equipment and the intensive patient care require dedicated staff who are able to provide continuous bedside treatment.

In most instances, patients receive anticoagulants, drugs that prevent clots in the blood. Frequent laboratory testing determines the proper amount of medication required to prevent blood clots. To mimic the lining of blood vessels, some surfaces of the device attract the body's cells, which stick to the device surface and eliminate the need for anticoagulation.

Blood flow generated by these devices is able to sustain blood pressure and flow to the heart, kidneys, liver, and brain. Temporary assist devices sustain vital organ tissues in situations where recovery of the heart function is anticipated. Long-term support devices

sustain patients until a donor heart is available for transplantation.

Short- to intermediate-term support devices

ECMO circulatory support provides cardiopulmonary bypass. Both cardiac and pulmonary (lung) function can be supplemented with this device. The complexity of care and the need for highly trained staff with specialized equipment limit the availability of ECMO to specialty care facilities. Surgical cannulation (placement of tubes) is required. **Postoperative care** in the critical care unit requires dedicated bedside staffing.

Blood flow to the lungs is reduced as blood is drained from the venous circulation. Blood pumped by the left ventricle is also reduced as blood is returned directly to the systemic circulation. The heart is allowed to rest, pumping less blood than needed to maintain pressure and flow to the vital organs. As cardiac function improves, flow from ECMO support is reduced, allowing the heart to gradually resume normal function. The cannulae are surgically removed from the patient once the heart can maintain adequate cardiac output. Systemic anticoagulation is required throughout the length of support, and often leads to complications of stroke and coagulapathies. Long-term use of ECMO is limited since the patient is immobilized and sedated during treatment.

Ease of insertion for placement in the aorta makes the intra-aorta balloon pump (IABP) the most often used **ventricular assist device**. Specialty care centers provide this service in the **cardiac catheterization** laboratory, **operating room**, critical care unit, and emergency room. Secondary-care-level hospitals can also employ this technology. Well-trained staff are required to monitor equipment at regular intervals and troubleshoot problems.

Left ventricular (the lower left chamber of the heart) support with the IABP reduces the workload of the heart and increases blood flow to the vital organs. The balloon inflates during diastole (the filling phase of the heart) to deliver increased oxygen-saturated blood to the heart; blood flow is also increased to the arteries. Deflation of the balloon occurs prior to systole (the emptying phase of the heart).

With recovery of the heart, the IABP device is timed to inflate with every second or third heart beat. The catheter is removed, non-surgically, when the heart can sustain blood pressure and systemic blood flow. Anticoagulation is achieved with minimal drugs throughout the treatment. The device can be in place up to several weeks, but duration is limited because the patient must be immobilized during the treatment.

Centrifugal pumps are able to provide support to one or both ventricles. Blood is removed from the left or right atrium (upper chamber) and returned to the aorta or pulmonary artery, respectively; therefore, surgery is required to place the device. Specialty care facilities have the staff and equipment to provide treatment to heart failure patients with the use of mechanical circulatory support devices. Postoperative care in critical care units requires continuous monitoring by dedicated staff.

The cannulae are passed through the chest wall to attach to a pump that draws blood into the device and propels it to the arterial cannula. As the heart recovers, blood flow is decreased from the centrifugal pump until the device can be removed. An anticoagulant drug is delivered continuously during treatment with a centrifugal pump, and patient immobilization limits the length of support to several weeks.

Intermediate- to long-term support devices

When short-term support devices such as ECMO, IABP, and the centrifugal pump are ineffective to sustain the patient to recovery or organ transplantation, a medium- or long-term device is required. An advantage of treatment with a medium- to long-term device is that it allows the patient to be mobile. In some instances, patients have been able to leave the hospital for continued treatment at home with the implanted device. Complete recovery of the heart has been demonstrated in 5–15% of patients being supported as a bridge to organ transplantation.

Pulsatile paracorporeal mechanical circulatory support devices provide pulsatile support for the left or right ventricle, or both. Cannulation of the left or right atrium, along with the aorta or pulmonary artery, respectively, requires a surgical approach. The heart is emptied of blood by the assist device, so there is little ejection from the body's heart.

Removal of the device occurs at the time of cardiac transplant, unless the body's heart has healed during support. Anticoagulation is achieved by low doses of drugs. Some patients regain mobility while assisted by these devices.

Destination therapies

Destination therapies intended to supplement or permanently replace the body's heart are provided by chronic implantation of the mechanical circulatory support system. For example, total artificial hearts (TAH) replace the body's heart. Upon removal of the native heart, the TAH will be attached to the major blood vessels, thereby supplying blood pressure and flow to both the pulmonary and systemic circulation. Destination therapies are currently in clinical

trials, offering those patients not eligible for organ transplantation a promising future.

Preparation

General anesthetic is given to the patient if a chest incision will be used to expose the heart or if blood vessels need to be exposed. Sedation with local anesthetic is sufficient if the vessels can be accessed with a needle stick. Cardiac monitoring will be performed, including electrocardiograph and cardiovascular pressures. Blood tests prior to surgery are used to measure blood elements and electrolytes. Once all sterile

- What type of implant will I require?
- Who will be performing the surgery? How many years of experience does this surgeon have? How many other implants has this surgeon performed?
- Can I take my medications the day of the surgery?
- Can I or drink the day of the surgery? If not, how long before the surgery should I stop eating or drinking?
- How long will I have to stay in the hospital after the surgery?
- After I go home from the hospital, how long will it take me to recover from surgery?
- What should I do if I experience symptoms similar to those I felt before surgery?
- What types of symptoms should I report to my doctor?
- What types of medications will I have to take after surgery?
- When will I be able I resume my normal activities, including work and driving?
- When will I find out if the surgery was successful?
- What if the surgery was not successful?
- If I have had the surgery once, will the pump ever need replacement?
- Will I have any pain or discomfort after the surgery? If so, how can I relieve this pain or discomfort?
- Are there any medications, foods, or activities I should avoid to prevent my symptoms from recurring?
- How often do I need to see my doctor for follow-up visits after the surgery?

connections are complete, the physician will request that mechanical circulatory support be initiated. Adjustments may be frequent initially, but decrease as the patient stabilizes.

Normal results

Once stable following device implant, the patient is cared for in the **intensive care unit** (ICU). Any change in patient status is reported to the physician. Around-the-clock bedside care is provided by trained nursing staff.

These patients are very ill when they require device implant, often suffering from multi-system organ failure as a result of poor blood flow. The long-term survival is superior at one year when compared to medical treatment alone. Patients that continue to improve on intermediate-, long-term, and TAH increase in activity level and begin a regular **exercise** program. Eventually, with proper training about device maintenance, they are able to leave the hospital to live at home, returning to a normal lifestyle, until further medical treatment is required.

Resources

BOOKS

Khatri, VP and JA Asensio. Operative Surgery Manual. 1st ed. Philadelphia: Saunders, 2003.

Libby, P. et al. Braunwald's Heart Disease. 8th ed. Philadelphia: Saunders, 2007.

Townsend, CM et al. Sabiston Textbook of Surgery. 17th ed. Philadelphia: Saunders, 2004.

PERIODICALS

Boehmer JP "Cardiac failure: mechanical support strategies." Critical Care Medicine (September 2006): S268–77.

ORGANIZATIONS

Commission on Accreditation of Allied Health Education Programs. 1740 Gilpin St., Denver, CO 80218. (303) 320-7701. http://www.caahep.org.

Extracorporeal Life Support Organization (ELSO). 1327 Jones Dr., Ste. 101, Ann Arbor, MI 48105. (734) 998-6600. http://www.elso.med.umich.edu/.

Joint Commission on Accreditation of Health Organizations. One Renaissance Boulevard, Oakbrook Terrace, IL 60181. (630) 792-5000. http://www.jcaho.org/.

OTHER

"Spare Hearts: A Houston Chronicle Four-Part Series." The Houston Chronicle October 1997. http://www.chron.com/content/chronicle/metropolitan/heart/index.html.

Allison Joan Spiwak, BS, CCP
Rosalyn Carson-DeWitt, MD

Mechanical debridement *see* Debridement

Mechanical ventilation

Definition

Mechanical ventilation is the use of a mechanical device (machine) to inflate and deflate the lungs.

Purpose

Mechanical ventilation provides the force needed to deliver air to the lungs in a patient whose own ventilatory abilities are diminished or lost.

Description

Breathing requires the movement of air into and out of the lungs. This is normally accomplished by the diaphragm and chest muscles. A variety of medical conditions can impair the ability of these muscles to accomplish this task, including:

- muscular dystrophies
- motor neuron disease, including ALS
- damage to the brain's respiratory centers
- polio
- myasthenia gravis
- myopathies affecting the respiratory muscles
- scoliosis

Mechanical ventilation may also be used when the airway is obstructed, especially at night in sleep apnea.

Mechanical ventilation may be required only at night, during limited daytime hours, or around the clock, depending on the patient's condition. Some patients require mechanical ventilation only for a short period, during recovery from traumatic nerve injury, for instance. Others require it chronically, and may increase the number of hours required over time as their disease progresses.

Mechanical ventilation is not synonymous with the use of an oxygen tank. Supplemental oxygen is used in patients whose gas exchange capacity has diminished, either through lung damage or obstruction of a major airway. For these patients, the muscles that deliver air work well, but too little oxygen can be exchanged in the remaining lung, and so a higher concentration is supplied with each breath. By the same token, many patients who require mechanical ventilation do not need supplemental oxygen. Their gas exchange capacity is normal, but they cannot adequately move air into and out of the lungs. In fact, excess oxygen may be dangerous, since it can suppress the normal increased respiration response to excess carbon dioxide in the lungs.

Mechanical ventilation systems come in a variety of forms. Almost all systems use a machine called a ventilator that pushes air through a tube for delivery to the patient's airways. The air may be delivered through a nasal or face mask, or through an opening in the trachea (windpipe), called a tracheostomy. Much rarer are systems that rhythmically change the pressure around a patient's chest when the pressure is low, air flows into the lungs, and when it increases, air flows out.

Ventilators

Ventilators can either deliver a set volume with each cycle, or can be set to a specific pressure regimen. Both are in common use. Volume ventilator settings are adjustable for total volume delivered, timing of delivery, and whether the delivery is mandatory or determined by the patient's initial inspiratory effort.

Pressure ventilators deliver one of two major pressure regimens. Continuous positive airway pressure (CPAP) delivers a steady pressure of air, which assists the patient's inspiration (breathing in) and resists expiration (breathing out). The pressure of CPAP is not sufficient to completely inflate the lungs; instead its purpose is to maintain an open airway, and for this reason it is used in sleep apnea, in which a patient's airway closes frequently during sleep.

Bilevel positive airway pressure (BiPAP) delivers a higher pressure on inspiration, helping the patient obtain a full breath, and a low pressure on expiration, allowing the patient to exhale easily. BiPAP is a common choice for neuromuscular disease.

The choice of ventilator type is partly determined by the knowledge and preferences of the treating physician. Settings are adjusted to maintain patient comfort and appropriate levels of oxygen and carbon dioxide in the blood.

Masks vs. tracheostomy

Delivery of air from a ventilator may be either through a mask firmly held to the face, or through a tube inserted into the trachea toward the bottom of the throat. A mask interface is called noninvasive ventilation, while a tracheostomy tube is called invasive ventilation.

Until the mid-1990s, invasive ventilation was the option used by virtually all patients requiring long-term mechanical ventilation. For some patients, tracheostomy continues to be a preferred option. It is commonly used when 24-hour ventilation assistance is required, and may be preferred by patients who find masks uncomfortable or unsightly. Some patients feel ventilation through a "trach tube" is more reassuring. Tracheostomy is also the preferred option for most patients with swallowing difficulties. The potential to choke and suffocate on improperly swallowed food is avoided with a tracheostomy.

Tracheostomies may require more frequent suctioning of airway secretions, produced in response to the presence of the tube and the inflatable cuff that some patients require to hold it in place. The risk of infection is higher, and air must be carefully humidified and cleaned, since these functions are not being served by the nasal passages. Tracheostomies do not prevent speech, despite misinformation to the contrary that even some doctors believe. Speech requires passage of air around the trach tube, which can occur either with an uncuffed tube, or with the presence of a special valve that allows air passage past the cuff.

Noninvasive interfaces come in a variety of forms. A simple mouthpiece may be used, which a patient bites down on to seal the lips around the tube as the pressure cycle delivers a breath. Most masks are individually fitted to the patient's face, and held in place with straps. A tight fit is essential, since the pressure must be delivered to the patient's lungs, and not be allowed to blow out the sides of the mask. Masks may be used around the clock. Nasal masks do not prevent speech, though the tone may change. Oral or full-face masks do interfere with speech, and are typically used at night or intermittently throughout the day, for patients who do not need continuous ventilation assistance.

Other alternatives

The iron lung was an early mechanical ventilation device, and is still in use in some hospitals. The patient's head remains outside of it, while the interior depressurizes. This allows air to push in to the lungs. Repressurizing deflates the lungs again.

A device that works on the same principle is the chest shell (something like a turtle's shell swung around to the front). The pneumobelt applies pressure to deflate, and relaxes it to allow inflation. A rocking bed is used for nighttime ventilation. Tilting the head of the bed down deflates the lungs by allowing the abdominal contents to press against the diaphragm. Reversing the angle reverses the process, allowing inflation.

Preparation

Patients with diseases in which mechanical ventilation may be required are advised to learn as much as possible about treatment options before they become necessary. In particular, it is important to learn about and make decisions about invasive vs. noninvasive ventilation before the time comes. Many patients who begin ventilation with emergency tracheostomy have a difficult time switching to noninvasive ventilation later on (though it is certainly possible).

It is often a good idea to try out different masks and other interfaces before their need arises, and to have these fitted in preparation for a planned transition to the ventilator. Patients can find support groups and other sources of information to learn more about the options and the features of each means of ventilation. Patients may have to help educate their doctors if they are not familiar with noninvasive options.

Patients with neuromuscular disease may have as much or more need for a deep cough as they do for ventilatory assistance, and many patients who undergo emergency tracheostomy do so because their airways have become clogged with mucus build up. Physical therapy cough assistance and a cough assist device are important options for full respiratory health.

Normal results

Mechanical ventilation is a life saver, and provides comfort and confidence to patients who require it. Proper ventilation restores levels of oxygen and carbon dioxide in the blood, improving sleep at night and increasing the ability to engage in activities during the day. When combined with proper respiratory hygiene, it can prolong life considerably. Patients with progressive diseases such as ALS may wish to consider end-of-life decisions before commencing mechanical ventilation, or before the ability to communicate is lost.

Resources

BOOKS

Khatri, VP and JA Asensio. Operative Surgery Manual. 1st ed. Philadelphia: Saunders, 2003.

Libby, P. et al. Braunwald's Heart Disease. 8th ed. Philadelphia: Saunders, 2007.

Mason, RJ et al. Murray & Nadel's Textbook of Respiratory Medicine. 4th ed. Philadelphia: Saunders, 2007.

Townsend, CM et al. Sabiston Textbook of Surgery. 17th ed. Philadelphia: Saunders, 2004.

PERIODICALS

Robinson, R. "Breathe Easy." Quest Magazine 5 (October 1998) [cited July 1, 2003]. http://www.mdausa.org/publications/Quest/q55breathe.html.

ORGANIZATIONS

ALS Association. 27001 Agoura Road, Suite 150 Calabasas Hills, CA 91301-5104. (800) 782-4747. http://www.alsa.org.

Muscular Dystrophy Association. 3300 E. Sunrise Drive Tucson, AZ 85718. (800) 572-1717. http://www.mdausa.org.

Richard Robinson

Meckel's diverticulectomy

Definition

Meckel's diverticulectomy is a surgical procedure that isolates and removes an abnormal diverticulum (Meckel's diverticulum) or pouch, as well as surrounding tissue, in the lining of the small intestine. It is performed to remove an obstruction, adhesions, infection, or inflammation.

Purpose

Meckel's diverticulum is an intestinal diverticulum (pouch) that results from the inability of the vitteline (umbilical) duct to close at five weeks of embryonic development. The vitteline duct is lined with layers of intestinal tissue containing cells that can develop into many different forms, called pluripotent cells. Meckel's diverticulum is a benign congenital condition that has no symptoms for some people, and develops complications in others.

Ninety percent of diverticula are close to the ileocecal valve in the upper intestine, and tissue made up predominantly of gastric and pancreatic cells is thought to cause chemical changes in the mucosa, or lining of the intestines.

The most common cells found in the mucosa of diverticula are gastric cells (present in 50% of all Meckel's diverticulum cases). The highly acidic secretions of gastric tissue may cause the early symptoms of Meckel's diverticulum. The alkaline secretions of pancreatic tissue are also thought to be a source of diverticula inflammation in a small number—about 5%—of cases.

Inflammation of the diverticula or infection of the intestines around the diverticula results in a condition known as **diverticulitis**, which may be treated with **antibiotics**. However, when it is acute and causes obstructions and bleeding, surgery is the treatment of choice.

Demographics

Meckel's diverticulum is present in approximately 2% of the population. It is the most commonly encountered congenital anomaly of the small intestine. Although the abnormality occurs in both sexes, men have more

KEY TERMS

Diverticulitis—Inflammation or infection of the diverticula of the intestines.

Diverticulum—Pouches or bulges of tissue in the lining of organs or canals that can become infected, especially in the intestines and esophagus.

Littre's hernia—A Meckel's diverticulum trapped in an inguinal hernia.

Merkel's diverticulum—Tissue faults in the lining of the intestines that are the result of a congenital abnormality originating in the umbilical duct's failure to close. Largely asymptomatic, the diverticula in some cases can become infected or obstructed.

Perforation—The rupture or penetration by injury or infection of the lining of an organ or canal that allows infection to spread into a body cavity, as in peritonitis, the infection of the lining of the stomach or intestines.

frequent complications with the condition and are more often diagnosed with it. One 15-year study set the complication risk of the abnormality at 4.2%. A recent 10-year study done retrospectively reported an even age distribution for complications of the diverticulum. Malignancy is found in only 0.5–4.9% of patients with complications of Meckel's diverticulum.

Description

Open surgery of the intestines is indicated in acute cases. In the surgery, the intestinal segment containing the diverticulum, usually the ileum or upper intestines, is removed. After the diverticulum is removed, the healthy portions of the intestine are joined together. Some debate exists about whether surgery for asymptomatic Meckel's diverticulum found incidentally is recommended. Some researchers have shown that preventive removal of the diverticulum is less risky than surgical complications, and point to the fact that 6.4% of patients with Meckel's diverticulum develop complications of the condition over their lifetime.

Depending on the surgeon's decision, the operation may be minimal, isolating and then removing the pouch containing the inflammation, or it may be more extensive. In the latter cases, surrounding tissue is removed due to the presence of pervasive inflammation, obstruction, or incarceration in an inguinal hernia (Littre's hernia). Removing additional tissue is done to prevent recurrences. Recent studies have demonstrated the

feasibility of laparoscopic, or minimally invasive diverticulectomy, utilizing small incisions and video imagery via tiny cameras. No long-term studies of this procedure have been conducted.

Surgery is performed under general anesthetic. The small intestine is isolated and the diverticulum is removed, sometimes with a small segment of the intestines. Operative techniques are used to conjoin the end sections of the intestines that have been severed. Some surgeons prefer to perform two surgeries, and do not join together the intestinal sections until some healing of the segments has occurred. In this case, a stoma, or temporary outlet for tubal connection to the intestines, is created in the wall of the abdomen where an external appliance, called an ostomy, can receive waste until the intestinal sections are rejoined.

Diagnosis/Preparation

The vast majority of Meckel's diverticulum diagnoses are incidental, that is, discovered during barium studies, abdominal surgery for other conditions, or autopsy. The most common symptom of the condition is intestinal bleeding, which occurs in 25–50% of patients who have complications. Hemorrhage is the most significant symptom in children two years old and younger. Intestinal obstructions are common, resulting from complications of the tissue surrounding the diverticula. Symptomatic Meckel's diverticulum has symptoms similar to appendicitis. Lower abdominable pain or diverculitits accounts for 10–20% of cases, and requires careful diagnosis to distinguish it from appendicitis. Left untreated, diverticulitis can lead to perforation of the intestine and peritonitis.

Patients who have diverticulitis symptoms, such as acute abdominal pain are given various imaging tests, including a CT scan, **colonoscopy**, or a **sigmoidoscopy** (view of the lower colon through a tiny video instrument placed in the rectum). For children, a special chemical diagnostic test of sodium Tc-pertechnetate, a radioisotope that reacts to the mucosa in the diverticulum, allows inflammation or infection to be viewed radiographically. In adult patients, barium studies may help with diagnosis. When acute hemorrhaging is present, MR imaging of blood vessels is an effective diagnostic tool.

If surgery is indicated for Meckel's diverticulum, an enema is given (unless contraindicated by complications) to completely clear the bowel and avoid infection during surgery.

Aftercare

Intestinal surgery is a serious procedure, and recovery may take two weeks. The number of

WHO PERFORMS THE
PROCEDURE AND WHERE IS IT
PERFORMED?

Surgery takes place in a hospital setting by a physician with advanced training in surgery and gastrointestinal surgery. If the surgery is minimally invasive, requiring only small incisions, it may be performed in an outpatient surgical area of the hospital.

QUESTIONS TO ASK THE
DOCTOR

- Is this surgery necessary or can changing the diet and medical treatment be just as effective?
- Because this surgery was performed on an emergency basis, how extensive was the surgery and how much of the intestine was removed?

postoperative days spent in the hospital depends on the extent of the diverticulum surgery and complications of the condition prior to surgery. Barring complications, patients usually stay in the hospital for about one week. Immediately after surgery, the patient is observed carefully, and given intravenous fluids and antibiotics. Surgical catheters, or stents, are removed over the next two days, with food by mouth offered once bowel sounds are heard.

Risks

Intestinal surgery has the surgical complications associated with any open surgery. These include lung and heart complications, as well as reactions to medications, bleeding, and infection.

Normal results

The usual results of this surgery are an end to obstruction, pain, and infection. Highly successful results include the return of bowel function and daily activities.

Morbidity and mortality rates

Patients with complications of Meckel's diverticulum have a 10–12% incidence of early postoperative complications such as an intestinal leak, a suture line leak or intra-abdominal abscess. Later complications occur in about 7% of patients, and include bowel obstructions and intestinal adhesions. The reported mortality rate for surgery on patients with symptomatic diverticulum is 2–5%. With asymptomatic patients who undergo incidental diverticulectomy, both early and late complications occur in 2% of cases, and the mortality rate is 1%.

Alternatives

Diverticulitis is routinely treated with a change in diet that includes increasing bulk with high-fiber foods and bulk additives like Metamucil. Recurrent attacks, perforation, tissue adhesions, or infections are initially treated with antibiotics, a liquid diet, and bed rest. If medical treatment does not clear the complications, **emergency surgery** may be required.

Resources

BOOKS

Townsend, Courtney M. "Diverticular Disease" In *Sabiston Textbook of Surgery* 16th ed. W. B. Saunders Company, 2001.

PERIODICALS

"Laparoscopy-assisted Resection of Complicated Meckel's Diverticulum in Adults." *Surgical Laparoscopy, Endoscopy and Percutaneous Techniques* 12(3) (June 1, 2000): 190-4.

"Meckel's Diverticulum." *American Family Physician* 61(4) (February 15, 2000).

ORGANIZATIONS

International Foundation for Functional Gastrointestinal Disorders (IFFGD). P.O. Box 170864, Milwaukee, WI 53217-8076. (888) 964-2001 or (414) 964-1799. fax: (414) 964-7176. http://www.iffgd.org.

National Digestive Diseases Information Clearinghouse. 2 Information Way, Bethesda, Maryland 20892-3570. http://www.niddk.nih.gov.

OTHER

"Meckel's diverticulectomy." *MedlinePlus*.http://www.nlm. nih/medlineplus.gov.

Nancy McKenzie, Ph.D.

Mediastinoscopy

Definition

Mediastinoscopy is a surgical procedure that allows physicians to view areas of the mediastinum, the cavity behind the sternum (breastbone) that lies between the lungs. The organs in the mediastinum

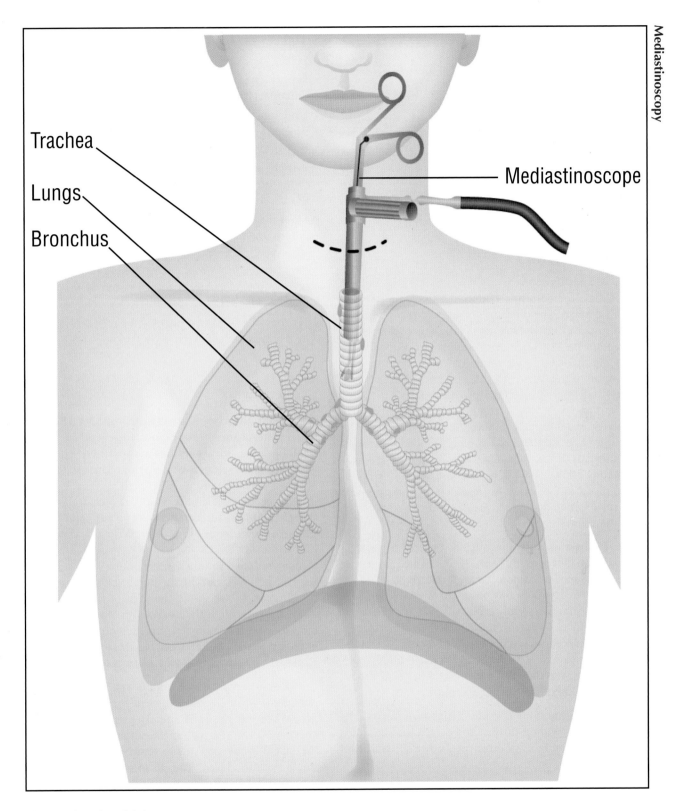

Trachea

Lungs

Bronchus

Mediastinoscope

(Cengage Learning, Gale.)

include the heart and its vessels, the lymph nodes, trachea, esophagus, and thymus.

Mediastinoscopy is most commonly used to detect or stage cancer. It is also ordered to detect infection, and to confirm diagnosis of certain conditions and diseases of the respiratory organs. The procedure involves insertion of an endotracheal (within the trachea) tube, followed by a small incision in the chest. A mediastinoscope is inserted through the incision. The purpose of this equipment is to allow the physician to directly see the organs inside the mediastinum, and to collect tissue samples for laboratory study.

Purpose

Mediastinoscopy is often the diagnostic method of choice for detecting lymphoma, including Hodgkin's disease. The diagnosis of sarcoidosis (a chronic lung disease) and the staging of lung cancer can also be accomplished through mediastinoscopy. Lung cancer staging involves a determination of the level or progression of the cancer into stages. These stages help a physician study cancer and provide consistent cancer definition levels and corresponding treatments. They also provide some guidance as to prognosis. The lymph nodes in the mediastinum are likely to reveal if lung cancer has spread beyond the lungs. Mediastinoscopy allows a physician to observe and extract a sample from the nodes for further study. Involvement of these lymph nodes indicates the diagnosis and stage of lung cancer.

Mediastinoscopy may also be ordered to verify a diagnosis that was not clearly confirmed by other methods, such as certain radiographic and laboratory studies. Mediastinoscopy may aid in some surgical biopsies of nodes or cancerous tissue in the mediastinum. In fact, a surgeon may immediately perform a surgical procedure if a malignant tumor is confirmed while the patient is undergoing mediastinoscopy. In these cases, the diagnostic exam and surgical procedure are combined into one operation.

Mediastinoscopy provides a diagnosis in 10–75% of cases, depending on histology, location, and size of cancer. The false positive rate, however can be as high as 20%.

Demographics

Approximately 130,000 new pulmonary nodules are diagnosed each year in the United States. Of those, half are malignant. The majority of pulmonary nodules are diagnosed via mediastinoscopy.

KEY TERMS

Endotracheal—Placed within the trachea, also known as the windpipe.

Hodgkin's disease—A malignancy of lymphoid tissue found in the lymph nodes, spleen, liver, and bone marrow.

Lymph nodes—Small round structures located throughout the body; contain cells that fight infections.

Pleural space—Space between the layers of the pleura (membrane lining the lungs and thorax).

Sarcoidosis—A chronic disease characterized by nodules in the lungs, skin, lymph nodes, and bones; however, any tissue or organ in the body may be affected.

Thymus—An unpaired organ in the mediastinal cavity that is important in the body's immune response.

Description

Mediastinoscopy is usually performed in a hospital under **general anesthesia**. Before the general anesthesia is administered, **local anesthesia** is applied to the throat while an endotracheal tube is inserted. Once the patient is under general anesthesia, a small incision is made, usually just below the neck or at the notch at the top of the sternum. The surgeon may clear a path and feel the person's lymph nodes first to evaluate any abnormalities within the nodes. Next, the physician inserts the mediastinoscope through the incision. The scope is a narrow, hollow tube with an attached light that allows the surgeon to see inside the area. The surgeon can insert tools through the hollow tube to help perform biopsies. A tissue sample from the lymph nodes or a mass can be removed and sent for study under a microscope, or to a laboratory for further testing.

In some cases, tissue sample analysis that shows malignancy will suggest the need for immediate surgery while the person is already prepared and under anesthesia. In other cases, the surgeon will complete the visual study and tissue removal, and stitch the small incision closed. The person will remain in the surgerical recovery area until the effects of anesthesia have lessened and it is safe to leave the area. The entire procedure should require about an hour, not counting preparation and recovery time. Studies have shown that mediastinoscopy is a safe, thorough, and cost-effective diagnostic tool with less risk than some other procedures.

Diagnosis/Preparation

Because mediastinoscopy is a surgical procedure, it should only be performed when the benefits of the exam's findings outweigh the risks of surgery and anesthesia. Individuals who previously had mediastinoscopy should not receive it again if there is scarring from the first exam.

Several other medical conditions, such as impaired cerebral circulation, obstruction or distortion of the upper airway, or thoracic aortic aneurysm (abnormal dilation of the thoracic aorta) may also preclude mediastinoscopy. Certain structures in a person's anatomy that can be compressed by the mediastinoscope may complicate these pre-existing medical conditions.

Patients are asked to sign a consent form after reviewing the risks of mediastinoscopy and known risks and reactions to anesthesia. The physician will normally instruct the patient to fast from midnight before the test until after the procedure is completed. A physician may also prescribe a sedative the night before the exam and again before the procedure. Often a local anesthetic will be applied to the throat to prevent discomfort during placement of the endotracheal tube.

Aftercare

Following mediastinoscopy, patients will be carefully monitored and watched for changes in **vital signs**, or symptoms of complications from the procedure or anesthesia. The patient may have a sore throat from the endotracheal tube, experience temporary chest pain, and have soreness or tenderness at the incision site.

Risks

Complications from the actual mediastinoscopy procedure are relatively rare. The overall complication rates in various studies have been reported in the range of 1.3–3%. However, the following complications, in decreasing order of frequency, have been reported:

- hemorrhage
- pneumothorax (air in the pleural space)
- recurrent laryngeal nerve injury, causing hoarseness
- infection
- tumor implantation in the wound
- phrenic nerve injury (injury to a thoracic nerve)
- esophageal injury
- chylothorax (chyle is milky lymphatic fluid in the pleural space)
- air embolism (air bubble)
- transient hemiparesis (paralysis on one side of the body)

WHO PERFORMS THE PROCEDURE AND WHERE IS IT PERFORMED?

A mediastinoscopy procedure is usually performed by a thoracic or general surgeon in a hospital setting.

The usual risks associated with general anesthesia also apply to this procedure.

Normal results

In the majority of procedures performed to diagnose cancer, a normal result indicates the presence of small, smooth lymph nodes with no abnormal tissue, growths, or signs of infection. In the case of lung cancer staging, results are related to the severity and progression of the cancer.

Abnormal findings may indicate lung cancer, tuberculosis, the spread of disease from one body part to another, sarcoidosis (a disease that causes nodules, usually affecting the lungs), lymphoma (abnormalities in the lymph tissues), and Hodgkin's disease.

Morbidity and mortality rates

Complications of mediastinoscopy include bleeding, pain, and post-procedure infection. These are relatively uncommon. Mortality is extremely rare.

Alternatives

A less invasive technique is **ultrasound**. However, it is not as specific as mediastinoscopy, and the information obtained is not as useful in making a diagnosis.

Although still performed, there is a decline in the use of mediastinoscopy as a result of advancements in computed tomography (CT), **magnetic resonance imaging** (MRI), and ultrasonography techniques. In addition, improved fine-needle aspiration (withdrawing fluid using suction) results of and core-needle biopsy (using a needle to obtain a small tissue sample) investigations, along with new techniques in thoracoscopy (examination of the thoracic cavity with a lighted instrument called a thoracoscope) offer additional options in examining masses in the mediastinum. Mediastinoscopy may be required when other methods cannot be used or when they provide inconclusive results.

QUESTIONS TO ASK THE DOCTOR

- Why is this test needed?
- Is the test dangerous?
- What test preparation is required?
- How long will the test take?
- When will the results be available?
- What form of anesthesia will be used?
- Is the surgeon board certified?
- How many mediastinoscopy procedures has the surgeon performed?
- What is the surgeon's complication rate?

Resources

BOOKS

Bland, K.I., W.G. Cioffi, M.G. Sarr. *Practice of General Surgery*. Philadelphia: Saunders, 2001.

Fischbach, F. and F. Talaska. *A Manual of Laboratory and Diagnostic Tests,* 6th ed. Philadelphia: Lippincott Williams and Wilkins, 2000.

Grace, P.A., A. Cuschieri, D. Rowley, N. Borley, A. Darzi. *Clinical Surgery,* 2nd ed. London: Blackwell Publishing, 2003.

Schwartz, S.I., J.E. Fischer, F.C. Spencer, G.T. Shires, J.M. Daly, J.M. *Principles of Surgery,* 7th ed. New York: McGraw Hill, 1998.

Townsend, C., K.L. Mattox, R.D. Beauchamp, B.M. Evers, D.C. Sabiston. *Sabiston's Review of Surgery,* 3rd ed. Philadelphia: Saunders, 2001.

PERIODICALS

Beadsmoore C.J., N.J. Screaton. "Classification, Ttaging and Prognosis of Lung Cancer." *European Journal of Radiology* 45, no 1 (2003): 8–17.

Choi, Y.S., Y.M. Shim, J. Kim, K. Kim. "Mediastinoscopy in Patients with Clinical Stage I Non-small Cell Lung Cancer." *Annals of Thoracic Surgery* 75, no. 2 (2003): 364–6.

Detterbeck, F.C., M.M. DeCamp, Jr., L.J. Kohman, G.A. Silvestri. "Lung cancer. Invasive staging: the guidelines." *Chest* 123, no. 1 Suppl (2003): 167S–175S.

Falcone F., F. Fois, D. Grosso. "Endobronchial Ultrasound." *Respiration* 70, no. 2 (2003): 179–94.

Sterman, D.H., E. Sztejman, E. Rodriguez, J. Friedberg. "Diagnosis and Staging of 'Other Bronchial Tumors'." *Chest Surgery Clinics of North America* 13, no. 1 (2003): 79–94.

ORGANIZATIONS

American Board of Surgery. 1617 John F. Kennedy Boulevard, Suite 860, Philadelphia, PA 19103. (215) 568-4000. Fax: (215) 563-5718. http://www.absurgery.org.

American Cancer Society. 1599 Clifton Rd. NE, Atlanta, GA 30329. (800) 227-2345. http://www.cancer.org.

American College of Surgeons. 633 North St. Clair Street, Chicago, IL 60611-32311. (312) 202-5000. Fax: (312) 202-5001. postmaster@facs.org. http://www.facs.org.

American Lung Association. 1740 Broadway, New York, NY 10019-4374. (800) 586-4872. http://www.lungusa.org.

American Medical Association. 515 N. State Street, Chicago, IL 60610. (312) 464-5000. http://www.ama-assn.org.

Society of Thoracic Surgeons. 633 N. Saint Clair St., Suite 2320, Chicago, IL 60611-3658. (312) 202-5800. Fax: (312) 202-5801. <sts@sts.org>. http://www.sts.org.

OTHER

Creighton University School of Medicine. [cited May 14, 2003]. <http://medicine.creighton.edu/forpatients/mediast/mediastin.html>.

Harvard University Medical School. [cited May 14, 2003]. http://www.health.harvard.edu/fhg/diagnostics/mediastinoscopy/mediastinoscopy.shtml.

Merck Manual. [cited May 14, 2003]. http://www.merck.com/pubs/mmanual/section6/chapter65/65i.htm.

University of Missouri. [cited May 14, 2003]. http://www.ellisfischel.org/thoracic/testing/mediastinoscopy.shtml.

L. Fleming Fallon, Jr., M.D., Dr.PH.

Medicaid

Definition

Medicaid is a federal-state entitlement program for low-income citizens of the United States. The Medicaid program is part of Title XIX of the Social Security Act Amendment that became law in 1965. Medicaid offers federal matching funds to states for costs incurred in paying health care providers for serving covered individuals. State participation is voluntary, but since 1982, all 50 states have chosen to participate in Medicaid.

Description

Medicaid benefits

Medicaid benefits cover basic health care and long-term care services for eligible persons. About 58% of Medicaid spending covers hospital and other acute care services. The remaining 42% pays for nursing home and long-term care.

States that choose to participate in Medicaid must offer the following basic services:

KEY TERMS

Categorically needy—A term that describes certain groups of Medicaid recipients who qualify for the basic mandatory package of Medicaid benefits. There are categorically needy groups that states participating in Medicaid are required to cover, and other groups that the states have the option to cover.

Department of Health and Human Service (DHHS)—It is a federal agency that houses the Centers for Medicare and Medicaid Services, and distributes funds for Medicaid.

Entitlement—A program that creates a legal obligation by the federal government to any person, business, or government entity that meets the legally defined criteria. Medicaid is an entitlement both for eligible individuals and for the states that decide to participate in it.

Federal poverty level (FPL)—The definition of poverty provided by the federal government, used as the reference point to determine Medicaid eligibility for certain groups of beneficiaries. The FPL is adjusted every year to allow for inflation.

Health Care Financing Administration (HCFA)—A federal agency that provides guidelines for the Medicaid program.

Medically needy—A term that describes a group whose coverage is optional with the states because of high medical expenses. These persons meet category requirements of Medicaid (they are children or parents or elderly or disabled) but their income is too high to qualify them for coverage as categorically needy.

Supplemental Security Income (SSI)—A federal entitlement program that provides cash assistance to low-income blind, disabled, and elderly people. In most states, people receiving SSI benefits are eligible for Medicaid.

- hospital care, both inpatient and outpatient
- nursing home care
- physician services
- laboratory and diagnostic x-ray services
- immunizations and other screening, diagnostic, and treatment services for children
- family planning
- health center and rural health clinic services
- nurse midwife and nurse practitioner services
- physician assistant services

Participating states may offer the following optional services and receive federal matching funds for them:

- prescription medications
- institutional care for the mentally retarded
- home- or community-based care for the elderly, including case management
- personal care for the disabled
- dental and vision care for eligible adults

Because participating states are allowed to design their own benefits packages as long as they meet federal minimum requirements, Medicaid benefits vary considerably from state to state. About half of all Medicaid spending covers groups of people and services above the federal minimum.

Eligibility for Medicaid

Medicaid covers three major groups of low-income Americans:

- All recipients. In 2006, Medicaid covered an estimated 46.5 million low-income persons in the United States.
- Parents and children. In 2005, Medicaid covered approximately 25.2 million low-income children, approximately one-fifth of all children in the United States. It provided coverage to an estimated 10.2 million low-income adults in families with children; most of these low-income adults were women.
- The elderly. In 2006, Medicaid covered an estimated 5.8 million adults over the age of 65. Medicaid is the largest single purchaser of long-term and nursing home care in the United States.
- The disabled. About 17% of Medicaid recipients are blind or disabled. Most of these persons are eligible for Medicaid because they receive assistance through the Supplemental Security Income (SSI) program.

All Medicaid recipients must have incomes and resources below specified eligibility levels. These levels vary from state to state depending on the local cost of living and other factors. For example, in 2006, the federal poverty level (FPL) was determined to be $16,600 for a family of three on the mainland of the United States, but $24,900 in Hawaii and $29,050 in Alaska.

In most cases, persons must be citizens of the United States to be eligible for Medicaid, although legal immigrants may qualify in some circumstances depending on their date of entry. Illegal aliens are not eligible for Medicaid, except for emergency care.

Persons must fit into an eligibility category to receive Medicaid, even if their income is low. Childless couples and single childless adults who are not disabled or elderly are not eligible for Medicaid.

Medicaid costs

Medicaid is by far the government's most expensive general welfare program. In 1966, Medicaid accounted for 1.4% of the federal budget, but by 2006, its share had risen to nearly 9.1%. Combined federal and state spending for Medicaid takes approximately 21 cents of every tax dollar. The federal government covers about 56% of costs associated with Medicaid. The states pay for the remaining 44%.

As of 2006, costs for Medicaid continued to rise at an average annual rate of approximately 8%. The states spent $303 billion in FY 2006 to cover Medicaid costs. These costs are projected to continue to increase.

Although more than half (54%) of all Medicaid beneficiaries are children, most of the money (more than 70%) goes for services for the elderly and disabled. The single largest portion of Medicaid money pays for long-term care for the elderly. Only 18% of Medicaid funds are spent on services for children.

There are several factors involved in the steep rise of Medicaid costs:

- The rise in the number of eligible individuals. As the lifespan of most Americans continues to increase, the number of elderly individuals eligible for Medicaid also rises. The fastest-growing age group in the United States is people over 85.
- The price of medical and long-term care. Advances in medical technology, including expensive diagnostic imaging tests, cause these costs to rise.
- The increased use of services covered by Medicaid.
- The expansion of state coverage from the minimum benefits package to include optional groups and optional services.

Normal results

The need to contain Medicaid costs is considered one of the most problematic policy issues facing legislators. In addition, the complexity of the Medicaid system, its vulnerability to billing fraud and other abuses, the confusing variety of the benefits packages available in different states, and the time-consuming paperwork are other problems that disturb both taxpayers and legislators.

Medicaid has increased the demand for health care services in the United States without greatly impacting or improving the quality of health care for low-income Americans. Medicaid is the largest health insurer in the United States. As such, it affects the employment of several hundred thousand health care workers, including health care providers, administrators, and support staff. Participation in Medicaid is optional for physicians and **nursing homes**. Many do not participate in the program because the reimbursement rates are low. As a result, many low-income people who are dependent on Medicaid must go to overcrowded facilities where they often receive substandard health care.

Resources

BOOKS

Atlantic Publishing Company. The Complete Guide to Medicaid and Nursing Home Costs: How to Keep Your Family Assets Protected - Up to Date Medicaid Secrets You Need to Know. Ocala, FL: Atlantic Pub Co, 2008.

Engel, J. Poor People's Medicine: Medicaid and American Charity Care since 1965. Durham, NC: Duke University Press, 2006.

Scott, S. W. The Medicaid Handbook 2007: Protecting Your Assets From Nursing Home Costs. 3rd ed. Largo, FL: Masveritas Publishing, 2007.

Smith, D., and J. D. Moore. Medicaid Politics and Policy. New Brunswick, NJ: Transaction Publishers, 2007.

PERIODICALS

Bhuridej, P., KR. A. Kuthy, S. D. Flach, K. E. Keller, D. V. Dawson, M. J. Kanellis, and P. C. Damiano. "Four-year cost-utility analyses of sealed and nonsealed first permanent molars in Iowa Medicaid-enrolled children." Journal of Public Health Dentistry 67, no. 4 (2007): 191–198.

Churchill, S. S., B. J. Williams, and N. L. Villareale. "Characteristics of publicly insured children with high dental expenses." Journal of Public Health Dentistry 67, no. 4 (2007): 199–207.

Goetzel, R. Z., D. Schecter, R. J. Ozminkowski, D. C. Stapleton, P. J. Lapin, J. M. McGinnis, C. R. Gordon, and L. Breslow. "Can health promotion programs save Medicare money?." Clinical Interventions in Aging 2, no. 1 (2007): 117–122.

Grabowski, D. C. " Medicare and Medicaid: conflicting incentives for long-term care." Milbank Quaterly 85, no. 4 (2007): 579–610.

Perry, C. D., and G. M. Kenney. "Preventive care for children in low-income families: how well do Medicaid and state children's health insurance programs do?" Pediatrics 120, no. 6 (2007): e1393–e1401.

ORGANIZATIONS

Kaiser Family Foundation. 2400 Sand Hill Road, Menlo Park, CA 94025, Phone: (650) 854-9400, Fax: (650) 854-4800 http://www.kff.org/.

National Center for Policy Analysis. 12770 Coit Rd., Suite 800, Dallas, TX 75251-1339, Phone: (972) 386-6272, Fax: (972) 386-0924. http://www.ncpa.org.

National Library of Medicine. http://www.nlm.nih.gov/medlineplus/medicaid.html.

United States Department of Health and Human Services. 200 Independence Avenue SW, Washington, DC 20201. http://www.hhs.gov.

OTHER

Centers for Medicare and Medicaid Services, US Department of Health and Human Services. Information about Medicaid. 2007 [cited December 26, 2007]. http://cms.hhs.gov/.

National Association of State Medicaid Directors. Information about Medicaid. 2007 [cited December 26, 2007]. http://www.nasmd.org/Home/home_news.asp.

National Governor's Association. Information about Medicaid. 2007 [cited December 26, 2007]. http://www.nga.org/portal/site/nga.

Social Security Administration. Information about Medicaid. 2007 [cited December 26, 2007]. http://www.ssa. gov/.

L. Fleming Fallon, Jr, MD, DrPH

Medical charts

Definition

A medical chart is a confidential document that contains detailed and comprehensive information on an individual and the care experience related to that person. It is commonly called a medical record.

Purpose

The purpose of a medical chart is to serve as both a medical and legal record of an individual's clinical status, care, history, and caregiver involvement. The specific information contained in the chart is intended to provide a record of a person's clinical condition by detailing diagnoses, treatments, tests and responses to treatment, as well as any other factors that may affect the person's health or clinical state.

Demographics

Every person who has a professional relationship with a health-care provider has a medical record. Because most people have such relationships with more than one health professional or caregiver, most people actually have more than one medical chart.

Description

The terms medical chart or medical record are a general description of a collection of information on a person. However, different clinical settings and systems utilize different forms of documentation to achieve this purpose. As technology progresses, more institutions are adopting computerized systems that aid in clearer documentation, enhanced access and searching, and more efficient storage and retrieval of individual records.

New uses of technology have also raised concerns about confidentiality. Confidentiality, or personal privacy, is an important principle related to the chart. Whatever system may be in place, it is essential that the health-care provider protect an individual's privacy by limiting access only to authorized individuals. Generally, physicians and nurses write most frequently in the chart. Documentation by the clinician who is leading treatment decisions (usually a physician) often focuses on diagnosis and prognosis, while the documentation by members of the nursing team generally focuses on individual responses to treatment and details of day-to-day progress. In many institutions, the medical and nursing staff may complete separate forms or areas of the chart specific to their disciplines.

Other health-care professionals that have access to the chart include physician assistants; social workers; psychologists; nutritionists; physical, occupational, speech, or respiratory therapists; and consultants. It is important that the various disciplines view the notes written by other specialties in order to form a complete picture of a person and provide continuity of care. Quality assurance and regulatory organizations, legal bodies, and insurance companies may also have access to the chart for specific purposes such as documentation, institutional audits, legal proceedings, or verification of information for care reimbursement. It is important to know about institutional policies regarding chart access in order to ensure the privacy of personal records.

The medical record should be stored in a pre-designated, secure area and discussed only in appropriate and private clinical areas. All individuals have a right to view and obtain copies of their own records. Special state statutes may cover especially sensitive information such as psychiatric, communicable disease

KEY TERMS

Consultation—Evaluation by an outside expert or specialist, someone other than the primary care provider.

Continuity—Consistency or coordination of details.

Discipline—In health care, a specific area of preparation or training such as social work, nursing, or nutrition.

Documentation—The process of recording information in the medical chart, or the materials contained in a medical chart.

Interdisciplinary—Consisting of several interacting disciplines that work together to care for an individual.

Objective—Not biased by personal opinion; repeatable.

Prognosis—Expected resolution or outcome of an illness or injury.

Regulatory organization—Organization designed to maintain or control quality in health care.

Subjective—Influenced by personal opinion, bias, or experience; not reliably repeatable.

(i.e., HIV), or substance abuse records. Institutional and government policies govern what is contained in the chart, how it is documented, who has access, and policies for regulating access to the chart and protecting its integrity and confidentiality. In those cases in which individuals outside of the immediate care system must access chart contents, an individual or personal representative is asked to provide permission before records can be released. Individuals are often asked to sign these releases so that caregivers in new clinical settings may review their charts.

Diagnosis/Preparation

Training

Thorough training is essential prior to independent use of the medical chart. Whenever possible, a new clinician should spend time reviewing the chart to get a sense of organization and documentation format and style. Training programs for health-care professionals often include practice in writing notes or flow charts in mock medical records. Notes by trainees are often initially cosigned by supervisors to ensure accurate and relevant documentation and document-appropriate supervision.

Operation

Documentation in the medical record begins when an individual enters the care system, which may be a specific place such as a hospital or professional office, or a program such as a home health-care service. Frequently, a facility will request permission to obtain copies of previous records so that they have complete information on the person. Although chart systems vary from institution to institution, there are many aspects of the chart that are universal. Frequently used chart sections include the following:

- Admission paperwork. Includes legal paperwork such as a living will or health care proxy, consents for admission to the facility or program, demographics, and contact information.
- History and physical. Contains comprehensive review of an individual's medical history and physical examinations.
- Orders. Contains medication and treatment orders by the doctor, nurse practitioner, physician assistant, or other qualified health-care team members.
- Medication record. Documents all medications administered.
- Treatment record. Documents all treatments received such as dressing changes or respiratory therapy.
- Procedures. Summarizes diagnostic or therapeutic procedures, i.e., colonoscopy or open-heart surgery.
- Tests. Provides reports and results of diagnostic evaluations, such as laboratory tests and electrocardiography tracings or radiography images or summaries of test results.
- Progress notes. Includes regular notes on the individual's status by members of the interdisciplinary care team.
- Consultations. Contains notes from specialized diagnosticians or external care providers.
- Consents. Includes permissions signed by the individual for procedures, tests, or access to chart. May also contain releases such as the release signed by any person when leaving the facility against medical advice (AMA).
- Flow records. Tracks specific aspects of professional care that occur on a routine basis, using tables or in a chart format.
- Care plans. Documents treatment goals and plans for future care within a facility or following discharge.
- Discharge. Contains final instructions for the person and reports by the care team before the chart is closed and stored following discharge.
- Insurance information. Lists health care benefit coverage and insurance provider contact information.

These general categories may be further divided by individual facilities for their own purposes. For example, a psychiatric facility may use a special section for psychometric testing, or a hospital may provide sections specifically for operations, x-ray reports, or electrocardiograms. In addition, certain details such as allergies or do not resuscitate orders may be displayed prominently (for instance, with large colored stickers or special chart sections) on the chart in order to communicate uniquely important information. It is important for health-care providers to become familiar with the charting systems in place at their specific facilities or programs.

It is important that the information in the chart be clear and concise, so that those utilizing the record can easily access accurate information. The medical chart can also aid in clinical problem solving by tracking an individual's baseline, or status on admission or entry into an office or health care system; orders and treatments provided in response to specific problems; and individual responses. Another reason for the standard of clear documentation is the possibility that the record may be used in legal proceedings, when documentation serves as evidence in exploring and evaluating a person's care experience. When medical care is being referred to or questioned by the legal system, chart contents are frequently cited in court. For all of these purposes, certain practices that protect the integrity of the chart and provide essential information are recommended for adding information and maintaining the chart. These practices include the following:

- Date and time should be included on all entries.
- A person's full name and other identifiers (i.e., medical record number, date of birth) on all records.
- Continued records should be marked clearly (i.e., if a note is continued on the reverse side of a page).
- Each page of documentation should be signed.
- Blue or black non-erasable ink should be used on handwritten records.
- Records should be maintained in chronological order.
- Disposal or obliteration of any records or portions of records should be prevented.
- Documentation errors and corrections should be noted clearly, i.e., by drawing one line through the error and noting the presence of an error, and then initialing the area.
- Excess empty space should be avoided on the page. A line should be drawn through any unused space, the initial, time, and date included.
- Only universally accepted abbreviations should be used.

- Unclear documentation such as illegible penmanship should be avoided.
- Contradictory information should be avoided. For example, if a nurse documents that a person has complained of abdominal pain throughout a shift, while a physician documents that the person is free of pain, these discrepancies should be discussed and clarified. The resolution should be entered into the chart and signed by all parties involved in the disagreement.
- Objective rather than subjective information should be included. For example, personality conflicts between staff should not enter into the notes. All events involving an individual should be described as objectively as possible, i.e., describe a hostile person by simply stating the facts such as what the person said or did and surrounding circumstances or response of staff, without using derogatory or judgmental language.
- Any occurrence that might affect the person should be documented. Documented information is considered credible in court. Undocumented information is considered questionable since there is no written record of its occurrence.
- Current date and time should be used in documentation. For example, a note is added after the fact, it should be labeled as an addendum and inserted in correct chronological order, rather than trying to insert the information on the date of the actual occurrence.
- Actual statements of people should be recorded in quotes.
- The chart should never be left in an unprotected environment where unauthorized individuals may read or alter the contents.

Several methods of documentation have arisen in response to the need to accurately summarize a person's experience. In the critical care setting, flow records are often used to track frequent personal evaluations, checks of equipment, and changes of equipment settings that are required. Flow records also offer the advantages of displaying a large amount of information in a relatively small space and allowing for quick comparisons. Flow records can also save time for a busy clinician by allowing for the completion of checklists versus requiring written narrative notes.

Narrative progress notes, while more time consuming, are often the best way to capture specific information about an individual. Some institutions require only charting by exception (CBE), which requires notes only for significant or unusual findings. While this method may decrease repetition and lower

WHO PERFORMS THE PROCEDURE AND WHERE IS IT PERFORMED?

All members of a health-care team or individuals who render professional health-care services usually make entries into medical records. Health-care records are maintained in hospitals or other clinical settings and professional offices. Insurance companies and corporations may maintain limited health-care records or obtain copies of records created by other health-care providers.

required documentation time, most institutions that use CBE notes also require a separate flow record that documents regular contact with a person. Many facilities or programs require notes at regular intervals even when there is no significant occurrence, i.e., every nursing shift. Frequently used formats in individual notes include SOAP (subjective, objective, assessment, plan) notes. SOAP notes use an individual's subjective statement to capture an important aspect of care, follow with a key objective statement regarding the person's status, a description of the clinical assessment, and a plan for how to address individual problems or concerns. Focus charting and PIE (problem-intervention-evaluation) charting use similar systems of notes that begin with a particular focus such as a nursing diagnosis or an individual concern. Nursing diagnoses are often used as guides to nursing care by focusing on individual care-recipient needs and responses to treatment. An example of a nursing diagnosis is fluid volume for someone who is dehydrated. The notes would then focus on assessment for dehydration, interventions to address the problem, and a plan for continued care such as measurement of input and output and intravenous therapy.

Aftercare

Current medical charts are maintained by members of the health-care team and usually require clerical assistance such as a unit clerk in the hospital setting or records clerk in a professional office. No alterations should be made to the record unless they are required to clarify or correct information and are clearly marked as such. After discharge, the medical records department of a facility checks for completeness and retains the record. Similar checks may be made in professional office settings. Sometimes, the record will be made available in another format, i.e., recording paper charts on microfilm or computer

QUESTIONS TO ASK THE DOCTOR

- In a particular setting, who has the authority to make entries in a medical chart?
- Who has access to the chart?
- How is security maintained for medical records?

imaging. Institutional policies and state laws govern storage of charts on- and off-site and length of storage time required.

Risks

A major potential risk associated with medical charts is breach of confidentiality. This must be safeguarded at all times. Other risks include loss of materials in a chart or incorrectly filing a chart so that subsequent retrieval is impeded or impossible.

Normal results

All members of a health-care team require thorough understanding of the medical chart and documentation guidelines in order to provide competent care and maintain a clear, concise, and pertinent record. Health care systems often employ methods to guarantee thorough and continuous use and review of charts across disciplines. For example, nursing staff may be required to sign below every new physician order to indicate that this information has been communicated, or internal quality assurance teams may study groups of charts to determine trends in missing or unclear documentation. In legal settings, health-care team members may be called upon to interpret or explain chart notations as they relate to a specific legal case.

Morbidity and mortality rates

Medical charts are made of paper or other materials. They are subject to deterioration or loss. Transporting them may cause lifting injuries, but not lead to disease or **death**.

Alternatives

There are no alternatives for medical charts. Alternative mediums exist for paper records. These include fixing images on plastic media (photographs or x rays) or electronic storage. The latter can include magnetic tape or computer disks.

Resources

BOOKS

Gartee, R. W. Electronic Health Records: Understanding and Using Computerized Medical Records. Upper Saddle River, NJ: Prentice Hall, 2006.

Goldstein, D., P. J. Groen, S. Ponkshe, and M. Wine. Medical Informatics 20/20: Quality And Electronic Health Records Through Collaboration, Open Solutions, And Innovation. Sudbury, MA: Jones and Bartlett, 2007.

Maki, S. E., and Patterson, B. Using the Electronic Health Record in the Healthcare Provider Practice. Florence, KY: CENGAGE Delmar, 2007.

Scott, T., T. G. Rundall, T. M. Vogt, and J. Hsu. Implementing an Electronic Medical Record System: Successes, Failtures, Lessons. Oxford, UK: Radcliffe Medical Press, 2007.

Walker, J. M., E. J. Bieber, F. Richards, and S. Buckley. Implementing an Electronic Health Record System. New York: Springer, 2006.

PERIODICALS

Arar, N. H., C. P. Wang, and J. A. Pugh. "Self-Care Communication during Medical Encounters: Implications for Future Electronic Medical Records." Perspectives in Health Information Management 24, no. 3 (2006): 3–11.

Callan, C. M., and C. V. DeSHazo. "How to navigate health care information technology and electronic medical records." Physician Executive 33, no. 6 (2007): 36–42.

Kizer, K. W. "The adoption of electronic health records: benefits and challenges." Annals of Health Care Law 16, no. 2 (2007): 323–334.

Recupero, P. R. "Ethics of medical records and professional communications." Child and Adolescent Psychiatric Clinics of North America 17, no. 1 (2008): 37–51.

ORGANIZATIONS

American Academy of Family Physicians. 11400 Tomahawk Creek Parkway, Leawood, KS 66211-2672. (913) 906-6000. <fp@aafp.org>. http://www.aafp.org.

American Academy of Pediatrics. 141 Northwest Point Boulevard, Elk Grove Village, IL 60007-1098. (847) 434-4000. Fax: (847) 434-8000. kidsdoc@aap.org. http://www.aap.org/default.htm.

American College of Physicians. 190 N Independence Mall West, Philadelphia, PA 19106-1572. (800) 523-1546, x2600, or (215) 351-2600. http://www.acponline.org.

American Hospital Association. One North Franklin, Chicago, IL 60606-3421. (312) 422-3000. http://www.aha.org/aha_app/index.jsp.

American Medical Association. 515 N. State Street, Chicago, IL 60610. (312) 464-5000. http://www.ama-assn.org.

American Medical Informatics Association. 4915 St. Elmo Avenue, Suite 401, Bethesda, MD 20814. (301) 657-1291. Fax: (301) 657-1296. http://www.amia.org.

OTHER

Electronic Privacy Information Center. Information about Electronic Medical Records. 2007 [cited December 27, 2007]. http://www.epic.org/privacy/medical/.

Privacy Rights Clearinghouse. Information about Medical Privacy Resources. 2007 [cited December 28, 2007]. http://www.privacyrights.org/medical.htm.

American Medical Association. Information about Electronic Medical Records. 2007 [cited December 27, 2007]. http://www.ama-assn.org/amednews/site/topic.htm.

Georgetown University Center on Medical Record Rights and Privacy. Information about Medical Record Privacy. 2007 [cited December 28, 2007]. http://ihcrp.georgetown.edu/privacy/records.html.

L. Fleming Fallon, Jr, MD, DrPH

Medical co-morbidities

Definition

Morbidity is the presence of a disease state or disorder within a patient. Co-morbidity is the presence of more than one individual disease or disorder within the same patient. It is a state of having multiple distinct medical conditions at the same time.

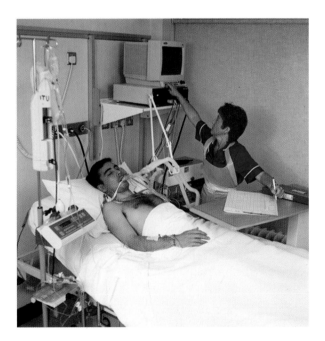

(Medical-on-Line / Alamy)

Demographic

Co-morbidities may be present in anyone regardless of age, but certain populations are more prone to having co-morbidities. Patients that are an advanced age are more vulnerable to medical problems than a younger patient demographic. Certain medical conditions are also prone to association with co-morbidities. For example, diabetes, psychiatric diseases, and cancer (especially in the elderly) are very frequently associated with co-morbid health conditions.

Description

Co-existing or co-morbid conditions are sometimes commonly associated with a particular disease. For example, cancer patients may frequently have co-existing major depression. Diabetes patients may frequently have co-morbidities involving the cardiovascular system, kidney, and the eye. Chronic diseases are often co-morbid with depression.

Having co-morbidities also increases the risks associated with some surgical procedures. Co-morbidities may complicate the diagnosis of a new disease, especially if there are overlapping symptoms between the two. Co-morbidities have an impact on the type of treatment chosen for a patient, as well as the patient's prognosis. A patient's disease burden may have a health impact that is greater than the sum of the impact of the individual diseases. The medical outcome of co-morbid conditions may be very severe.

The Charlson Co-morbidity Index

There are many systems that endeavor to standardize the "weight" of the medical impact of different co-morbidities. The end result is to predict the medical outcome or mortality that may result from the presence of specific co-morbidities. There are no systems that have currently been developed that accurately and completely assess this issue and are considered a true medical standard. However, one commonly used system is the Charlson Index, which has been validated and is the most widely accepted of the assessments.

The Charlson Co-morbidity Index attempts to predict the one-year mortality for patients with more than one medical disease or disorder. Each medical condition is categorized according to a set of codes known as the International Statistical Classification of Diseases and Related Health Problems, or ICD Codes. Each ICD Code represents a medical condition and is assigned a specific number that represents the medical weight of the disease. The score assigned to each disease is based on the risk of fatality within one

year associated with the disease. Additional points may be added for age, with each decade over forty being one point. The sum of the scores for each co-morbidity gives a total score that represents the risk of **dying**. The higher the score, the greater the risk of dying. This score assists physicians in determining how to treat patients with multiple co-morbidities. For example, if one patient has cancer, but also very severe co-morbidities, it may not be appropriate to subject the patient to difficult treatments because of the reduced likelihood of survival associated with the co-morbidity.

Co-morbidity of Psychiatry

In psychiatry, a co-morbidity is defined as a diagnosis that exists simultaneously with another diagnosis. However, psychiatric co-morbidities may not represent the presence of multiple disorders. Rather they represent the number of diagnoses necessary to accurately describe the full range of the patient's symptoms. The severity of a patient's mental illness has a strong association with the number of co-morbid disorders present. Treatment of psychiatric diseases and disorders are impacted by co-morbidity, as the co-morbidity may render the normal treatment of an illness inappropriate. For example, some pharmaceutical treatments may cause symptoms of anxiety as a side effect. In a patient with an anxiety disorder as a co-morbidity, using this treatment for their primary illness would be inappropriate. Pharmaceutical treatments that have addictive potential are not appropriate for treatment of a primary illness in a patient with drug abuse as a co-morbidity. Drug abuse is often co-morbid with psychiatric disorders, and may be a consequence of the initial illness. Studies have shown that proper treatment of some psychiatric disorders may prevent the development of drug abuse problems.

Providing treatment for patients with co-morbidities that address and do not aggravate all the aspects of their various disorders can be challenging for health care providers. Co-morbidities in psychiatry can be controversial to diagnose as distinct disorders. For example, does a patient with drug abuse problems as well as bulimia (binging on food and then purging through vomiting) have two separate illnesses, or do they have a single disorder involving impulse control? Whether some co-morbidities are truly separate diagnoses or all part of one disorder can be difficult to judge.

Co-morbidity of Diabetes

Diabetes is associated with many different co-morbidities. The increased blood glucose that is part

QUESTIONS TO ASK YOUR DOCTOR

- Do I have co-morbid health conditions?
- Are my co-morbidities truly distinct from each other, or could they be related?
- What can I do to address health concerns regarding my co-morbid conditions?
- Do any of my treatments for primary illness have an adverse impact on one of my co-morbid health conditions?
- Do any of my co-morbidities have an adverse impact on treatment for my primary illness?

KEY TERMS

Bulimia—Psychiatric disorder involving eating large amounts of food in a short time period and then vomiting to purge the contents of the stomach.

Cardiovascular System—The physiological system including the heart and the blood vessels.

Metabolic Syndrome—A combination of medical disorders including diabetes, high blood pressure, and heart disease.

Pulmonary Disease—Disease involving the lungs.

of the disease process can be very damaging to the blood vessels and the organ systems. Some of the co-morbidities associated with diabetes were previously believed to be separate from the course of the diabetes disease. It is controversial whether the co-morbidities associated with diabetes are distinct diseases or are a result of the diabetes itself, which is increasingly referred to as "metabolic syndrome". Regardless of their source, the co-morbidities associated with diabetes have a significant impact on the overall health profile of the patient.

Patients with diabetes often develop vascular complications, which are medical problems of the blood vessels. Damaged blood vessels are a serious complication, as they affect all the organ systems. Excess blood glucose can also directly damage organs. In diabetics, there are often medical complications seen with the kidneys, the retina of the eye, the peripheral nervous system, heart disease, and stroke or peripheral artery disease. Tight control of blood glucose levels may help to prevent the development of complications and these co-morbidities of diabetes.

Co-morbidity of Cancer in Elderly Patients

Patients above 65 years of age statistically bear a large proportion of cancer cases seen in the United States. In addition to cancer, the elderly are vulnerable to many different health conditions such as pulmonary disease, heart disease, and hypertension. Having co-morbidities with cancer has a great impact on decisions made by the patient and the physician regarding treatment choices. When an elderly person is newly diagnosed with cancer and has other existing medical conditions, each health problem needs to be evaluated in the context of its predicted impact on the course of the cancer. Awareness and evaluation of co-

morbidities is crucial to optimize care of a cancer patient, and may alter the appropriateness of treatment options. Quality of life, limiting the potential complications seen with treatment, and preventing recurrence of cancer are all impacted by how the co-morbidities are managed.

The existence of co-morbidities with cancer also affects the patient's prognosis for survival. Because of this, physicians must often make treatment choices in the context of the likelihood of survival. For example a physician and patient may need to decide whether it is worth putting the patient through the rigors of chemotherapy, when congestive heart failure may already be severely limiting the patient's life span in the short term. In some cases, the cancer treatment may cause mortality because of the co-morbidities. The co-morbidity may increase and amplify the adverse effects normally seen with some types of cancer treatment. This may limit the amount of medical assistance available to a cancer patient. Depending on their nature and severity, co-morbidities in cancer may create a far more severe overall health profile and prognosis for a patient.

Resources

BOOKS

Diagnostic and Statistical Manual of Mental Disorders, Fourth Edition, Text Revision (DSM-IV-TR). Washington, DC: American Psychiatric Association; 2000.

Kumar, Vinay, Nelson Fausto, and Abul Abbas. *Robbins & Cotran: Pathologic Basis of Disease,* Seventh Edition. Saunders, Elsevier, 2005.

The Merck Manual of Diagnosis and Therapy, Eighteenth Edition. 2006.

PERIODICALS

Hall, H., R. Ramachandran, S. Narayan, A. B. Jani, and S. Vijayakumar. "An electronic application for rapidly calculating Charlson comorbidity score." *BMC Cancer* 2004; 4(94)doi:10.1186/1471-2407-4-94

Pincus, H. A., J. D. Tew, M. B. First. "Psychiatric comorbidity: is more less?" *World Psychiatry* 2004;3(1):18-23.

Yancik, R., P. A. Ganz, C. G. Varricchio, B. Conley. "Perspectives on Comorbidity and Cancer in Older Patients: Approaches to Expand the Knowledge Base." *J Clin Oncol* 2001;19:1147-51.

OTHER

Bankhead, Charles. "Comorbidity Can Confound Prostate Cancer Treatment." MedPage Today. January 22, 2008. http://www.medpagetoday.com/urology/prostatecancer/tb/8061 [Accessed April 15, 2008].

Maria Basile, PhD

Medical errors

Introduction and definitions

The subject of medical errors is not a new one. However, it did not come to widespread attention in the United States until the 1990s, when government-sponsored research about the problem was undertaken by two physicians, Lucian Leape and David Bates. In 1999, a report compiled by the Committee on Quality of Health Care in America and published by the Institute of Medicine (IOM) made headlines with its findings. As a result of the IOM report, President Clinton asked the Quality Interagency Coordination Task Force (QuIC) to analyze the problem of medical errors and patient safety, and make recommendations for improvement. The Report to the President on Medical Errors was published in February 2000.

It is important to understand the terms used by the government and health care professionals in describing medical errors in order to distinguish between injury or **death** resulting from mistakes made by people on the one hand, and unfortunate results of treatment on the other. Some allergic reactions to medications or failures to respond to cancer treatment, for example, result from physical differences among patients or the known side effects of certain treatments, and not from prescribing the wrong drug or therapy for the patient's condition. This type of negative outcome is called an adverse event in official documents. Adverse events can be defined as undesirable and unintentional, though not necessarily unexpected, results of medical treatment. An example of an adverse event is discomfort in an artificial joint that continues after the expected recovery period, or a chronic headache following a spinal tap.

A medical error, on the other hand, is an adverse event that could be prevented given the current state of medical knowledge. The QuIC task force expanded the IOM's working definition of a medical error to cover as many types of mistakes as possible. Their definition of a medical error is as follows: "The failure of a planned action to be completed as intended or the use of a wrong plan to achieve an aim. Errors can include problems in practice, products, procedures, and systems." The National Patient Safety Foundation (NPSF) prefers the term "healthcare error" to "medical error," and defines such errors as follows: "An unintended healthcare outcome caused by a defect in the delivery of care to a patient. Healthcare errors may be errors of commission (doing the wrong thing), omission (not doing the right thing), or execution (doing the right thing incorrectly)." A useful brief definition of a medical error is that it is a preventable adverse event.

Statistics

The statistics contained in the IOM report were startling. The authors of the report stated that between 45,000 and 98,000 Americans die each year as the result of medical errors. If the lower figure is used as an estimate, deaths in hospitals resulting from medical errors are the eighth leading cause of mortality in the United States, surpassing deaths attributable to motor vehicle accidents (43,458), breast cancer (42,297), and AIDS (16,516). Moreover, these figures refer only to hospitalized patients; they do not include people treated in outpatient clinics, **ambulatory surgery centers**, doctors' or dentists' offices, college or military health services, or **nursing homes**. Medical errors certainly occur outside hospitals; in 1999, the Massachusetts State Board of Registration in Pharmacy estimated that 2.4 million prescriptions are filled incorrectly each year in that state—which is only one of 50 states.

In terms of health-care costs, the IOM report estimated that medical errors cost the United States about $37.6 billion each year; about half this sum pays for direct health care.

Medical errors also carry a high psychological cost; according to a poll conducted by the National Patient Safety Foundation, 42% of the respondents had been affected personally by a medical error or had a friend or family member affected by one. The respondents rated the American health care system overall as only moderately safe, giving it a score of 4.9 on a 1–7 point scale, in which 7 was defined as very safe and 1 as very unsafe.

KEY TERMS

Adverse event—An undesirable and unintended result of a medical treatment or intervention.

Medical error—A preventable adverse event.

Systems analysis—An approach to medical errors and other management issues that looks for problems in the work process rather than singling out individuals as bad or incompetent.

The United States is not unique in having a high rate of medical errors. The United Kingdom, Australia, and Sweden are presently undertaking studies of their respective health-care systems. British experts estimate that 40,000 patients die each year in the United Kingdom as the result of medical errors. Australia has been testing a new system for reporting errors since 1995.

Description

There is no single universally accepted method of classifying medical errors in order to describe them more fully. The 2000 QuIC report lists five different classification schemes that have been used:

- type of health care given (medication, surgery, diagnostic imaging, etc.)
- severity of the injury (minor discomfort, serious injury, death, etc.)
- legal definitions (negligence, malpractice, etc.)
- setting (hospital, emergency room, intensive care unit, nursing home, etc.)
- persons involved (physician, nurse, pharmacist, patient, etc.)

The importance of these different ways to classify medical errors is their indication that different types of errors require different approaches to prevention and problem solving. For example, medication errors are often related to such communication problems as misspelled words or illegible handwriting, whereas surgical errors are often related to unclear or misinterpreted diagnostic images.

Causes of medical errors

The causes of medical errors are complex and not yet completely understood. Some causes that have been identified include the following:

- Communication errors. One widely publicized case from 1994 involved the death of a Boston newspaper columnist from an overdose of chemotherapy for breast cancer due to misinterpretation of the doctor's prescription; the patient was given four times the correct daily dose, when the doctor intended the dosage to be administered instead over a four-day period. Other cases involve medication mix-ups due to drugs with very similar names. The Food and Drug Administration (FDA) has identified no fewer than 600 pairs of look-alike or sound-alike drug names since 1992.
- The increasing specialization and fragmentation of health care. The more people involved in a patient's treatment, the greater the possibility that important information will be missing along the chain.
- Human errors resulting from overwork and burnout. For some years, hospital interns, residents, and nurses have attributed many of the errors made in patient care to the long hours they are expected to work, many times with inadequate sleep. With the coming of managed care, many hospitals have cut the size of their nursing staff and require those that remain to work mandatory overtime shifts. A study published in the *Journal of the American Medical Association* in October 2002 found a clear correlation between higher-than-average rates of patient mortality and higher-than-average ratios of patients to nurses.
- Manufacturing errors. Instances have been reported of blood products being mislabeled during the production process, resulting in patients being given transfusions of an incompatible blood type.
- Equipment failure. A typical example of equipment failure might be intravenous pump with a malfunctioning valve, which would allow too much of the patient's medication to be delivered over too short a time period.
- Diagnostic errors. A misdiagnosed illness can lead the doctor to prescribe an inappropriate type of treatment. Errors in interpreting diagnostic imaging have resulted in surgeons operating on the wrong side of the patient's body. Another common form of diagnostic error is failure to act on abnormal test results. As of 2006, studies of autopsies in the United States indicated that doctors misdiagnosed fatal illnesses about 20% of the time.
- Poorly designed buildings and facilities. Hallways that end in sharp right angles, for example, increase the likelihood of falls or collisions between people on foot and patients being wheeled to an operating room.

Ways of thinking about medical errors

One subject that has been emphasized in recent reports on medical errors is the need to move away from a search for individual culprits to blame for medical errors. This judgmental approach has sometimes been called the "name, shame, and blame game." It is characterized by the belief that medical errors result from inadequate training or from a few "bad apples" in the system. It is then assumed that medical errors can be reduced or eliminated by identifying the individuals at fault, and firing or disciplining them. The major drawback of this judgmental attitude is that it makes health-care workers hesitate to report errors for fear of losing their own jobs or fear of some other form of reprisal. As a result of underreporting, hospital managers and others concerned with patient safety often do not have an accurate picture of the frequency of occurrence of some types of medical errors.

Both the IOM report and the QuIC report urge the adoption of a model borrowed from industry that incorporates systems analysis. This model emphasizes making an entire system safer rather than punishing individuals; it assumes that most errors result from problems with procedures and work processes rather than bad or incompetent people; and it analyzes all parts of the system in order to improve them. The industrial model is sometimes referred to as the continuous quality improvement model (CQI). Hospitals that are implementing error-reduction programs based on the CQI model have found that a non-punitive procedure for reporting medical errors has improved morale among the staff as well as significantly reduced the number of medical errors. At Columbia-Presbyterian Hospital, for example, patients as well as staff can report medical errors via the Internet, a telephone hotline, or paper forms.

Proposals for improvement

Current proposals for reducing the rate of medical errors in the American health-care system include the following:

- Adopt stricter standards of acceptable error rates. One reason that industrial manufacturers have made great strides in product safety and error reduction is their commitment to improving the quality of the work process itself.
- Standardize medical equipment and build in mechanical safeguards against human error. Anesthesiology is the outstanding example of a medical specialty that has cut its error rate dramatically by asking medical equipment manufacturers to design ventilators with standardized controls and valves to prevent the oxygen content from falling below that of room air. These changes were the result of studies that showed that many medical errors resulted from doctors having to use unfamiliar ventilators and accidentally turning off the oxygen flow to the patient.

- Improve the working conditions for nurses and other hospital staff. Recommendations in this area include redesigning hospital facilities to improve efficiency and minimize falls and other accidents, as well as reducing the length of nursing shifts below 12.5 hours. Since 2003, residency programs for physicians have been redesigned to lower the risk of medical errors caused by human fatigue. These changes resulted from rules imposed in July 2003 by the Accreditation Council for Graduate Medical Education (ACGME). The rules limit residents to an 80-hour work week and 24 continuous hours on call, and guarantee one day off each week.
- Make use of new technology to improve accuracy in medication dosages and recording patients' vital signs. Innovations in this field include giving nurses and residents handheld computers for recording patient data so that they do not have to rely on human memory for so many details. Another innovation that helped Veterans Administration (VA) hospitals cut the rate of medication errors was the introduction of a handheld wireless bar-coding system. After the system went into operation at the end of 1998, the number of medication errors in VA hospitals dropped by 70%.
- Develop a nationwide database for error reporting and analysis. At present, there is no unified system for tracking different types of medical errors. An error in liver transplantation in August 2002 that cost the life of a baby led several researchers to recognize that there is still no national registry recording transplant mismatches. As a result, no one knows how many cases occur each year, let alone find ways to improve the present system.
- Encourage patients to become more active participants in their own health care. This recommendation includes asking more questions and requesting adequate explanations from health-care professionals, as well as reporting medical errors.
- Address the fact that both patients and physicians have emotional as well as knowledge-related needs around the issue of medical errors. A report published in the *Journal of the American Medical Association* in February 2003 stated that patients clearly want emotional support from their doctors following an error, including an apology. The researchers also found, however, that doctors are as upset when an error occurs and, additionally, are unsure where to turn for emotional support.
- Adopt a teamwork rather than an individualistic approach to medical care. According to an article

published in 2005 in the *Annals of Internal Medicine*, health care teams make fewer mistakes than individuals.

What patients can do

Patients are an important resource in lowering the rate of medical errors. The QuIC task force has put together some fact sheets to help patients improve the safety of their health care. One of these fact sheets, entitled "Five Steps to Safer Health Care," gives the following tips:

- Do not hesitate to ask questions of your health-care provider, and ask him or her for explanations that you can understand.
- Keep lists of all medications, including over-the-counter items as well as prescribed drugs.
- Ask for the results of all tests and procedures, and find out what the results mean for you.
- Find out what choices are available to you if your doctor recommends hospital care.
- If your doctor suggests surgery, ask for information about the procedure itself, the reasons for it, and exactly what will happen during the operation.

This fact sheet, as well as a longer and more detailed patient fact sheet on medical errors, is available for free download from the Agency for Health Research and Quality (AHRQ) Website, or by telephone order from the AHRQ Publications Clearinghouse at (800) 358-9295. In addition, the AHRQ has set up a patient safety network website at <http://www.psnet.ahrq.gov/index.aspx.> The website has an extensive list of resources ranging from online articles and fact sheets to links to audiovisual materials, journal articles, government reports, and other online materials. The site is produced and maintained by a team of editors at the University of California, San Francisco.

Resources

BOOKS

Committee on Quality of Health Care in America, Institute of Medicine. To Err Is Human: Building a Safer Health System. Washington, DC: National Academy Press, 2000.

Dhillon, B. S. Reliability Technology, Human Error, and Quality in Health Care. Boca Raton, FL: Taylor and Francis, 2007.

Peters, George A., and Barbara J. Peters. Medical Error and Patient Safety: Human Factors in Medicine. Boca Raton, FL: CRC Press/Taylor and Francis, 2008.

Woods, Michael S. Healing Words: The Power of Apology in Medicine, 2nd ed. Oakbrook Terrace, IL: Joint Commission Resources, 2007.

PERIODICALS

Aiken, Linda H., et al. "Hospital Nurse Staffing and Patient Mortality, Nurse Burnout, and Job Dissatisfaction." Journal of the American Medical Association 288 (October 23–30, 2002): 1987–1993.

Amalberti, René, Yves Auroy, Don Berwick, and Paul Barach. "Five System Barriers to Achieving Ultrasafe Health Care." Annals of Internal Medicine 142 (May 3, 2005): 756–764.

Cottrill, Ken. "Mistaken Identity: Barcoding Recommended to Combat Medical Errors." Traffic World (July 2, 2001).

Farley, Peter. "Redesigning the Residency." Yale Medicine 39 (Fall/Winter 2004): 22–24.

Friedman, Richard A. "Do Spelling and Penmanship Count? In Medicine, You Bet." New York Times March 11, 2003.

Gallagher, T. H., et al. "Patients' and Physicians' Attitudes Regarding the Disclosure of Medical Errors." Journal of the American Medical Association 289 (February 26, 2003): 1001–1007.

Gawande, Atul. "Annals of Medicine: The Checklist." New Yorker, December 10, 2007. Available online at http://www.newyorker.com/reporting/2007/12/10/071210fa_fact_gawande [cited January 7, 2008].

Grady, Denise, and Lawrence K. Altman. "Suit Says Transplant Error Was Cause in Baby's Death in August." New York Times March 12, 2003.

Hsia, David C. "Medicare Quality Improvement: Bad Apples or Bad Systems?" Journal of the American Medical Association 289 (January 15, 2003): 354–356.

Leonhardt, David. "Why Doctors So Often Get It Wrong." New York Times, February 22, 2006. Available online at http://www.nytimes.com/2006/02/22/business/22leonhardt.html [cited January 7, 2008].

Lockley, S. W., L. K. Barger, N. T. Ayas, et al. "Effects of Health Care Provider Work Hours and Sleep Deprivation on Safety and Performance." Joint Commission Journal on Quality and Patient Safety 33 (November 2007): 7–18.

Olden, P. C., and W. C. McCaughrin. "Designing Healthcare Organizations to Reduce Medical Errors and Enhance Patient Safety." Hospital Topics 85 (Fall 2007): 4–9.

Pyzdek, Thomas. "Motorola's Six Sigma Program." Quality Digest (December, 1997).

ORGANIZATIONS

Agency for Healthcare Research and Quality (AHRQ). 540 Gaither Road, Rockville, MD 20850. (301) 427-1364. <http://www.ahrq.gov/>.

Institute of Medicine (IOM). The National Academies. 500 Fifth Street, NW, Washington, DC 20001. www.iom. edu.

National Patient Safety Foundation (NPSF). 132 MASS MoCA Way, North Adams, MA 01247. (413) 663-8900. <http://www.npsf.org/>.

United States Food and Drug Administration (FDA). 5600
Fishers Lane, Rockville, MD 20857-0001. (888) 463-
6332. www.fda.gov.

OTHER

Agency for Healthcare Research and Quality (AHRQ) Fact
Sheet. Medical Errors: The Scope of the Problem.
Publication No. AHRQ 00-PO37.

Agency for Healthcare Research and Quality (AHRQ)
Patient Fact Sheet. 20 Tips to Help Prevent Medical
Errors. Publication No. AHRQ 00-PO38.

Burton, Susan. "The Biggest Mistake of Their Lives." New
York Times, March 16, 2003. www.nytimes.com/2003/
03/16/magazine/16MISTAKE.html.

Quality Interagency Coordination Task Force (QuIC)
Patient Fact Sheet. Five Steps to Safer Health Care,
January 2001 [cited March 17, 2003]. www.ahrq.gov/
consumer/5steps.htm.

Report of the Quality Interagency Coordination Task Force
(QuIC) to the President. Doing What Counts for
Patient Safety: Federal Actions to Reduce Medical
Errors and Their Impact, 2000.

Rebecca Frey, PhD

Medical history *see* **Health history**

Medicare

Definition

Medicare is a national health insurance program
created and administered by the federal government in
the United States to address the medical needs of older
American citizens. Medicare is available to U.S. citizens 65 years of age and older and some people with
disabilities under age 65.

Description

Medicare is the largest health insurance program
in the United States. The program was created as part
of the Social Security Act Amendment in 1965 and was
put into effect in 1966. At the end of 1966, Medicare
served approximately 3.9 million individuals. As of
2003, it serves about 41 million people. There are 5.6
million Medicare beneficiaries enrolled in managed
care programs.

In 1973, the Medicare program was expanded to
include people who have permanent kidney failure and
need dialysis or transplants and people under the age of
65 who have specific types of disabilities. Medicare was
originally administered by the Social Security Administration, but in 1977, the program was transferred to

KEY TERMS

DHHS—The Department of Health and Human
Service. This federal agency houses the Centers
for Medicare and Medicaid Services and distributes
funds for Medicaid.

Entitlement—A program that creates a legal obligation by the federal government to any person,
business, or government entity that meets the
legally defined criteria. Medicare is an entitlement
for eligible individuals.

HCFA—Health Care Financing Administration. A
federal agency that provides guidelines for the
Medicaid program.

Medicare Part A—Hospital insurance provided by
Medicare, provided free to persons aged 65 and
older.

Medicare Part B—Medical insurance provided by
Medicare that requires recipients to pay a monthly
premium. Part B pays for some medical services
Part A does not.

the Health Care Financing Administration (HCFA),
which is part of the United States Department of
Health and Human Services (DHHS). The Centers for
Medicare and **Medicaid** Services, an agency of the
DHHS, is the administrative agency. This agency also
administers Medicaid programs.

Medicare is an entitlement program similar to
Social Security and is not based on financial need.
Medicare benefits are available to all American citizens over the age of 65 because they or their spouses
have paid Social Security taxes through their working
years. Since Medicare is a federal program, the rules
for eligibility remain constant throughout the nation
and coverage remains constant regardless of where an
individual receives treatment in the United States.

Medicare benefits are divided into two different
categories referred to as Part A and Part B. Medicare
Part A is hospital insurance that provides basic coverage for hospital stays and post-hospital nursing facilities, home health care, and **hospice** care for terminally
ill patients. Most people automatically receive Part A
when they turn 65 and do not have to pay a premium
because they or their spouse paid Medicare taxes while
they were working.

Medicare Part B is medical insurance. It covers
most fees associated with basic doctor visits and laboratory testing. It also pays for some outpatient medical

services such as medical equipment, supplies, and home health care and physical therapy. However, these services and supplies are only covered by Part B when medically necessary and prescribed by a doctor. Enrollment in Part B is optional and the Medicare recipient pays a premium of approximately $65 per month for these added benefits. The amount of the premium is periodically adjusted. Not every person who receives Medicare Part A enrolls in Part B.

Although Medicare provides fairly broad coverage of medical treatment, neither Part A nor B pays for the cost of prescription drugs or other medications.

Medicare is funded solely by the federal government. States do not make matching contributions to the Medicare fund. Social Security contributions, monthly premiums paid by program participants, and general government revenues generate the money used to support the Medicare program. Insurance coverage provided by Medicare is similar to that provided by private health insurance carriers. Medicare usually pays 50–80% of the medical bill, while the recipient pays the remaining balance for services provided.

Normal results

As the population of the United States ages, concerns about health care and the financing of quality health care for all members of the elderly population grow. One concern is that health insurance provided by the Medicare program will become obsolete or will be cut from the federal budget in an attempt to save money. Another concern is that money provided by the Social Security Administration for Medicare will be depleted before the aging population of the United States can actually benefit from the taxes they are now paying. A third concern is coverage for prescription medications.

During the Clinton administration, several initiatives were started that saved funds for Medicare. The DHHS also supports several initiatives to save and improve the program. However, continuance of the federal health insurance program is still a problem that American citizens expect legislators to resolve.

During the George W. Bush administration, there has been debate concerning coverage for prescription drugs. Health-care reformers suggest that prescription drugs be made available through the Medicare program due to the high cost of such medications. This debate has not been resolved as of early 2003, and legislation has not been enacted.

Some of the successful initiatives undertaken since 1992 include:

- Fighting fraud and abuse. Much attention has focused on Medicare abuse, fraud, and waste. As a result, overpayments were stopped, fraud was decreased, and abuse was investigated. This has saved the Medicare program approximately $500 million per year.

- Preserving the Medicare benefit. Due to aggressive action by the federal government, it is estimated that funds have been appropriated to keep Medicare viable through 2026.

- Supporting Preventive Medicine and the Healthy Aging Project. Medicare programs are supporting preventive medicine and diagnostic treatments in anticipation that preventive measures will improve the health of older Americans and thereby reduce health-care costs.

Medicare benefits and health care financing are major issues in the United States. Legislators and federal agencies continue to work on initiatives that will keep health-care programs in place and working for the good of American citizens.

Resources

BOOKS

Blumenthal, David and Jon Erickson. *Long-Term Care and Medicare Policy: Can We Improve the Continuity of Care?* Washington, DC: Brookings Institution Press, 2003.

Marmor, Theodore R. *The Politics of Medicare.* Second edition. Hawthorne, NY: Aldine de Gruyter, 2000.

Oberlander, Jonathan. *Political Life of Medicare.* Chicago: University of Chicago Press, 2003.

Pratt, David A. and Sean K. Hornbeck. *Social Security and Medicare Answer Book.* Gaithersburg, MD: Aspen, 2002.

Stevens, Robert and Rosemary Stevens. *Welfare Medicine in America: A Case Study of Medicaid.* Somerset, NJ: Transaction Publishers, 2003.

PERIODICALS

Charatan, Fred. "Bush proposes Medicare reform." *British Medical Journal* 326, no. 7389 (March 15, 2003): 570–572.

Hyman, David A. "Does Medicare care about quality? " *Perspectives in Biology and Medicine* 46, no. 1 (Winter 2003): 55–68.

Pulec, Jack L. "Medicare: all or nothing." *Ear Nose and Throat Journal* 82, no. 1 (January 2003): 7–8.

Smith, John J., and Leonard Berlin. "Medicare fraud and abuse." *American Journal of Roentgenology* 180, no. 3 (2003): 591–595.

ORGANIZATIONS

American College of Physicians, 190 North Independence Mall West, Philadelphia, PA 19106-1572. (800) 523-1546 x2600 or (215) 351-2600. http://www.acponline.org.

American College of Surgeons, 633 North St. Clair Street, Chicago, IL 60611-32311. (312) 202-5000 fax: (312) 202-5001. http://www.facs.org.

American Hospital Association, One North Franklin, Chicago, IL 60606-3421. (312) 422-3000 fax: (312) 422-4796. http://www.aha.org.

American Medical Association, 515 North State Street, Chicago, IL 60610. (312) 464-5000. http://www.ama-assn.org.

Center for Medicare Advocacy, P.O. Box 350, Willimantic, CT 06226. (860) 456-7790 or (202) 216-0028. http://www.medicareadvocacy.org.

OTHER

Centers for Medicare and Medicaid Services, U.S. Department of Health and Human Services. <http://cms.hhs.gov>.

Medicare Information Center, http://www.medicare.org.

Medicare Rights Center, http://www.medicarerights.org.

United States Government Medicare Information, http://www.medicare.gov.

L. Fleming Fallon, Jr., MD, DrPH

Medication Monitoring

Definition

Medication monitoring is the process of monitoring prescription medications to check that blood levels are within the expected and desired range, or the process of measuring the effects of a prescription medication in the blood.

Description

Medication monitoring is done by measuring blood levels of a drug or some aspect of a drug's effects. Some prescription drugs are very beneficial for health and may even be life saving, yet are very dangerous if even a small overdose is given. Because of this danger, drugs that are associated with severe or life threatening medical effects after a small overdose would not be available for use in medicine without a method by which to monitor their blood levels or their effects. Medication monitoring is a critical tool in the administration of these medications.

Therapeutic Index of Medications

All drugs may be dangerous if taken in great enough quantity. However for some drugs, the difference between a therapeutic dose and a dangerous or poisonous dose is smaller than others. The figurative "distance" between a medically effective and safe dose of a medication and its toxic dose is known as the therapeutic index or therapeutic window. Drugs with wide therapeutic windows require a greatly increased dose before they are toxic and are therefore safer to use than drugs with narrow therapeutic windows. Drugs with narrow therapeutic windows have a smaller difference in dose amount between their beneficial and harmful effects. If the therapeutic index of a drug is small enough, that drug may require medication monitoring techniques to be added as part of the treatment regimen to ensure that it is used safely.

Monitoring the Effects of Anticoagulants

Anticoagulant drugs are administered to inhibit the ability of the blood to form a blood clot, a process known as blood coagulation. Anticoagulants are not administered to dissolve existing blood clots, but rather to prevent the clotting process from forming a new blood clot or increasing an existing one. The most common health condition that may require anticoagulation drug therapy is a cardiac arrhythmia (abnormal heart rhythm) called atrial fibrillation. Atrial fibrillation is a rapid arrhythmia in a portion of the heart known as the atria, that may lead to a stroke. A stroke is a condition involving the inability of blood vessels in the brain to provide oxygen to brain tissue. A stroke may be caused by a blood clot blocking the blood vessel that supplies a part of the brain, thereby depriving the brain of oxygen and causing **death** of brain tissue. In atrial fibrillation, blood clots are sometimes knocked off of the heart tissue and travel through the blood to the brain, causing a stroke. Anticoagulant therapy may prevent a stroke by preventing the formation of blood clots. It may also prevent blood clots that could damage heart tissue or lead to a heart attack. The anticoagulant drug warfarin (coumadin) is most commonly used for this purpose.

While anticoagulant drugs have great benefit for prevention of stroke in atrial fibrillation, they can also be very dangerous. If the blood is kept too "thin" (via a decreased ability to clot), small wounds or a bump on the head may cause life threatening internal bleeding. Under normal conditions, these minor injuries would not cause excessive bleeding because the blood would clot and close the wound. With too great a dose of warfarin, minor injuries may become catastrophes. Even without injury, dangerous internal bleeding such as gastrointestinal bleeding or brain hemorrhages may occur. For this reason, the amount of warfarin given must only be the minimum necessary for treatment.

There is no one dose of warfarin that is safe and standardized for all patients. It must be individually determined, and the amount that is necessary may change frequently even within an individual. The effects of warfarin must be monitored at least weekly

QUESTIONS TO ASK YOUR DOCTOR

- Which of my medications needs to be routinely monitored?
- Why does this medication require monitoring?
- Why is this medication the best treatment option for my health condition?
- What are the effects of too much of this medication?
- How often do I need to come have my blood levels checked?
- Is the drug being measured in my blood, or an effect of the drug?

KEY TERMS

Atria—Plural for atrium.

Atrial Fibrillation—A dangerous heart condition involving a rapid, irregular heartbeat.

Atrium—Chamber of the heart that contains specialized heart cells that set the heartbeat.

Blood Serum—The fluid portion of the blood.

Cardiac Arrhythmia—An irregular heartbeat.

Coagulation—Blood clotting.

Epilepsy—A neurological disorder that involves uncontrolled seizures.

Gastrointestinal Tract—The path in the body from the mouth, through the stomach, intestines, rectum, and the anus.

Phlebitis—Inflammation of a vein.

Stroke—An event causing impairment of blood circulation to the brain, causing death of brain tissue and potentially drastically affecting mental functioning.

to ensure that too much has not been given (avoiding dangerous blood conditions) or that too little has been given to provide the therapeutic effect. Warfarin is not directly measured from blood samples, but rather the blood is examined for the degree of change in its blood clotting mechanisms. By measuring the effect of warfarin on the blood, doses can be tailored up or down to maintain a therapeutic but safe level. There is a very narrow window in which warfarin's effects are desirable, and it is very close to dangerous doses. Without medication monitoring techniques, warfarin could not be used to save lives in patients with heart conditions.

Monitoring Anticonvulsant Drugs

Anticonvulsant drugs are used to treat epilepsy, a type of neurological seizure disorder. The goal of anticonvulsant therapy is to provide seizure prevention without causing too many adverse side effects of drug treatment. Anticonvulsants such as phenytoin (dilantin) are beneficial for seizure patients, but also have a relatively narrow therapeutic index. Additionally, there is great variability in the way different patients metabolize the drug. Studies have shown that different patients taking the same dose of phenytoin may have up to a 50-fold difference in blood levels. There is also variability in the amount of drug needed to control seizure disorders in different patients within a safe range of doses. For all these reasons, there is no one dose that is standardized for all patients. Rather, the dose used for each patient varies widely, and needs to be individually tailored and monitored. The level of phenytoin may be directly measured in blood serum to make sure that blood levels are within the therapeutic range, and that they are not toxic levels. If blood levels of phenytoin are below what is considered a therapeutic range, doses are usually increased within safe limits even if the patient has not been experiencing seizures since initiating therapy.

Anticonvulsant drugs may be monitored when a patient first starts the drug to make sure they reach therapeutic levels, after a patient has been on the drug to make sure they are maintaining therapeutic and not toxic levels, or to explore symptoms of toxicity that may potentially be caused by the drug. Anticonvulsant drugs may also be monitored when the patient is experiencing seizures despite drug therapy. If levels of the current anticonvulsant are within the established therapeutic range of doses, then there may be need to assess whether to add other medications to the treatment regimen or switch to another medication entirely.

Risks of Medication Monitoring

There is very little risk associated with having blood drawn for medication monitoring. Most people have no side effects or a small bruise. However, with any blood draw there is a small chance that the area around the punctured vein may develop phlebitis, the inflammation of a vein. Phlebitis may also involve a bacterial infection if the site of the blood draw was not appropriately cleaned before the needle was inserted. Phlebitis can be locally painful but usually resolves in a short period of time.

Resources

BOOKS

Kumar, Vinay, Nelson Fausto, and Abul Abbas. *Robbins & Cotran: Pathologic Basis of Disease,* Seventh Edition. Saunders, Elsevier, 2005.

OTHER

"Anticoagulant Drugs." American Heart Association. October 22, 2007. http://www.americanheart.org/presenter.jhtml?identifier = 155 [Accessed April 15, 2008].

"Stroke." American Heart Association. http://www.americanheart.org/presenter.jhtml?identifier = 4755 [Accessed April 15, 2008].

Olson, K. R. "Toxicity, Warfarin and Superwarfarins." eMedicine. January 17, 2008. http://www.emedicine.com/emerg/topic872.htm [Accessed April 15, 2008].

Maria Basile, PhD

Meningocele repair

Definition

A meningocele repair is a surgical procedure performed to repair an abnormal opening in the spinal column (called spina bifida) by draining excess fluid and closing the opening.

Purpose

The surgery is necessary to close this abnormal opening in order to decrease the risk of infection and protect the integrity of the spinal column and the tissue inside.

Demographics

According to the Spina Bifida Association of America, spina bifida is both the most common neural tube defect and the most common birth defect resulting in permanent disability. It is estimated that about 40% of Americans have spina bifida occulta. However, some people who have it may have no symptoms and may therefore be unaware of their condition, so the percentage is an approximation. Meningocele and myelomeningocele are noticeable at birth and are paired together as spina bifida manifesta. Spina bifida manifesta occurs in about one in 1,000 births, with 4–5% occurring as meningocele and 95–96% occurring as myelomeningocele.

KEY TERMS

Folic acid—A water-soluable vitamin belonging to the B-complex group of vitamins.

Meninges—The membrane covering neural tissue.

Shunt—A shunt is a tube than is used to drain excess fluid. It is surgically implanted. The shunt drains the fluid from around the brain and sends it into the abdomen.

Description

The term meningocele may be used to refer to more than one condition. Spina bifida is a neural tube birth defect involving an abnormal opening in the spine. It occurs when the fetus's spine does not close properly during the first month of fetal development. In spina bifida occulta an opening in the spinal bones exists, but the neural tissue and membrane covering the spine (the meninges) are not exposed. Because there is no opening, the defect may appear as a dimple, or depression, at the base of the spine (the sacrum). Another sign of spina bifida occulta is the presence of tufts of hair at the sacrum. It is possible that while there is no opening, vertebrae are missing and there is damage to nerve tissue.

A meningocele is a sac protruding from the spinal column, which contains some of the spinal fluid and meninges. The sac may be covered with skin or with the meninges, and does not contain neural tissue. It may be located near the brain or along the spinal column. Hydrocephalus is rarely present, and the neurological examination may be normal. Because the neural tissue remains intact, it can be repaired by the experienced neurosurgeon, with excellent results.

A myelomeningocele is the most severe type of spina bifida because the spinal cord has herniated into the protruding sac. Neural tissue and nerves may be exposed. About 80% of myelomeningoceles occur at the lower back, where the lumbar and sacral regions join. Some people refer to myelomeningocele as spina bifida. Because of the exposed neural tissue, significant symptoms may be present. These symptoms may include:

- muscle weakness or paralysis in the hips and lower limbs
- no sensation in the part of the body below the defect
- lack of bowel and bladder function
- fluid build-up in the brain, known as hydrocephalus

Because of the risk of neural tissue damage, swelling, and infection into the spinal fluid and brain with an opening in the spinal column, surgery to repair the meningocele or myelomeningocele is usually done within 24 hours of birth. However, although the opening is closed, whatever damage has already been done to the neural tissue is permanent. If hydrocephalus is developing, the meningocele repair may be done first. Then, a few days later, a shunt can be inserted to resolve the hydrocephalus. If the hydrocephalus is present at birth, the two surgeries may be done at the same time to decrease the risks associated with increasing pressure on the brain. To prevent drying of the sac, it may be kept moist with sterile **dressings** until surgery is begun. Once the anesthesia has put the baby to sleep and the surgery is pain-free, a surgical incision is made into the sac. Excess fluid is drained, and the meninges is wrapped around the spine to protect it. The opening is then closed with sutures.

Diagnosis/Preparation

If an individual has spina bifida occulta, with no outward signs of a neural tube defect and no symptoms, the condition may go undetected. The protruding sacs associated with meningocele and myelomeningocele are quite noticeable at birth. To understand the extent of the defect x rays, **ultrasound**, computed tomography (CT) scans, or **magnetic resonance imaging** (MRI) of the spine may be taken.

Spina bifida may be diagnosed while the mother is still pregnant, through prenatal screening. If spina bifida is indicated, a blood test will show an elevated alpha fetoprotein. However, elevated levels can be present without spina bifida, so further testing should be done if the test is positive. There is an elevated alpha fetoprotein level in about 85% of women with a fetus with spina bifida. An ultrasound can reliable reveal the spinal structure of the fetus. An **amniocentesis** may be done to check for chromosomal abnormalities. In amniocentesis, a long syringe is used to draw amniotic fluid out from the uterus through the mother's abdomen. Because the protruding sac of the meningocele and myelomeningocele can look the same on the outside, it is important to have a clear diagnosis, as the anticipated outcome of the two conditions is very different.

Aftercare

The infant will first spend some time in the **recovery room**, and then be transferred to an **intensive care unit**. The infant will be monitored for signs of excess bleeding and infection. Temperature will be closely monitored. **Antibiotics** will be given to decrease the

WHO PERFORMS THE PROCEDURE AND WHERE IS IT PERFORMED?

Surgery on the spine is a very delicate procedure and needs to be done by a surgeon specializing in pediatric neurosurgery. It is best performed in a hospital with a pediatric intensive care unit available to closely monitor the infant after the surgery.

risk of infection, and the infant will be positioned to lie flat on the stomach to avoid pressure on the surgical wound. Extreme care is taken to keep the wound clean of urine and stool.

Risks

Surgical risks include infection and bleeding. Anesthesia risks include a reaction to the medications used, including difficulty breathing. During meningocele and myelomeningocele repair, there are additional risks of damage to the spinal column and infection of the spinal fluid surrounding the spine and brain. Damage to the neural tissue could result in paralysis, or loss of nerve function (for example, loss of bowel and bladder control). There may also be an increased risk of an urinary tract infection. An infection of the meninges is called meningitis. However, further damage would be expected if surgery were not done, and serious infection would be likely. As in all surgery, one must weigh the potential risks against the expected benefits.

Normal results

Results depend greatly on the extent of involvement of exposed neural tissue and the condition of the infant prior to surgery. A meningocele repair can have excellent results, as neural tissue does not extend into the protruding sac. In myelomeningocele, the amount of exposed neural tissue will determine the extent of lower limb weakness, or paralysis. The infant will usually spend a few weeks in the hospital after surgery before being able to be discharged home. As the child grows, it may be necessary to use braces, crutches, or a wheelchair for mobility. If surgery for hydrocephalus is successful, the prognosis is better. Children with a repaired myelomeningocele may be able to go to school, but will benefit from special education and associated services. There may be varying degrees of learning problems, and difficulties with the child's attention span. An effective bowel and bladder-training program can help make attending school easier. Because of muscle

QUESTIONS TO ASK THE DOCTOR

- What is the extent of the neurological damage?
- Is my child likely to walk?
- What experience do you have with this procedure?
- What complications have your patients experienced with this procedure?
- How long is my child likely to stay in the hospital?

weakness or paralysis, a child with spina bifida will need physical therapy and may require future surgeries.

Morbidity and mortality rates

With current medical and surgical treatments, about 85% of infants survive, and about 50% will be able to walk. Bowel and bladder disorders contribute significantly to morbidity and mortality in those with spina bifida who survive past the age of two years.

Alternatives

There is no alternative to surgical repair. Risk of infection and damage to the spine and brain is high with an opening to the spine, so surgery is necessary to close the opening and drain the excess fluid that could put pressure on the brain. The Spina Bifida Association of America recommends that all women of childbearing age take 0.4 mg of folic acid daily, as this amount has been shown to decrease the likelihood of neural tube defects. Once a woman is aware of being pregnant, the critical first month of neural tube development has already past, and folic acid cannot cure any damage that has been done.

Resources

BOOKS

Senisi, Ellen B. *All Kinds of Friends, Even Green!* Woodbine House, November 2002.

ORGANIZATIONS

March of Dimes Birth Defects Foundation. 1275 Mamaroneck Avenue; White Plains, NY. Telephone (914) 428-7100. <http://wwwmodimes.org>.

National Library of Medicine. http://www.nlm.nih.gov.

Spina Bifida Association of America. 4590 MacArthur Boulevard, NW, Suite 250; Washington, DC 20007-4226. Telephone (800) 621-3141, (202)944-3285. sbaa@sbaa.org. http://www.sbaa.org.

Esther Csapo Rastegari, R.N., B.S.N., Ed.M.

Mental health assessment

Definition

A mental health assessment is an examination used to ascertain whether or not a patient is functioning on a healthy psychological, social, or developmental level. A mental health assessment can also be used to aid diagnosis of some neurological disorders, specific diseases, or possible drug abuse.

Purpose

Mental health assessments are performed to screen for mental health disorders such as depression or anxiety, or as part of their continuing evaluation. They can also be used to help diagnose neurological pathology, such as Alzheimer's disease. A mental health assessment may be indicated if a person is having difficulty at work, school, or in social situations. For example, a diagnosis of Attention Deficit Hyperactivity Disorder (ADHD) or a personality disorder may begin with a mental health assessment as part of their discovery. Mental health assessments may also be done if substance abuse is suspected.

Demographics

A mental health assessment can be done for patients of any age or gender. The mental health assessment of a child or adolescent is based on developmental stage as appropriate for age. An adult mental health assessment may be done to screen for new diagnoses, assess patients with an existing diagnosis for changes in severity, or to assess the need to modify current a treatment plan.

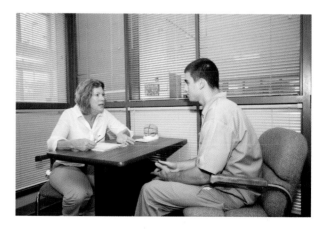

(Mikael Karlsson / Alamy)

WHO PERFORMS THE PROCEDURE?

A general practitioner may perform a brief mental health assessment during a routine examination. However, if there are symptoms of a mental disorder present, the patient may be referred to a specialist for a more thorough mental health assessment. A specialist for a mental health assessment may be a psychologist or a psychiatrist.

A psychologist is a health care professional who is not a medical doctor. A psychologist may have a degree called a PsyD (doctor of psychology), or a PhD (doctor of philosophy) in psychology. Psychologists can evaluate and counsel patients, and need to be licensed to practice. However in most states, psychologists cannot prescribe medication.

A psychiatrist is a medical doctor who specializes in the diagnosis and treatment of mental health problems. Psychiatrists can evaluate, counsel, and prescribe medications to treat mental health problems. Some psychiatrists further specialize in specific areas of mental health, such as psychiatry for adolescents. Psychiatrists need to be licensed to practice. They should be board-certified through the Board of Psychiatry and Neurology, a board that is validated by the American Board of Medical Specialties.

Description

Patient History

History taking is an important component of the mental health assessment. The **health history** of a patient includes their medical health history, family health history, medications they are currently on, and social history. Social history is a critical component, including history of drug use, physical or emotional abuse, and exposure to traumatic situations. It also covers the "chief complaint," or description of the patient's current issue in the context of the patient's life, both past and present. Health care professionals who perform a mental health assessment need to obtain a thorough health history from the patient, because it places the current situation into the context of the patient's overall health. For the current chief complaint, the health care provider will ask questions to form an overall picture of how the patient is feeling and any distressing emotions the patient is experiencing. A pertinent health history also includes information on

QUESTIONS TO ASK YOUR DOCTOR

- Why do I need a mental health assessment?
- Who will perform the assessment?
- How will the assessment be performed?
- How long is the assessment expected to take?
- What tests are involved in my mental health assessment?
- Are there any specific preparations I need to make before or after the assessment?
- What will the results of the assessment specifically indicate?
- When will the results be available?
- What are the risks of the assessment?
- Who else has access to the results of the assessment?
- Do any of my prescription medications, non-prescription medications, nutritional, or herbal supplements potentially affect the results of my mental health assessment?

any previous psychiatric illness, for both the patient and the patient's family. It is important that the health care provider be made aware of not only current prescription medications, but also non-prescription medications, nutritional supplements, and herbal supplements or teas the patient is currently taking, as they may affect the patient's mental status. History of suicide attempts or thoughts may be initially discussed during the history portion of the assessment.

Mental Status Examination

The mental status examination explores multiple aspects of the patient's ability to function in a healthy, normal manner. The health care provider will assess the multiple components of the patient's mental status through both direct questioning and objective observation.

GENERAL APPEARANCE. General appearance is assessed by observation on the part of the health care provider. Patient hygiene, grooming, excessive nervousness or physical activity, and apparent nutritional state are all pertinent to the mental status examination. General alertness, facial expressions, and eye contact are noted. The patient's attitude toward the health care provider is also an important component, including whether the patient seems hostile, guarded, friendly, or cooperative.

Affect—The external manifestation of a mood or state of mind. Affect is usually observed in facial expression or other body language.

Attention Deficit Hyperactivity Disorder (ADHD)—A disorder involving a developmentally inappropriate degree of inattention and impulsivity. Hyperactivity may or may not be a component. This disorder usually appears in childhood and manifests itself as difficulty at home or school. It sometimes persists into adulthood where it may affect work, relationships, and other social situations.

Alzheimer's Disease—A disease of the elderly involving progressive mental deterioration including loss of memory, judgment, and intellect; disorientation; confusion; general inability to mentally function in social situations. The disease may begin as early as late mid-life and results in eventual death. It is associated with specific physical changes to the brain that can be visualized using medical imaging techniques.

Autism—A childhood disorder that manifests as an inability to communicate with or relate to others, or interact in social situations in a healthy, normal manner. Autism may range from mild to severe and includes repetitive behaviors, the inability to cope with changes from routine activities, and obsessions with specific objects. Autism is sometimes associated with below-normal intelligence or anxiety.

Brain Lesion—Physical damage done to a specific part or location of the brain, that may result in

specific symptoms or behaviors associated with that brain lesion.

Chemical Toxicity—State of physical illness induced by poisoning with toxic chemicals. Chemical toxicities may affect a person's behavior or mental function.

Cognition—The mental activity of thinking, learning, and memory.

Compulsion—The uncontrollable impulse to perform specific acts. In mental health disorders, compulsions are often repetitive and carried out by the person in order to avoid feelings of anxiety.

Computed Tomography (CT scan)—A computer uses x-rays across many different directions on a given cross section of the body, and combines all the cross sections to create one image. CT scans can be used to visualize bodily organs including the brain, blood vessels, bones, and the spinal cord. Contrast dye is sometimes administered to the patient to help visualize structures.

Delusion—Conviction of a false belief or wrong judgment despite obvious evidence to the contrary.

Dementia—The progressive loss of cognitive and intellectual function of the brain including impaired memory, judgment, and disorientation, without the impairment of perception or consciousness. It is usually associated with a structural brain disease such as Alzheimer's disease.

Developmental Disorder—A disorder or disability that occurs because of prenatal or early childhood

---

MOOD AND AFFECT. Mood is the internal set of sustained emotions that the patient experiences, while affect is the external manifestation of mood as body language and facial expression. Patients are questioned as to what moods they have experienced for lengths of time, such as depression, tiredness, or anxiety. Affect may be described as normal; blunted or flat where the patient has little expression; expansive and inappropriate where the patient seems to be experiencing extremes of emotion that may not be appropriate to the setting.

SPEECH AND THOUGHT PROCESSES. Speech is examined for clarity, general coherence, appropriate inflection (not monotone), quantity that is unusually large or small, a rate that is unusually fast or slow, and appropriate volume. While asking questions during the examination, the health care provider will also monitor

the responses given by the patient for specific thought processes or patterns of speech. The following examples may be observed by the health care provider or described by the patient: flight of ideas where the patient randomly changes from one topic to another; looseness of association where the patient makes irrelevant connections between seemingly unrelated topics; racing thoughts; excessively trailing off onto tangents; nonsensical speech; rhyming or creation of new words; halting speech; paucity of speech; or speaking in riddles.

THOUGHT CONTENT. Thought content may be evaluated through both direct questioning and observation of topics brought up by the patient. There are many types of thought content that may be pertinent to this section of the mental health assessment. Thought aspects of mental disorders may include the following: hallucinations that may be auditory, visual, events that affect cognition, language, motor, or social skills.

Flight of Ideas—A psychiatric term describing a thought disorder where streams of unrelated words or ideas enter a patient's mind too quickly to be properly vocalized despite the rushed and rapid rate of the patient's speech.

Hallucination—The perception of a person, object, event, or sensory stimulus that is not truly there. Hallucinations can be visual (seen), auditory (heard), olfactory (smelled), tactile (felt), gustatory (tasted), or a combination thereof.

Looseness of Association—A psychiatric term describing a thought disorder where a patient makes irrelevant connections between seemingly unrelated topics. In a mental health assessment the patient's responses may not seem to correspond to the question asked by the health care provider.

Magnetic Resonance Imaging (MRI)—A diagnostic test where a magnetic field is applied to atoms within a patient's body, aligns the atoms, and reads the energy pulses given off by the atoms in a manner that creates a three-dimensional picture of the patient's internal structures. There is no exposure to radiation. An MRI is especially useful for visualizing soft tissue and for neurological imaging.

Metabolic Disturbance—A disturbance in the general function of the body's basic life processes such as energy production. The body's ability to provide the brain with appropriate nourishment can affect the mental status of the individual.

Obsession—A recurrent and persistent idea, thought, or impulse that the individual cannot repress.

Parkinson's Disease—A neurological disease resulting from a deficiency of the neurotransmitter dopamine that is associated with specific recognizable movements, affects, and behavior patterns.

Personality Disorder—Group of behavioral disorders characterized by maladaptive patterns of behavior, social interactions, or lifestyles that deviate from the healthy normal. Personality disorders are distinct from psychotic disorders.

Phobia—An irrational and unfounded fear of a situation, place, or object that causes a state of panic.

Psychiatrist—A medical doctor (MD) who specializes in the treatment of mental health problems and can prescribe medication.

Psychologist—A health care professional (PsyD or PhD) who is not a medical doctor but can evaluate or provide counseling for patients with mental health issues.

Thyroid Dysfunction—A physical state that involves the failure of the thyroid gland to function properly. Thyroid dysfunction not only affects a person's physical state, but may have secondary effects on their mental state as well.

---

tactile, or olfactory; auditory hallucinations involving commands for the patient to carry out specific actions; delusions of having special powers, status, or persecution by others; paranoid thinking; obsessions, compulsions, and ritualistic behaviors; phobias; thoughts of self-harm or suicide; homicidal thoughts.

COGNITION. An important aspect of the mental status examination is assessment of the patient's cognitive state. Elements of this section include the following: assessment of general awareness and level of consciousness; orientation to person, current location, current date and time, and situation; ability to pay attention and concentrate; general memory tests; ability to follow directions; language comprehension and appropriate usage of language; ability to perform abstract reasoning by interpreting proverbs supplied by the health care provider.

Written and Verbal Tests

Written or verbal tests are used as part of a mental health assessment when there is a reason to apply the test to explore a specific potential diagnosis. There are standardized tests for many different mental disorders and disturbances. For example, depression is sometimes assessed using a specific set of standards or measurements called a rating scale. Other tests may evaluate intelligence levels, and aid in the diagnosis of dementia or developmental disorders such as learning disabilities or autism. These types of tests are controversial and do not stand alone to make a diagnosis, but rather may be used in addition to the other components of the mental health assessment. Each test may take from thirty minutes to several hours to complete, and be may administered over multiple days.

Adjunctive Tests

PHYSICAL EXAMINATION. Mental health assessments are sometimes helpful in diagnosing certain neurological disorders, and may be performed in the larger context of a neurological examination. The neurological examination includes a mental status exam, as well as assessing motor function, reflexes, sensory perception, posture, and gait. Diseases such as Parkinson's disease or Alzheimer's disease may initially be suspected as a result of the mental health assessment.

CLINICAL TESTS. Clinical tests may be necessary as an adjunct to the mental health assessment, to aid in diagnosis of specific neurological or neuropsychiatric disorders. For example, a patient with Alzheimer's disease may require **Magnetic Resonance Imaging** (MRI) as an adjunct to the mental health assessment for a successful diagnosis. Clinical tests may also be used rule out non-mental health related illnesses. Some drugs of abuse, thyroid dysfunction, hormonal imbalances, prescription medications, chemical toxicities, metabolic disturbances, selective brain lesions, or types of tumors may all manifest in ways that affect the mental status assessment. Blood laboratory testing, Computed Tomography (CT scan), or an MRI may help to assess the presence or absence of these physical states.

Follow-up after the Assessment

Whether or not a patient requires further inpatient care, outpatient care, or medication is dependent upon the final diagnosis. Inpatient care is always indicated if the patients are unable to suitably care for themselves, suicidal, or homicidal.

Risks

The mental health assessment is a valuable tool in the diagnosis of mental health problems. However, some mental health problems are very difficult to diagnose. Mental health assessments may need to be performed multiple times before any medical conclusion is reached. Even with multiple mental health assessments and adjunctive tests, there is risk that an accurate diagnosis may still be missed.

Resources

BOOKS

Bickley LS. *Bates Guide to Physical Examination and History Taking.* Eighth Edition. Lippincott Williams & Wilkins: 2003.

Davidson T, Gulli LF, Nasser B.*Gale Encyclopedia of Children's Health.*Thomson Gale, Detroit. 2006.

Diagnostic and Statistical Manual of Mental Disorders Fourth Edition, Text Revision (DSM-IV-TR). Washington, DC: American Psychiatric Association; 2000.

OTHER

Brannon, Guy E. "History and Mental Status Examination." Emedicine (February 4, 2008). http://www.emedicine.com/Med/topic3358.htm [accessed April 3, 2008].

Practice Guideline for the Psychiatric Evaluation of Adults. Second Edition. American Psychiatric Association; 2006

ORGANIZATIONS

American Psychiatric Association, 1000 Wilson Boulevard, Suite 1825, Arlington, Virginia, 22209-3901, 703-907-7300, apa@psych.org, http://www.psych.org/.

Maria Basile, PhD

Mentoplasty

Definition

Mentoplasty is a term that refers to **plastic surgery** procedures for the chin. It comes from the Latin word *mentum*, which means chin, and the Greek verb *plassein*, which means "to form" or "to shape." Mentoplasty is also known as genioplasty or chinplasty.

Purpose

Mentoplasty may be done for several reasons:

- To correct malformations of the chin resulting from developmental abnormalities of the bones in the jaw. Sometimes the jawbones continue to grow on one side of the face but not the other, leading to facial asymmetry. In other instances a part of the jawbone is missing; this condition is known as congenital agenesis of the jaw.

- To reshape a chin that is out of proportion to other facial features.

- As part of gender reassignment surgery. The size and shape of the chin and lower jawline are somewhat different in men and women. Some people choose to have mentoplasty as part of their gender transition.

- As part of craniofacial reconstruction following trauma or cancer surgery.

- As part of orthognathic surgery. Orthognathic surgery involves repositioning the facial bones in order to correct deformities that affect the patient's ability to speak or chew normally.

KEY TERMS

Aesthetic—Pertaining to beauty. Plastic surgery done to improve the patient's appearance is sometimes called aesthetic surgery.

Agenesis—The absence of an organ or body part due to developmental failure.

Alloplast—An implant made of an inert foreign material such as silicone or hydroxyapatite.

Congenital—Present at the time of birth.

Extrusion—Pushing out or expulsion. Extrusion of a chin implant is one possible complication of mentoplasty.

Genioplasty—Another word for mentoplasty. It comes from the Greek word for "chin."

Hematoma—A localized collection of blood in an organ or tissue due to broken blood vessels.

Intraoral—Inside the mouth.

Malocclusion—Malpositioning and defective contact between opposing teeth in the upper and lower jaws.

Microgenia—An extremely small chin. It is the most common deformity of the chin.

Orthognathic surgery—Surgery that corrects deformities or malpositioning of the bones in the jaw. The term comes from two Greek words meaning straight and jaw.

Sliding genioplasty—A complex plastic surgery procedure in which the patient's jawbone is cut, moved forward or backward, and repositioned with metal plates and screws.

Submental—Underneath the chin.

Insurance coverage for mentoplasty depends on its purpose. Chin reshaping that is done to improve personal appearance is not usually covered by insurance. Mentoplasty that is performed as a reconstructive procedure after trauma, genetic deformity, or orthognathic surgery may be covered by insurance.

The cost of mentoplasty varies considerably according to the complexity of the procedure. The average surgeon's fee for a chin implant was $1,612 in 2002. The average fee for a sliding genioplasty, however, was $4,000–$6,000.

Demographics

In spite of the fact that chin deformities are the most common facial abnormality, mentoplasty is not one of the more frequently performed procedures in plastic surgery. In 2002, there were 18,352 mentoplasties performed in the United States, compared to 117,831 face lifts and 282,876 liposuctions. Most mentoplasties are done in combination with rhinoplasties.

Mentoplasty is primarily performed in adult patients; it is not usually done in children until all permanent teeth have come in and the jaw is close to its adult size. According to the American Society of Plastic Surgeons, 7% of patients who had mentoplasties in the United States in 2002 were 18 or younger; 35% were between the ages of 19 and 34; 40% were between the ages of 35 and 50, while another 15% were between 51 and 64. Only 3% were over 65.

With respect to sex, women account for 69% of mentoplasty patients; only 31% are men.

Description

Mentoplasties fall into two large categories: procedures that augment (increase) small or receding chins; and those that reduce large or protruding chins. Chin augmentation is done more frequently than chin reduction, reflecting the fact that microgenia (small chin) is the most common abnormality of the chin.

Chin augmentation

Chin augmentation can be performed by inserting an implant under the skin of the chin or by performing a sliding genioplasty. Insertion of an implant takes 30–60 minutes, while a sliding genioplasty takes slightly longer, 45–90 minutes. If the mentoplasty is done together with orthognathic surgery, the operation may take as long as three hours.

Chin implants are used in patients with mild or moderate microgenia. At one time they were made of cartilage taken from donors or from other sites on the patient's body, but as of 2003 alloplastic implants (made from inert foreign materials) are used more often because they reduce the risk of infection. To insert the implant, the surgeon can choose to make the incision under the chin (submental) or inside the mouth (intraoral). In either case, the surgeon cuts through several layers of tissue, taking care to avoid damaging the major nerve in the chin. The surgeon makes a pocket in the connective tissue inside the chin and washes it out with an antiseptic solution. The sterile implant is then inserted in the pocket and positioned properly. The incision is closed and the wound covered with Steri-Strips.

A sliding genioplasty may be performed if the patient's chin is too small for augmentation with an implant, or if the deformity is more complex. In this procedure, the surgeon cuts through the jawbone with an oscillating saw and removes part of the bone. He or she then moves the bone segment forward, holding it in place with metal plates and screws. After the bone segment has been fixed in place, the incision is closed and the patient's head is wrapped with a pressure dressing.

Chin reduction

Reduction of an overly large or protruding chin may be done either by direct reduction or a sliding genioplasty. In a direct reduction, the surgeon makes either a submental or an intraoral incision and removes excess bone from the chin with a burr. A sliding genioplasty reduction is similar to a genioplasty to augment the chin, except that the bone segment is moved backward rather than forward.

Diagnosis/Preparation

Diagnosis

Diagnostic evaluation consists of a facial analysis as well as a complete dental and medical history. The chin is one of the three most significant parts of the face from an aesthetic standpoint, the others being the forehead and the nose. Many patients who are concerned about the size of their nose, for example, can be helped by having a too-small chin augmented as well as having the nose reshaped. In the facial analysis, the face is divided into thirds, with the mouth and chin in the lowest third. The surgeon compares the proportions of the features in each third in order to determine the most suitable procedure for restoring balance. The patient will be photographed from several angles to document the condition of the chin before surgery.

The dental history and x-ray studies of the head and jaw are necessary in order to determine whether the facial disproportion can be corrected by an implant or simple reduction, or whether orthognathic surgery is required. Patients who have severe malocclusion (irregular contact between the teeth in the upper and lower jaws) or deformities of the facial bones are usually referred to a maxillofacial specialist for **reconstructive surgery**.

Lastly, the surgeon will evaluate the patient for any signs of psychological instability, including unrealistic expectations of the results of surgery.

Preparation

Patients should stop smoking and discontinue all medications containing **aspirin** or NSAIDs for two weeks prior to mentoplasty. If the surgeon is planning to make a submental incision, the patient should use an antibacterial facial cleanser for two days before surgery. Patients scheduled for an intraoral approach should rinse the mouth with mouthwash three times a day for two days before surgery. They should not eat or drink anything for eight hours prior to the procedure.

Aftercare

Patients should have someone drive them home after the procedure. They are given medication for discomfort and a one-week course of antibiotic medication to reduce the risk of infection. Most patients can return to work in seven to 10 days.

Other aspects of aftercare include the following:

- a soft or liquid diet for four to five days
- raising the head of the bed or using two to three pillows
- rinsing the mouth with a solution of hydrogen peroxide and warm water two to three times daily
- avoiding sleeping on the face and unnecessary touching of the chin area
- avoiding vigorous physical exercise for about two weeks

Risks

In addition to infection, bleeding, and an allergic reaction to the anesthetic, the risks of insertion of a chin implant include:

- deformity of the chin following an infection
- injury to the major nerve in the chin, leading to loss of feeling or paralysis of the chin muscles
- erosion of the bone beneath the implant
- moving around or dislocation of the implant
- extrusion (pushing out) of the implant

Specific risks associated with sliding genioplasties include:

- under- or overcorrection of the defect
- injury to the major nerve in the chin
- failure of the bone segment to reunite properly with the other parts of the jaw
- damage to the roots of the teeth
- hematoma (a collection of blood within a body organ or tissue caused by leakage from broken blood vessels; it can damage the results of a mentoplasty by causing pressure that distorts the final shape of the chin)

WHO PERFORMS THE PROCEDURE AND WHERE IS IT PERFORMED?

Mentoplasties may be performed by plastic surgeons, oral surgeons, or maxillofacial surgeons. Fat injections and facial liposuction are usually performed by plastic surgeons.

Chin implant insertions or direct reductions are usually performed as outpatient procedures in the surgeon's office or an ambulatory surgery center. The patient may be given either general or local anesthesia. Sliding genioplasties can be done as outpatient procedures; however, they are usually performed in hospitals under general anesthesia, particularly if the patient is having orthognathic surgery at the same time.

Normal results

Normal results of either augmentation or reduction mentoplasty include correction of facial asymmetry and disproportion. The functioning of the jaw is also often improved. Patients who have had a mentoplasty are usually very satisfied with the results.

Morbidity and mortality rates

The rate of complications with chin implants as well as sliding genioplasties is about 5%.

Alternatives

Fat injections

In some cases, fat may be injected into the area below the chin to plump up the skin and minimize the apparent size of the chin. This technique, however, is limited to minor disproportions of chin size. In addition, fat injections must be repeated periodically as the fat is gradually absorbed by the body.

Liposuction

Facial **liposuction** can be used together with or instead of mentoplasty to improve the patient's profile. In particular, removal of fatty tissue below the chin can make a receding chin look larger or more prominent.

QUESTIONS TO ASK THE DOCTOR

- Would you recommend a chin implant or a sliding genioplasty in my case?
- Would you use a submental or an intraoral approach to a chin augmentation?
- How many mentoplasties have you performed?
- Should I consider a mentoplasty in combination with another facial procedure?

Resources

BOOKS

Sargent, Larry, MD. *The Craniofacial Surgery Book*. Chattanooga, TN: Erlanger Health System, 2000.

"Temporomandibular Disorders." In *The Merck Manual of Diagnosis and Therapy*, edited by Mark H. Beers, MD, and Robert Berkow, MD. Whitehouse Station, NJ: Merck Research Laboratories, 1999.

PERIODICALS

Abraham, Manoj T., MD, and Thomas Romo III, MD. "Liposuction of the Face and Neck." *eMedicine*, January 8, 2003 [cited April 22, 2003]. http://www.emedicine.com/ent/topic581.htm.

Chang, Edward, MD, DDS, Samuel M. Lam, MD, and Edward Farrior, MD. "Genioplasty." *eMedicine*, June 7, 2002 [cited April 20, 2003]. http://www.emedicine.com/ent/topic106.htm.

Chang, E. W., S. M. Lam, M. Karen, and J. L. Donlevy. "Sliding Genioplasty for Correction of Chin Abnormalities." *Archives of Facial Plastic Surgery* 3 (January-March 2001): 8–15.

Danahey, D. G., S. H. Dayan, A. G. Benson, and J. A. Ness. "Importance of Chin Evaluation and Treatment to Optimizing Neck Rejuvenation Surgery." *Facial Plastic Surgery* 17 (May 2001): 91–97.

Galli, Suzanne K. D., MD, and Philip J. Miller, MD. "Chin Implants." *eMedicine*, May 15, 2002 [cited April 22, 2003]. http://www.emedicine.com/ent/topic628.htm.

Grossman, John A., MD. "Facial Alloplastic Implants, Chin." *eMedicine*, July 5, 2001 [cited April 21, 2003]. http://www.emedicine.com/plastic/topic56.htm.

Jafar, M., and R. A. Younger. "Screw Fixation Mentoplasty." *Journal of Otolaryngology* 29 (October 2000): 274–278.

Meszaros, Liz. "Sliding Genioplasty Successful in Correcting Chin Abnormalities." *Cosmetic Surgery Times* September 1, 2001.

Patel, Pravin K., MD, Hongshik Han, MD, and Nak-Heon Kang, MD. "Craniofacial, Orthognathic Surgery." *eMedicine*, December 27, 2001 [cited April 21, 2003]. http://www.emedicine.com/plastic/topic177.htm.

Siwolop, Sana. "Beyond Botox: An Industry's Quest for Smooth Skin." *New York Times* March 9, 2003 [cited March 9, 2003]. http://www.nytimes.com/2003/03/09/business/09FACE.html.

ORGANIZATIONS

American Academy of Facial Plastic and Reconstructive Surgery (AAFPRS). 310 South Henry Street, Alexandria, VA 22314. (703) 299-9291. http://www.facemd. org.

American Society of Plastic Surgeons (ASPS). 444 East Algonquin Road, Arlington Heights, IL 60005. (847) 228-9900. http://www.plasticsurgery.org.

FACES: The National Craniofacial Association. P. O. Box 11082, Chattanooga, TN 37401. (800) 332-2373. http://www.faces-cranio.org.

OTHER

American Academy of Facial Plastic and Reconstructive Surgery. *2001 Membership Survey: Trends in Facial Plastic Surgery*. Alexandria, VA: AAFPRS, 2002.

American Academy of Facial Plastic and Reconstructive Surgery. *Procedures: Understanding Mentoplasty Surgery*. [cited April 20, 2003]. http://www.facial-plastic-surgery.org/patient/procedures/mentoplasty.html.

American Society of Plastic Surgeons. *Procedures: Facial Implants*. [cited April 20, 2003]. http://www.plasticsurgery.org/public_education/procedures/FacialImplants.cfm.

Rebecca Frey, Ph.D.

Microalbumin test *see* **Urinalysis**

Microsurgery

Definition

Microsurgery is surgery that is performed on very small structures, such as blood vessels and nerves, with specialized instruments under a microscope.

Purpose

Microsurgical procedures are performed on parts of the body that are best visualized under a microscope. Examples of such structures are small blood vessels, nerves, and tubes. Microsurgery uses techniques that have been performed by surgeons since the early twentieth century, such as blood vessel repair and organ transplantation, but under conditions that make traditional **vascular surgery** difficult or impossible.

The first microvascular surgery, using a microscope to aid in the repair of blood vessels, was described by Jules Jacobson of the University of Vermont in 1960. The first successful replantation (reattachment of an amputated body part) was reported in 1964 by Harry Bunke. This replantation of a rabbit's ear was significant because blood vessels smaller than 0.04 inch (1 mm)—similar in size to the blood vessels found in a human hand—were successfully attached. Two years later, the successful replantation of a toe to the hand of a monkey was made possible using microsurgical techniques. Soon thereafter, microsurgery began being used in a number of clinical settings.

Numerous surgical specialties utilize the techniques of microsurgery. Otolaryngologists (ear, nose, and throat doctors) perform microsurgery on the small, delicate structures of the inner ear or the vocal cords. Cataracts are removed by ophthalmologists (eye doctors), who also perform corneal transplants and treat eye conditions like glaucoma. Urologists can reverse vasectomies (male sterilization), and gynecologists can reverse tubal ligations (female sterilization), giving people new choices about having children. Microsurgical techniques are used by plastic surgeons to reconstruct damaged or disfigured skin, muscles, or other tissues, or to transplant tissues from other parts of the body. And, importantly, a number of specialties can collaborate to treat patients who have limbs or other body parts; under certain circumstances, amputated parts can be reattached, or another body part can be replanted in the place of one lost (for example, a great toe replacing a lost or damaged thumb).

Today, microsurgery can be lifesaving. Neurosurgeons can treat vascular abnormalities found in the brain, and cancerous tumors can be removed.

Description

Equipment

Microsurgical equipment magnifies the operating field, provide instrumentation precise enough to

---

KEY TERMS

Capillaries—Tiny blood vessels that deliver oxygen to tissues.

Peripheral nerves—The nerves outside of the brain and spinal cord.

Vascular surgery—A branch of medicine that deals with the surgical repair of disorders of or injuries to the blood vessels.

Venous valves—Folds on the inner lining of the veins that prevent the backflow of blood.

---

maneuver under high magnification, and allow the surgeon to operate on structures barely visible to the human eye. The most important tools used by the microsurgeon are the microscope, microsurgical instruments, and microsuture materials.

MICROSCOPE. While operating microscopes may differ according to their specific use, certain features are standard. The microscope may be floor- or ceiling-mounted, with a moveable arm that allows the surgeon to manipulate the microscope's position. A view of the surgical site is afforded by a set of lenses and a high-intensity light source. This lighting is enhanced by maintaining a low level of light in the rest of the **operating room**. Two or more sets of lenses allow a surgeon and an assistant to view the operating field and focus and zoom independently. A video camera allows the rest of the **surgical team** to view the operating field on a display screen. Features that come on some microscopes include foot and/or mouth switch controls and motorized zoom and focus.

A magnification of five to forty times (5–40x) is generally required for microsurgery. A lower magnification may be used to identify and expose structures, while a higher magnification is most often used for microsurgical repair. Alternatively, surgical loupes (magnifying lenses mounted on a pair of eyeglasses) may be used for lower magnifications (2–6x).

INSTRUMENTS. Microsurgical instruments differ from conventional instruments in a number of ways. They must be capable of delicately manipulating structures barely visible to the naked eye, but with handles large enough to hold comfortably and securely. They must also take into account the tremor of the surgeon's hand, greatly amplified under magnification.

Some of the various instruments that are used in microsurgery include:

- forceps
- needle holders (for suturing)
- scissors
- vascular clamps (for controlling bleeding) and clamp applicators
- irrigators (for washing structures in the surgical field)
- vessel dilators (for opening up the cut end of a blood vessel)
- various standard surgical tools

SUTURE MATERIALS. Suturing, or stitching, is done by means of specialized thread and needles. The diameter (gauge) of suture thread ranges in size and depends on the procedure and tissue to be sutured. Conventional suturing usually requires gauges of 2-0 (0.3 mm) to 6-0 (0.07 mm). Conversely, gauges of 9-0 (0.03 mm) to 12-0 (0.001 mm) are generally used for microsurgery. Suture thread may be absorbable (able to be broken down in the body after a definite amount of time) or non-absorbable (retaining its strength indefinitely), natural (made of silk, gut, linen, or other natural material) or synthetic (made of nylon, polyester, wire, or other man-made material). The type of suture thread used depends on the procedure and tissue to be sutured.

The suture needle comes in various sizes (diameters and length) and shapes (straight or curved), and also with different point types (rounded, cutting, or blunt). It comes with suture thread preattached to one end; this is called the swage. As in the case of suture thread, the type of needle used depends on the procedure and tissue to be sutured; generally, needles with a diameter of less than 0.15 mm are used for microsurgery.

Training

For a surgeon to perform microsurgery in a clinical setting, extensive training and practice are required. A basic knowledge of anatomy and surgical techniques is essential. After a thorough introduction to the operating microscope and other microsurgical equipment, basic techniques are introduced using small animals as the experimental model. Specifically, surgeons must be taught how to maintain correct posture and to maintain constant visual contact with the microscope during surgery, how to properly hold and use the instruments, how to minimize the amount of hand tremor, and how to perform basic techniques, such as suturing. After becoming proficient at these skills, more advanced techniques can be taught, including procedures regarding how to treat specific conditions.

Extensive and ongoing practice is necessary for a surgeon to maintain adequate proficiency at microsurgical techniques. For this reason, a microsurgical laboratory is made available to surgeons for training and practice.

Techniques

Most microsurgical procedures utilize a set of basic techniques that must be mastered by the surgeon. These include blood vessel repair, vein grafting, and nerve repair and grafting.

BLOOD VESSEL REPAIR. Blood vessel, or vascular anastomosis, is the connection of two cut or separate blood vessels to form a continuous channel. Anastomoses may be end-to-end (between two cut ends of a blood vessel) or end-to-side (a connection of one cut end of a blood vessel to the wall of another vessel).

The first step of creating an anastomosis is to identify and expose the blood vessel by isolating it from surrounding tissues. Each end of the vessel is irrigated (washed) and secured with clamps for the duration of the procedure. A piece of contrast material is placed behind the surgical site so that the tiny vessel can be more easily visualized. The magnification is then increased for the next segment of surgery. The first suture is placed through the full thickness of the vessel wall; the second and third sutures are then placed at 120° from the first. Subsequent sutures are placed evenly in the remaining spaces. Arteries 1 millimeter in diameter generally require between five and eight **stitches** around the perimeter, and veins of the same size between seven and 10. Once the last suture has been placed, the clamps are released and blood is allowed to flow through the anastomosis. If excessive bleeding occurs between the stitches, the vessel is reclamped and additional sutures are placed.

The procedure for an end-to-side anastomosis is similar, except that an oval-shaped hole is cut in the wall of the recipient vessel. Sutures are first placed at each of the oval to connect the attaching vessel to the recipient vessel, and then placed evenly to fill in the remaining spaces.

VEIN GRAFTING. Vein grafting is an alternative procedure to end-to-end anastomosis and may be pursued if cut ends of a blood vessel cannot be attached without tension. Nonessential veins similar in diameter to the recipient blood vessel can be removed from the hand, arm, or foot. If the graft is to be used to reconstruct an artery, its direction is reversed so that the venous valves do not interfere with blood flow. End-to-end anastomosis is then performed on each end of the graft, using the suture techniques described above.

NERVE REPAIR. The process of connecting two cut ends of a nerve is called neurorrhaphy, or nerve anastomosis. Peripheral nerves are composed of bunches of nerve fibers called fascicles that are enclosed by a layer called the perineurium; the epineurium is the outer layer of the nerve that encases the fascicles. Nerve repair may involve suturing of the epineurium only, the perineurium only, or through both layers.

Many of the techniques used for blood vessel anastomoses are also used for nerves. The cut ends of the nerve are exposed, then isolated from surrounding tissues. The ends are trimmed so that healthy nerve tissue is exposed, and a piece of contrast material placed behind the nerve for better visualization. Each nerve end is examined to determine the pattern of fascicles; the nerve ends are then rotated so that the fascicle patterns align. Sutures may be placed around

the circumference of the epineurium; this is called epineurial neurorrhaphy. The perineurium of each cut fascicle end may be stitched with excess epineurium removed (perineurial neurorrhaphy), or both layers may be sutured (epiperineurial neurorrhaphy).

NERVE GRAFTING. If there is a large gap between the cut ends of a nerve, neurorrhaphy cannot be performed without creating tension in the nerve, which can interfere with postsurgical function. A piece of nerve from another part of body may be used to create a nerve graft, which is stitched into place using anastomosis techniques. A disadvantage to nerve grafting is that a loss of function or sensation is experienced from the donor nerve site. A common nerve used for grafting is the sural nerve, which innervates parts of the lower leg.

Diagnosis/Preparation

In an emergency situation, such as an **amputation** or crushing injury, a number of steps must be taken immediately to improve the odds that replantation or reconstruction will be successful. An IV line is placed so that fluids and **antibiotics** can be administered. The injured area is x rayed so that the extent of the injury can be determined, and the amputated body part is wrapped in sterile gauze and placed on ice, so that the tissues are preserved. To prevent freezing, the body part must not be packed below the ice. The patient is transported by ambulance or helicopter to the nearest surgical center capable of microsurgical repair.

In other cases, a patient may suffer from a chronic condition or wound, and microsurgery can be scheduled as an elective procedure. Prior to surgery, the patient will be instructed to refrain from tobacco use because it interferes with healing. In addition, the patient will be told not to eat after midnight the day of surgery. It is important that the patient inform the doctor completely about any prior surgeries, medical conditions, or medications taken on a regular basis, including **nonsteroidal anti-inflammatory drugs** (NSAIDs), such as **aspirin**. Patients taking blood thinners, such as Coumadin or Heparin (generic name: warfarin), should not adjust their medication themselves, but should speak with their prescribing doctors regarding their upcoming surgery). Patients should never adjust dosage without their doctors' approval. This is especially important for elderly patients, asthmatics, those with hypertension, or those who are on ACE inhibitors.

The patient will be placed under **general anesthesia** for the duration of the procedure. The advantages to general anesthesia are that the patient remains unconscious and completely relaxed during the procedure, imperative because of the precise nature and extended duration of the surgery. The patient must be able to tolerate the long surgery and therefore must be relatively stable condition; complex surgeries may take up to 12 hours or more.

Microsurgery makes possible a number of reconstructive procedures that would be more difficult or impossible with conventional surgery. Some of the more frequently performed microsurgical procedures include:

- Replantation. This emergency surgery is performed to reattach an amputated body part such as a finger, arm, or foot. Replantation surgery requires a series of time- and energy-intensive steps to reattach all of the structures while the amputated part is still viable. The cut bone must be shortened slightly so that blood vessels and nerves can be reattached without tension. Anastomoses are created between cut arteries and veins and blood flow is reestablished to the amputated part. Tendons (if present) are then repaired, followed by nerves and soft tissues. Further procedures may be necessary to completely the reconstruction depending on the extent of the injury.

- Transplantation. In some cases an amputated part cannot be reattached, or tissue is deformed because of a congenital defect or an injury. Transplantation may then be an option. The great toe or second toe may be removed from a patient's foot and transplanted to the hand to replace a missing finger. A segment of rib along with its blood supply can be used to reconstruct bones in the face and jaw.

- Free-tissue transfers. Also called free flaps, free-tissue transfers may be used to reconstruct damaged tissues that cannot be treated with skin grafts, closed by traditional methods such as suturing, or allowed to heal without intervention. This includes tissues that have constricted after a burn, injuries in which there is not sufficient skin to properly close the wound, or tissues that have been removed as a result of treatment for cancer. Examples of tissues that may be transferred with microsurgical techniques are skin, muscle, fat, bone, and intestine.

Afterare

Following surgery, the patient is given intravenous fluids and usually progresses to a liquid diet within 12 to 24 hours, and a regular diet soon thereafter. The patient must be kept warm and adequately hydrated, and the surgical site is elevated if possible to help drain excess fluids. Medications are administered to help manage pain. The color, temperature, quality of capillary refill, and tissue turgor (fullness) of the surgical site are closely monitored. Skin should be pink, warm, and have one-to two-second capillary refill. Conversely, tissue that is pale or blue, cool, with no refill or rapid refill may indicate a problem with blood flow.

Certain tests may be recommended to further evaluate the surgical site. These include:

- Doppler ultrasound. This technology uses high-frequency sound waves to evaluate the flow of blood to and from the surgical site.

- Intravenous fluorescein. After a chemical dye called fluorescein is administered to the patient, a specialized machine called a fluorimeter is used to determine how much blood is flowing through the surgical site.

- Pulse oximetry. A pulse oximeter measures the amount of oxygen in the blood and tracks the patient's pulse.

- Arteriography. X rays are taken of the surgical site after a contrast dye has been injected into the bloodstream to determine the condition of vascular anastomoses.

When the patient is discharged from the hospital, he or she will receive instructions for aftercare. Exposure to tobacco must be limited for at least six weeks following the surgery, as nicotine interferes with circulation. The patient must remain warm as **body temperature** also affects circulation. Bed rest may be prescribed for a period of days to weeks after surgery, depending on the procedure. Patients who have had a hand, finger, or multiple fingers replanted must keep the part elevated at heart level to help blood flow and decrease swelling.

Some form of rehabilitation is often recommended after microsurgery. This includes a program of individualized exercises used to restore function to a replanted or transplanted body part. In some cases where problems with circulation occur after surgery, leech therapy may be recommended. Leeches are worms that attach to the skin and draw blood while also injecting substances into the skin that act as a local anesthetic and an anticoagulant (preventing the formation of blood clots). Therapy involves attaching a leech to the replanted part or tissue flap and allow it to feed for 15 to 30 minutes, several times a day, until blood flow is established.

Resources

BOOKS

Canale, ST, ed. Campbell's Operative Orthopaedics. 10th ed. St. Louis: Mosby, 2003.

Cummings, CW, et al. Otolayrngology: Head and Neck Surgery. 4th ed. St. Louis: Mosby, 2005.

Khatri, VP and JA Asensio. Operative Surgery Manual. 1st ed. Philadelphia: Saunders, 2003.

Townsend, CM et al. Sabiston Textbook of Surgery. 17th ed. Philadelphia: Saunders, 2004.

Wein, AJ et al. Campbell-Walsh Urology. 9th ed. Philadelphia: Saunders, 2007.

ORGANIZATIONS

American Society for Reconstructive Microsurgery. 20 North Michigan Ave., Suite 700, Chicago, IL 60602. (312) 456-9579. http://www.microsurg.org.

OTHER

Buncke, Harry J. Microsurgery: Transplantation-Replantation. 2002 [cited April 25, 2003]. <http://buncke.org/book/contents.html>.

Chang, James. "Principles of Microsurgery." eMedicine. August 5, 2002 [cited April 25, 2003]. http://www.emedicine.com/plastic/topic262.htm.

"Microsurgery." California Pacific Medical Center. [cited April 25, 2003]. http://www.cpmc.org/advanced/microsurg/.

"Online Atlas of Microsurgery." Microsurgeon.org. March 20, 2003 [cited April 25, 2003]. http://www.microsurgeon.org.

Stephanie Dionne Sherk

Minimally invasive heart surgery

Definition

Minimally invasive heart surgery refers to surgery performed on the beating heart to provide coronary artery bypass grafting. This technique is often referred to as MIDCAB, minimally invasive direct coronary artery bypass; or OPCAB, off-pump CABG.

Purpose

Minimally invasive heart surgery is performed on the diseased heart to reroute blood around clogged arteries and improve the blood and oxygen supply to the heart. This approach provides patients some benefit in that cardiopulmonary bypass (use of a heart-lung machine) may be avoided. In addition, smaller incisions can be used instead of the standard sternotomy (incision through the sternum, or breastbone) approach. Faster recovery time, decreased procedure costs, and reduced morbidity and mortality are the goals of this technique.

Minimally invasive technique is not new to the field of cardiac surgery. It was performed as early as the 1950s, although the technology associated with

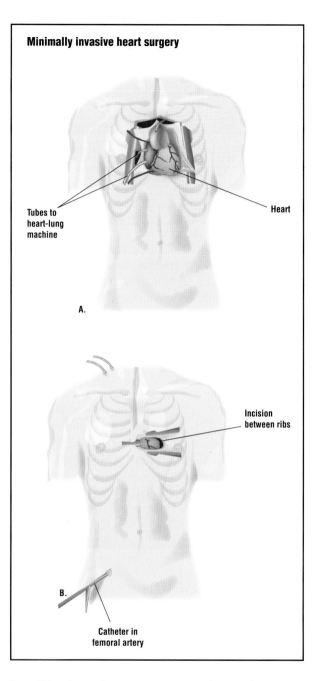

Minimally invasive heart surgery

Tubes to heart-lung machine

Heart

A.

Incision between ribs

B.

Catheter in femoral artery

In traditional open heart surgery, a large incision is made in the chest, and the sternum must be broken (A). Minimally invasive surgery uses a much smaller incision between the ribs to access the heart (B). *(Illustration by GGS Information Services. Cengage Learning, Gale.)*

stabilizing the cardiac structure during the procedure has become more sophisticated. Also, the anesthesiologist and perfusionist (person monitoring blood flow) have developed better techniques to preserve cardiac function during the procedure to help the surgeon achieve the desired outcome. During the 1990s these new techniques were named: off-pump CABG

Anastomosis—Connection of the bypassing blood vessel to the blocked blood vessel by surgical suture. The stitches may be made in continuous manner or individual, with continuous being more common. The disadvantage of continuous suture can be purse-stringing or cinching of the graft opening during knotting of the suture.

Angiography—Injecting dye into blood vessels so they can be seen on an x ray.

Arrhythmia—Cardiac electrical signaling that generates an ECG rhythm other than normal sinus rhythm.

Balloon angioplasty—A procedure used to open an obstructed blood vessel. A small, balloon-tipped catheter is inserted into the vessel and the balloon is inflated to widen the vessel and push the obstructing material against the vessel's walls. The result is improved blood flow through the vessel.

Cannula—A small, flexible tube.

Cardioplegic arrest—Halting the electrical activity of the heart by delivery of a high potassium solution to the coronary arteries. The arrested heart provides a superior surgical field for operation.

Cardiopulmonary bypass—Use of the heart-lung machine to provide systemic circulation cardiac output and ventilation of the blood.

Coronary occlusion—Obstruction of an artery that supplies the heart. When the artery is completely blocked, a myocardial infarction (heart attack) results; an incomplete blockage may result in angina.

Coronary stent—An artificial support device used to keep a coronary vessel open.

Electrocardiography—A testing technique used to measure electrical impulses from the heart in order to gain information about its structure or function.

Myocardial infarction—Heart attack.

Stabilizer—A device used to depress the movement of the area around the coronary artery where the anastomosis is made. The stabilizer is used to provide a still, motionless field for suturing.

Sternotomy—A surgical opening into the thoracic cavity through the sternum (breastbone).

Thoracotomy—A surgical opening into the thoracic cavity.

(OPCAB) and minimally invasive direct coronary artery bypass (MIDCAB). The MIDCAB procedure includes procedures done both with and without cardiopulmonary bypass, the later being referred to as off-pump MIDCAB. Unless otherwise specified, MIDCAB refers to both types of procedures.

Minimally invasive valve surgery has been an outgrowth of the success with minimally invasive coronary artery bypass grafting. Incisions other then the traditional sternotomy allow access to the heart. Minimally invasive valve surgery still requires cardiopulmonary bypass, since this is a true open-heart procedure (i.e. this is not surgery that is done while the heart is beating). New tools in managing cardioplegic cardiac arrest allow for the smaller incision unobstructed by the required instrumentation. Cannulation of the femoral vessels instead of the larger vessels of the heart also improves visualization.

Demographics

Patients under the age of 70, but not limited by age, with a history of coronary artery disease can be evaluated for this procedure. High risk patients with advanced age, at risk for stroke, or suffering peripheral vascular disease, renal disease, or with poor lung function may benefit from OPCAB and MIDCAB.

Typically, disease of the left anterior descending coronary artery is treated with the technique called off-pump MIDCAB. With sternotomy, disease of the right and left coronary arteries can also be addressed by OPCAB. The significance and location of the coronary artery lesions may limit the success of the MIDCAB or OPCAB procedure. Most practices have at least one surgeon skilled in performing revascularizations without cardiopulmonary bypass. Of all coronary artery bypass grafting procedures, approximately 10–20% are performed in this manner.

Description

The patient receives cardiac monitoring during **general anesthesia**. Systemic anticoagulation is given to avoid clot formation from foreign surfaces and any periods of artery blockage (occlusion).

MIDCAB

If cardiopulmonary bypass is not employed, the procedure is called an off-pump MIDCAB. The surgeon performs an alternative incision (rather than a midline sternotomy), typically a left anterior **thoracotomy**. The left internal mammary artery is dissected from the left chest wall. A stabilizer device is placed on the heart to provide support of the left anterior descending artery as the heart continues to beat. This device applies gentle pressure or suction, mildly limiting cardiac function. The left internal mammary artery is sutured to the left anterior descending artery to bypass the blockage (anastomosis).

If cardiopulmonary bypass is indicated, the surgeon inserts cannulae (small, flexible tubes) into the femoral vessels. Aortic occlusion and cardioplegia are administered through a catheter advanced through the contralateral femoral artery into the aortic root (ascending aorta). This catheter has a balloon tip that stops blood flow to the coronary arteries when inflated, but allows selective administration of cardioplegia (a solution that stops the heart) to the coronary arteries. **Angiography** is performed to provide visualization of catheter placement.

The surgeon performs an alternative incision (rather than a midline sternotomy), typically a left anterior thoracotomy. The left internal mammary artery is dissected from the left chest wall. Cardiopulmonary bypass can be instituted with or without cardioplegic arrest. Cardioplegic arrest requires cardiopulmonary bypass. The use of cardioplegic arrest makes this a non-beating heart procedure, but it is still considered MIDCAB. Cardioplegic arrest of the heart occurs as the balloon tip of the catheter is inflated. The left internal mammary artery is sutured to the left anterior descending artery to bypass the blockage (anastomosis). Once the anastomosis is complete the balloon is deflated, allowing the heart to begin to beat. Cardiopulmonary bypass is discontinued once cardiac function is stabilized. The cannulae and catheter are removed, and the groin wounds are closed with sutures.

OPCAB

The OPCAB procedure does not use cardiopulmonary bypass. The incision of choice can be a midline sternotomy or a left anterior thoracotomy (incision in the side). The midline sternotomy allows access to both the right and left internal mammary arteries. Additional vascular bypass conduits may be acquired by harvesting the saphenous vein (in the leg), gastroepiploic artery (near the stomach), or radial artery (in the arm). A stabilizing device is used to secure the coronary artery of choice. This device applies gentle pressure or suction, mildly limiting cardiac function, but providing better access to posterior and inferior vessels of the heart. The surgeon makes the necessary anastomosis to the targeted coronary arteries. If conduits other then the mammary arteries are used they are connected to the ascending aorta to provide systemic blood flow.

If an anticoagulant was administered, drugs are given to reverse the anticoagulant. Upon completion of the off-pump MIDCAB, MIDCAB, or OPCAB procedure, the chest is closed. If a midline sternotomy was performed, stainless steel wires are implanted to hold the sternal bone together. Sutures are used to close the skin wound, and sterile **bandages** are applied as a wound dressing.

Diagnosis/Preparation

An **electrocardiogram** detects the presence of acute coronary blockage (occlusion). A history of myocardial infarction can also be detected by electrocardiogram. Patients with a history of angina also are evaluated for coronary artery disease. Coronary angiography provides the best diagnostic information about the extent and location of the coronary artery disease.

Aftercare

The patient receives continued cardiac monitoring in the **intensive care unit**. Once the patient is able to breathe on his/her own, the breathing tube is removed (extubation), if it is not removed immediately postoperatively. Any medications to treat poor cardiac function or manage blood pressure are discontinued as cardiac function improves and blood pressure stabilizes. Blood drainage tubes protruding from the chest cavity are removed once internal bleeding decreases. The patient also may be equipped with external cardiac pacing to maintain heart rate. The pacing is terminated once the heart is beating at an adequate rate free of arrhythmia. A warming blanket may be used to warm the patient's core temperature that was decreased by the surgical exposure.

The duration of the post-operative hospital stay is reduced by one to two days in these procedures. Pain also should be reduced. **Home care** for the wound is described prior to discharge, and instructions for responding to adverse events after discharge also are given. Patients who have undergone these procedures should expect to return to normal activities sooner than those who have undergone traditional coronary artery bypass grafting.

Risks

MIDCAB can result in a higher rate of restenosis (recurrence of narrowing of the arteries) then traditional coronary artery bypass grafting, but these numbers continue to decrease as experience with the

WHO PERFORMS THE PROCEDURE AND WHERE IS IT PERFORMED?

Medical centers performing cardiac surgical procedures are equipped to perform this procedure. A cardiothoracic, cardiovascular, or cardiac surgeon receives additional training to successfully complete this procedure. Special technology in stabilizer design is purchased by the institution and made available for the surgeon to master. Within most clinical practices one surgeon becomes skilled in the technique. This one surgeon completes most procedures off-pump with MIDCAB or OPCAB techniques as necessary to revascularize the patient.

QUESTIONS TO ASK THE DOCTOR

- Is there a surgeon associated with this practice skilled with OPCAB or MIDCAB procedures?
- Can the surgeon skilled in these procedures evaluate the patient for an OPCAB or MIDCAB procedure?
- How many procedures has the surgeon performed in the last year? In the last five years?
- What is the surgeon's reoperation rate in regards to length of graft patency?

procedure improves. Some patients may have to have the procedure converted to a standard sternotomy with cardiopulmonary bypass, if the anastomosis can not be completed from the MIDCAB approach. Rib fracture is the most common adverse event. Pericarditis also is a possible complication. Supraventricular arrhythmias and ST segment elevation also may develop.

In the event of systemic blood pressure abnormalities, arrhythmia, poor surgical anastomosis, or poor exposure of the coronary blood vessels, OPCAB patients may require conversion to cardiopulmonary bypass for completion of the anastomosis. Post-operatively some patients may need additional surgery to control bleeding or to address poor sternal healing. This is related to the increased use of both internal mammary arteries for these procedures. Cerebral complications and atrial fibrillation also may be experienced. These post-operative complications are comparable to those seen in patients who have undergone traditional coronary artery bypass grafting.

Normal results

Patency (openness) of the grafted vessels is expected to be the same as what is seen in traditional coronary artery bypass grafting. When compared to traditional coronary artery bypass grafting, minimally invasive heart surgery also is expected to result in a shorter hospital stay, less pain, fewer blood transfusions, and quicker return to normal activity.

Morbidity and mortality rates

MIDCAB

Conversion to a full sternotomy or sternotomy with cardiopulmonary bypass is expected in 1–2% of

patients. Redo procedures and **reoperation** can occur in over 5% of patients, which is still lower than the risk of a second procedure associated with balloon **angioplasty** and stent placement. Over 90% of all patients are expected to be free of adverse events. Complications most frequently involve rib fracture (over 10% of patients). Mortality associated with MICAB is low and is not seen during the surgical procedure in most instances, but is associated with post-operative complications.

OPCAB

Conversion to cardiopulmonary bypass may be required in patients if anastomosis cannot be completed due to unstable blood pressure, arrhythmia, ischemia, poor anastomosis, or poor surgical access. The same operative mortality is expected when compared to cardiopulmonary bypass patients. The expected decrease in neurological events, renal dysfunction, pulmonary complications, or arrhythmias has not yet been shown to be a consistent benefit, therefore all of these complications can still occur.

Alternatives

Percutaneous balloon angioplasty and **coronary stenting** of the left anterior descending artery are successful alternative procedures. MIDCAB may be a preferred treatment when compared to balloon angioplasty and stenting because fewer repeat interventions are required. An additional alternative is traditional on-pump, cardiopulmonary bypass; coronary artery bypass grafting is a powerful technique with a long record of safety and effectiveness since the 1960s.

Resources

BOOKS

Libby, P. et al. Braunwald's Heart Disease. 8th ed. Philadelphia: Saunders, 2007.

Townsend, CM et al. Sabiston Textbook of Surgery. 17th ed. Philadelphia: Saunders, 2004.

Allison Joan Spiwak, MSBME

Minor tranquilizers *see* **Antianxiety drugs**

Mitral valve repair

Definition

Mitral valve repair is a surgical procedure used to improve the function of a stenotic (narrowed), prolapsed (slipped from its normal position), or insufficient (weakened) mitral valve of the heart.

Purpose

The mitral valve controls the blood flow between the left atrium (upper chamber) and left ventricle (lower chamber) of the heart. When the mitral valve functions correctly, blood flows in one direction only— from the atrium to the ventricle. Then the valve becomes diseased or weakened, blood can backflow from the ventricle to the atrium when the ventricle contracts (systole). The mitral valve also can become narrowed, preventing the flow of blood from the left atrium into the left ventricle during ventricular filling (diastole). In mitral valve prolapse, one or more of the mitral valve's cusps protrude back into the left atrium during ventricular contraction. Mitral valve repair is performed to improve the function of the diseased valve so that it correctly controls the amount and direction of blood flow.

Demographics

Mitral valve prolapse is the most common heart valve defect. In the United States it is present in about 2–6% of the population. The defect is believed to have an inherited component and is seen twice as often in women as in men. Having this condition does not automatically mean that mitral insufficiency will develop. Patients with a history of rheumatic fever, coronary artery disease, infective endocarditis, or collagen vascular disease also may develop mitral insufficiency.

Mitral valve stenosis almost always is the result of having rheumatic fever in childhood. Rheumatic fever occurs in some people after a group A streptococcal throat infection (commonly called strep throat). Genetics appears to play a role in determining who develops rheumatic fever after a strep infection, with women more likely than men to progress to the disease. After rheumatic fever subsides, there is usually a latency period of 10–20 years before symptoms of mitral valve stenosis appear. The prevalence of mitral valve stenosis has declined in the United States because there has been a decline in the number of cases of rheumatic fever. In the United States in 2005, about one case of rheumatic fever occurred for every 100,000 people. Rheumatic fever is much more common in developing countries (100–150 cases per 100,000 in India, for example), and thus the rate of mitral valve stenosis is also higher. Mitral valve stenosis may be present at birth (congenital); however, it rarely occurs alone but rather in conjunction with other heart defects.

Description

Mitral valve repair is done under **general anesthesia** with continuous cardiac monitoring. Uncomplicated mitral valve surgery normally takes 2–3 hours. In traditional mitral repair, the surgeon uses a sternotomy to access the heart and large blood vessels. Anticoagulation drugs are given as cannulae are inserted into the large veins. Cardiopulmonary bypass (use of a heart-lung machine) is instituted. The heartbeat is stopped as blood vessels are clamped to prevent blood flow through the heart. The surgeon opens the heart to see the mitral valve. He/she may expose the mitral valve by opening the right atrium and then opening the atrial septum (tissue dividing the atria). Another approach requires a large left atrium that can be opened directly, making the mitral valve visible.

Mitral commissurotomy

Mitral commissurotomy is used to repair mitral stenosis associated with rheumatic fever. The commissures—openings between the valve leaflets—are manually separated by the surgeon. Fused chordae tendineae (cords of connective tissue that connect the mitral valve to the papillary muscle of the heart's left ventricle) are separated, along with papillary muscles. Calcium deposits may be removed from the valve leaflets. The left atrial appendage is removed to reduce the risk of future thromboemboli (blood clot) generation.

Chordae tendineae repair

The chordae tendineae can become lengthened or rupture, resulting in mitral valve prolapse (the valve slipping out of place). A skilled surgeon repairs the mitral valve structure by placing sutures in the valve

Mitral valve repair

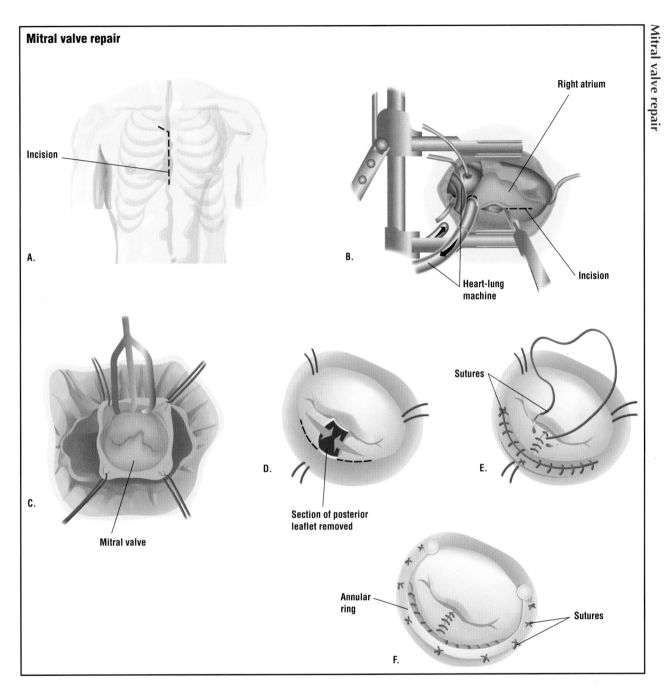

A.

B.

Right atrium

Incision

Heart-lung
machine

Incision

C.

Mitral valve

D.

Section of posterior
leaflet removed

Sutures

E.

Annular
ring

Sutures

F.

During a mitral valve repair, the patient's chest is opened along the sternum (A). The heart is connected to a heart-lung machine, and an incision is made into the right atrium, or upper chamber of the heart (B), exposing the mitral valve (C). A section of the valve is removed, and the area is repaired with sutures (D and E). A flexible fabric ring may be stitched to the outside of the valve to strengthen it, in a procedure called an annuloplasty (F). *(Illustration by GGS Information Services. Cengage Learning, Gale.)*

leaflets to stabilize the valve structure. Typically the posterior leaflet requires this type of repair.

Annuloplasty

A flexible fabric ring is sutured to the valve annulus to provide support and reconstruction for the patient's valve annulus. The size of the ring is selected to match the patient's own valve size. This repair allows the valve to function normally.

The heart is closed with sutures. De-airing of the heart is performed before removal of the clamps. When the clamps are removed, de-airing continues to

KEY TERMS

Acute—Rapid onset.

Annulus—A ring-shaped structure.

Anticoagulants—Drugs that are given to slow blood clot formation.

Atrium (plural Atria)—The right or left upper chamber of the heart.

Cannula (plural cannulae)—A small, flexible tube.

Cardiac catheterization—A diagnostic procedure (using a catheter inserted through a vein and threaded through the circulatory system to the heart) which does a comprehensive examination of how the heart and its blood vessels function.

Cardiopulmonary bypass—Use of the heart-lung machine to provide systemic circulation cardiac output and ventilation of the blood.

Chordae tendineae—The strands of connective tissue that connect the mitral valve to the papillary muscle of the heart's left ventricle.

Chronic—Long-term.

Commissures—The normal separations between the valve leaflets.

Doppler echocardiography—A testing technique that uses Doppler ultrasound technology to evaluate the pattern and direction of blood flow in the heart.

Endocarditis—Infection of the heart endocardium tissue, the inner most tissue and structures of the heart.

NYHA heart failure classification—A classification system for heart failure developed by the New York Heart Association. It includes the following four categories: I, symptoms with more than ordinary activity; II, symptoms with ordinary activity; III, symptoms with minimal activity; IV, symptoms at rest.

Rheumatic carditis—Inflammation of the heart muscle associated with acute rheumatic fever.

Rheumatic fever—An inflammatory disease that arises as a complication of untreated or inadequately treated strep throat infection. Rheumatic fever can seriously damage the heart valves.

Sternotomy—A surgical opening into the thoracic cavity through the sternum (breastbone).

Systemic circulation—Circulation supplied by the aorta including all tissue and organ beds, except the alveolar sacs of the lungs used for gas exchange and respiration.

Thromboemboli—Blood clots that develop in the circulation and lodge in capillary beds of tissues and organs.

Transesophageal echocardiography—A diagnostic test using an ultrasound device that is passed into the esophagus of the patient to create a clear image of the heart muscle and other parts of the heart.

---

ensure that no air enters the systemic circulation. At this time a transesophageal echocardiogram (TEE) may be used to test that the valve is functioning correctly and that the heart is free of air. If the surgeon is not satisfied with the repair, **mitral valve replacement** is performed. Once the surgeon is satisfied that the valve is working correctly, cardiopulmonary bypass is terminated, anticoagulation is reversed, and the cannulae are removed from the blood vessels. The sternotomy is closed. Permanent stainless steel wires are used to hold the sternum bone together. The skin incision is closed with sutures, and sterile **bandages** are applied to the wound.

Minimally invasive mitral valve repair

In the mid-2000s, some cardiac surgery centers began performing robot-assisted minimally invasive mitral valve repair. In minimally invasive repair, a 2–3 inch (5–8 cm) opening is made in the side of the chest instead of reaching the heart by breaking the sternum.

Then, with the assistance of a robotic arm, the valve is repaired. Minimally invasive mitral valve repair may not be appropriate for all patients, but when it is, it offers the advantages of less chance of infection and blood loss, a shorter hospital stay, and a faster, less painful recovery.

Diagnosis/Preparation

Mitral valve stenosis is diagnosed by history, **physical examination**, listening to the sounds of the heart (cardiac auscultation), **chest x ray**, and ECG. Patients may have no symptoms of a valve disorder or may have shortness of breath (dyspnea), fatigue, or pulmonary edema (fluid in the lungs). Other patients present with atrial fibrillation (a cardiac arrhythmia) or an embolic event (result of a blood clot, i.e., heart attack or stroke). Doppler **echocardiography** is the preferred diagnostic tool for evaluation of mitral valve stenosis, and can be performed in conjunction with non-invasive **exercise** testing by treadmill or bicycle. **Cardiac catheterization** is reserved for patients who demonstrate discrepancies in Doppler testing. Both left- and right-heart catheterization should be performed in the presence of elevated pulmonary artery pressures.

A diagnosis of mitral insufficiency requires a detailed patient history. Listening to the heart (auscultation) reveals the presence of a third heart sound. Chest x ray and ECG provide additional information. Again, Doppler echocardiography provides valuable information. Exercise testing with Doppler echocardiography can show the true severity of the disease.

After initial findings, patients may be followed with repeat visits and testing to monitor disease progress. If the patient has reached NYHA Class III or IV, replacement is considered. Severe pulmonary hypertension with pulmonary artery systolic pressures greater than 60 mm Hg is considered an indication for surgery. Left ventricular ejection fraction less than 60% also is an indication for surgery.

Aftercare

The patient receives continued cardiac monitoring in the **intensive care unit** and usually remains in intensive care for 24–48 hours after surgery. Ventilation support is discontinued when the patient is able to breathe on his/her own. If mechanical circulatory support and inotropic drugs (substances that stimulate heart muscle contractions, e.g. digitalis) were needed during the surgical procedure, they are discontinued as cardiac function recovers. Tubes draining blood from the chest cavity are removed as bleeding from the surgical procedure decreases. Prophylactic **antibiotics** are given to prevent infective endocarditis and prevent the recurrence of rheumatic carditis.

If the patient recovers normally, **discharge from the hospital** occurs within a week of surgery. At discharge, the patient is given specific instructions about **wound care** and infection recognition, as well as contact information for the physician and guidelines about when a visit to the emergency room is indicated. Within three to four weeks after discharge, the patient is seen for a follow-up office visit with the physician, at which time physical status will have improved for evaluation. Thereafter, asymptomatic, uncomplicated patients are seen at yearly intervals. Few limitations are placed on patient activity once recovery is complete.

Risks

There are always risks associated with general anesthesia and cardiopulmonary bypass. Risks specifically

WHO PERFORMS THE PROCEDURE AND WHERE IS IT PERFORMED?

Cardiothoracic and cardiovascular surgeons perform mitral valve repair. Surgeons are trained during their residency to perform these procedures, although a certain level of skill is required for perfection of the technique. Medical centers that perform cardiac surgery are able to provide mitral valve repair.

associated with mitral valve repair include embolism, bleeding, or operative valvular endocarditis. When valve repair does not produce adequate results, then increased operative time is required to replace the mitral valve. If the patient's mitral valve is replaced with a mechanical valve, the patient must take an anticoagulation drug, such as Coumadin, for the rest of his/her life. An inadequately repaired valve, if left untreated, results in continued myocardial dysfunction resulting in pulmonary edema, congestive heart failure, and systemic thromboemboli generation.

Normal results

Patients treated by mitral valve repair for mitral insufficiency can expect improved myocardial function and relief of symptoms. Oxygen consumption by skeletal muscle continues to improve. Cardiac output improves and pulmonary hypertension resolves over several months after the initial decrease in left atrial pressure, pulmonary artery pressure, and pulmonary arteriolar resistance.

Excellent results in terms of improved cardiac function and symptom relief also are expected for patients that undergo mitral valve repair for mitral stenosis.

Morbidity and mortality rates

Operative mortality associated with mitral valve repair for stenosis is 1–3%. The prognosis for restenosis (re-narrowing) is 30% at five years and 60% at nine years; additional surgery is required in 4–7% of patients at five years. Eighty to 90% of patients whose mitral valve stenosis was repaired by commissurotomy are complication free at five years after surgery.

Mitral valve repair for mitral insufficiency is the preferred approach because it preserves the valvular apparatus and left ventricular function. It also eliminates the risk of mechanical valve failure and the need for lifelong anticoagulation.

QUESTIONS TO ASK THE DOCTOR

- Is mitral valve repair the best treatment choice for my condition?
- Am I a candidate for minimally invasive mitral valve repair?
- How many of these procedures has the surgeon performed in the last year? in the last five years?
- What is the surgeon's morbidity and mortality rate with mitral valve repair?
- What will happen if the repair fails?
- What type of follow-up care is required during the first year after surgery and throughout the rest of my life?
- What type of complications can be encountered both acute and chronic?

Alternatives

The asymptomatic patient with a history of rheumatic fever can be treated with prophylactic antibiotics and followed until symptoms are appear. If atrial fibrillation develops antiarrhythmic medications can be used for treatment. Atrial **defibrillation** may relieve atrial fibrillation. Anticoagulants may be prescribed to prevent the occurrence of systemic embolization.

Mitral valve repair for mitral regurgitation is not as successful if the anterior leaflet is involved. Rheumatic, ischemic, or calcific diseases decrease the likelihood of repair in even the most skilled hands. In the absence of mitral valve replacement, mitral valve repair is indicated.

Resources

BOOKS
ICON Health Publications. *The Official Patient's Sourcebook on Mitral-Valve Prolapse.* San Diego, CA: ICON Health Publications, 2006.

PERIODICALS
Bonow, R., et al. "ACC/AHA 2006 Guidelines for the Management of Patients with Valvular Heart Disease." Circulation. 114 (2006) e84-e231. http://circ.ahajournals.org/cgi/reprint/114/5/e84.

ORGANIZATIONS
American Heart Association. 7272 Greenville Avenue, Dallas, TX 75231. (800) 242-8721. http://www.americanheart.org .
Mitral Valve Repair Center at Mount Sinai Hospital. 1190 Fifth Avenue, New York, NY 10029 (212) 659-6820. http://www.mitralvalverepair.org.

OTHER
Gillinov, A, Marc. "Mitral Valve Repair." *Cleveland Clinic Heart and Vascular Institute.*http://www.clevelandclinic.org/heartcenter/ [accessed May 16, 2008].
"Mitral Valve Repair Using Robotic Surgery." *St. Joseph' Hospital (Atlanta) Center for Robotic Surgery.* [cited February 5, 2008]. http://www.stjosephsatlanta.org/center-for-robotic-surgery/heart/mitral-valve-repair-robotic-surgery.html.

Allison Joan Spiwak, MSBME
Tish Davidson, A. M.

Mitral valve replacement

Definition

Mitral valve replacement is surgical procedure in which the diseased mitral valve of the heart is replaced by a mechanical valve or biological tissue valve.

Purpose

The mitral valve controls the blood flow between the left atrium (upper chamber) and left ventricle (lower chamber) of the heart. When the mitral valve functions correctly, blood flows in one direction only— from the atrium to the ventricle. When the valve becomes diseased or weakened, blood can backflow from the ventricle to the atrium when the ventricle contracts (systole). The mitral valve also can become narrowed, preventing the flow of blood from the left atrium into the left ventricle during ventricular filling (diastole). In mitral valve prolapse, one or more of the mitral valve's cusps protrude back into the left atrium during ventricular contraction. **Mitral valve repair** is the preferred operation to correct these conditions and improve the function of the diseased valve so that it correctly controls the amount and direction of blood flow. When mitral valve repair is not possible, mitral valve replacement is performed. The defective mitral valve is surgically removed and a new mechanical valve or biological tissue valve (from a pig, cow, or human cadaver) is put into place to correctly control blood flow.

Demographics

Mitral valve prolapse is the most common heart valve defect. In the United States it is present in about 2–6% of the population. The defect is believed to have an inherited component and is seen twice as often in women as in men. Having this condition does not

Annulus—A ring-shaped structure.

Anticoagulants—Drugs that are given to slow blood clot formation.

Biological tissue valve—An autograft is a valve that comes from the patient, usually the pulmonary valve. An autologous pericardial valve is constructed from the patient's pericardium (the fibrous sac that surrounds the heart and the roots of the great vessels and also forms the outer layer of the heart wall) at the time of surgery. A homograft (or allograft) valve is a valve harvested from a human cadaver. A porcine (pig) or bovine (cow) heterograft is animal tissue valve that is made acceptable to the body by destroying antigenicity so that the body will not reject the foreign tissue.

Cardiac catheterization—A diagnostic procedure (using a catheter inserted through a vein and threaded through the circulatory system to the heart) which does a comprehensive examination of how the heart and its blood vessels function.

Cardiopulmonary bypass—Use of the heart-lung machine to provide systemic circulation cardiac output and ventilation of the blood.

Doppler echocardiography—A testing technique that uses Doppler ultrasound technology to evaluate the pattern and direction of blood flow in the heart.

Endocarditis—Infection of the heart endocardium tissue, the inner most tissue and structures of the heart.

Mechanical valve—There are three types of mechanical valve: ball valve, disk valve, and bileaflet valve.

NYHA heart failure classification—A classification system for heart failure developed by the New York Heart Association. It includes the following four categories: I, symptoms with more than ordinary activity; II, symptoms with ordinary activity; III, symptoms with minimal activity; IV, symptoms at rest.

Rheumatic carditis—Inflammation of the heart muscle associated with acute rheumatic fever.

Rheumatic fever—An inflammatory disease that arises as a complication of untreated or inadequately treated strep throat infection. Rheumatic fever can seriously damage the heart valves.

Sternotomy—A surgical opening into the thoracic cavity through the sternum (breastbone).

Systemic circulation—Circulation supplied by the aorta including all tissue and organ beds, except the alveolar sacs of the lungs used for gas exchange and respiration.

Thromboemboli—Blood clots that develop in the circulation and lodge in capillary beds of tissues and organs.

Transesophageal echocardiography—A diagnostic test using an ultrasound device that is passed into the esophagus of the patient to create a clear image of the heart muscle and other parts of the heart.

automatically mean that mitral insufficiency will develop, and even when it does, mitral valve repair is often preferable to valve replacement. Patients with a history of rheumatic fever, coronary artery disease, infective endocarditis, or collagen vascular disease also may develop mitral insufficiency.

Mitral valve stenosis almost always is the result of having rheumatic fever in childhood. Rheumatic fever occurs in some people after a group A streptococcal throat infection (commonly called strep throat). Genetics appears to play a role in determining who develops rheumatic fever after a strep infection, with women more likely than men to progress to the disease. After rheumatic fever subsides, there is usually a latency period of 10–20 years before symptoms of mitral valve stenosis appear. The prevalence of mitral valve stenosis has declined in the United States because there has been a decline in the number of

cases of rheumatic fever. In the United States in 2005, about one case of rheumatic fever occurred for every 100,000 people. Rheumatic fever is much more common in developing countries (100–150 cases per 100,000 in India, for example), and thus the rate of mitral valve stenosis is also higher. Mitral valve stenosis may be present at birth (congenital); however, it rarely occurs alone but rather in conjunction with other heart defects. Again, repair is preferable to replacement of the mitral valve.

Description

A heart valve is a structure within the heart that prevents the backflow of blood by opening and closing with each heartbeat. Replacement heart valves are either mechanical or biological tissue valves. For patients under the age of 65, the mechanical valve offers superior longevity, but the use of this type of valve requires that the patient take an anticoagulation drug for the rest of his/her life. The biological tissue valve does not require anticoagulation therapy, but this type of valve is prone to deterioration leading to re-operation after about 10–15 years. Women who may want to have children after a valve replacement should usually receive a biological tissue valve, because the anticoagulant warfarin (Coumadin) most often prescribed for patients with mechanical valves is associated with fetal birth defects. **Aspirin** can be substituted for warfarin in certain circumstances.

Mitral valve replacement is done under **general anesthesia** with continuous cardiac monitoring. Uncomplicated mitral valve surgery normally takes 2–3 hours. To replace the mitral valve, the surgeon breaks the breastbone (sternum) to gain access to the heart and large blood vessels. Anticoagulation drugs are given as cannulae are inserted into the large veins. Cardiopulmonary bypass (use of a heart-lung machine) is instituted. The heartbeat is stopped as blood vessels are clamped to prevent blood flow through the heart. The surgeon opens the heart to see the mitral valve. He/she may expose the mitral valve by opening the right atrium and then opening the atrial septum (tissue dividing the atria). Another approach requires a large left atrium that can be opened directly, making the mitral valve visible.

Next, the surgeon cuts the diseased valve away from the valve annulus (outer ring). The annulus is sized so that the proper size of valve can be selected for the patient's anatomy. Sutures are applied around the valve annulus, the valve is sutured into place, and tied into position. The atrial septum is closed with suture or left to heal naturally, and the heart is closed with sutures.

De-airing of the heart is performed before removal of the clamps. When the clamps are removed, de-airing continues to ensure that no air enters the systemic circulation. At this time a transesophageal echocardiogram (TEE) may be used to test that the valve is functioning correctly and that the heart is free of air. If the surgeon is not satisfied with the repair, mitral valve replacement is performed. Once the surgeon is satisfied that the valve is working correctly, cardiopulmonary bypass is terminated, anticoagulation is reversed, and the cannulae are removed from the blood vessels. The sternotomy is closed. Permanent stainless steel wires are used to hold the sternum bone together. The skin incision is closed with sutures, and sterile **bandages** are applied to the wound.

Diagnosis/Preparation

Mitral valve stenosis is diagnosed by history, **physical examination**, listening to the sounds of the heart (cardiac auscultation), **chest x ray**, and ECG. Patients may have no symptoms of a valve disorder or may have shortness of breath (dyspnea), fatigue, or frank pulmonary edema. Other patients present with atrial fibrillation (a cardiac arrhythmia) or an embolic event. Doppler **echocardiography** is the preferred diagnostic tool for evaluation of mitral valve stenosis, and it can be performed in conjunction with non-invasive **exercise** testing by treadmill or bicycle. **Cardiac catheterization** is reserved for patients who demonstrate discrepancies in Doppler testing. Both left- and right-heart catheterization should be performed in the presence of elevated pulmonary artery pressures.

A diagnosis of mitral insufficiency requires a detailed patient history. Listening to the heart (auscultation) reveals the presence of a third heart sound. Chest x ray and ECG provide additional information. Again, Doppler echocardiography provides valuable information. Exercise testing with Doppler echocardiography can show the true severity of the disease.

After initial findings, patients may be followed with repeat visits and testing to monitor disease progress. If the patient has reached NYHA Class III or IV, replacement is considered. Severe pulmonary hypertension with pulmonary artery systolic pressures greater than 60 mm Hg is considered an indication for surgery. Left ventricular ejection fraction (a measure of blood output with each heartbeat) less than 60% normal also is an indication for surgery.

Aftercare

The patient receives continued cardiac monitoring in the **intensive care unit** and usually remains in intensive care for 24–48 hours after surgery. Ventilation support is discontinued when the patient is able to breathe on his/her own. If mechanical circulatory support and inotropic agents (a substance that influences the force of muscle contractions, e.g. digitalis) were needed during the surgical procedure, they are discontinued as cardiac function recovers. Tubes draining blood from the chest cavity are removed as bleeding from the surgical procedure decreases. Prophylactic **antibiotics** are given to prevent infective endocarditis and the recurrence of rheumatic carditis.

Both mechanical and biological tissue valves require anticoagulation therapy after surgery, and while patients are hospitalized their anticoagulant status is monitored and dosages are adjusted accordingly. Patients with biological tissue valves can discontinue anticoagulation therapy within three months of valve replacement surgery, but those with mechanical valves must take an anticoagulant (aspirin, warfarin, or a

WHO PERFORMS THE PROCEDURE AND WHERE IS IT PERFORMED?

Cardiothoracic and cardiovascular surgeons provide surgical treatment. Surgeons are trained during the residency to perform these procedures. Medical centers that perform cardiac surgery are able to provide mitral valve replacement.

combination of the two) for the rest of their lives. These patients are regularly monitored for INR values (a measure of the clotting potential of their blood).

If the patient recovers normally, **discharge from the hospital** occurs within a week of surgery. At discharge, the patient is given specific instructions about **wound care** and infection recognition, as well as contact information for the physician and guidelines about when a visit to the emergency room is indicated. Within three to four weeks after discharge, the patient is seen for follow-up office visit with the physician, at which time physical status will have improved for evaluation. Thereafter, asymptomatic, uncomplicated patients are seen at yearly intervals. Few limitations are placed on patient activity once recovery is complete.

Risks

There are always risks associated with general anesthesia and cardiopulmonary bypass. Risks specifically associated with mitral valve replacement include embolism, bleeding, and operative valvular endocarditis. Hemolysis (the breakdown of red blood cells) is associated with certain types of mechanical valves, but is not a contraindication for implantation.

Normal results

Patients treated by mitral valve replacement for mitral insufficiency can expect relief of symptoms. For patients who received mechanical valves, anticoagulation therapy is continued for life. Since thromboembolic complications are associated with initial implant of biological tissue valves, patients who received this type of valve take an anticoagulant for three months after surgery. If non-cardiac surgery or dental care is needed, the anticoagulation therapy is adjusted to prevent bleeding complications.

Patients who undergo mitral valve replacement for mitral stenosis can expect excellent improvement of symptoms. Those patients with symptoms consistent with NYHA class IV before surgery have better

QUESTIONS TO ASK THE DOCTOR

- Is mitral valve replacement the best treatment option for my condition? Why is it preferable to mitral valve repair?
- How many of these procedures has the surgeon performed in the last year? in the last five years?
- What is the surgeon's morbidity and mortality rate with mitral valve replacement?
- What type of replacement valve, biological tissue or mechanical, is best for me?
- What are the pros and cons of each valve type?
- What type of follow-up care is required during the first year after valve implant and for the rest of my life?
- What types of complications are associated with this surgery?

outcome after mitral valve replacement compared to no treatment.

Morbidity and mortality rates

Mitral valve replacement carries a 5% risk of **death** in young, healthy patients. With increased age, additional medical problems, or pulmonary hypertension the risk of death increases substantially. Postreplacement the five-year survival is 80%. Patients over the age of 75 have poorer outcomes when mitral valve replacement is used to treat mitral insufficiency.

Alternatives

Mitral valve replacement is considered only after mitral valve repair has proved inadequate or inappropriate. An asymptomatic patient with a history of rheumatic fever can be treated with prophylactic antibiotics and followed until symptoms are appear. If atrial fibrillation develops, drugs may be used to regulate heart rhythm. Anticoagulation therapy is employed to avoid systemic emboli during periods of atrial fibrillation.

Resources

BOOKS

ICON Health Publications. *The Official Patient's Sourcebook on Mitral-Valve Prolapse.* San Diego, CA: ICON Health Publications, 2006.

PERIODICALS

Bonow, R., et al. "ACC/AHA 2006 Guidelines for the Management of Patients with Valvular Heart Disease." Circulation. 114 (2006) e84-e231. http://circ.ahajour nals.org/cgi/reprint/114/5/e84.

ORGANIZATIONS

American Heart Association. 7272 Greenville Avenue, Dallas, TX 75231. (800) 242-8721. http://www.american heart.org .

Mitral Valve Repair Center at Mount Sinai Hospital. 1190 Fifth Avenue, New York, NY 10029 (212) 659-6820. http://www.mitralvalverepair.org.

Allison Joan Spiwak, MSBME
Tish Davidson, A. M.

Modified radical mastectomy

Definition

A surgical procedure that removes the breast, surrounding tissue, and nearby lymph nodes that are affected by cancer.

Purpose

The purpose for modified radical **mastectomy** is the removal of breast cancer (abnormal cells in the breast that grow rapidly and replace normal healthy tissue). Modified radical mastectomy is the most widely used surgical procedure to treat operable breast

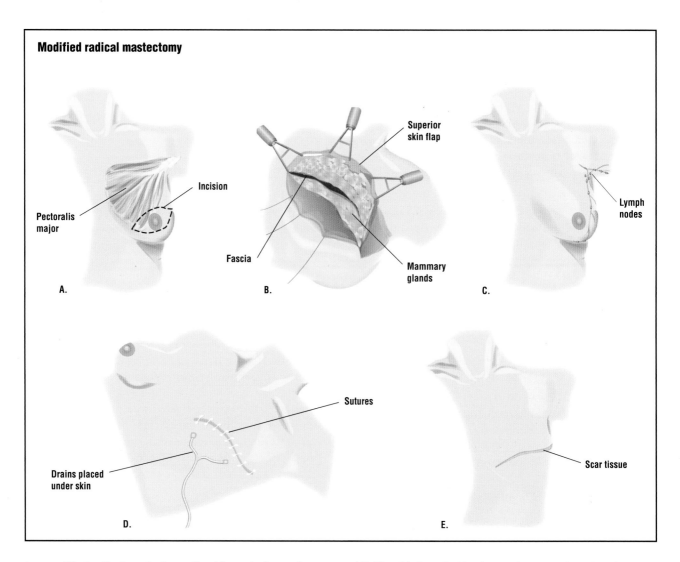

Modified radical mastectomy

A. Pectoralis major, Incision

B. Superior skin flap, Fascia, Mammary glands

C. Lymph nodes

D. Sutures, Drains placed under skin

E. Scar tissue

In a modified radical mastectomy, the skin on the breast is cut open (A). The skin is pulled back, and the tumor, lymph nodes, and breast tissue is removed (B and C). The incision is closed (D). *(Illustration by GGS Information Services. Cengage Learning, Gale.)*

cancer. This procedure leaves a chest muscle called the pectoralis major intact. Leaving this muscle in place will provide a soft tissue covering over the chest wall and a normal-appearing junction of the shoulder with the anterior (front) chest wall. This sparing of the pectoralis major muscle will avoid a disfiguring hollow defect below the clavicle. Additionally, the purpose of modified radical mastectomy is to allow for the option of **breast reconstruction**, a procedure that is possible, if desired, due to intact muscles around the shoulder of the affected side. The modified radical mastectomy procedure involves removal of large multiple tumor growths located underneath the nipple and cancer cells on the breast margins.

Demographics

The highest rates of breast cancer occur in Western countries (more than 100 cases per 100,000 women) and the lowest among Asian countries (10–15 cases per 100,000 women). Men can also have breast cancer, but the incidence is much less when compared to women. There is a strong genetic correlation since breast cancer is more prevalent in females who had a close relative (mother, sister, maternal aunt, or maternal grandmother) with previous breast cancer. Increased susceptibility for development of breast cancer can occur in females who never breastfed a baby, had a child after age 30, started menstrual periods very early, or experienced menopause very late.

The American Cancer Society estimated that in 2007, 240,510 new cases of breast cancer would be diagnosed in the United States and 40,460 women would die as a result of the disease. Approximately one in eight women will develop breast cancer at some point in her life. The risk of developing breast cancer increases with age: women aged 30 to 40 have a one in 252 chance of developing breast cancer; women aged 40 to 50 have a one in 68 chance; women aged 50 to 60 have a one in 35 chance; and women aged 60 to 70 have a one in 27 chance—and these statistics do not even account for genetic and environmental factors.

Description

The surgeon's goal during this procedure is to minimize any chance of local/regional recurrence; avoid any loss of function; and maximize options for breast reconstruction. Incisions are made to avoid visibility in a low neckline dress or bathing suit. An incision in the shape of an ellipse is made. The surgeon removes the minimum amount of skin and tissue so that remaining healthy tissue can be used for possible reconstruction. Skin flaps are made carefully and as

KEY TERMS

Lymphatic system—A system that filters excess tissue fluids through lymph nodes to return to the bloodstream.

thinly as possible to maximize removal of diseased breast tissues. The skin over a neighboring muscle (pectoralis major fascia) is removed, after which the surgeon focuses in the armpit (axilla, axillary) region. In this region, the surgeon carefully identifies vital anatomical structures such as blood vessels (veins, arteries) and nerves. Accidental injury to specific nerves like the medial pectoral neurovascular bundle will result in destruction of the muscles that this surgery attempts to preserve, such as the pectoralis major muscle. In the armpit region, the surgeon carefully protects the vital structures while removing cancerous tissues. After axillary surgery, breast reconstruction can be performed, if desired by the patient.

Diagnosis/Preparation

Modified radical mastectomy is a surgical procedure to treat breast cancer. In order for this procedure to be an operable option, a definitive diagnosis of breast cancer must be established. The first clinical sign for approximately 80% of women with breast cancer is a mass (lump) located in the breast. A lump can be discovered by monthly self-examination or by a health professional who can find 10–25% of breast cancers that are missed by yearly mammograms (a low radiation x ray of the breasts). A biopsy can be performed to examine the cells from a lump that is suspicious for cancer. The diagnosis of the extent of cancer and spread to regional lymph nodes determines the treatment course (i.e., whether surgery, chemotherapy, or radiation therapy, either singly or in combinations). Staging the cancer can estimate the amount of tumor, which is important not only for diagnosis but for prognosis (statistical outcome of the disease process). Patients with a type of breast cancer called ductal carcinoma in situ (DCIS), which is a stage 0 cancer, have the best outcome (nearly all these patients are cured of breast cancer). Persons who have cancerous spread to other distant places within the body (metastases) have stage IV cancer and the worst prognosis (potential for survival). Persons affected with stage IV breast cancer have essentially no chance for cure.

Persons affected with breast cancer must undergo the staging of the cancer to determine the extent of cancerous growth and possible spread (metastasis) to distant organs. Patients with stage 0 disease have non-invasive cancer with a very good outcome. Stages I and II are early breast cancer, without lymph node involvement (stage I) and with node positive results (stage II). Persons with stage III disease have locally advanced disease and about a 50% chance for five-year survival. Stage IV disease is the most severe since the breast cancer cells have spread through lymph nodes to distant areas and/or other organs in the body. It is very unlikely that persons with stage IV metastatic breast cancer survive 10 years after diagnosis.

It is also imperative to assess the degree of cancerous spread to lymph nodes within the armpit region. Of primary importance to stage determination and regional lymph node involvement is identification and analysis of the sentinel lymph node. The sentinel lymph node is the first lymph node to which any cancer would spread. The procedure for sentinel node biopsy involves injecting a radioactively labeled tracer (technetium 99) or a blue dye (isosulphan blue) into the tumor site. The tracer or dye will spread through the lymphatic system to the sentinel node, which should be surgically removed and examined for the presence of cancer cells. If the sentinel node and one or two other neighboring lymph nodes are negative, it is very likely that the remaining lymph nodes will not contain cancerous cells, and further surgery may not be necessary.

Once a breast lump (mass) has been identified by **mammography** or **physical examination**, the patient should undergo further evaluation to histologically (studying the cells) identify or rule out the presence of cancer cells. A procedure called fine-needle aspiration allows the clinician to extract cells directly from the lump for further evaluation. If a diagnosis cannot be established by fine-needle biopsy, the surgeon should perform an open biopsy (surgical removal of the suspicious mass). Preparation for surgery is imperative. The patient should plan for both direct care and recovery time after modified radical mastectomy. Preparation immediately prior to surgery should include no food or drink after midnight before the procedure. Post-surgical preparation should include caregivers to help with daily tasks for several days.

Aftercare

After breast cancer surgery, women should undergo frequent testing to ensure early detection of cancer recurrence. It is recommended that annual mammograms, physical examination, or additional tests (biopsy) be performed annually. Aftercare can also include psychotherapy since mastectomy is emotionally

WHO PERFORMS THE PROCEDURE AND WHERE IS IT PERFORMED?

The procedure is typically performed by a surgeon who has received five years of general surgery training and additional training in the specialty of surgical oncology. A surgeon who specializes in the area has expertise in removing cancerous tissues or areas. The procedure is performed in a hospital and requires that the hospital have a surgical care unit. In the surgical care unit, the patient will be treated by a team of professionals that includes, but is not limited to, physicians, nurses, physician assistants, and medical assistants.

traumatic. Affected women may be worried or have concerns about appearance, the relationship with their sexual partner, and possible physical limitations. Community-centered support groups usually made up of former breast cancer surgery patients can be a source of emotional support after surgery. Patients may stay in the hospital for one to two days. For about five to seven days after surgery, there will be one or two drains left inside to remove any extra fluid from the area after surgery. Usually, the surgeon will prescribe medication to prevent pain. Movement restriction should be specifically discussed with the surgeon.

Risks

There are several risks associated with modified radical mastectomy. The procedure is performed under **general anesthesia**, which itself carries risk. Women may have short-term pain and tenderness. The most frequent risk of breast cancer surgery (with extensive lymph node removal) is edema, or swelling of the arm, which is usually mild, but the presence of fluid can increase the risk of infection. Leaving some lymph nodes intact instead of removing all of them may help lessen the likelihood of swelling. Nerves in the area may be damaged. There may be numbness in the arm or difficulty moving shoulder muscles. There is also the risk of developing a lump scar (keloid) after surgery. Another risk is that surgery did not remove all the cancer cells and that further treatment may be necessary (with chemotherapy and/or radiotherapy). By far, the worst risk is recurrence of cancer. However, immediate signs of risk following surgery include fever, redness in the incision area, unusual drainage from the incision, and

QUESTIONS TO ASK THE DOCTOR

- What is the prognosis for the stage (0, I, II, III, IV) of my type of cancer?
- Will my movement be restricted after surgery?
- What care will I need on a daily basis following surgery?
- When should we set up a follow-up consultation/ examination?
- Will I require other treatment (chemotherapy and/ or radiation therapy) following surgery?
- What kind of mental-health treatment should I pursue (psychotherapy, community-centered support groups, etc.) following surgery?
- What options do I have for breast reconstruction? When would that treatment begin?

increasing pain. If any of these signs develop, it is imperative to call the surgeon immediately.

Normal results

If no complications develop, the surgical area should completely heal within three to four weeks. After mastectomy, some women may undergo breast reconstruction (which can be done during mastectomy). Recent studies have indicated that women who desire cosmetic **reconstructive surgery** have a higher quality of life and better sense of well-being than those who do not utilize this option.

Morbidity and mortality rates

The outcome of breast cancer is very dependent of the stage at the time of diagnosis. For stage 0 disease, the five-year survival is almost 100%. For stage I (early/lymph node negative), the five-year survival is alsom almost 100%. For stage II (early/ lymph node positive), the five-year survival decreases to 81-92%. For stage III disease (locally advanced), the five-year survival is 54-67%. For women with stage IV (metastatic) breast cancer, the five-year survival is about 20%.

Approximately 17% of patients develop lymphedema after axillary lymph node dissection, while only 3% of patients develop lymphedema after sentinel node biopsy. Five percent of women are unhappy with the cosmetic effects of the surgery.

Alternatives

There are no real alternatives to mastectomy. Surgical requirement is clear since mastectomy is recommended for tumors with dimensions over 2 in (5 cm). Additional treatment (adjuvant) is typically recommended with chemotherapy and/or radiation therapy to destroy any remaining cancer during surgery. Modified radical mastectomy is one of the standard treatment recommendations for stage III breast cancer.

Resources

BOOKS

Abeloff, MD et al. Clinical Oncology. 3rd ed. Philadelphia: Elsevier, 2004.

Khatri, VP and JA Asensio. Operative Surgery Manual. 1st ed. Philadelphia: Saunders, 2003.

Townsend, CM et al. Sabiston Textbook of Surgery. 17th ed. Philadelphia: Saunders, 2004.

ORGANIZATIONS

American Cancer Society. (800) ACS-2345. http://www.cancer.org.

Cancer support groups. http://www.cancernews.com.

Y-ME National Breast Cancer Organization. http://www.y-me.org.

Laith Farid Gulli, MD
Nicole Mallory, MS, PA-C

Mohs surgery

Definition

Mohs surgery, also called Mohs micrographic surgery, is a precise surgical technique that is used to remove all parts of cancerous skin tumors while preserving as much healthy tissue as possible.

Purpose

Mohs surgery is used to treat cancers of the skin, such as basal cell carcinoma, squamous cell carcinoma, and melanoma.

Malignant skin tumors may occur in strange, asymmetrical shapes. The tumor may have long finger-like projections that extend across the skin (laterally) or down into the skin. Because these extensions may be composed of only a few cells, they cannot be seen or felt. Standard surgical removal (excision) may miss these cancerous cells leading to recurrence of the tumor. To assure removal of all cancerous tissue, a large piece of skin needs to be removed. This causes a cosmetically unacceptable result, especially if the cancer is located on

KEY TERMS

Carcinoma—Cancer that begins in the cells that cover or line an organ.

Fixative—A chemical that preserves tissue without destroying or altering the structure of the cells.

Fixed—A term used to describe chemically preserved tissue. Fixed tissue is dead so it does not bleed or sense pain.

Mohs excision—Referring to the excision of one layer of tissue during Mohs surgery. Also called stage.

the face. Mohs surgery enables the surgeon to precisely excise the entire tumor without removing excessive amounts of the surrounding healthy tissue.

Mohs surgery is performed when:

- The cancer was treated previously and recurred.
- Scar tissue exists in the area of the cancer.
- The cancer is in at least one area where it is important to preserve healthy tissue for maximum functional and cosmetic result, such as on the eyelids, the nose, the ears, and the lips.
- The edges of the cancer cannot be clearly defined.
- The cancer grows rapidly or uncontrollably.

Demographics

According to the American Cancer Society, about one million people in the United States are diagnosed with non-melanoma skin cancer every year. Another 59,940 people are diagnosed with melanoma. The two most common types of skin cancer are basal cell carcinoma and squamous cell carcinoma, with basal cell carcinoma accounting for more than 90% of all of skin cancers.

Melanoma is the most serious type of skin cancer. Each year in the United States more than 59,940 people are diagnosed with melanoma, and it is becoming more and more common, especially among Western countries. In the United States, the percentage of people who develop melanoma has more than doubled in the past 30 years.

Description

There are two types of Mohs surgery: fresh-tissue technique and fixed-tissue technique. Of the surgeons who perform Mohs surgery, 72% use only the fresh-tissue technique. The remaining surgeons (18%) use both techniques. However, the fixed-tissue technique is used in fewer than 5% of patients. The main difference between the two techniques is in the preparatory steps.

Fresh-tissue technique

Fresh-tissue Mohs surgery is performed under **local anesthesia** for tumors of the skin. The area to be excised is cleaned with a disinfectant solution and a sterile drape is placed over the site. The surgeon may outline the tumor using a surgical marking pen, or a dye. A local anesthetic (lidocaine plus epinephrine) is injected into the area. Once the local anesthetic has taken effect, the main portion of the tumor is excised (debulked) using a spoon-shaped tool (curette). To define the area to be excised and to allow for accurate mapping of the tumor, the surgeon makes identifying marks around the lesion. These marks may be made with **stitches**, **staples**, fine cuts with a scalpel, or temporary tattoos. One layer of tissue is carefully excised (first Mohs excision), cut into smaller sections, and taken to the laboratory for analysis.

If cancerous cells are found in any of the tissue sections, a second layer of tissue is removed (second Mohs excision). Because only the sections that have cancerous cells are removed, healthy tissue can be spared. The entire procedure, including surgical repair of the wound, is performed in one day. Surgical repair may be performed by the Mohs surgeon, a plastic surgeon, or another specialist. In certain cases, wounds may be allowed to heal naturally.

Fixed-tissue technique

With fixed-tissue Mohs surgery, the tumor is debulked, as described previously. Trichloracetic acid is applied to the wound to control bleeding, followed by a preservative (fixative) called zinc chloride. The wound is dressed and the tissue is allowed to fix for six to 24 hours, depending on the depth of the tissue involved. This period, called the fixation period, can be painful to the patient. The first Mohs excision is performed as described; however, anesthesia is not required because the tissue is dead. If cancerous cells are found, fixative is applied to the affected area for an additional six to 24 hours. Excisions are performed in this sequential process until all cancerous tissue is removed. Surgical repair of the wound may be performed once all fixed tissue has sloughed off—usually a few days after the last excision.

Diagnosis/Preparation

An oncologist will have diagnosed the skin cancer of the patient using standard cancer diagnostic tools, such as biopsy of the tumor.

WHO PERFORMS THE PROCEDURE AND WHERE IS IT PERFORMED?

Mohs surgery is performed in a hospital setting by highly trained surgeons who are specialists both in dermatology and pathology. With their extensive knowledge of the skin and unique pathologic skills, they are able to remove only diseased tissue, preserving healthy tissue and minimizing the cosmetic impact of the surgery. Only physicians who have also completed a residency in dermatology are qualified for Mohs surgical training. The surgery is very often performed on an outpatient basis, usually in one day.

To prepare for surgery, and under certain conditions (such as the location of the skin tumor or health status of the patient), **antibiotics** may be given to the patient prior to the procedure; this is known as prophylactic antibiotic treatment. Patients are encouraged to eat prior to surgery and also to bring along snacks in case the procedure become lengthy. To reduce the risk of bleeding, the use of **nonsteroidal anti-inflammatory drugs** (NSAIDs), alcohol, vitamin E, and fish oil tablets should be avoided prior to the procedure. The patient who uses over-the-counter **aspirin** or the prescription blood-thinners, brands Coumadin (warfarin, generically) and heparin, should consult with the prescribing physician before adjusting the dosage of any drug.

Aftercare

Patients should expect to receive specific **wound care** instructions from their physician or surgeon. Generally, however, wounds that have been repaired with absorbable stitches or skin grafts should be kept covered with a bandage for one week. Wounds that have been repaired using nonabsorbable stitches should also be covered with a bandage that should be replaced daily until the stitches are removed one to two weeks later. Signs of infection (e.g., redness, pain, drainage) should be reported to the physician immediately.

Risks

Using the fresh-tissue technique on a large tumor requires large amounts of local anesthetic that can be toxic. Complications of Mohs surgery include infection, bleeding, scarring, and nerve damage.

Tumors spread in unpredictable patterns. Sometimes a seemingly small tumor is found to be quite

QUESTIONS TO ASK THE DOCTOR

- How long have you been performing Mohs surgery?
- Will you use the fresh-tissue or fixed-tissue technique?
- Will I have to alter the use of my current medications for this procedure?
- What will you do if you don't find the border of the cancerous lesion?
- How will the wound be repaired?
- Will I need a plastic surgeon to repair the wound?
- What is the cure rate for this type of cancer when treated by Mohs surgery?
- What is the chance that the tumor will recur?
- How often will I have follow-up appointments?

large and widespread, resulting in a much larger excision than was anticipated.

Normal results

Most skin cancers treated by Mohs surgery are completely removed with minimal loss of normal skin.

Morbidity and mortality rates

Mohs surgery provides high cure rates for malignant skin tumors. For instance, the five-year recurrence rate for primary basal cell carcinomas treated by Mohs surgery is about 1%. Five-year recurrence rates for other techniques are as follows: surgical excision, 10.1%; curettage and desiccation, 7.7%, radiation therapy, 8.7%, and **cryotherapy**, 7.5%. For squamous cell carcinoma treated by Mohs surgery, the five-year recurrence rate is 3.1% for lesions involving the skin and lip, 5.3% for lesions involving the ear. Other modalities have a 10.9% five-year recurrence rate for lesions involving the skin and lip, and a 18.7% five-year recurrence rate for lesions involving the ear.

Alternatives

Mohs surgery is a specialized technique that is not indicated for the treatment of every type of skin cancer, and is most appropriately used under specific, well-defined circumstances. The majority of basal cell carcinomas can be treated with very high cure rates by standard methods, including electrodessication and curettage (ED&C), local excision, cryosurgery (freezing), and irradiation.

Resources

BOOKS

Habif TP. Clinical Dermatology. 4th ed. St. Louis: Mosby, 2004.

PERIODICALS

Cook, J. L., and J. B. Perone. "A prospective evaluation of the incidence of complications associated with Mohs micrographic surgery." Archives of Dermatology 139 (February 2003): 143–152.

Jackson, E. M., and J. Cook. "Mohs micrographic surgery of a papillary eccrine adenoma." Dermatologic Surgery 28 (December 2002): 1168–1172.

Smeets, N. W., Stavast-Kooy, A. J., Krekels, G. A., Daemen, M. J., and H. A. Neumann. "Adjuvant Cytokeratin Staining in Mohs Micrographic Surgery for Basal Cell Carcinoma." Dermatologic Surgery 29 (April 2003): 375–377.

ORGANIZATIONS

American Society for Mohs Surgery. Private Mail Box 391, 5901 Warner Avenue, Huntington Beach, CA 92649-4659. (714) 840-3065. (800) 616-ASMS (2767). www.mohssurgery.org.

OTHER

"About Mohs Micrographic Surgery." Mohs College. www.mohscollege.org/AboutMMS.html.

Belinda Rowland, Ph.D.
Monique Laberge, Ph.D.

Mometasone *see* **Corticosteroids**

MR *see* **Magnetic resonance imaging**

MRA *see* **Magnetic resonance angiogram; Magnetic resonance imaging**

MRI *see* **Magnetic resonance imaging**

MRS *see* **Magnetic resonance imaging**

MUGA scan *see* **Multiple-gated acquisition (MUGA) scan**

Multiple-gated acquisition (MUGA) scan

Definition

The multiple-gated acquisition (MUGA) scan, also called a cardiac blood pool study, is a non-invasive nuclear medicine test that enables clinicians to obtain information about heart muscle activity. The scan displays the distribution of a radioactive tracer in the heart. The images of the heart are obtained at intervals throughout the cardiac cycle, and are used to calculate ejection fraction (an important measure of heart performance) and evaluate regional myocardial wall motion.

Purpose

A MUGA scan may be done while the patient is at rest and again with stress. The resting study is usually performed to obtain the ejection fraction of the right and left ventricles, evaluate the left ventricular regional wall motion, assess the effects of cardiotoxic drugs (i.e., chemotherapy), and differentiate the cause of shortness of breath (pulmonary vs. cardiac). Ejection fraction and wall motion are also important measurements made during a stress study, but the stress study is performed primarily to detect coronary artery disease and evaluate angina.

Description

The MUGA scan is a series of images that demonstrate the flow of blood through the heart, providing information about heart muscle activity. Before images are taken, a radionuclide is injected into the bloodstream, a process that requires two injections in most health care facilities. The first injection contains a chemical that adheres to red blood cells, and the second contains a radioactive tracer (Tc99m) that attaches to that chemical. Alternatively, the two chemicals can be mixed together first and then injected, but the material tends to accumulate in bone and may obscure the heart.

The pictures are taken via gamma camera driven by a computer program that times the images, processes the information, and performs the mathematical calculations to provide ejection fraction and demonstrate wall motion. Images are obtained at various intervals during the cardiac cycle. Electrodes are placed on the patient so that a time frame can be established, for example, the time period between each "wave" (a part of the cardiac cycle seen on an EKG). The time frame is divided into several intervals, or "multiple gates." The result is a series of pictures showing the left and right ventricles at end-diastole (when the heart is dilated and filled with blood) and end-systole (when the heart is contracted and blood is being pumped out), and a number of stages in between.

A MUGA scan is performed in a hospital nuclear medicine department or in an outpatient facility. It takes approximately 30 minutes to one hour. The patient lies down on a bed alongside the gamma camera, receives the radionuclide injections, and multiple

KEY TERMS

Ejection fraction—The fraction of blood in the ventricle that is ejected during each beat. One of the main advantages of the MUGA scan is its ability to measure ejection fraction, one of the most important measures of the heart's performance.

Electrocardiogram—Also known as an EKG, less often as an ECG. A test in which electrodes are placed on the body to record the heart's electrical activities.

Ischemia—A decreased supply of oxygenated blood to a body part or organ, often marked by pain and organ dysfunction, as in ischemic heart disease.

Non-invasive—A procedure that does not penetrate the body.

images are taken. If a stress study is indicated, the rest study is performed first. In a stress study, the patient usually lies on a special bed fitted with a bicycle apparatus. While an image is being recorded, the patient is asked to cycle for about two minutes, then the resistance of the wheels is increased. After two more minutes of **exercise**, another image is obtained and the resistance is increased again. Blood pressure and ECG are monitored during the procedure. After the stress portion is finished, one more resting, or recovery, study is obtained.

Preparation

Standard preparation for an ECG is required. Special handling of nuclear materials by a nuclear medicine technologist may be required for the injections.

Aftercare

The patient may resume normal activities immediately following the test.

Normal results

A normal MUGA scan should not demonstrate areas of akinesis (lack of movement), or hypokinesis (decreased movement) of the heart muscle walls. Abnormal motion, especially in the left ventricle, is suggestive of an infarct or other myocardial defect. The ejection fraction is a measure of heart function, and should be within the normal limits established by the testing facility.

Resources

BOOKS

DeBakey, Michael E. and Gotto, Antonio M., Jr. "Non-invasive Diagnostic Procedures." In *The New Living Heart.* Holbrook, MA: Adams Media Corporation, 1997, pp. 59–70.

Klingensmith III, M.D., Wm. C., Dennis Eshima, Ph.D., John Goddard, Ph.D. *Nuclear Medicine Procedure Manual 2000-2001.*

"Radionuclide Angiography." In *Cardiac Stress Testing & Imaging,* edited by Thomas H. Marwick. New York: Churchill Livingstone, 1996, pp. 517–21.

Raizner, Albert E. "Nuclear Cardiology Testing." In: *Indications for Diagnostic Procedures: Topics in Clinical Cardiology.* New York, Tokyo: Igaku-Shon, 1997, pp. 44–47.

Texas Heart Institute. "Diagnosing Heart Diseases." In *Texas Heart Institute Heart Owner's Handbook.* New York: John Wiley & Sons, 1996, p. 333.

Ziessman, Harvey, ed. *The Radiologic Clinics of North America, Update on Nuclear Medicine.* Philadelphia: W.B. Saunders Company, 2001.

ORGANIZATIONS

American Heart Association. National Center. 7272 Greenville Avenue, Dallas, TX 75231-4596. (214) 373-6300. http://www.medsearch.com/pf/profiles/amerh/.

Texas Heart Institute Heart Information Service. P.O. Box 20345, Houston, TX 77225-0345. (800) 292-2221. http://www.tmc.edu/thi/his.html.

Christine Miner Minderovic, B.S., R.T., R.D.M.S.
Lee A. Shratter, M.D.

Muscle relaxants

Definition

Skeletal muscle relaxants are drugs that relax striated muscles (those that control the skeleton). They are a separate class of drugs from the muscle relaxant drugs used during intubations and surgery to reduce the need for anesthesia and facilitate intubation.

Purpose

Skeletal muscle relaxants may be used for relief of spasticity in neuromuscular diseases such as multiple sclerosis, as well as for spinal cord injury and stroke. They may also be used for pain relief in minor strain injuries and control of the muscle symptoms of tetanus. Dantrolene (Dantrium) has been used to prevent or treat malignant hyperthermia in surgery.

KEY TERMS

Central nervous system (CNS)—The brain and spinal cord.

Intrathecal—Introduced into or occurring in the space under the arachnoid membrane that covers the brain and spinal cord.

Pregnancy category—A system of classifying drugs according to their established risks for use during pregnancy: category A: controlled human studies have demonstrated no fetal risk; category B: animal studies indicate no fetal risk, and there are no adequate and well-controlled studies in pregnant women; category C: no adequate human or animal studies, or adverse fetal effects in animal studies, but no available human data; category D: evidence of fetal risk, but benefits outweigh risks; category X: evidence of fetal risk, which outweigh any benefits.

Sedative—Medicine used to treat nervousness or restlessness.

Spasm—Sudden, involuntary tensing of a muscle or a group of muscles.

Tranquilizer (minor)—A drug that has a calming effect and is used to treat anxiety and emotional tension.

Description

The muscle relaxants are divided into two groups: centrally acting and peripherally acting. The centrally acting group appears to act on the central nervous system (CNS), and contains 10 drugs that are chemically different. Only dantrolene has a direct action at the level of the nerve-muscle connection.

Baclofen (Lioresal) may be administered orally or intrathecally (introduced into the space under the arachnoid membrane that covers the brain and spinal cord) for control of spasticity due to neuromuscular disease.

Several drugs, including carisoprodol (Soma), chlorphenesin (Maolate), chlorzoxazone (Paraflex), cyclobenzaprine (Flexeril), diazepam (Valium), metaxalone (Skelaxin), methocarbamol (Robaxin), and orphenadrine (Norflex), are used primarily as an adjunct for rest in management of acute muscle spasms associated with sprains. Muscle relaxation may also be an adjunct to physical therapy in rehabilitation following stroke, spinal cord injury, or other musculoskeletal conditions.

Diazepam and methocarbamol are also used by injection for relief of tetanus.

Recommended dosage

Dose varies with the drug, route of administration, and purpose. There may be individual variations in absorption that require doses higher than those usually recommended (particularly with methocarbamol). The consumer is advised to consult specific references or ask a doctor for further information.

Precautions

All drugs in the muscle relaxant class may cause sedation. Baclofen, when administered intrathecally, may cause severe CNS depression with cardiovascular collapse and respiratory failure.

Diazepam may be addictive, and is a controlled substance under federal law.

Dantrolene has a potential for hepatotoxicity. The incidence of symptomatic hepatitis is dose related, but may occur even with a short period of doses at or above 800 mg per day, which greatly increases the risk of serious liver injury. Overt hepatitis has been most frequently observed between the third and twelfth months of therapy. Risk of liver injury appears to be greater in women, in patients over 35 years of age, and in patients taking other medications in addition to dantrolene.

Tizanidine may cause low blood pressure, but this may be controlled by starting with a low dose and increasing it gradually. Rarely, the drug may cause liver damage.

Methocarbamol and chlorzoxazone may cause harmless color changes in urine—orange or reddish purple with chlorzoxazone; and purple, brown, or green with methocarbamol. The urine will return to its normal color when the patient stops taking the medicine.

Most drugs in the muscle relaxant class are well tolerated, but not all of these drugs have been evaluated for safety in pregnancy and breastfeeding.

Baclofen is pregnancy category C. It has caused fetal abnormalities in rats at doses 13 times above the human dose. Baclofen passes into breast milk, so breastfeeding while taking baclofen is not recommended.

Diazepam is category D. All benzodiazepines cross the placenta. Although the drugs appear to be safe for use during the first trimester of pregnancy, use later in pregnancy may be associated with cleft lip and palate. Diazepam should not be taken while breastfeeding. It was found that infants who were breastfed while their mothers took diazepam were excessively sleepy and lethargic.

Dantrolene is category C. In animal studies, it has reduced the rate of survival of the newborn when given in doses seven times the normal human dose. Mothers should not breastfeed while receiving dantrolene.

Interactions

Skeletal muscle relaxants have many potential drug interactions. It is recommended that individual references be consulted.

Because these drugs cause sedation, they should be used with caution when taken with other drugs that may also cause drowsiness.

The activity of diazepam may be increased by drugs that inhibit its metabolism in the liver. These include cimetidine, oral contraceptives, disulfiram, fluoxetine, isoniazid, ketoconazole, metoprolol, propoxyphene, propranolol, and valproic acid.

Dantrolene may have an interaction with estrogens. Although no interaction has been demonstrated, the rate of liver damage in women over the age of 35 who were taking estrogens is higher than in other groups.

Resources

BOOKS

Ford MD et al. Clinical Toxicology. 1st ed. Philadelphia: Saunders, 2001.

Frontera, WR and Silver J. Essentials of Physical Medicine and Rehabilitation. 1st ed. Philadelphia: Hanley and Belfus, 2002.

Miller RD. Miller's Anesthesia. 6th ed. Philadelphia: Elsevier, 2006.

OTHER

"Muscle Relaxants." Hendrick Health System. http://www.hendrickhealth.org/healthy/000923.htm.

"Neurological, Neuromuscular Junction, Muscle Disorders." Continuing Education Committee of Anaesthetists of New Zealand. http://www.anaesthesia.org.nz/Files/Help41A.pdf.

Samuel D. Uretsky, PharmD
Rosalyn Carson-DeWitt, MD

Myelography

Definition

Myelography is an x-ray examination of the spinal canal. A contrast agent is injected through a needle into the space around the spinal cord to display the spinal cord, spinal canal, and nerve roots on an x ray.

Purpose

The purpose of a myelogram is to evaluate the spinal cord and nerve roots for suspected compression. Pressure on these delicate structures causes pain or other symptoms. A myelogram is performed when precise detail about the spinal cord is needed to make a definitive diagnosis. In most cases, myelography is used after other studies, such as **magnetic resonance imaging** (MRI) or a computed tomography scan (CT), have not provided enough information to be certain of the diagnosis. Sometimes myelography followed by CT scan is an alternative for patients who cannot have an MRI scan, because they have a pacemaker or other implanted metallic device.

A herniated or ruptured intervertebral disc, or related condition such as disc bulge or protrusion, popularly known as a slipped disc, is one of the most common causes for pressure on the spinal cord or nerve roots. The condition is popularly known as a pinched nerve. Discs are pads of fiber and cartilage that contain rubbery tissue. They lie between the vertebrae, or individual bones, which make up the spine.

Discs act as cushions, accommodating strains, shocks, and position changes. A disc may rupture suddenly, due to injury or a sudden strain with the spine in an unnatural position. In other cases, the problem may come on gradually as a result of progressive deterioration of the discs with aging. The lower back is the most common area for this problem, but it sometimes occurs in the neck, and rarely in the upper back. A myelogram can help accurately locate the disc or discs involved.

Myelography may be used when a tumor is suspected. Tumors can originate in the spinal cord or in tissues surrounding the cord. Cancers that have started in other parts of the body may spread or metastasize in the spine. It is important to precisely locate the mass causing pressure so effective treatment can be undertaken. Patients with known cancer who develop back pain may require a myelogram for evaluation.

Other conditions that may be diagnosed using myelography include arthritic bony growths (spurs), narrowing of the spinal canal (spinal stenosis), or malformations of the spine.

Description

Myelograms can be performed in a hospital x-ray department or in an outpatient radiology facility. The patient lies face down on the x-ray table. The radiologist first looks at the spine under fluoroscopy, and the images appear on a monitor screen. This is done to

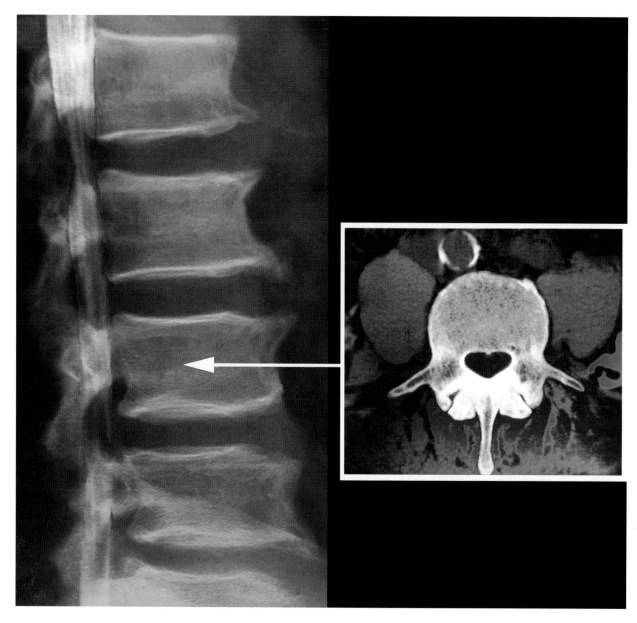

Myelogram of the lumbar spine. *(ISM/Phototake. Reproduced by permission.)*

find the best location to position the needle. The skin is cleaned, numbed with local anesthetic, and then the needle is inserted. Occasionally, a small amount of cerebrospinal fluid, the clear fluid that surrounds the spinal cord and brain, may be withdrawn through the needle and sent for laboratory studies. Contrast material (dye that shows up on x rays) is then injected.

The x-ray table is tilted slowly, allowing the contrast material to reach different levels in the spinal canal. The flow is observed under fluoroscopy, and x rays are taken with the table tilted at various angles. A footrest and shoulder straps or supports keep the patient from sliding.

In many instances, a CT scan of the spine is performed immediately after a myelogram, while the contrast material is still in the spinal canal. This helps outline internal structures more clearly.

A myelogram takes approximately 30–60 minutes. A CT scan adds about another hour to the examination. If the procedure is done as an outpatient exam, some facilities prefer the patient to stay in a recovery area up to four hours.

Patients who are unable to lie still or cooperate with positioning should not have this examination. Severe congenital spinal abnormalities may make the

KEY TERMS

Contrast agent—Also called a contrast medium, this is usually a barium or iodine dye that is injected into the area under investigation. The dye makes the interior body parts more visible on an x-ray film. For myelograms, an iodine based contrast agent is used.

examination technically difficult to carry out. Patients with a history of severe allergic reaction to contrast material (x-ray dye) should report this to their physician prior to having myelography. Medications to minimize the risk of severe reaction may be recommended before the procedure. Given the invasive nature and risks of myelograms and increased anatomic detail provided by MRI or CT, myelograms are generally not used as the first imaging test.

Preparation

Patients should be well-hydrated at the time they are undergoing a myelogram. Increasing fluids the day before the study is usually recommended. All food and fluid intake should be stopped approximately four hours before the procedure.

Certain medications may need to be stopped for one to two days before myelography is performed. These include some antipsychotics, antidepressants, blood thinners, and diabetic medications. Patients should discuss this with their physician or the staff at the facility where the study is to be done.

Patients who smoke may be asked to stop the day before the test. This helps decrease the chance of nausea or headaches after the myelogram. Immediately before the examination, patients should empty their bowels and bladder.

Aftercare

After the examination is complete, the patient usually rests for several hours, with the head elevated. Extra fluids are encouraged, to help eliminate the contrast material and prevent headaches. A regular diet and routine medications may be resumed. Strenuous physical activities, especially those that involve bending over, may be discouraged for one or two days. The physician should be notified if the patient develops a fever, excessive nausea and vomiting, severe headache, or a stiff neck.

Risks

Headache is a common complication of myelography. It may begin several hours to several days after the examination. The cause is thought to be changes in cerebrospinal fluid pressure, not a reaction to the dye. The headache may be mild and easily alleviated with rest and increased fluids. Sometimes, nonprescription medicines are recommended. In some instances, the headache may be more severe and require stronger medication or other measures for relief. Many factors influence whether the patient develops this problem, including the type of the needle used and his or her age and gender. Patients with a history of chronic or recurrent headaches are more likely to develop a headache after a myelogram.

The chance of a reaction to the contrast material is a very small, but potentially significant risk. It is estimated that only 5–10% of patients experience any effect from contrast exposure. The vast majority of reactions are mild, such as sneezing, nausea, or anxiety. These usually resolve by themselves. A moderate reaction, like wheezing or hives, may be treated with medication, but is not considered life threatening. Severe reactions, such as heart or respiratory failure, occur very infrequently, and require emergency medical treatment.

Rare complications of myelography include injury to the nerve roots from the needle or from bleeding into the spaces around the roots. Inflammation of the delicate covering of the spinal cord, called arachnoiditis, or infections, can also occur. Seizures are another very uncommon complication reported after myelography.

Normal results

A normal myelogram shows nerves that appear normal, and a spinal canal of normal width, with no areas of constriction or obstruction.

A myelogram may also reveal a herniated disk, tumor, bone spurs, or narrowing of the spinal canal (spinal stenosis).

Resources

BOOKS

Daffner, Richard. *Clinical Radiology, The Essentials.* Baltimore: Williams and Wilkins, 1993.

Pagana, Kathleen Deska. *Mosby's Manual of Diagnostic and Laboratory Tests.* St. Louis: Mosby, Inc., 1998.

Torres, Lillian. *Basic Medical Techniques and Patient Care in Imaging Technology.* Philadelphia: Lippincott, 1997.

ORGANIZATIONS

Spine Center. 1911 Arch St., Philadelphia, PA 19103. (215) 665-8300. http://www.thespinecenter.com

Ellen S. Weber, M.S.N.
Lee A. Shratter, M.D.

Myocardial resection

Definition

Myocardial resection is a surgical procedure in which a portion of the heart muscle is removed.

Purpose

Myocardial resection is done to improve the stability of the heart function or rhythm. Also known as endocardial resection, this open-heart surgery is done to destroy or remove damaged areas. These areas can generate life-threatening heart rhythms. Conditions resulting in abnormal heart rhythms caused by re-entry pathways or aberrant cells are corrected with this treatment.

Areas of the heart involved in a myocardial infarction change in contractility and function, becoming scar tissue that thins and hinders its ability to contract. Removing this diseased area can improve myocardial contractility reversing the severity of chronic heart failure. This procedure has shown promise for patients with chronic heart failure, in order to improve cardiac output and quality of life.

Demographics

Patients are not limited by age, race or sex when being evaluated for myocardial resection surgery. Patients who experience angina, congestive heart failure, arrhythmias, and pulmonary edema (fluid on the lungs) are candidates for this procedure. Contraindications—conditions in which the surgery is not recommended—include right heart failure, high pressure in the blood coming from left ventricle (lower chamber), and pulmonary hypertension (high blood pressure in the circulation around the lungs).

Description

After receiving a general anesthetic, an incision will be made in the chest to expose the heart. Cardiopulmonary bypass (to a heart-lung machine) will be instituted since this procedure requires direct visualization of the heart muscle. Since this is a true open

---

KEY TERMS

Arrhythmia—An abnormal heart rhythm. Examples are a slow, fast, or irregular heart rate.

Cardiac catheterization—A diagnostic procedure in which a thin tube is inserted into an artery or vein and guided to the heart using x rays. The function of the heart and blood vessels can be evaluated using this technique.

Dacron graft—A synthetic material used in the repair or replacement of blood vessels.

Ejection fraction—The amount of blood pumped out at each heartbeat, usually referred to as a percentage.

Implantable cardioverter-defibrillator—A device placed in the body to deliver an electrical shock to the heart in response to a serious abnormal rhythm.

Infarction—Tissue death resulting from a lack of oxygen to the area.

Intra-aortic balloon pump—A temporary device inserted into the femoral artery and guided up to the aorta. The small balloon helps strengthen heart contractions by maintaining improved blood pressure.

Radiofrequency ablation—A procedure in which a catheter is guided to an area of heart where abnormal heart rhythms originate. The cells in that area are killed using a mild radiofrequency energy to restore normal heart contractions.

Wolff-Parkinson-White syndrome—An abnormal, rapid heart rhythm, due to an extra pathway for the electrical impulses to travel from the atria to the ventricles.

---

heart procedure, the heart will be unable to pump blood during the surgery.

Arrhythmias

When the exact source of the abnormal rhythm is identified, it is removed. If there are areas around the source that may contribute to the problem, they can be frozen with a special probe. The amount of tissue removed is so small, usually only 2–3 mm, that there is no damage to the structure of the heart.

Ventricular reconstruction

Weakened myocardium (heart muscle) allows the heart to remodel and become less efficient at pumping blood. The goal is to remove the damaged region of the free wall of the left ventricle along with any involved septum. The heart is then reconstructed to provide a more elliptical structure that pumps blood more efficiently. In some instances a Dacron graft is used to replace the removed myocardium to aid in the reconstruction.

Diagnosis/Preparation

Diagnosis of arrhythmias begins with a Holter monitor that can identify the type of arrhythmia. This is followed by a **cardiac catheterization** to find the aberrant cells generating the arrhythmia. The patient is then recommended for open-heart surgery to remove the cells generating the arrhythmia.

Diagnosis of chronic heart failure is demonstrated by a cardiac catheterization or nuclear medicine study. During cardiac catheterization, the patient's cardiac function will be measured by cardiac output, ejection fraction and cardiovascular pressures. A nuclear medicine study can demonstrate areas of myocardium that are damaged. Muscle that is akinetic (does not move) will be identified. This information allows the surgeon to identify candidates for myocardial resection.

This is major surgery and should be the treatment of choice only after medications have failed and the use of an **implantable cardioverter-defibrillator** (a device that delivers electrical shock to control heart rhythm) has been ruled out along with medical therapy.

Prior to surgery, the physician will explain the procedure and order blood tests of the formed blood elements and electrolytes.

Aftercare

Immediately after surgery, the patient will be transferred to the **intensive care unit** for further cardiac monitoring. Any medications to improve cardiac performance will be weaned as necessary to allow the native heart function to return. The patient will be able to leave the hospital within five days, assuming there are no complications. Complications may include the need for intra-aortic balloon pump **ventricular assist device**, surgical bleeding, and infection.

Risks

The risks of myocardial resection are based in large part on the patient's underlying heart condition and, therefore, vary greatly. The procedure involves opening the heart, so the person is at risk for the complications associated with major heart surgery, such as stroke, shock, infection, and hemorrhage. Since the amount

WHO PERFORMS THIS PROCEDURE AND WHERE IS IT PERFORMED?

Electrophysiologists, cardiac surgeons and cardiologists, specially trained in cardiac electrical signaling and ventricular reconstruction have undergone specific training in these procedures. The number of patients suitable for these procedures are limited so experienced physicians should be sought to provide medical treatment.

of myocardium to remove is not precise, a patient may demonstrate little benefit in cardiac performance. If not enough or too much tissue is rmoved, the patient will continue to have heart problems.

General anesthetic with inhalation gases should be avoided as they can promote arrhythmias. Therefore, anesthesia should be limited to intravenous medications.

Normal results

Postoperative treatment for arrhythmias demonstrates 90% of patients are arrhythmia-free at the end of one year. A study of 245 patients published in 2001, demonstrated a 98% event free survival rate for patients after one year. After five years, 80% of patients had remained event free.

Morbidity and mortality rates

Cardiopulmonary bypass has an associated risk of complications separate from myocardial resection, with age greater than 70 years of age being a predictor for increased morbidity and mortality. In 1999, over 350,000 total procedures were performed using cardiopulmonary bypass.

In the study of 245 patients, ventricular reconstruction by myocardial resection was found to have an associated in-hospital mortality rate of 78.1%.

Alternatives

If myocardial resection is being performed to prevent arrhythmia generation, new techniques allow for minimally invasive procedures to be performed, including radiofrequency ablation performed in an electrophysiology laboratory with mild sedation, instead of general anesthetic.

If ventricular restoration is contraindicated, medical treatment will be continued. Mechanical

QUESTIONS TO ASK THE DOCTOR

- In the past year, how many of these procedures have been performed by the physician?
- What is the standard of care for a patient with arrhythmias/congestive heart failure/angina/pulmonary edema?
- What alternative therapies can be suggested, and what is the difference in survival outcomes at one and five years?
- Where can additional information be found about this procedure?
- What new technologies are available to assist in completing the procedure successfully?
- What are the risks associated with cardiopulmonary bypass?
- What type of post-operative course can be expected?
- How long will it be before normal activities can be reinstituted, such as driving, exercise and returning to work?

circulatory assist with a ventricular assist device may be a suitable option. Heart transplant and total artificial heart should also be explored as alternative therapies.

Resources

BOOKS

Hensley, Frederick Jr., et al. A Practical Approach to Cardiac Anesthesia, 3rd ed. Philadelphia: Lippincott Williams & Wilkins, 2003.

Libby, P. et al. Braunwald's Heart Disease. 8th ed. Philadelphia: Saunders, 2007.

PERIODICALS

Kawaguchi AT, et al. "Left ventricular volume reduction surgery: The 4th International Registry Report 2004." Journal of Cardiac Surgery 20, no. 6 (November 2005): 468–475.

ORGANIZATIONS

American Heart Association. 7320 Greenville Avenue, Dallas, TX 75231. (800) 242-8721 or (888) 478-7653. http://www.americanheart.org.

Dorothy Elinor Stonely
Allison J. Spiwak, MSBME

Myoglobin test see **Cardiac marker tests**

Myomectomy

Definition

Myomectomy is the removal of fibroids (non-cancerous tumors) from the wall of the uterus. Myomectomy is the preferred treatment for symptomatic fibroids in women who want to keep their uterus. Larger fibroids must be removed with an abdominal incision, but small fibroids can be taken out by **laparoscopy** or **hysteroscopy**.

Purpose

A myomectomy can remove uterine fibroids that are causing symptoms such as abnormal bleeding or pain. It is an alternative to surgical removal of the whole uterus (**hysterectomy**). The procedure can relieve fibroid-induced menstrual symptoms that have not responded to medication. Myomectomy also may be an effective treatment for infertility caused by the presence of fibroids.

Demographics

Uterine fibroids are more common among African-American women than among women of other ethnicities. Fibroids affect 20–40% of all women over the age of 35, and 50% of African-American women. A 2001 study by the National Institute of Environmental Health Sciences found that the incidence of fibroids among African-American women in their late 40s was as high as 80%, while approximately 70% of white women of that age were diagnosed as having fibroids. Women who are obese, are older, or started menstruating at an early age are also at an increased risk of developing uterine fibroids. Another study published in 2003 indicated that women with less education were more likely to have a hysterectomy performed to treat fibroids, instead of a less-invasive procedure such as myomectomy.

Description

Usually, fibroids are buried in the outer wall of the uterus, and abdominal surgery is required. If they are on the inner wall of the uterus, uterine fibroids can be removed using hysteroscopy. If they are on a stalk (pedunculated) on the outer surface of the uterus, laparoscopy can be performed.

Removing fibroids through abdominal surgery is a more difficult and slightly more risky operation than a hysterectomy. This is because the uterus bleeds from the sites where the fibroids were removed, and it may be difficult or impossible to stop the bleeding. This

Myomectomy

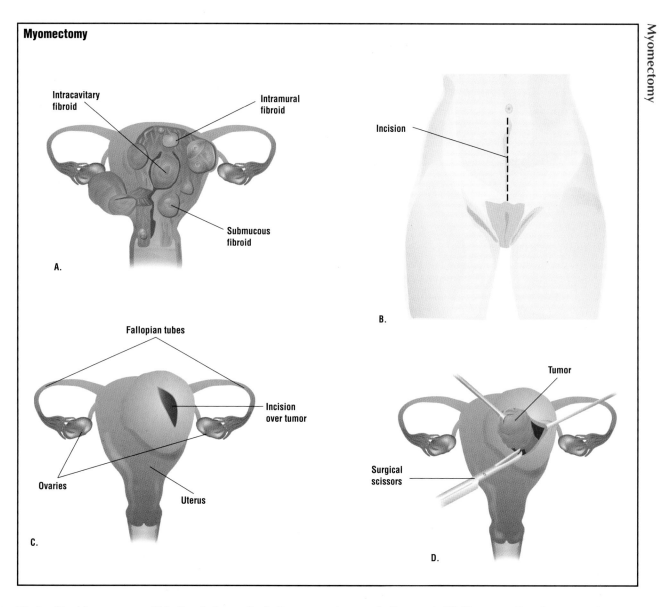

A.

B.

C.

D.

Uterine fibroids can occur within the uterine cavity, in the mucous layer, or in the muscle (A). To remove them by myomectomy, an incision is made into the woman's lower abdomen (B). An incision is made in the uterus over the tumor (C), and it is removed (D). *(Illustration by GGS Information Services. Cengage Learning, Gale.)*

surgery is usually performed under **general anesthesia**, although some patients may be given a spinal or epidural anesthesia.

The incision may be horizontal (the "bikini" incision) or a vertical incision from the navel downward. After separating the muscle layers underneath the skin, the surgeon makes an opening in the abdominal wall. Next, the surgeon makes an incision over each fibroid, grasping and pulling out each growth.

Every opening in the uterine wall is then stitched with sutures. The uterus must be meticulously repaired in order to eliminate potential sites of bleeding or

infection. The surgeon then sutures the abdominal wall and muscle layers above it with absorbable **stitches**, and closes the skin with clips or non-absorbable stitches.

When appropriate, a laparoscopic myomectomy may be performed. In this procedure, the surgeon removes fibroids with the help of a viewing tube (laparoscope) inserted into the pelvic cavity through an incision in the navel. The fibroids are removed through a tiny incision under the navel that is much smaller than the 4–5 in (10–13 cm) opening required for a standard myomectomy.

KEY TERMS

Adhesions—Bands of scar tissue between organs that can form after surgery or trauma.

Cesarean section—A surgical procedure in which incisions are made through a woman's abdomen and uterus to deliver her baby.

Epidural anesthesia—A method of pain relief for surgery in which local anesthetic is injected into the epidural space in the middle and lower back.

If the fibroids are small and located on the inner surface of the uterus, they can be removed with a thin, telescope-like device called a hysteroscope. The hysteroscope is inserted into the vagina through the cervix and into the uterus. This procedure does not require any abdominal incision, so hospitalization is shorter.

Diagnosis/Preparation

Surgeons often recommend hormone treatment with a drug called leuprolide (Lupron) two to six months before surgery in order to shrink the fibroids. This makes the fibroids easier to remove. In addition, Lupron stops menstruation, so women who are anemic have an opportunity to build up their blood count. While the drug treatment may reduce the risk of excess blood loss during surgery, there is a small risk that smaller fibroids might be missed during myomectomy, only to enlarge later after the surgery is completed.

Aftercare

Patients may need four to six weeks of recovery following a standard myomectomy before they can return to normal activities. Women who have had laparoscopic or hysteroscopic myomectomies, however, can usually recover completely within one to three weeks.

Risks

The risks of a myomectomy performed by a skilled surgeon are about the same as hysterectomy (one of the most common and safest surgeries). Removing multiple fibroids is more difficult and slightly more risky. Possible complications include:

- infection
- blood loss
- weakening of the uterine wall to the degree that future deliveries need to be performed via cesarean section

WHO PERFORMS THE PROCEDURE AND WHERE IS IT PERFORMED?

Myomectomies are usually performed in a hospital operating room or an outpatient setting by a gynecologist, a medical doctor who has specialized in the areas of women's general health, pregnancy, labor and childbirth, prenatal testing, and genetics.

- adverse reactions to anesthesia
- internal scarring (and possible infertility)
- reappearance of new fibroids

There is a risk that removal of the fibroids may lead to such severe bleeding that the uterus itself will have to be removed. Because of the risk of blood loss during a myomectomy, patients may want to consider banking their own blood before surgery (**autologous blood donation**).

Normal results

Removal of uterine fibroids will usually improve any side effects that the patient may have been suffering from, including abnormal bleeding and pain. Under normal circumstances, a woman who has had a myomectomy will be able to become pregnant, although she may have to deliver via **cesarean section** if the uterine wall has been weakened.

Morbidity and mortality rates

Depending on the surgical approach, the rate of complications for myomectomy is about the same as those for hysterectomy (anywhere between 3% and 9%). The rate of fibroid reoccurrence is approximately 15%. Adhesions (bands of scar tissue between organs that can form after surgery or trauma) occur in 15–53% of women postoperatively.

Alternatives

Hysterectomy (partial or full removal of the uterus) is a common alternative to myomectomy. The most frequent reason for hysterectomy in the United States is to remove fibroid tumors, accounting for 30% of all hysterectomies. A subtotal (or partial) hysterectomy is the preferable procedure because it removes the least amount of tissue (i.e., the opening to the cervix is left in place).

QUESTIONS TO ASK THE DOCTOR

• Why is a myomectomy being recommended?

• How many myomectomies do you perform a year?

• What type of myomectomy will be performed?

• What are the risks if I decide against the myomectomy?

• What alternatives to myomectomy are available to me?

Fibroid embolization is a relatively new, less-invasive procedure in which blood vessels that feed the fibroids are blocked, causing the growths to shrink. The blood vessels are accessed via a catheter inserted into the femoral artery (in the upper thigh) and injected with tiny particles that block the flow of blood. The fibroids subsequently decrease in size and the patient's symptoms improve.

Resources

BOOKS

Connolly, Anne Marie and William Droegemueller. "Leiomyomas." In *Conn's Current Therapy 2003*. Philadelphia: Elsevier Science, 2003.

Ludmir, Jack and Phillip G. Stubblefield. "Surgical Procedures in Pregnancy: Myomectomy." (Chapter 19). In *Obstetrics: Normal & Problem Pregnancies*. Philadelphia: Churchill Livingstone, 2002.

ORGANIZATIONS

American College of Obstetricians and Gynecologists. 409 12th St., SW, P.O. Box 96920, Washington, DC 20090-6920. http://www.acog.org.

Center for Uterine Fibroids, Brigham and Women's Hospital. 623 Thorn Building, 20 Shattuck Street, Boston, MA 02115. (800) 722-5520. http://www.fibroids.net.

OTHER

de Candolle, G., and D. M. Walker. "Myomectomy." *Practical Training and Research in Gynecologic Endoscopy*. February 17, 2003 [cited March 13, 2003]. http://www.gfmer.ch/Books/Endoscopy_book/Ch14_Myomectomy.html.

"High Efficacy Rate Shown in Minimally Invasive Treatment of Uterine Fibroids." *Doctor's Guide*. January 13, 2003 [cited March 14, 2003]. http://www.pslgroup.com/dg/2271BA.htm.

Indman, Paul D. "Myomectomy: Removal of Uterine Fibroids." *All About Myomectomy*. 2002 [cited March 14, 2003]. http://www.myomectomy.net.

Toaff, Michael E. "Myomectomy." *Alternatives to Hysterectomy Page*. [cited March 14, 2003]. http://www.netreach.net/~hysterectomyedu/myomecto.htm.

"Uterine Fibroids: Disproportionate Number of Black Women with More, Larger Tumors." National Institute of Environmental Sciences. March 2001 [cited March 14, 2003]. http://www.niehs.nih.gov/oc/crntnws/2001mar/fibroids.htm.

Carol A. Turkington
Stephanie Dionne Sherk

Myringotomy and ear tubes

Definition

Myringotomy is a surgical procedure in which a small incision is made in the eardrum (the tympanic membrane), usually in both ears. The English word is derived from *myringa,* modern Latin for drum membrane, and *tomē,* Greek for cutting. It is also called myringocentesis, tympanotomy, tympanostomy, or **paracentesis** of the tympanic membrane. Fluid in the middle ear can be drawn out through the incision.

Ear tubes, or tympanostomy tubes, are small tubes open at both ends that are inserted into the incisions in the eardrums during myringotomy. They come in various shapes and sizes and are made of plastic, metal, or both. They are left in place until they fall out by themselves or until they are removed by a doctor.

Purpose

Myringotomy with the insertion of ear tubes is an optional treatment for inflammation of the middle ear with fluid collection (effusion) that lasts longer than three months (chronic otitis media with effusion) and does not respond to drug treatment. This condition is also called **glue** ear. Myringotomy is the recommended treatment if the condition lasts four to six months. Effusion refers to the collection of fluid that escapes from blood vessels or the lymphatic system. In this case, the effusion collects in the middle ear.

Initially, acute inflammation of the middle ear with effusion is treated with one or two courses of **antibiotics**. Antihistamines and decongestants have been used, but they have not been proven effective unless there is also hay fever or some other allergic inflammation that contributes to the problem. Myringotomy with or without the insertion of ear tubes is *not* recommended for initial treatment of otherwise healthy children with middle ear inflammation with effusion.

Myringotomy and ear tubes

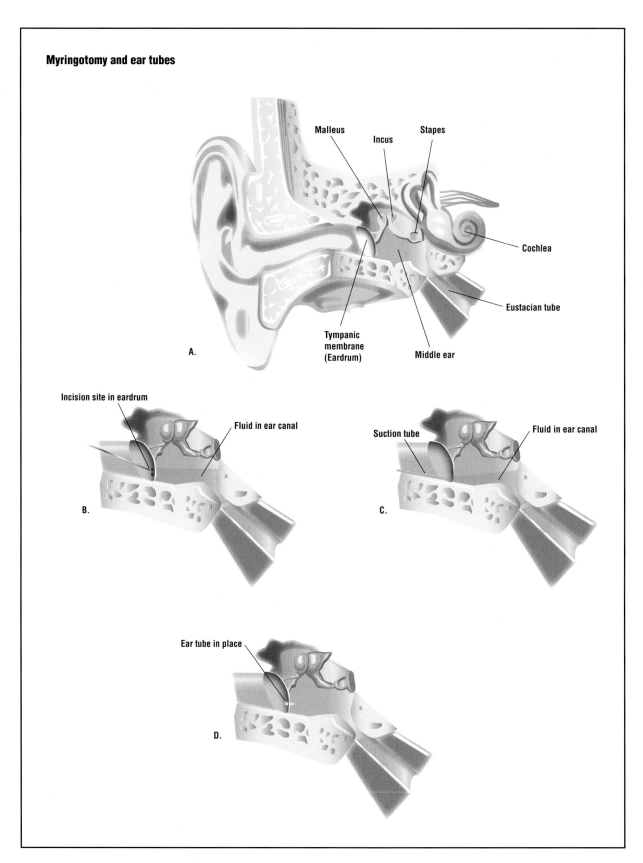

During a myringotomy, an incision is made into the ear drum, or tympanic membrane (B). The fluid in the ear canal is suctioned out (C), and a small tube is put in place to allow future drainage in the event of an infection (D). *(Illustration by GGS Information Services. Cengage Learning, Gale.)*

KEY TERMS

Acute otitis media—Inflammation of the middle ear with signs of infection lasting less than three months.

Adenoids—Clusters of lymphoid tissue located in the upper throat above the roof of the mouth. Some doctors think that removal of the adenoids may lower the rate of recurrent otitis media in high-risk children.

Barotrauma—Ear pain caused by unequal air pressure on the inside and outside of the ear drum. Barotrauma, which is also called pressure-related ear pain or barotitis media, is the most common reason for myringotomies in adults.

Chronic otitis media—Inflammation of the middle ear with signs of infection lasting three months or longer.

Effusion—The escape of fluid from blood vessels or the lymphatic system and its collection in a cavity, in this case, the middle ear.

Eustachian tube—A canal that extends from the middle ear to the pharynx.

Insufflation—Blowing air into the ear as a test for the presence of fluid in the middle ear.

Middle ear—The cavity or space between the eardrum and the inner ear. It includes the eardrum, the three little bones (hammer, anvil, and stirrup) that transmit sound to the inner ear, and the Eustachian tube, which connects the inner ear to the nasopharynx (the back of the nose).

Otolaryngologist—A surgeon who specializes in treating disorders of the ears, nose, and throat.

Tympanic membrane—The eardrum. A thin disc of tissue that separates the outer ear from the middle ear.

Tympanostomy tube—Ear tube. A small tube made of metal or plastic that is inserted during myringotomy to ventilate the middle ear.

In about 10% of children, the effusion lasts for three months or longer, when the disease is considered chronic. In children with chronic disease, systemic steroids may help, but the evidence is not clear, and there are risks.

When medical treatment doesn't stop the effusion after three months in a child who is one to three years old, is otherwise healthy, and has hearing loss in both ears, myringotomy with insertion of ear tubes becomes an option. If the effusion lasts for four to six months, myringotomy with insertion of ear tubes is recommended.

The purpose of myringotomy is to relieve symptoms, to restore hearing, to take a sample of the fluid to examine in the laboratory in order to identify any microorganisms present, or to insert ear tubes.

Ear tubes can be inserted into the incision during myringotomy and left there. The eardrum heals around them, securing them in place. They usually fall out on their own in six to 12 months or are removed by a doctor.

While the tubes are in place, they keep the incision from closing, keeping a channel open between the middle ear and the outer ear. This allows fresh air to reach the middle ear, allowing fluid to drain out, and preventing pressure from building up in the middle ear. The patient's hearing returns to normal immediately and the risk of recurrence diminishes.

Demographics

In the United States, myringotomy and tube placement have become a mainstay of treatment for recurrent otitis media in children. More than 500,000 procedures are performed annually, making myringotomy the most common pediatric, ambulatory operation performed in the U.S.

Myringotomy in adults is a less common procedure than in children, primarily because adults benefit from certain changes in the anatomy of the middle ear that occur after childhood. In particular, the adult ear is less likely to accumulate fluid because the Eustachian tube, which connects the middle ear to the throat area, lies at about a 45-degree angle from the horizontal. This relatively steep angle means that the force of gravity helps to keep fluids from the throat containing disease organisms out of the middle ear. In children, however, the Eustachian tube is only about 10 degrees above the horizontal, which makes it relatively easy for disease organisms to migrate from the nose and throat into the inner ear. Myringotomies in adults are usually performed as a result of barotrauma, which is also known as pressure-related ear pain or barotitis media. Barotrauma refers to earache caused by unequal air pressure on the inside and outside of the eardrum. Adults with very narrow Eustachian tubes may experience barotrauma in relation to scuba diving, using elevators, or frequent flying. A myringotomy with tube insertion may be performed if the condition is not helped by decongestants or antibiotics.

Most myringotomies in children are performed in children between one to two years of age. One Canadian study found that the number of myringotomies performed was 12.8 per thousand for children 11 months old or younger; 54.2 per thousand for children between 12 and 23 months old; and 11.1 per thousand for children between three and 15 years old. Sex and race do not appear to affect the number of myringotomies in any age group, although boys are reported to have a slightly higher rate of ear infections than girls.

Description

When a conventional myringotomy is performed, the ear is washed, a small incision made in the eardrum, the fluid sucked out, a tube inserted, and the ear packed with cotton to control bleeding.

Recent developments include the use of medical acupuncture to control pain during the procedure, and the use of carbon dioxide lasers to perform the myringotomy itself. Laser-assisted myringotomy can be performed in a doctor's office with only a local anesthetic. It has several advantages over the older technique: it is less painful; less frightening to children; and minimizes the need for tube insertion because the hole in the eardrum produced by the laser remains open longer than an incision done with a scalpel.

Another technique to keep the incision in the eardrum open without the need for tube insertion is application of a medication called mitomycin C, which was originally developed to treat bladder cancer. The mitomycin prevents the incision from sealing over. As of 2007, however, this approach is still being studied.

There has also been an effort to design ear tubes that are easier to insert or to remove, and to design tubes that stay in place longer. As of 2003, ear tubes come in various shapes and sizes.

Diagnosis/Preparation

The diagnosis of otitis media is based on the doctor's visual examination of the patient's ear and the patient's symptoms. Patients with otitis media complain of earache and usually have a fever, sometimes as high as 105°F (40.5°C). There may or may not be loss of hearing. Small children may have nausea and vomiting. When the doctor looks in the ear with an otoscope, the patient's eardrum will look swollen and may bulge outward. The doctor can evaluate the presence of fluid in the middle ear either by blowing air into the ear, known as insufflation, or by tympanometry, which is an indirect measurement of the mobility of the eardrum. If the eardrum has already ruptured, there may be a watery, bloody, or pus-streaked discharge.

Fluid removed from the ear can be taken to a laboratory for culture. The most common bacteria that cause otitis media are *Pneumococcus*, *Haemophilus influenzae*, and *Moraxella catarrhalis*. Some cases are caused by viruses, particularly respiratory syncytial virus (RSV).

A child scheduled for a myringotomy should not have food or water for four to six hours before anesthesia. Antibiotics are usually not needed.

If **local anesthesia** is used, a cream containing lidocaine and prilocaine is applied to the ear canal about 30 minutes before the myringotomy. If medical acupuncture is used for pain control, the acupuncture begins about 40 minutes before surgery and is continued during the procedure.

Aftercare

The use of antimicrobial drops is controversial. Water should be kept out of the ear canal until the eardrum is intact. A doctor should be notified if the tubes fall out.

Risks

The risks include:

- cutting the outer ear
- formation at the myringotomy site of granular nodes due to inflammation
- formation of a mass of skin cells and cholesterol in the middle ear that can grow and damage surrounding bone (cholesteatoma)
- permanent perforation of the eardrum

It is also possible that the incision won't heal properly, leaving a permanent hole in the eardrum. This result can cause some hearing loss and increases the risk of infection.

The ear tube may move inward and get trapped in the middle ear, rather than move out into the external ear, where it either falls out on its own or can be retrieved by a doctor. The exact incidence of tubes moving inward is not known, but it could increase the risk of further episodes of middle-ear inflammation, inflammation of the eardrum or the part of the skull directly behind the ear, formation of a mass in the middle ear, or infection due to the presence of a foreign body.

The surgery may not be a permanent cure. As many as 30% of children undergoing myringotomy

WHO PERFORMS THE PROCEDURE AND WHERE IS IT PERFORMED?

Myringotomies are performed by family practitioners, pediatricians, and otolaryngologists, who are surgeons who specialize in treating disorders of the ears, nose, and throat.

A conventional myringotomy is usually done in an ambulatory surgical unit under general anesthesia, although some physicians do it in the office with sedation and local anesthesia, especially in older children and adults. In either case, it is considered same-day surgery. Laser-assisted myringotomies are usually performed in doctors' offices or outpatient surgery clinics.

QUESTIONS TO ASK THE DOCTOR

- What alternatives to myringotomy might work for my child?
- How can I lower my child's risk of recurrent ear infections?
- Do you perform laser-assisted myringotomies?
- What is your opinion of removing my child's adenoids to lower the risk of future hospitalizations?

with insertion of ear tubes need to undergo another procedure within five years.

The other risks include those associated with sedatives or **general anesthesia**. Some patients may prefer acupuncture for pain control in order to minimize these risks.

An additional element of **postoperative care** is the recommendation of many doctors that the child use ear plugs to keep water out of the ear during bathing or swimming to reduce the risk of infection and discharge.

Normal results

Parents often report that children talk better, hear better, are less irritable, sleep better, and behave better after myringotomy with the insertion of ear tubes. Normal results in adults include relief of ear pain and ability to resume flying or deep-sea diving without barotrauma.

Morbidity and mortality rates

Morbidity following myringotomy usually takes the form of either otorrhea, which is a persistent discharge from the ear, or changes in the size or texture of the eardrum. The risk of otorrhea is about 13%. If the procedure is repeated, the eardrum may shrink, retract, or become flaccid. The eardrum may also develop an area of hardened tissue. This condition is known as tympanosclerosis. The risk of hardening is 51%; its effects on hearing aren't known, but they appear to be insignificant.

A report published in 2002 indicates that morbidity following myringotomy in the United States is highest among children from families of low socioeconomic status. The study found that children from poor urban families had more episodes of otorrhea following tube insertion then children from suburban families. In addition, the episodes of otorrhea in the urban children lasted longer.

Mortality rates are extremely low; case studies of fatalities following myringotomy are rare in the medical literature, and most involve adults.

Alternatives

Preventive measures

There are several lifestyle issues related to high rates of middle ear infection. One of the most serious is parental smoking. One study of the effects of passive smoking on children's health estimated that as many as 165,000 of the myringotomies performed each year on American children are related to the use of tobacco in the household.

Studies have shown that children in daycare have a higher risk of chronic ear infection, and therefore a higher risk of needing myringotomy..

A third factor that affects a child's risk of recurrent middle ear infection is breastfeeding. Toddlers who were breastfed as infants for at least four months have a lower risk of ear infection than those who were bottlefed.

Other surgical approaches

Because the adenoids may harbor infection, when myringotomy and tube placement fails, **adenoidectomy** may be performed in order to resolve chronic otitis media.

Alternative medicine

According to Dr. Kenneth Pelletier, former director of the program in complementary and alternative medicine at Stanford University, there is some evidence that homeopathic treatment is effective in reducing the pain of otitis media in children and lowering the risk of recurrence.

Resources

BOOKS

Behrman RE, et al. Nelson Textbook of Pediatrics. 17th ed. Philadelphia: Saunders, 2004.

Cummings, CW, et al. Otolayrngology: Head and Neck Surgery. 4th ed. St. Louis: Mosby, 2005.

Pelletier, Kenneth R., MD. The Best Alternative Medicine, Part II: CAM Therapies for Specific Conditions: Otitis Media. New York: Simon & Schuster, 2002.

PERIODICALS

Desai, S. N., J. D. Kellner, and D. Drummond. "Population-Based, Age-Specific Myringotomy with Tympanostomy Tube Insertion Rates in Calgary, Canada." Pediatric Infectious Disease Journal 21 (April 2002): 348–350.

Lin, Yuan-Chi, MD. "Acupuncture Anesthesia for a Patient with Complex Congenital Anomalies." Medical Acupuncture 13 (Fall/Winter 2002) [cited February 22, 2003]. http://www.medicalacupuncture.org/aama_marf/journal/vol13_2/poster3.html.

Perkins, J. A. "Medical and Surgical Management of Otitis Media in Children." Otolaryngology Clinics of North America 35 (August 2002): 811-825.

Siegel, G. J., and R. K. Chandra. "Laser Office Ventilation of Ears with Insertion of Tubes." Otolaryngology—Head and Neck Surgery 127 (July 2002): 60–66.

ORGANIZATIONS

American Academy of Medical Acupuncture (AAMA). 4929 Wilshire Boulevard, Suite 428, Los Angeles, CA 90010. (323) 937-5514. http://www.medical acupuncture.org.

American Academy of Otolaryngology, Head and Neck Surgery, Inc. One Prince Street, Alexandria, VA 22314-3357. (703) 836-4444. http://www.entnet.org.

American Academy of Pediatrics (AAP). 141 Northwest Point Boulevard, Elk Grove Village, IL 60007. (847) 434-4000. http://www.aap.org.

Mary Zoll, PhD
Rebecca Frey, PhD

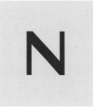

N

Narcotics *see* **Analgesics, opioid**

Nasal septum surgery *see* **Septoplasty**

Necessary surgery

Definition

Necessary surgery is a term that refers both to a medical requirement for the surgery determined by a physician and to an insurance plan's inclusion of the surgery in the covered conditions. For the most part, these two ways of talking about required surgery coincide. When they do not, the physician is asked to demonstrate to the insurance plan that the surgery is necessary by reference to the medical condition to be treated and the customary medical practice that deems it required as opposed to optional or elective.

Purpose

Not all surgery is an emergency. Not all surgery is medically required. Some surgeries are for cosmetic or for aesthetic enhancements and are deemed optional or elective, both by physicians and by insurance plans.

Necessary surgery refers to surgical procedures that pertain to a condition that cannot be treated by other methods and, if left untreated, would threaten the life of the patient, fail to repair or improve a body function, increase the patient's pain, or prevent the diagnosis of a serious or painful condition. The emphasis here is that, according to medical judgment, surgery is mandated.

Not all necessary surgery is absolutely required until the patient is satisfied that he or she has all the information needed to opt for surgery. All surgery has risks and the decision to have surgery is one that needs to be made by both the physician and the patient.

Description

The decision to have surgery should be made by the patient after:

- complete evaluation by a physician to determine if the surgery is medically indicated
- discussion with the physician about alternative treatments
- discussion that allows the patient to understand why the surgery is necessary, what the surgery involves, and why the particular procedure has been chosen by the surgeon
- discussion of the complete risks and benefits of the procedure
- second opinion has been enlisted about the surgery and its components and/or alternatives (Many health insurance plans require this step and will pay for the second opinion.)

Only after a physician has taken the condition and symptoms into account with a complete evaluation of alternatives, will surgery be judged to be necessary. During the course of this evaluation, and after non-surgical treatments have failed, the patient needs to be actively involved in understanding the actual procedure that might mitigate the condition, the full array of risks and benefits of the surgery, and why the surgeon has arrived at the particular procedure. The patient should understand the likelihood of danger or risk if he or she foregoes the surgery and the patient needs to understand that there may be a possibility of improvement, given sufficient time, without the surgery. Before choosing to undergo a particular surgical procedure, the patient should get a **second opinion** about the wisdom, efficacy, risk, and benefits of the procedure.

Diagnosis/Preparation

Preparation for surgery should include knowing:

OTHER

Wax, C. M. "Preparation for Surgery." <http://www/HealthIsNumberOne.com>.

Nancy McKenzie, PhD

Neck dissection *see* **Radical neck dissection**

KEY TERMS

Alternatives to surgery —Other treatments for the condition or illness that do not involve surgery; these are usually tried before surgery is an option.

Elective surgery—Surgery chosen by someone over 18 and/or a guardian for a patient that is not medically required for an illness, condition, or pain relief.

Surgical alternatives—Surgical options within a range of surgical procedures used to treat a specific condition.

- Where surgery will take place and the length of stay in the hospital. Some insurance companies may press for shorter hospital stays.

- What pain medication will be used, and how medications for home use will be ordered for discharge. The physician should know all medications that are currently being taken.

- Who will make decisions on the patient's behalf and with what legal authority, should the patient be unable to make a decision in the hospital. The physician and the nursing team need to know who this "patient advocate" is.

- What the visiting hours, rules, and limits on children are.

- That the hospital plans to accommodate any dietary restrictions the patient may have.

- That there is sufficient at-home assistance and resources for the patient upon discharge.

- The dietary and behavioral requirements for the days just preceding surgery.

Resources

BOOKS

Khatri, VP and JA Asensio. Operative Surgery Manual. 1st ed. Philadelphia: Saunders, 2003.

Townsend, CM et al. Sabiston Textbook of Surgery. 17th ed. Philadelphia: Saunders, 2004.

ORGANIZATIONS

Patient Rights and Responsibilities. Agency for Health Care Research and Quality. http://www.consumer.gov/qualityhealth/rights.htm/.

Questions To Ask Your Doctor Before You Have Surgery. Agency for Health Care Research and Quality. http://www.ahcpr.gov/consumer/surgery.htm#head2/.

Needle bladder neck suspension

Definition

Needle bladder neck suspension, also known as needle suspension, or paravaginal surgery, is performed to support the hypermobile, or moveable urethra using sutures to attach it to tissues covering the pelvic floor. Of the three popular surgical procedures for urethral instability and its results in urinary stress incontinence, needle bladder neck suspension is the quickest and easiest to perform. It has many variants, such as the Raz, Stamey, modified Pereyra, or Gattes procedures, but its long-term results are less impressive than other, more extensive, anti-incontinent surgeries.

Purpose

Fifty years of work to treat incontinence, especially in women, has resulted in three types of surgery tied to essentially three causes of a particular type of incontinence related to muscle weakening of the urethra and the "gate-keeping" sphincter muscles. Stress urinary incontinence, the uncontrollable leakage of urine when pressure is put on the bladder during sneezing, coughing, laughing, or exercising, is very common in women. It is estimated to affect 50% of elderly women in long-term care facilities. The inability to hold urine has two causes. One has to do with support for the urethra and bladder, known as genuine stress incontinence (GSI), and the other is related to the inability of sphincter muscles, or intrinsic sphincter deficiency (ISD), to keep the opening of the bladder closed.

In GSI, weak muscles supporting the urethra allow it to be displaced and/or descend into the pelvic-floor fascia (connective tissues) and create cystoceles, or pockets. The goal of surgery for GSI is to stabilize the suburethral fascia to prevent the urethra from being overly mobile during increased abdominal pressure.

The other major source of stress incontinence is due to weakening of the internal muscles of the sphincter, as they affect closure of the bladder. These muscles, called the intrinsic sphincter muscles, regulate the opening and

KEY TERMS

Genuine stress incontinence (GSI)—A specific term for a type of incontinence that has to do with the instability of the urethra due to weakened support muscles.

Hypermobile urethra—A term that denotes the movement of the urethra that allows for leakage or spillage of urine.

Intrinsic sphincter deficiency—A type of incontinence caused by the inability of the sphincter muscles to keep the bladder closed.

Urinary stress incontinence—The involuntary release of urine due to pressure on the abdominal muscles during exercise or laughing or coughing.

closing of the bladder when a decision is made to urinate. Deficiency of the intrinsic sphincter muscles causes the opening to remain open and thus leads to chronic incontinence. ISD is a source of severe stress incontinence and may be combined with urethral hypermobility.

The challenge of surgery for stress incontinence is to adequately evaluate the actual source of incontinence, whether GSI or ISD, and also to determine the likelihood of cystoceles that may need repair. Under good diagnostic conditions, surgery for stress incontinence will utilize a suprapubic (above the pubic area) procedure, or Burch procedure, to secure the hypermobile urethra and stabilize it in a neutral position. Surgery for ISD uses what is known as a **sling procedure**, or "hammock" effect, that uses auxiliary tissue to undergird the urethra and provide contractive pressure to the sphincter. Most stress incontinence surgeries fall into one of these two procedures and their variants.

Needle neck bladder suspension, the third most utilized procedure for stress incontinence, simply attempts to attach the urethra neck to the posterior pelvic wall through the vagina or abdomen in order to stabilize the urethra. It is, however, considered a poor choice in comparison to the other two procedures because of its lack of long-term efficacy and its high incidence of urinary retention as an operative complication.

Demographics

More than 13 million people in the United States, both males and females, have urinary incontinence. Women experience it twice as often as men due to pregnancy, childbirth, menopause, and the structure of the female urinary and gynecological systems. Anyone can become incontinent due to neurological injury, birth

WHO PERFORMS THE PROCEDURE AND WHERE IS IT PERFORMED?

Surgery is performed by a urological surgeon who has a medical degree with advanced training in urology and in surgery. Surgery is performed in a general hospital.

defects, cardiac conditions, multiple sclerosis, and chronic conditions in later life. Incontinence does not naturally accompany old age but is associated with many chronic conditions that occur as age increases. Incontinence is highly associated with obesity and lack of **exercise**. As many as 15–30% of adults over 60 have some form of urinary incontinence. Stress incontinence is, by far, the most frequent form of incontinence and is the most common type of bladder control problem in younger and middle-age women.

Description

Needle bladder neck suspension surgery can be performed as open abdominal or vaginal surgery, or laproscopically, which allows for small incisions, video magnification of the operative field, and precise placement of sutures. Under a general anesthetic, the patient is placed in a position on her back with legs in stirrups allowing access to the suprapubic area. A Foley catheter is inserted into the bladder. The open procedure involves the passage of a needle from the suprapubic area to the vagina with multiple sutures through looping. Cytoscopic monitoring (using an endoscope passed into the urethra) prevents passage of the needle through the bladder or the urethra. The laparoscopic method allows visualization of the needle pass made from the suprapubic area to the vagina and the looping technique. The vagina and the surrounding areas are thoroughly irrigated with an antibiotic solution throughout the procedure. The patient is discharged the same evening or the next morning with the catheter in place. She is kept on **antibiotics** and examined on the fourth day after surgery with the removal of the catheter. The follow-up examination includes wound inspection and a evaluation of residual urine. A pelvic examination is performed to check for bleeding or injury.

Diagnosis/Preparation

Stress urinary incontinence can have a number of causes. It is important that patients confer with their physicians to rule out medication-related, psychological, and/or behavioral sources of incontinence as well as physical and neurological causes. This involves complete medical history, as well as medication, clinical,

QUESTIONS TO ASK THE DOCTOR

- Is surgery my only alternative to living with urinary incontinence?
- Are there other surgical procedures that are more effective for my incontinence?
- Can you recommend any literature I can read that explains my surgical options for incontinence?
- Can you explain why this procedure is preferable to what is known as a "sling procedure?"

neurological, and radiographic evaluations. Once these are completed, urodynamic tests that evaluate the urethra, bladder, flow, urine retention, and leakage, are performed and allow the physician to determine the primary source of the stress incontinence. Patients who are obese and/or engage in high-impact exercise are not good candidates for this surgery. Patients with ISD may not be cured with this procedure, since it is primarily intended to treat the hypermobile urethra.

Morbidity and mortality rates

Urologic surgery has inherent morbidity and mortality risks related primarily to **general surgery**, with lung conditions, blood clots, infections, and cardiac events occurring in a small percentage of surgeries, independent of the type of procedure. In addition, the American Urological Association (AUA) has concluded that needle suspension surgery has a number of complications related directly to suturing in the suprapulic area. These complications include:

- a 5% incidence of bladder injury
- urethral injury, although rare, in a small percentage of cases
- bleeding, with an incidence of 3–5%, primarily from the area below the pubic area
- nerve entrapment (8–16% of cases) due to lateral placement of the sutures into the fascia at the back of the suprapubic area (This has improved with a change in the placement of sutures.)
- wound infections in about 7% of cases, with higher rates among those with diabetes or obesity

These operative complications, coupled with the procedure's high rate (10%) of reported pain after surgery, and its relatively high rate (5%) of urinary retention lasting longer than four weeks, have resulted in needle neck suspension having a limited role in the management of stress urinary incontinence.

Normal results

Despite modifications in the needle suspension procedure, the long-term outcome of the procedure does not indicate its lasting efficacy. According to a recent report by the AUA, a study of the effects of needle suspension found only a 72-91% cure, or "dry rate," after 48 months, with delayed failures of sutures in a very high percentage (33-80%) of cases.

Resources

BOOKS

Katz VL et al. Comprehensive Gynecology. 5th ed. St. Louis: Mosby, 2007.

Wein, AJ et al. Campbell-Walsh Urology. 9th ed. Philadelphia: Saunders, 2007.

PERIODICALS

Bodell, D. M. and G. E. Leach. "Needle Suspension Procedures for Female Incontinence." Urologic Clinics 29 (August 2002).

Takahashi, S., et al. "Complications of Stamey Needle Suspension for Female Stress Urinary Incontinence." Urology International 86 (January 2002): 148–151.

ORGANIZATIONS

American Foundation for Urologic Diseases. The Bladder Health Council. 300 West Pratt Street, Suite 401, Baltimore, MD 21201.

American Urological Association. 1120 North Charles Street, Baltimore, MD 21201.(410) 727-1100. Fax: 410-223-4370. http://www.urologyhealth.org.

The Simon Foundation for Continence. P.O. Box 835, Wilmette, IL 60091. (800) 237-simon or (800) 237-4666. Toll-free (847) 864-3913. (847) 864-9758.

OTHER

"Urinary Incontinence." MD Consult Patient Handout. January 2, 2003 [cited July 7, 2003]. http://www. MDConsult.com.

Nancy McKenzie, PhD

Needle suspension *see* **Needle bladder neck suspension**

Needles *see* **Syringe and needle**

Negative pressure rooms

Definition

A negative pressure room is a volumetric space in which the internal atmospheric pressure is lower than the spaces into which it opens.

WHO PERFORMS THE PROCEDURE AND WHERE IS IT PERFORMED?

An infectious disease or emergency physician usually admits patients to negative pressure rooms in hospitals or other healthcare facilities.

Purpose

The purpose of a negative pressure room is to confine pathogens to sa single closed environment and to prevent the release of pathogens into other adjacent spaces.

Demographics

Official counts of negative pressure rooms do not exist. Experts estimate that approximately 4000-5000 negative pressure rooms exist in hospitals throughout the United States.

Description

A negative pressure room is designed to confine pathogens to a small volume of space. It is also intended to prevent the accidental release of pathogens into a greater space thereby protecting workers and employees in a hospital or other healthcare facility.

All communications between a negative pressure room and adjacent spaces are controlled. Communications include doors and ventilations ducts. These are sealed. Air flow is controlled by airlocks for human travel and vacuum pumps for ventilation systems.

Diagnosis/Preparation

Negative pressure rooms require special construction. All points if entrance or egress must be able to be tightly sealed so that air cannot pass by the seals. The room ventilation system must be equipped with a vacuum pump that must create a constant but relatively low level vacuum. This creates the negative pressure.

In operation, the vacuum created stops the outflow of air, thus containing

Two doors, separated by at least 6 feet, must be installed to create an airlock. Only one door is opened at a time. This preserves the vacuum, maintains the negative pressure and prevents pathogens from escaping.

QUESTIONS TO ASK YOUR DOCTOR

- Why am I being confined in a negative pressure room?
- What treatment options do I have?

All air exhausted from the room is routed through special filters that are designed to trap and contain pathogens.

Negative pressure rooms are used when the presence of an airborne pathogen such as tuberculosis is suspected.

Aftercare

Entrance and egress protocols must be followed by all people that enter or leave a negative pressure room.

Seals on vents and airlocks must be checked on a regular basis.

Negative pressure rooms must be decontaminated before being cleaned after being occupied.

Risks

Seal, pump or protocol failure destroys the negative pressure and increases the chances that pathogens will be released.

Inadequate cleaning after occupancy puts subsequent occupants at risk of exposure to a potentially dangerous pathogen.

Normal results

In a properly operating negative pressure room, the expected and normal result is containment of a potentially dangerous pathogen.

Morbidity and mortality rates

Data on morbidity and mortality related to negative pressure rooms is not available.

Alternatives

The only feasible alternative to a negative pressure room is quarantine and isolation. This practice is very difficult to enforce. Even when enforced, it is not as microbiologically efficient.

KEY TERMS

Anthrax—A dangerous pathogen that should contained in a negative pressure room.

Ebola virus—A dangerous pathogen that should contained in a negative pressure room.

Tuberculosis—A dangerous pathogen that should contained in a negative pressure room.

Resources

BOOKS

Fischbach, F. T. and M. B. Dunning. *A Manual of Laboratory and Diagnostic Tests*. 8th ed. Philadelphia: Lippincott Williams & Wilkins, 2008.

McGhee, M. *A Guide to Laboratory Investigations*. 5th ed. Oxford, UK: Radcliffe Publishing Ltd, 2008.

Price, C. P. *Evidence-Based Laboratory Medicine: Principles, Practice, and Outcomes*. 2nd ed. Washington, DC: AACC Press, 2007.

Scott, M.G., A. M. Gronowski, and C. S. Eby. *Tietz's Applied Laboratory Medicine*. 2nd ed. New York: Wiley-Liss, 2007.

Springhouse, A. M. *Diagnostic Tests Made Incredibly Easy!*. 2nd ed. Philadelphia: Lippincott Williams & Wilkins, 2008.

PERIODICALS

Chow, T. T., A. Kwan, Z. Lin, and W. Bai. "A computer evaluation of ventilation performance in a negative-pressure operating theater." *Anesthesia and Analgesia* 103, no. 4 (2006): 913–918.

Humphreys, H. "Control and prevention of healthcare-associated tuberculosis: the role of respiratory isolation and personal respiratory protection." *Journal of Hospital Infection* 66, no. 1 (2007): 1–5.

NIska, R. W., and C. W. Burt. "Emergency response planning in hospitals, United States: 2003-2004." *Advance Data* 391 (2007): 1–13.

Rydock, J. P. "On the need for a separate standard for performance testing of negative-pressure isolation rooms." *Infection Control and Hospital Epidemiology* 27, no. 5 (2006): 531–532.

Walker, J. T., P. Hoffman, A. M. Bennett, M. C. Vos, M. Thomas, and N. Tomlinson. "Hospital and community acquired infection and the built environment–design and testing of infection control rooms." *Journal of Hospital Infection* 65, Supplement 2 (2007): 43–49.

ORGANIZATIONS

American Academy of Family Physicians. 11400 Tomahawk Creek Parkway, Leawood, KS 66211-2672. (913) 906-6000. E-mail: fp@aafp.org. http://www.aafp.org.

American Academy of Pediatrics. 141 Northwest Point Boulevard, Elk Grove Village, IL 60007-1098. (847) 434-4000, Fax: (847) 434-8000. E-mail: kidsdoc@aap. org. http://www.aap.org/default.htm.

American College of Physicians. 190 N. Independence Mall West, Philadelphia, PA 19106-1572. (800) 523-1546, x2600, or (215) 351-2600. http://www.acponline.org.

American Medical Association. 515 N. State Street, Chicago, IL 60610. (312) 464-5000. http://www.ama-assn.org.

OTHER

Centers for Disease Control and Prevention. Information about negative pressure rooms. 2008 [cited February 25, 2008]. http://www.cdc.gov/mmwR/preview/mmwrhtml/00020788.htm.

Scientific American. Information about negative pressure rooms. 2008 [cited February 22, 2008]. http://www.sciam.com/article.cfm?id=er-of-future-fights-threa.

University of Pennsylvania Medical Center. Information about negative pressure rooms. 2008 [cited February 24, 2008]. http://www.uphs.upenn.edu/bugdrug/antibiotic_manual/infctl%20tuber.htm.

Yale-New Haven Hospital. Information about negative pressure rooms. 2008 [cited February 24, 2008]. http://www.med.yale.edu/ynhh/infection/airborne/negrooms.html.

L. Fleming Fallon, Jr, MD, DrPH

Nephrectomy

Definition

A nephrectomy is a surgical procedure for the removal of a kidney or section of a kidney.

Purpose

Nephrectomy, or kidney removal, is performed on patients with severe kidney damage from disease, injury, or congenital conditions. These include cancer of the kidney (renal cell carcinoma); polycystic kidney disease (a disease in which cysts, or sac-like structures, displace healthy kidney tissue); and serious kidney infections. It is also used to remove a healthy kidney from a donor for the purposes of **kidney transplantation**.

Demographics

The HCUP Nationwide Inpatient Sample from the Agency for Healthcare Research and Quality (AHRQ) reports that 46,130 patients underwent partial or radical nephrectomy surgery for non-transplant-related indications in the United States in 2000. Patients with kidney cancer accounted for over half of those procedures. About 51,190 new cases of renal cell

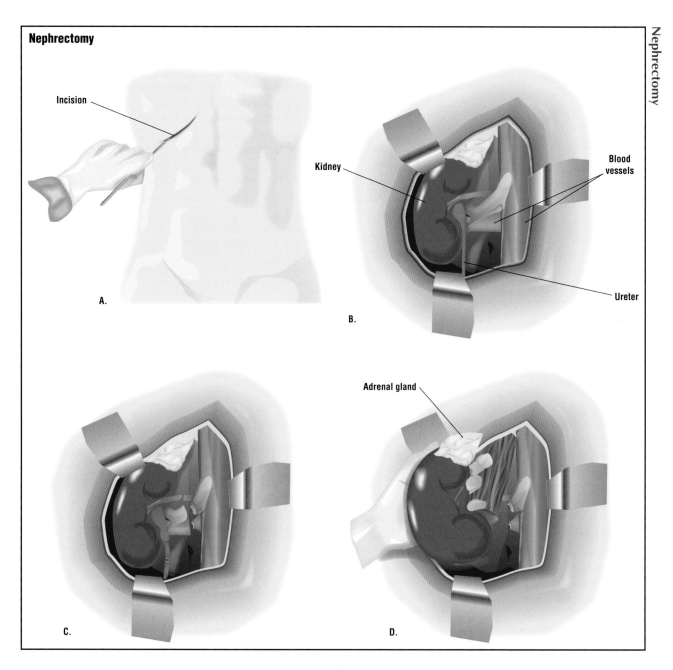

Nephrectomy

A. Incision

B. Kidney — Blood vessels — Ureter

C.

D. Adrenal gland

To remove a kidney in an open procedure, an incision is made below the ribcage (A). The kidney is exposed (B) and connections to blood vessels and the ureter are severed (C). The kidney is removed in one piece (D). *(Illustration by GGS Information Services. Cengage Learning, Gale.)*

carcinoma were expected to be diagnosed in 2007, per the American Cancer Society.

According to the United Network for Organ Sharing (UNOS), 5,086 people underwent nephrectomy to become living kidney donors in 2007. Of these, 2,911were male and 2,975 were female. Related donors were more common than non-related donors, with full siblings being the most common relationship

between living donor and kidney recipients (28.5% of living donors).

Description

Nephrectomy may involve removing a small portion of the kidney or the entire organ and surrounding tissues. In partial nephrectomy, only the diseased or

KEY TERMS

Cadaver kidney—A kidney from a brain-dead organ donor used for purposes of kidney transplantation.

Polycystic kidney disease—A hereditary kidney disease that causes fluid- or blood-filled pouches of tissue called cysts to form on the tubules of the kidneys. These cysts impair normal kidney function.

Renal cell carcinoma—Cancer of the kidney.

infected portion of the kidney is removed. Radical nephrectomy involves removing the entire kidney, a section of the tube leading to the bladder (ureter), the gland that sits atop the kidney (adrenal gland), and the fatty tissue surrounding the kidney. A simple nephrectomy performed for living donor transplant purposes requires removal of the kidney and a section of the attached ureter.

Open nephrectomy

In a traditional, open nephrectomy, the kidney donor is administered **general anesthesia** and a 6–10 in (15.2–25.4 cm) incision through several layers of muscle is made on the side or front of the abdomen. The blood vessels connecting the kidney to the donor are cut and clamped, and the ureter is also cut between the bladder and kidney and clamped. Depending on the type of nephrectomy procedure being performed, the ureter, adrenal gland, and/or surrounding tissue may also be cut. The kidney is removed and the vessels and ureter are then tied off and the incision is sutured (sewn up). The surgical procedure can take up to three hours, depending on the type of nephrectomy being performed.

Laparoscopic nephrectomy

Laparoscopic nephrectomy is a form of minimally invasive surgery that utilizes instruments on long, narrow rods to view, cut, and remove the kidney. The surgeon views the kidney and surrounding tissue with a flexible videoscope. The videoscope and **surgical instruments** are maneuvered through four small incisions in the abdomen, and carbon dioxide is pumped into the abdominal cavity to inflate it and improve visualization of the kidney. Once the kidney is isolated, it is secured in a bag and pulled through a fifth incision, approximately 3 in (7.6 cm) wide, in the front of the abdominal wall below the navel. Although this surgical technique takes slightly longer than a traditional nephrectomy, preliminary studies have shown that it promotes a faster recovery time, shorter hospital stays, and less post-operative pain.

A modified laparoscopic technique called hand-assisted laparoscopic nephrectomy may also be used to remove the kidney. In the hand-assisted surgery, a small incision of 3–5 in (7.6–12.7 cm) is made in the patient's abdomen. The incision allows the surgeon to place his hand in the abdominal cavity using a special surgical glove that also maintains a seal for the inflation of the abdominal cavity with carbon dioxide. This technique gives the surgeon the benefit of using his hands to feel the kidney and related structures. The kidney is then removed by hand through the incision instead of with a bag.

Diagnosis/Preparation

Prior to surgery, blood samples will be taken from the patient to type and crossmatch in case **transfusion** is required during surgery. A catheter will also be inserted into the patient's bladder. The surgical procedure will be described to the patient, along with the possible risks.

Aftercare

Nephrectomy patients may experience considerable discomfort in the area of the incision. Patients may also experience numbness, caused by severed nerves, near or on the incision. Pain relievers are administered following the surgical procedure and during the recovery period on an as-needed basis. Although deep breathing and coughing may be painful due to the proximity of the incision to the diaphragm, breathing exercises are encouraged to prevent pneumonia. Patients should not drive an automobile for a minimum of two weeks.

Risks

Possible complications of a nephrectomy procedure include infection, bleeding (hemorrhage), and post-operative pneumonia. There is also the risk of kidney failure in a patient with impaired function or disease in the remaining kidney.

Normal results

Normal results of a nephrectomy are dependent on the purpose of the procedure and the type of nephrectomy performed. Immediately following the procedure, it is normal for patients to experience pain near the incision site, particularly when coughing or breathing deeply. Renal function of the patient is monitored carefully after surgery. If the remaining kidney is

WHO PERFORMS THE PROCEDURE AND WHERE IS IT PERFORMED?

If nephrectomy is required for the purpose of kidney donation, it will be performed by a transplant surgeon in one of over 200 UNOS-approved hospitals nationwide. For patients with renal cell carcinoma, nephrectomy surgery is typically performed in a hospital setting by a surgeon specializing in urologic oncology.

healthy, it will increase its functioning over time to compensate for the loss of the removed kidney.

Length of hospitalization depends on the type of nephrectomy procedure. Patients who have undergone a laparoscopic radical nephrectomy may be discharged two to four days after surgery. Traditional open nephrectomy patients are typically hospitalized for about a week. Recovery time will also vary, on average from three to six weeks.

Morbidity and mortality rates

Survival rates for living kidney donors undergoing nephrectomy are excellent; mortality rates are only 0.03%—or three deaths for every 10,000 donors. Many of the risks involved are the same as for any surgical procedure: risk of infection, hemorrhage, blood clot, or allergic reaction to anesthesia.

For patients undergoing nephrectomy as a treatment for renal cell carcinoma, survival rates depend on several factors, including the stage of the cancer and the patient's overall **health history**. According to the American Cancer Society, the five-year survival rate for patients with stage I renal cell carcinoma is 96 percent, while the five-year survival rate for stage II kidney cancer is 82 percent. Stage III and IV cancers have metastasized, or spread, beyond the kidney and have a lower survival rate, 64 percent for stage III and about 23 percent for stage IV. Chemotherapy, radiation, and/or immunotherapy may also be required for these patients.

Alternatives

Because the kidney is responsible for filtering wastes and fluid from the bloodstream, kidney function is critical to life. Nephrectomy candidates diagnosed with serious kidney disease, cancer, or infection usually have few treatment choices aside from this

QUESTIONS TO ASK THE DOCTOR

- How many procedures of this type have you performed, and what are your success rates?
- Will my nephrectomy surgery be performed with a laparoscopic or an open technique?
- Will my nephrectomy be partial or radical, and what are the risks involved with my particular surgery?
- What will my recovery time be after the procedure?
- What are the chances that the transplant will be successful? (For those undergoing a nephrectomy to donate a kidney.)
- What are the odds of success, and will I require adjunctive treatment such as chemotherapy or immunotherapy? (For those undergoing a nephrectomy to treat kidney cancer.)

procedure. However, if kidney function is lost in the remaining kidney, the patient will require chronic dialysis treatments or transplantation of a healthy kidney to sustain life.

Resources

BOOKS

Brenner, BM et al Brenner & Rector's The Kidney. 7th ed. Philadelphia: Saunders, 2004.

Wein, AJ et al. Campbell-Walsh Urology. 9th ed. Philadelphia: Saunders, 2007.

PERIODICALS

Johnson, Kate. "Laparoscopy is Big Hit With Living Donors." Family Practice News 31 (January 2001): 12.

ORGANIZATIONS

American Cancer Society. (800) 227-2345. http://www.cancer.org.

National Kidney Foundation. 30 East 33rd St., Suite 1100, New York, NY 10016. (800) 622-9010. http://www.kidney.org.

United Network for Organ Sharing (UNOS). 700 North 4th St., Richmond, VA 23219. (888) 894-6361. UNOS Transplant Connection: http://www.transplantliving.org.

OTHER

Living Donors Online. http://www.livingdonorsonline.org.

Paula Anne Ford-Martin

Nephrolithotomy, percutaneous

Definition

Percutaneous nephrolithotomy, or PCNL, is a procedure for removing medium-sized or larger renal calculi (kidney stones) from the patient's urinary tract by means of an nephroscope passed into the kidney through a track created in the patient's back. PCNL was first performed in Sweden in 1973 as a less invasive alternative to open surgery on the kidneys. The term "percutaneous" means that the procedure is done through the skin. Nephrolithotomy is a term formed from two Greek words that mean "kidney" and "removing stones by cutting."

Purpose

The purpose of PCNL is the removal of renal calculi in order to relieve pain, bleeding into or obstruction of the urinary tract, and/or urinary tract infections resulting from blockages. Kidney stones range in size from microscopic groups of crystals to objects as large as golf balls. Most calculi, however, pass through the urinary tract without causing problems.

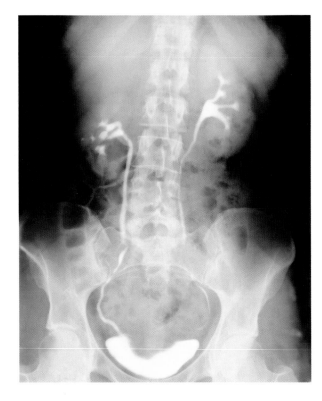

Intravenous pyelogram (IVP) of kidneys, ureters, and urinary bladder. *(Scott Camazine / Phototake. Reproduced by permission.)*

Renal calculi are formed when the urine becomes supersaturated (overloaded) with mineral compounds that can form stones. This supersaturation may occur because the patient has low urinary output, is excreting too much salt, or has very acid urine. Urolithiasis is the medical term for the formation of kidney stones; the word is also sometimes used to refer to disease conditions associated with kidney stones.

There are several different types of kidney stones, in terms of chemical composition:

- Calcium oxalate calculi. About 80% of calculi found in patients in the United States are formed from calcium combined with oxalate, which is a salt formed from oxalic acid. Some foods, such as rhubarb and spinach, are high in oxalic acid. Oxalic acid is also formed in the body when vitamin C is broken down. Oxalic acid is ordinarily excreted through the urine but may be absorbed in large amounts due to chronic pancreatic disease or surgery involving the small intestine.

- Uric acid calculi. These stones develop from crystals of uric acid that form in highly acidic urine. Uric acid calculi account for about 5% of kidney stones. In addition, some kidney stones are a combination of calcium oxalate and uric acid crystals.

- Cystine calculi. Cystine calculi represent about 2% of kidney stones. Cystine is an amino acid found in proteins that may form hexagonal crystals in the urine when it is excreted in excessive amounts. Kidney stones made of cystine indicate that the patient has cystinuria, a hereditary condition in which the kidneys do not reabsorb this amino acid.

- Struvite calculi. Struvite is a hard crystalline form of magnesium aluminum phosphate. Kidney stones made of this substance are formed in patients with urinary tract infections caused by certain types of bacteria. Struvite calculi are also known as infection calculi for this reason.

- Staghorn calculi. Staghorn calculi are large branched calculi composed of struvite. They are often discussed separately because their size and shape complicate their removal from the urinary tract.

Some people are more likely than others to develop renal calculi. Risk factors for kidney stones include:

- Male sex.

- Family history. Having a first-degree relative with urolithiasis increases a person's risk of developing kidney stones.

- Age over 30.

Percutaneous nephrolithotomy

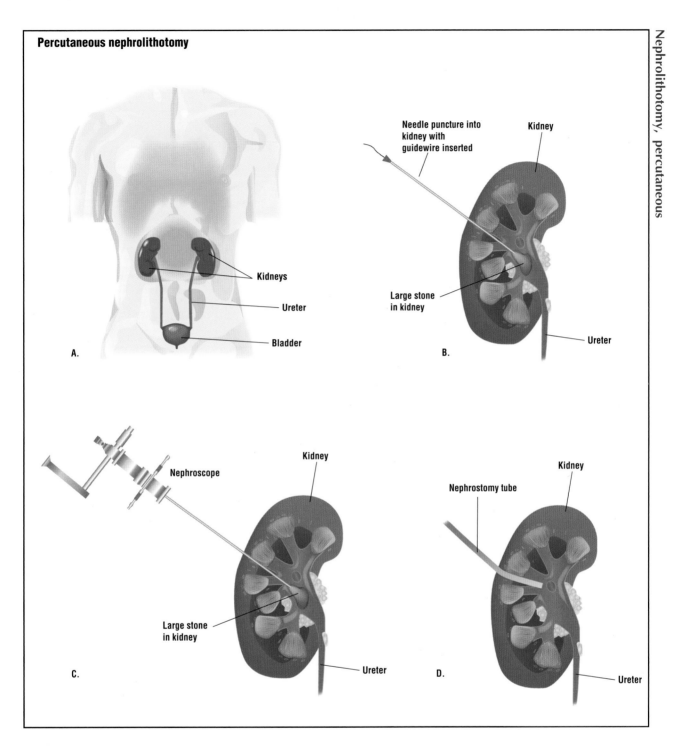

During a percutaneous nephrolithotomy, the surgeon inserts a needle through the patient's back directly into the kidney (B). A nephroscope uses an ultrasonic or laser probe to break up large kidney stones (C). Pieces of the stones are suctioned out with the scope, and a nephrostomy tube drains the kidney of urine (D). *(Illustration by GGS Information Services. Cengage Learning, Gale.)*

- Diet. People whose diet is high in protein or who eat foods rich in oxalate are more likely to develop kidney stones.

- Dehydration. People who do not drink enough fluid each day to replace what is lost through perspiration and excretion produce very concentrated urine. It is

Nephrolithotomy, percutaneous

Bougie—A slender, flexible tube or rod inserted into the urethra in order to dilate it.

Calculus (plural, calculi)—The medical term for a kidney or gallbladder stone.

Cystine—An amino acid found in protein molecules that may form kidney stones when excreted in excessive amounts in the urine.

Cystinuria—A hereditary condition characterized by chronic excessive excretion of cystine and three other amino acids.

Infection calculi—Another name for struvite calculi.

Lithotripsy—A technique for breaking up kidney stones within the urinary tract, followed by flushing out the fragments.

Nephrolithotomy—The removal of renal calculi by an incision through the kidney. The term by itself usually refers to the standard open procedure for the surgical removal of kidney stones.

Nephroscope—An instrument used to view the inside of the kidney during PCNL. A nephroscope has channels for a fiberoptic light, a telescope, and an irrigation system for washing out the affected part of the kidney.

Percutaneous—Through the skin.

Staghorn calculus—A kidney stone that develops a branched shape resembling the antlers of a stag. Staghorn calculi are composed of struvite.

Struvite—A crystalline form of magnesium ammonium phosphate. Kidney stones made of struvite form in urine with a pH above 7.2.

Ureter—The tubelike structure that carries urine from the kidney to the bladder.

Ureteroscope—A special type of endoscope that allows a surgeon to remove kidney stones from the lower urinary tract without the need for an incision.

Urolithiasis—The medical term for the formation of kidney stones. It is also used to refer to disease conditions related to kidney stones.

easier for crystals to form in concentrated than in dilute urine, and to grow into kidney stones.

- Metabolic disorders affecting the body's excretion of salt or its absorption of calcium or oxalate. Most cases of urolithiasis in children are related to metabolic disorders.

- Intestinal bypass surgery and ostomies. People who have had these surgical procedures lose larger than average amounts of water from the digestive tract.

Demographics

Calculi in the urinary tract are common in the general United States population. Between seven and 10 of every 1,hopsitalizations each year are due to urolithiasis; in addition, kidney stones are found in about 1% of bodies at autopsy. An estimated 10% of the population will suffer from kidney stones at some point in life. 12% of men and 6% of women will have kidney stones at some point over the course of their lifetimes.

In terms of age groups, most people with urolithiasis are between the ages of 20 and 40; kidney stones are rare in children. A person who develops one kidney stone has a 50% chance of developing another.

With regard to race, Caucasians are more likely to develop kidney stones than African Americans.

Description

Standard PCNL

A standard percutaneous nephrolithotomy is performed under **general anesthesia** and usually takes about three to four hours to complete. After the patient has been anesthetized, the surgeon makes a small incision, about 0.5 in (1.3 cm) in length in the patient's back on the side overlying the affected kidney. The surgeon then creates a track from the skin surface into the kidney and enlarges the track using a series of Teflon dilators or bougies. A sheath is passed over the last dilator to hold the track open.

After the track has been enlarged, the surgeon inserts a nephroscope, which is an instrument with a fiberoptic light source and two additional channels for viewing the inside of the kidney and irrigating (washing out) the area. The surgeon may use a device with a basket on the end to grasp and remove smaller kidney stones directly. Larger stones are broken up with an ultrasonic or electrohydraulic probe, or a holmium laser lithotriptor. The holmium laser has the advantage of being usable on all types of calculi.

A catheter is placed to drain the urinary system through the bladder and a **nephrostomy** tube is placed in the incision in the back to carry fluid from the kidney into a drainage bag. The catheter is removed after 24 hours. The nephrostomy tube is usually removed while the patient is still in the hospital but may be left in after the patient is discharged.

Mini-percutaneous nephrolithotomy

A newer form of PCNL is called mini-percutaneous nephrolithotomy (MPCNL) because it is performed with a miniaturized nephroscope. MPCNL has been found to be 99% effective in removing calculi between 0.4 and 1 in (1 and 2.5 cm) in size. Although it cannot be used for larger kidney stones, MPCNL has the advantage of fewer complications, a shorter operating time (about one and a half hours), and a shorter recovery time for the patient.

Diagnosis/Preparation

Diagnosis

Kidney stones may be discovered during a routine x-ray study of the patient's abdomen. These stones, which would ordinarily pass through the urinary tract unnoticed, are sometimes referred to as silent stones. In most cases, however, the patient seeks medical help for sudden intense pain in the lower back, usually on the side of the affected kidney. The pain is caused by the movement of the stone in the urinary tract as it irritates the tissues or blocks the passage of urine. If the stone moves further downward into the ureter (the tube that carries urine from the kidney to the bladder), pain may spread to the abdomen and groin area. The patient may also have nausea and vomiting, blood in the urine, pain on urination, or a need to urinate frequently. If the stone is associated with a UTI, the patient may also have chills and fever. The doctor will order both laboratory studies and imaging tests in order to rule out such other possible causes of the patient's symptoms as appendicitis, pancreatitis, peptic ulcer, and dissecting aneurysm.

The imaging studies most commonly performed are x ray and **ultrasound**. Pure uric acid and cystine calculi, however, do not show up well on a standard x ray, so the doctor may also order an intravenous pyelogram, or IVP. In an IVP, the radiologist injects a radioactive contrast material into a vein in the patient's arm, and records its passage through the urinary system in a series of x-ray images. Blood and urine samples will be taken to test for indications of a urinary tract infection. If the patient passes the kidney stone, it is saved and sent to a laboratory for analysis.

Preparation

Most hospitals require patients to have the following tests before a PCNL: a complete **physical examination**;

complete **blood count**; an **electrocardiogram** (EKG); a comprehensive set of metabolic tests; a urine test; and tests that measure the speed of blood clotting.

Aspirin and arthritis medications should be discontinued seven to 10 days before a PCNL because they thin the blood and affect clotting time. Some surgeons ask patients to take a laxative the day before surgery to minimize the risk of constipation during the first few days of recovery.

The patient is asked to drink only clear fluids (chicken or beef broth, clear fruit juices, or water) for 24 hours prior to surgery, with nothing by mouth after midnight before the procedure.

Aftercare

A standard PCNL usually requires hospitalization for five to six days after the procedure. The urologist may order additional imaging studies to determine whether any fragments of stones are still present. These can be removed with a nephroscope if necessary. The nephrostomy tube is then removed and the incision covered with a bandage. The patient will be given instructions for changing the bandage at home.

The patient is given fluids intravenously for one to two days after surgery. Later, he or she is encouraged to drink large quantities of fluid in order to produce about 2 qt (1.2 l) of urine per day. Some blood in the urine is normal for several days after PCNL. Blood and urine samples may be taken for laboratory analysis of specific risk factors for calculus formation.

Risks

There are a number of risks associated with PCNL:

- Inability to make a large enough track to insert the nephroscope. In this case, the procedure will be converted to open kidney surgery.
- Bleeding. Bleeding may result from injury to blood vessels within the kidney as well as from blood vessels in the area of the incision.
- Infection.
- Fever. Running a slight temperature (101.5°F; 38.5°C) is common for one or two days after the procedure. A high fever or a fever lasting longer than two days may indicate infection, however, and should be reported to the doctor at once.
- Fluid accumulation in the area around the incision. This complication usually results from irrigation of the affected area of the kidney during the procedure.
- Formation of an arteriovenous fistula. An arteriovenous fistula is a connection between an artery and

a vein in which blood flows directly from the artery into the vein.

- Need for retreatment. In general, PCNL has a higher success rate of stone removal than extracorporeal shock wave lithotripsy (ESWL), which is described below. PCNL is considered particularly effective for removing stones larger than 1 in (0.5 cm); staghorn calculi; and stones that have remained in the body longer than four weeks. Retreatment is occasionally necessary, however, in cases involving very large stones.
- Injury to surrounding organs. In rare cases, PCNL has resulted in damage to the spleen, liver, lung, pancreas, or gallbladder.

Normal results

PCNL has a high rate of success for stone removal, over 98% for stones that remain in the kidney and 88% for stones that pass into the ureter.

Morbidity and mortality rates

Standard PCNL has a higher rate of complications than extracorporeal shock wave **lithotripsy**; however, it is more successful in removing calculi. The overall rate of complications following PCNL is reported as 5.6% in one recent study and 6.5% in a second article. About 20% of patients scheduled for PCNL require a blood **transfusion** during the procedure, with 2.8% needing treatment for bleeding after the procedure. The rate of fistula formation is about 2.5%.

Alternatives

Patients with kidney stones may be treated with one or more of the following procedures in addition to PCNL, depending on the size of their renal calculi and possible complications. One frequently used combination, known as sandwich therapy, is extracorporeal shock wave lithotripsy for smaller stones followed by PCNL to remove larger calculi.

Conservative approaches

Conservative forms of treatment include the following:

- Watchful waiting.
- Hydration. Increasing the patient's fluid intake (to seven or more glasses of fluid each day) is a major component of treatment intended to prevent the formation of kidney stones. At least half of the fluid should be water.
- Dietary modification. Depending on the type of stone that has formed, the patient may benefit from

WHO PERFORMS THE PROCEDURE AND WHERE IS IT PERFORMED?

A PCNL or mini-PCNL is performed under general anesthesia in a hospital by a urologist, who is a surgeon with specialized training in treating disorders of the urinary tract. ESWL may be done as an outpatient procedure in an ambulatory surgery facility.

eating less animal protein, avoiding vegetables with high oxalate content, cutting down on table salt and vitamin C intake, etc.

- Medications. Patients who tend to form uric acid stones may be given allopurinol, which decreases the formation of uric acid; those who form calcium oxalate stones may be given thiazide diuretics; and those who develop infection stones can be treated with oral antibiotics.

Open surgery

Open surgery is the most invasive form of treatment for urolithiasis. As of 2003, it is performed primarily to remove very large and complex staghorn calculi or extremely hard stones that cannot be broken down by lithotripsy. Other indications for open surgery are extreme obesity, an anatomically abnormal kidney, or an infected and nonfunctioning kidney requiring complete removal. Patients are usually hospitalized for a week after open kidney surgery and take about six weeks to recover at home.

Extracorporeal shock wave lithotripsy (ESWL)

ESWL is a noninvasive procedure that was developed in the 1980s as a less invasive alternative to PCNL. It is presently used more often than PCNL to treat smaller renal calculi. In ESWL, the patient is given a local anesthetic and placed in a water bath or on a soft cushion while shock waves are transmitted through the tissues of the back to the stones inside the kidney. The shock waves cause the calculi to break up into smaller pieces that can be passed easily in the urine.

Although patients need less time to recuperate from ESWL, it has several disadvantages. It has lower success rates (50–90%) than PCNL. Moreover, it cannot be used to treat cystine calculi or calculi larger than 1.2 in (3 cm). An additional concern with shock wave lithotripsy is its safety in treating small or anatomically abnormal kidneys; it has been reported

QUESTIONS TO ASK THE DOCTOR

- Am I a candidate for a mini-PCNL?
- Do you consider the higher success rate of a PCNL a greater advantage than the lower rate of complications with ESWL?
- What can I do to prevent recurrence of kidney stones?
- What are the chances of my needing another operation?

to cause temporary damage to kidney tubules in smaller-than-average kidneys.

Ureteroscopy

Ureteroscopy refers to removal of calculi that have moved downward into the ureter with the help of a special instrument. A ureteroscope is a small fiberoptic endoscope that can be passed through the patient's urethra and bladder into the ureter. The ureteroscope allows the surgeon to locate and remove stones in the lower urinary tract without the need for an incision.

Complementary and alternative (CAM) approaches

Vegetarian and other low-protein diets have been found helpful in preventing kidney stone formation. In addition, recent ethnobotanical studies of ammi visnaga (toothpick weed), a plant belonging to the parsley family, and *Phyllanthus niruri*, a traditional Brazilian folk remedy for kidney stones, indicate that extracts from these plants are effective in increasing urinary output and inhibiting the development of calcium oxalate calculi.

Resources

BOOKS

Brenner, BM et al Brenner & Rector's The Kidney. 7th ed. Philadelphia: Saunders, 2004.

Pelletier, Kenneth R., MD. "CAM Therapies for Specific Conditions: Kidney Stones." In The Best Alternative Medicine. New York: Simon & Schuster, 2002.

Wein, AJ et al. Campbell-Walsh Urology. 9th ed. Philadelphia: Saunders, 2007.

PERIODICALS

Battino, B. S., W. DeFoor, F. Coe, et al. "Metabolic Evaluation of Children with Urolithiasis: Are Adult References for Supersaturation Appropriate?" Journal of Urology 168 (December 2002): 2568–2571.

Jin, Chua Wei, and Chin Chong Min. "Management of Staghorn Calculus." Medical Progress (February 2003): 1–6.

Kim, S. C., R. L. Kuo, and J. E. Lingeman. "Percutaneous Nephrolithotomy: An Update." Current Opinion in Urology 13 (May 2003): 235–241.

ORGANIZATIONS

American Foundation for Urologic Disease (AFUD). 1128 North Charles Street, Baltimore, MD 21201. (800) 242-2383. http://www.afud.org.

American Urological Association (AUA). 1120 North Charles Street, Baltimore, MD 21201. (410) 727-1100. http://www.auanet.org.

National Kidney Foundation. 30 East 33rd Street, Suite 1100, New York, NY 10016. (800) 622-9010 or (212) 889-2210. http://www.kidney.org.

National Kidney and Urologic Diseases Information Clearinghouse (NKUDIC). 3 Information Way, Bethesda, MD 20892-3580.

OTHER

National Kidney and Urologic Diseases Information Clearinghouse (NKUDIC). Kidney Stones in Adults. February 1998 [cited April 30, 2003]. NIH Publication No. 94-2495. http://www.niddk.nih.gov/health/urolog/pubs/stonadul/stonadul.htm.

Rebecca Frey, Ph.D.

Nephrostomy

Definition

A nephrostomy is a surgical procedure by which a tube, stent, or catheter is inserted through the skin and into the kidney.

Purpose

The ureter is the fibromuscular tube that carries urine from the kidney to the bladder. When this tube is blocked, urine backs up into the kidney. Serious, irreversible kidney damage can occur because of this backflow of urine. Infection is also a common consequence in this stagnant urine.

Nephrostomy is performed in several different circumstances:

- The ureter is blocked by a kidney stone.
- The ureter is blocked by a tumor, abscess, or fluid collection.
- There is a hole in the ureter or bladder and urine is leaking into the body. These may occur after trauma

KEY TERMS

Catheter—A tubular, flexible, surgical instrument for withdrawing fluids from a cavity of the body, especially one for introduction into the bladder through the urethra for the withdraw of urine.

Ostomy—General term meaning a surgical procedure in which an artificial opening is formed to either allow waste (stool or urine) to pass from the body, or to allow food into the GI tract. An ostomy can be permanent or temporary, as well as single-barreled, double-barreled, or a loop.

Septicemia—Systemic disease associated with the presence and persistence of pathogenic microorganisms or their toxins in the blood.

Stent—A tube made of metal or plastic that is inserted into a vessel or passage to keep it open and prevent closure.

Ureter—The fibromuscular tube that conveys the urine from the kidney to the bladder.

or accidental injury during surgery (iatrogenic injury), or severe hemorrhagic cystitis.

• The ureter is obstructed during pregnancy.

• Access is needed in order to infuse materials/medications directly into the kidney, such as antibiotics, antifungal agents, chemotherapeutic agents, or chemicals that will dissolve stones.

• As a diagnostic procedure to assess kidney anatomy.

• As a diagnostic procedure to assess kidney function.

Demographics

For unknown reasons, the number of people in the United States with kidney and ureter stones has been increasing over the past 20 years. White Americans are more prone to develop kidney stones than African Americans. Stones occur more frequently in men. The condition strikes most typically between the ages of 20 and 40. Once a person gets more than one stone, others are likely to develop.

Upper tract tumors develop in the renal pelvis (tissue in the kidneys that collects urine) and in the ureters. These cancers account for less than 1% of cancers of the reproductive and urinary systems. Upper tract tumors are often associated with bladder cancer.

Description

First, the patient is given an anesthetic to numb the area where the catheter will be inserted. The doctor then inserts a needle into the kidney. There are several imaging technologies such as **ultrasound** and computed tomography (CT) that are used to help the doctor guide the needle into the correct place.

Next, a fine guide wire follows the needle. The catheter, which is about the same diameter as intravenous (IV) tubing, follows the guide wire to its proper location. The catheter is then connected to a bag outside the body that collects the urine. The catheter and bag are secured so that the catheter will not pull out. The procedure usually takes one to two hours.

Diagnosis/Preparation

Either the day before or the day of the nephrostomy, blood samples are taken. Other diagnostic tests done before the procedure may vary, depending on why the nephrostomy is being done, but the patient may have a CT scan or ultrasound to help the treating physician locate the blockage.

Patients should not eat for eight hours before a nephrostomy. On the day of the procedure, the patient will have an IV line placed in a vein in the arm. Through this line, the patient will receive **antibiotics** to prevent infection, medication for pain, and fluids. The IV line will remain in place after the procedure for at least several hours, and often longer.

People preparing for a nephrostomy should review with their doctor all the medications they are taking. People taking anticoagulants (blood thinners such as Coumadin) may need to stop their medication. People taking metformin (Glucophage) may need to stop taking the medication for several days before and after nephrostomy. Diabetics should discuss modifying their insulin dose because fasting is required before the procedure.

Aftercare

Outpatients are usually expected to stay in the clinic or hospital for eight to 12 hours after the procedure to make sure the nephrostomy tube is functioning properly. They should plan to have someone drive them home and stay with them for at least the first 24 hours after the procedure. Inpatients may stay in the hospital several days. Generally, people feel sore where the catheter is inserted for about a week to 10 days.

Care of the nephrostomy tube is important. It is located on the patient's back, so it may be necessary to have someone help with its care. The nephrostomy

WHO PERFORMS THE PROCEDURE AND WHERE IS IT PERFORMED?

A nephrostomy is performed by an interventional radiologist or urologist with special training in the procedure. It can be done either on an inpatient or outpatient basis, depending on why it is required. For most cancer patients, nephrostomy is an inpatient procedure. Specially trained nurses called wound, ostomy continence nurses (WOCN) are commonly available for consultation in most major medical centers to assist patients.

QUESTIONS TO ASK THE DOCTOR

- Why am I having a nephrostomy?
- How do I prepare for surgery?
- How long will I have to stay in the hospital?
- How long do you expect the nephrostomy tube to stay in?
- How much help will I need in caring for the nephrostomy tube?

tube should be kept dry and protected from water when taking showers. The skin around it should be kept clean, and the dressing over the area changed frequently. It is the main part of the urine drainage system, and it should be treated very carefully to prevent bacteria and other germs from entering the system. If any germs get into the tubing, they can easily cause a kidney infection. The drainage bag should not be allowed to drag on the floor. If the bag should accidentally be cut or begin to leak, it must be changed immediately. It is not recommended to place the drainage bag in a plastic bag if it leaks.

Risks

A nephrostomy is an established and generally safe procedure. As with all operations, there is always a risk of allergic reaction to anesthesia, bleeding, and infection.

Bruising at the catheter insertion site occurs in about half of people who have a nephrostomy. This is a minor complication. Major complications include the following:

- injury to surrounding organs, including bowel perforation, splenic injury, and liver injury
- infection, leading to septicemia
- significant loss of functioning kidney tissue ($<1\%$)
- delayed bleeding, or hemorrhage ($<0.5\%$)
- blocking of a kidney artery ($<0.5\%$)

Normal results

In a successful nephrostomy, the catheter is inserted, and urine drains into the collection bag. How long the catheter stays in place depends on the reason for its insertion. In people with pelvic cancer or bladder cancer where the ureter is blocked by a tumor, the catheter will stay in place until the tumor is surgically removed. If the cancer is inoperable, the catheter may have to stay in place for the rest of the patient's life.

Morbidity and mortality rates

The mortality rate of nephrostomies is of the order of less than 0.05% and the incidence of the specific complications listed above ranges between less than 0.05% (hemorrhage, kidney arterial blocking, and loss of kidney tissue) to $<1\%$ (injury to surrounding organs and septicemia).

Alternatives

In the treatment of ureter stones, extracorporeal shock wave **lithotripsy** (ESWL) has been most widely performed and has become the preferred treatment for this condition. ESWL is a new technique that offers an alternative to surgery for patients with kidney or ureter stones. ESWL works by pulverizing the stones into sand-like particles that can be excreted with little or no pain. This is achieved by the ESWL procedure approximately 90% of the time. The shock waves are a form of high-energy pressure that can travel in air or water. When generated outside the body, they pass through the tissues of the body without damaging them, but can destroy a stone inside a kidney or urethra. The shock waves pass through both without injury. A stone has a greater density and, when the shock wave hits it, the waves scatter and break it up.

Resources

BOOKS

Brenner, BM et al Brenner & Rector's The Kidney. 7th ed. Philadelphia: Saunders, 2004.

Khatri, VP and JA Asensio. Operative Surgery Manual. 1st ed. Philadelphia: Saunders, 2003.

Townsend, CM et al. Sabiston Textbook of Surgery. 17th ed. Philadelphia: Saunders, 2004.

Wein, AJ et al. Campbell-Walsh Urology. 9th ed. Philadelphia: Saunders, 2007.

PERIODICALS

Cozens, N. J. "How Should We Deliver an Out of Hours Nephrostomy Service?" Clinical Radiology 58 (May 2003): 410.

Dyer, R. B., J. D. Regan, P. V. Kavanagh, E. G. Khatod, M. Y. Chen, and R. J. Zagoria. "Percutaneous Nephrostomy with Extensions of the Technique: Step by Step." Radiographics 22 (May–June 2002): 503–524.

Koral, K., M. C. Saker, F. P. Morello, C. K. Rigsby, and J. S. Donaldson. "Conventional versus Modified Technique for Percutaneous Nephrostomy in Newborns and Young Infants." Journal of Vascular and Interventional Radiology 14 (January 2003): 113–116.

Little, B., K. J. Ho, S. Gawley, and M. Young. "Use of Nephrostomy Tubes in Ureteric Obstruction from Incurable Malignancy." International Journal of Clinical Practice 57 (April 2003): 180–0181.

ORGANIZATIONS

American Cancer Society. National Headquarters. 1599 Clifton Road NE, Atlanta, GA 30329. (800) ACS-2345. http://www.cancer.org.

American College of Radiology (ACR). 1891 Preston White Drive, Reston, VA 20191-4397. (800) 227-5463. http://www.acr.org.

American Urological Association (AUA). 1120 North Charles Street, Baltimore, MD 21201. (410) 727-1100. http://www.auanet.org.

United Ostomy Association (UOA). 19772 MacArthur Blvd., #200, Irvine, CA 92612-2405. (800) 826-0826. http://www.uoa.org.

OTHER

"Extracorporeal Shock Wave Lithotripsy (ESWL)." Family Practice Notebook May 28, 2003 [cited July 7, 2003]. http://www.fpnotebook.com/SUR46.htm.

"Nephrostomy." Mid-South Imaging and Therapeutics [cited July 7, 2003]. http://www.msit.com.

"Percutaneous Nephrostomy." WFUSM Division of Radiologic Sciences. May 8, 2003 [cited July 7, 2003]. http://www.rad.bgsm.edu/patienteduc/percutaneous_nephrostomy.htm.

Tish Davidson, AM
Monique Laberge, PhD

Neurosurgery

Definition

Neurosurgery is a specialized field of surgery for the treatment of diseases or conditions of the central nervous system (CNS) and spine.

Description

Neurosurgery is the specialized field of surgery that treats diseases that affect the CNS—the brain and the spine. A neurosurgeon is a medical doctor who has received extensive training in the surgical and medical management of neurological diseases. The field of neurosurgery is one of the most sophisticated surgical specialties and encompasses advanced surgical and imaging technology and new research in molecular neurosurgery and gene therapy. There are five general categories of neurosurgical diseases that are commonly managed by neurosurgeons: cerebrovascular (hemorrhage [bleeding] and aneurysms); traumatic head injury (THI, traumatic injury caused by accident); degeneration diseases of the spine; tumors in the CNS; functional neurosurgery; surgery for congenital abnormalities; and neurosurgical management of the CNS.

Cerebrovascular diseases that usually require surgery include spontaneous intracranial hemorrhage (bleeding within the skull), spontaneous subarachnoid hemorrhage (bleeding beneath the outer membranous covering of the brain), spontaneous intracerebral hemorrhage (bleeding within the brain), cerebral aneurysms (outpouchings of the blood vessel), hypertensive intracerebral hemorrhage (due to high blood pressure), and angiomatous malformations.

Brain hemorrhage

Spontaneous intracranial hemorrhage is a condition characterized by hemorrhage in the brain (hemorrhagic stroke) that results in a sudden onset of neurologically worsening symptoms (that include focal neurologic deficits and loss of consciousness). **CT scans** are helpful in identifying the intracranial hemorrhage, of which there are two types—subarachnoid hemorrhage and intracerebral hematoma.

The subarachnoid space is an area that exists between two layers of coverings (membranes) that wrap around the brain. A spontaneous subarachnoid hemorrhage is defined as blood (not caused by trauma), in the subarachnoid space. The amount of blood in the subarachnoid space can be a focal (small area) amount or a larger, more diffuse hemorrhage, which can be further complicated by having an intraventricular hemorrhage or intracerebral hematoma at the same time.

The incidence of subarachnoid hemorrhage is 10 per 100,000 persons per year; approximately 30% of Americans will sustain a subarachnoid hemorrhage annually. Smoking is a major factor in increasing the odds of sustaining a subarachnoid hemorrhage.

KEY TERMS

Angiomatous malformations—Tumors in blood vessels.

Cerebral aneurysms—A sac in a blood vessel in the brain that can rupture and cause bleeding in the brain.

Craniosynostosis—Premature closure of the skull, which results in skull deformities.

Craniotomy—Procedure to remove a lesion in the brain through an opening in the skull.

Desiccation—Tissue death.

Encephaloceles—Protrusion of the brain through a defect in the skull.

Germinoma—A tumor of germ cells (ovum and sperm cells that participate in production of the developing embryo).

Hydrocephalus—A defect characterized by an increase in cerebrospinal fluid (CSF), which bathes and nourishes the brain and spinal cord.

Intraventricular hemorrhage—Hemorrhage in the ventricles of the brain.

Lymphoma—A tumor of lymph glands or lymph tissues.

Meninges—Membranes that cover the brain.

Myelomeningoceles (MMC)—A protrusion in the vertebral column containing spinal cord and meninges.

Subarachnoid space—A space between membranes that covers and protects the brain.

Subarachnoid hemorrhage can affect adults of all ages, but usually peaks in the fourth and fifth decades of life. Approximately 60% of patients are female. Approximately 30% of subarachnoid hemorrhages occur during sleep.

The most frequent cause of spontaneous subarachnoid hemorrhage is rupture of an intracranial aneurysm. The symptoms of subarachnoid hemorrhage are a sudden onset of severe headache that worsens over time, nausea, loss of consciousness (with or without seizure), and vomiting. Depending on the severity of bleeding, additional symptoms can also include visual sensitivity to light (photophobia), a stiff neck, and minor (low-grade) fever. Symptoms occur before rupture of the aneurysm in 40% of patients, usually in those with a minor hemorrhage. These symptoms can also include headache or dizziness, and tend to go unnoticed.

After a subarachnoid hemorrhage, most patients are hypertensive (have high blood pressure) and experience changes in heart rate and rhythm. CT scans are the best diagnostic tool for subarachnoid hemorrhage. The hemorrhage can be visualized in the first 24 hours after onset in 90% of patients and in more than 50% in the first week. Spinal taps to sample the cerebrospinal fluid (CSF) may be required to evaluate some patients who have the potential to suffer a subarachnoid hemorrhage. This procedure involves the insertion of a thin needle between the lumbar vertebral bodies (L–4 and L–5) to allow the removal of a small amount of fluid to look for either red or white blood cells (WBCs). Once the aneurysm has been identified, the patient is taken for surgery. A **craniotomy** is performed using microsurgical techniques. The operative microscope helps to identify the aneurysm, which is then clipped. Berry, or congenital aneurysm, is the reason for over half of all cases of spontaneous subarachnoid hemorrhage.

A spontaneous intracerebral hemorrhage (or hematoma) (SICH) is a blood clot in brain tissue that can arise abruptly and is strongly correlated with hypertension. There are approximately 40,000 new cases of SICH in the United States annually. Stroke is the third leading cause of **death** in the United States, and SICH accounts for 10% of all stroke cases. Advancing age is a major predisposing factor for SICH: The incidence of SICH is two per 1,000 persons per year by age 45, and rises to 350 per 100,000 persons per year in those aged 80 years or more. Hypertensive intracerebral hemorrhage can occur in different areas within the brain. Damage to some areas may be associated with a very high death rate. Treatment includes comprehensive ICU (**intensive care unit**) management of hypertension and maintenance of adequate cerebral perfusion (oxygenated blood going to the brain).

Accidental head injury is a major public health problem. Trauma causes approximately 150,000 deaths annually in the United States; approximately half of these deaths were caused by fatal head trauma. Additionally, there are 10,000 new spinal cord injuries annually. The cost of disability (e.g., chronic long-term care, lost wages, and work) is very high. Approximately 200,000 persons in the United States are living with disabilities associated with head and spinal cord trauma.

Severe head injury is defined as an injury that produces coma (patient will not open eyes even to painful stimulus; incapable of following simple commands; and inability to utter words). These clinical criteria are defined on the well-established Glasgow Coma Scale (GCS). A **physical examination** and neurologic assessment by a neurosurgeon and brain scan imaging (CT scan) are necessary for the initial evaluation. Additionally, a special catheter to monitor intracranial pressure (due to brain swelling) is necessary. A blood clot larger than 25 to 30 cubic centimeters is considered clinically large enough to cause progressive brain injury.

Tumors inside the brain (intracranial tumors) are typically of two types, primary and secondary intracranial tumors. Primary intracranial tumors (PICT) rarely metastasize and usually originate in the brain, coverings (membranes) of the brain, or the pituitary gland. The incidence of primary intracranial tumors is 11.5 per 100,000, or approximately 35,000 persons per year.

Secondary intracranial tumors arise from outside the brain coverings (meninges). Quite commonly, secondary intracranial tumors are bloodborne metastatic disease from primary malignant cancer outside the brain (i.e., cancer from some other location that has spread to the brain). Approximately 250,000 persons per year are affected by secondary intracranial tumors. A tumor in the brain can cause increased intracranial pressure, or cause symptoms associated with localized compression of the brain (i.e., a tumor grows and compresses part of the brain against the skull). One common cause of increased intracranial pressure is growth of a tumor that obstructs the duct system of cerebrospinal fluid (CSF), which bathes and nourishes the brain and spinal cord. Common symptoms can include nausea, vomiting, headache that is worse in the morning, and a reduced level of consciousness that causes drowsiness. Tumors causing focal compression on or irritation of the brain usually result in loss of neurologic function. This progressive loss of neurologic function can manifest as tinnitus (ringing in the ears) or aphasia (language problems).

Technical advancement has made surgical removal of brain tumors more effective and safer. Surgical management of intracranial tumors focuses on diagnosis and reduction of tumor mass. Depending on tumor location and patient health status, the neurosurgeon may perform a needle biopsy (called image-directed stereotactic needle biopsy) or a craniotomy to extract a piece of tumor for pathologic analysis. If the tumor is located in an area where surgery can be performed, the neurosurgeon generally will remove the mass if the patient can tolerate **general anesthesia**. Exceptions to a surgical option may be exercised to treat malignant tumors that are very sensitive to chemotherapy or radiation therapy (i.e., to manage lymphoma or germinoma). One of the most common types of tumors is the glioma, which accounts for 50% of all primary brain tumors.

Degenerative disorders of the spine

Degenerative disorders of the spine are a common problem. Between 50% and 90% of the population will experience back pain at some point in their lifetime. Most of these symptoms subside on their own within a few weeks; the cost, however, is realized in decreased productivity and lost wages—a public health problem. Pain in the lumbar spine is the most common reason adults seek medical attention. The lumbar spine comprises five lumbar vertebra and supports the weight of the entire vertebral column and head. Lower back disorders are among the most frequent reasons for referral to a neurosurgeon. Lumbar discs are prone to herniation and desiccation (drying out) as a result of the heavy load they bear and the motion to which they are subject. Nerves that run from the vertebrae extend out to distant body parts, and degeneration of the discs may change bony structures in such a manner that can cause nerve compression. Typically, patients with degenerative disorders of the spine may experience pain, numbness, paresthesia (tingling), and restriction of neck movement (if the affected vertebra is in the cervical spine, which is located in the back of the neck).

Surgery for congenital abnormalities

Congenital abnormalities arise during embryonic development. Important changes in growth and chemistry occur during the second week of human gestation; these changes contribute to the development of the nervous system. Several different types of cells proliferate as they move together or separate into other structures according to an orchestrated, natural timeline. Defects can occur at different stages of development. Among the defects with which infants can be born include myelomeningoceles, encephaloceles, hydrocephalus, and craniosynostosis.

Central nervous system infections

Solitary or multiple brain abscesses can occur as a result of infection in the brain. Patients present with clinical symptoms such as focal (a specific area is affected) neurologic signs, seizures, altered mental status, and increased intracranial pressure. CT scans and **magnetic resonance imaging** (MRI) are helpful for identification of brain abscesses. Surgery is usually indicated if the abscess fails to resolve or worsens following antibiotic treatment, or if there are signs of mass effect and brain herniation. Although rare, a spinal epidural abscess can occur. Typically, bacteria can spread in patients who have acute bacterial meningitis (infection of the subarachnoid spaces and meninges). The specific type of bacteria varies according to the patient's age.

WHO PERFORMS THE PROCEDURE AND WHERE IS IT PERFORMED?

A neurosurgeon performs the procedure in a major hospital. The neurosurgeon is a medical doctor who has obtained two years of general surgery training, plus an additional five years of training in neurosurgery.

QUESTIONS TO ASK THE DOCTOR

- What the potential side effects that can arise as a result of surgery?
- How likely are complications to develop?
- How long will recovery take?
- Will I undergo rehabilitation, and if so, for how long?

Functional neurosurgery

Functional neurosurgery is a special type of surgical procedure used to manage movement disorder, epilepsy, and pain. Stereotactic neurosurgery makes use of a coordinate system that provides accurate navigation to a specific point or region in the brain. This is usually done by placing and fixing into position a frame on the scalp (using four threaded pins that penetrate the outer skull to stabilize the frame in position) under **local anesthesia**. A special box and sterotactic arc are placed to precisely determine X, Y, and Z coordinates of any point within the frame.

Epilepsy surgery

Approximately 70 per 100,000 population in the United States takes antiepileptic medications for seizure disorders. The risk of developing epilepsy over a lifetime is 3%, and there are 100,000 new cases per year. The majority of cases (approximately 60,000) are epilepsy of the temporal lobe (the brain lobes located on the sides of the head). Approximately 25% of temporal lobe seizure patients who are prescribed antiepileptic drugs continue to have seizures that are not controlled or that can be controlled, but the side effects of the medication outweigh the therapeutic benefits. Approximately 5,000 new cases per year require epilepsy surgery (partial **anterior temporal lobectomy**). The patient and neurosurgeon should consider surgery if continued seizures cause injuries due to repeated falls; driving restrictions; limitation of social interactions; problems related to education and learning; and employment limitations.

The future of neurosurgery

Neurosurgery as a field is faced with many new opportunities and challenges, based on advanced technological approaches and molecular approaches to neurosurgical problems. Advances in technology have allowed the neurosurgeon to precisely locate abnormal tissue in the brain and spinal cord, thereby preserving normal tissues from surgical trauma. In addition to cardiovascular neurosurgery, functional neurosurgery, neuro-oncologic neurosurgery (surgical removal of brain tumors), and spinal surgery, the future holds many new research innovations. In the new millennium, the field of molecular neurosurgery can make it possible to introduce genetic material into nerve cells and to redirect protein synthesis—to work toward reversing the disease process, in general.

Resources

BOOKS
Goetz, CG. Goetz's Textbook of Clinical Neurology. 3rd ed. Philadelphia: Saunders, 2007.
Khatri, VP and JA Asensio. Operative Surgery Manual. 1st ed. Philadelphia: Saunders, 2003.
Townsend, CM et al. Sabiston Textbook of Surgery. 17th ed. Philadelphia: Saunders, 2004.

PERIODICALS
Freese, A., Simeone, F. "Ocular Surgery for the New Millennium." and "Treatment of Neurosurgical Disease in the New Millennium." Ophthalmology Clinics of North America 12, no. 4 (December 1999).

ORGANIZATIONS
The American Board of Neurological Surgery. 6550 Fannin Street, Suite 2139 Houston, TX 77030. (713) 441-6015. http://www.abns.org.

Laith Farid Gulli, M.D., M.S.
Miguel A. Melgar, M.D.,Ph.D.
Nicole Mallory, M.S.,PA-C

Nissen fundoplication *see* **Gastroesophageal reflux surgery**

Nitrite test *see* **Urinalysis**

NMR *see* **Magnetic resonance imaging**

Nonmelanoma skin cancer surgery *see* **Curettage and electrosurgery**

Nonsteroidal anti-inflammatory drugs

Definition

Nonsteroidal anti-inflammatory drugs (NSAIDs) are medications other than **corticosteroids** that relieve pain, swelling, stiffness, fever, and inflammation. The most commonly used NSAIDs, including **aspirin**, ibuprofen, and naproxen, are available as over-the-counter (OTC) preparations; most, however, are prescription drugs. The use of NSAIDs for inflammation and low-grade pain is steadily increasing; in the early 2000s, these drugs accounted for 70 million prescriptions and 30 billion OTC purchases every year in the United States alone. They are one of the oldest classes of pain relievers, aspirin having been introduced for human use in 1829. One important reason why NSAIDs are so widely prescribed and recommended is that they have a very low rate of addiction.

Purpose

Nonsteroidal anti-inflammatory drugs are prescribed for a variety of painful conditions, including arthritis, bursitis, tendinitis, gout, menstrual cramps, sprains, strains, and other injuries. They may be used for treatment of postsurgical pain that is either too mild to require narcotic **analgesics** or follows a period of use of stronger analgesics. Ketorolac (Toradol) may be used in place of narcotics for treatment of acute pain in patients who should not receive narcotics.

Description

The nonsteroidal anti-inflammatory drugs are a group of agents that inhibit prostaglandin synthetase, thereby reducing the process of inflammation. As a group, they are all effective analgesics. Some, including the salicylates, ibuprofen, and naproxen, are also useful antipyretics (fever-reducers).

Although NSAIDs fall into discrete chemical classes, they are usually divided into the nonselective NSAIDs and the COX-2 specific agents. Among the nonspecific NSAIDs are diclofenac (Voltaren), etodolac (Lodine), flurbiprofen (Ansaid), ibuprofen (Motrin, Advil, Rufen), ketoprofen (Orudis), ketorolac (Toradol), nabumetone (Relafen), naproxen (Naprosyn), naproxen sodium (Aleve, Anaprox, Naprelan), and oxaprozin (Daypro). The only COX-2 specific drug remaining on the market in the United States as of 2007 is celecoxib (Celebrex); four other drugs in this class were withdrawn in the United States in 2004 because of reports that they increased patients' risks

KEY TERMS

Ankylosing spondylitis—An autoimmune disorder of the joints in the spinal column, usually marked by pain and stiffness in the lower part of the spine.

Antipyretic—A medication that lowers fever.

Bursitis—Inflammation of the tissue around a joint.

Inflammation—Pain, redness, swelling, and heat that usually develop in response to injury or illness.

Metabolites—The chemicals produced in the body after nutrients, drugs, enzymes or other materials have been changed (metabolized).

Salicylates—A group of drugs that includes aspirin and related compounds; used to relieve pain, reduce inflammation, and lower fever.

Tendinitis—Inflammation of a tendon—a tough band of tissue that connects muscle to bone.

of heart attack and stroke, and a fifth in Australia in 2007 because of reports of increased risk of liver failure.

Nonselective NSAIDS inhibit both cyclooxygenase 1 and cyclooxygenase 2 (COX-2). Cyclooxygenase 1 is important for such body processes as platelet aggregation, the regulation of blood flow in the kidney and stomach, and the regulation of gastric acid secretion. The inhibition of cyclooxygenase 1 is considered the primary cause of NSAID toxicity, including gastric ulceration and bleeding disorders. COX-2 is the primary cause of pain and inflammation. Celecoxib is a relatively selective COX-2 agent; it may cause the same adverse effects as the nonselective drugs, although with somewhat reduced frequency.

The analgesic activity of NSAIDs has not been fully explained. Antipyretic activity may be caused by the inhibition of prostaglandin E2 (PGE2) synthesis.

Although not all NSAIDs have approved indications for all uses, as a class, they are used for:

- ankylosing spondylitis
- bursitis
- dental pain
- fever
- gout
- headache
- juvenile arthritis
- pain from metastatic bone cancer
- mild-to-moderate postoperative pain
- osteoarthritis

- premenstrual syndrome (PMS)
- primary dysmenorrhea (painful menstrual periods)
- renal colic
- rheumatoid arthritis
- tendinitis

As of the early 2000s, NSAIDs have been studied for their potential effectiveness in lowering the risk of certain types of cancer, particularly colon, prostate, and ovarian cancers. More research needs to be done, however, to confirm the drugs' ability to protect against cancer.

Recommended dosage

Recommended doses vary, depending on the patient, the type of nonsteroidal anti-inflammatory drug prescribed, the condition for which the drug is prescribed, and the form in which it is used. The patient is advised to consult specific sources for detailed information or ask a physician.

Precautions

The most common hazard associated with NSAID use is gastrointestinal intolerance and ulceration. This may occur without warning and is a greater risk among patients over the age of 65. The risk appears to rise with increasing length of treatment and increasing dose. Patients should be aware of the warning signs of gastrointestinal (GI) bleeding.

Allergic reactions are rare, but may be severe. Patients who have allergic reactions to aspirin should not be treated with NSAIDs.

Because NSAID metabolites are eliminated by the kidney, renal toxicity should be considered. Clinicians should monitor kidney function before and during NSAID use.

Among the NSAIDs that are classed as pregnancy category B are ketoprofen, naproxen, naproxen sodium, flurbiprofen, and diclofenac. Category C NSAIDs include Etodolac, ketorolac, mefenamic acid, meloxicam, nabumetone, oxaprozin, tolmetin, piroxicam, and celecoxib. Breastfeeding is not advised while taking NSAIDs.

Many other rare but potentially serious adverse effects have been reported with NSAIDs. The consumer should consult specific references.

Interactions

Many drug interactions have been reported with NSAID therapy. The most serious are those that may affect the bleeding hazards associated with NSAIDs. Consumers are advised to consult specific references for further information. A partial list of interacting drugs includes:

- blood-thinning drugs such as warfarin (Coumadin)
- other nonsteroidal anti-inflammatory drugs
- heparin
- tetracycline antibiotics
- cyclosporine
- digitalis drugs
- lithium
- methotrexate
- phenytoin (Dilantin)
- zidovudine (AZT, Retrovir)

Resources

BOOKS

AHFS: Drug Information. Washington, DC: American Society of Healthsystems Pharmacy, 2002.

Howardell, Maynard J. *Trends in COX-2 Inhibitor Research.* New York: Nova Science Publishers, 2006.

Karch, A. M. *Lippincott's Nursing Drug Guide.* Springhouse, PA: Lippincott Williams & Wilkins, 2003.

McCleane, Gary, and Howard Smith, eds. *Clinical Management of Bone and Joint Pain.* New York: Haworth Medical Press, 2007.

Neal, Michael J. *Medical Pharmacology at a Glance*, 5th ed. Malden, MA: Blackwell Publishing, 2005.

PERIODICALS

Barron, M. C., and B. R. Rubin. "Managing Osteoarthritic Knee Pain." *Journal of the American Osteopathic Association* 107 (November 2007): ES21–ES27.

Funk, C. D., and G. A. Fitzgerald. "COX-2 Inhibitors and Cardiovascular Risk." *Journal of Cardiovascular Pharmacology* 50 (November 2007): 470–479.

Green, G. A. "Understanding NSAIDs: From Aspirin to COX-2." *Clinical Cornerstone* 3 (May 2001): 50–60.

Slattery, M. L., W. Samowitz, M. Hoffman, et al. "Aspirin, NSAIDs, and Colorectal Cancer: Possible Involvement in an Insulin-Related Pathway." *Cancer Epidemiology, Biomarkers and Prevention* 13 (April 2004): 538–545.

Stock, D., P. A. Groome, and D. R. Siemens. "Inflammation and Prostate Cancer: A Future Target for Prevention and Therapy?" *Urologic Clinics of North America* 35 (February 2008): 117–130.

ORGANIZATIONS

U.S. Food and Drug Administration (FDA). 5600 Fishers Lane, Rockville, MD 20857-0001. (888) INFO-FDA (1-888-463-6332). http://www.fda.gov/ (accessed April 1, 2008).

U.S. Pharmacopoeia (USP). 12601 Twinbrook Parkway, Rockville, MD 20852–1790. (800) 227–8772. http://www.usp.org/ (accessed April 1, 2008).

Samuel D. Uretsky, PharmD
Rebecca Frey, PhD

Norepinephrine *see* **Adrenergic drugs**

Nose job *see* **Rhinoplasty**

Nosocomial infections *see* **Hospital-acquired infections**

NSAIDs *see* **Nonsteroidal anti-inflammatory drugs**

Nuclear magnetic resonance *see* **Magnetic resonance imaging**

Nursing homes

Definition

A nursing home is a long-term care facility licensed by the state that offers 24-hour room and board and health care services, including basic and skilled nursing care, rehabilitation, and a full range of other therapies, treatments, and programs. Other names for nursing homes are skilled nursing facilities (SNFs) and skilled nursing units (SNUs). There were about 16,100 nursing homes in the United States as of 2005. People who live in nursing homes are referred to as residents.

Description

Slightly over 5% of people 65 years and older occupy nursing homes, congregate housing, assisted living communities, and board-and-care homes. At any given time, approximately 4% of the population of the United States is in nursing homes with the rate of nursing home use increasing with age from 1.4% of the young-old to 24.5% of the oldest-old. Some SNFs accept younger adults (anyone over the age of 18) who need physical or occupational therapy following an

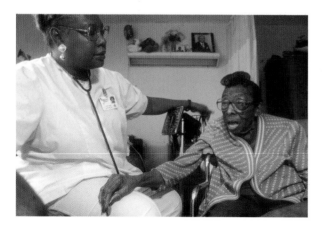

(Jim West/Alamy)

accident or illness. Nearly 50% of those 95 years old and older live in nursing homes. Nursing homes must meet the physical, emotional, and social needs of its residents.

Required care plans

There are federal laws regarding the care given in a nursing home, and it is essential that staff members become aware of these regulations. Staff members are required to conduct a thorough assessment of each new resident during the first two weeks following admission. The assessment includes the resident's ability to move, his or her rehabilitation needs, the status of the skin, any medical conditions that are present, nutritional state, and abilities regarding activities of daily living.

In some cases, the nursing home residents are unable to communicate their needs to the staff. Therefore, it is particularly important for nurses and other professionals to look for problems during their assessments. Signs of malnutrition and dehydration are especially important when assessing nursing home residents.

It is not normal for an elderly person to lose weight. However, some people lose their ability to taste and smell as they age and may lose interest in food. This can result in malnutrition, which can lead to confusion and impaired ability to fight off disease.

Older people are also more susceptible to dehydration. Their medications may lead to dehydration as a side effect, or they may limit fluids because they are too afraid of uncontrolled urination. It is very dangerous to be without adequate fluid, so the nurse and other staff must be able to recognize early signs of dehydration.

When the assessment is complete, a care plan is developed. This plan is subject to change as changes in the resident's condition occur.

Nursing homes are often the only alternative for patients who require nursing care over an extended period of time. Such persons are too ill to remain at home, with families, or in less structured long-term facilities. These individuals are unable to live independently and need assistance with activities of daily living (ADLs). Some nursing homes offer specialized care for certain medical conditions such as Alzheimer's disease.

Commonly, nursing home residents are no longer able to participate in the activities they once enjoyed. However, it is required by law that these facilities help residents achieve their highest possible quality of life.

KEY TERMS

Activities of daily living (ADLs)—Self-care activities performed during the course of a normal day such as eating, bathing, dressing, toileting, etc.

Assisted living—A type of facility for people who are not able to live independently but do not require the level of skilled nursing provided by a nursing home.

Congregate housing—A type of housing arrangement for seniors that offers independent living in separate apartments as well as opportunities to share activities of daily living with other residents. Congregate housing does not usually involve assisted living or skilled nursing care, however.

Culture change—A term that refers to a movement in the United States to make nursing homes more resident-centered and less like hospitals.

Long-term care—Residential care over a period of time. A nursing home is a type of long-term care facility that offers nursing care and assistance with daily living tasks.

Medicaid—The federally funded program in the United States for state-operated programs that provide medical assistance to permanently disabled patients and to low-income people. Medicaid is the medical assistance provided in Title XIX of the Social Security Act.

Medicare—The federally-funded national health insurance program, provided for by Title XVIII of the Social Security Act in the United States for all people over the age of 65.

Restraint—A physical device or a medication designed to restrict a person's movement.

Skilled nursing facility (SNF)—Another name for a nursing home.

It is important for residents to have as much control as possible over their everyday lives. Laws and regulations exist to raise nursing home quality of life and care standards.

By law, nursing homes cannot use chemical or physical restraints unless they are essential for treating a medical problem. There are many dangers associated with the use of restraints, including the chance of a fall if a resident tries to walk while restrained. The devices may also lead to depression and decreased self-esteem. A doctor's order is necessary before restraints can be used in a nursing home.

Licensing

The Joint Commission (formerly the Joint Commission on the Accreditation of Health Care Organizations) offers accreditation to nursing homes through the Long Term Care Accreditation Program established in 1966. This group helps nursing homes improve their quality of care. The commission periodically surveys nursing homes to check on quality issues.

A nursing home may be certified by **Medicare** or **Medicaid** if it meets the criteria of these organizations; 98.5% of nursing homes in the United States were certified to participate in one or both programs as of 2005. Families should be informed of the certifications a nursing home holds. Medicare and Medicaid are the main sources of financial income for nursing homes in the United States.

The state in which a nursing home is located conducts inspections every nine to 15 months. Fines and other penalties may be enforced if the inspection reveals areas where the nursing home does not meet requirements set by that state and the federal government. Problem areas are noted in terms of scope and severity. The scope of a problem is how widespread it is, and the severity is the seriousness of its impact on the residents. When a nursing home receives an inspection report, it must post it in a place where it can be easily seen by residents and their guests.

Contract

When a resident checks into a nursing home, a contract is drawn up between the patient and the facility. This document includes information regarding the rights of the residents. It also provides details regarding services provided and discharge policies.

Resident decision-making

Decisions are made by each nursing home resident unless he or she has signed an advanced directive giving this authority to someone else. In order for health care decisions to be made by another person, the resident must have signed a document called a durable **power of attorney** for health care.

Costs

Nursing **home care** is costly. The rate normally includes room and board, housekeeping, bedding, nursing care, activities, and some personal items. Additional fees may be charged for haircuts, telephones, and other personal items.

Medicare covers the cost of some nursing home services, such as skilled nursing or rehabilitative care.

This payment may be activated when the nursing home care is provided after a Medicare qualifying stay in the hospital for at least three days. It is common for nursing homes to have only a few beds available for Medicare or Medicaid residents. Residents relying solely on these types of coverage must wait for a Medicare or Medicaid bed to become available.

Medicare supplemental insurance, such as Medigap, assists with the payment of nursing home expenses that are not covered by Medicare.

Medicaid qualifications vary in each state. Families of potential residents should check with their state government to determine coverage options. According to a federal law, a nursing home that drops out of the Medicaid program cannot evict current residents whose care is supported by Medicaid.

Private insurance, such as long-term insurance, may cover costs associated with a nursing home. People may enroll in these plans through their employers or other group insurance policies.

In many cases, nursing homes are paid for by the residents' personal funds. When these funds are exhausted, the residents sometimes become eligible for Medicaid assistance.

Patients' rights

It is important for the professionals working in nursing homes to be aware of the residents' rights. Residents are informed of their rights when they are admitted. Residents have the right to:

- manage their finances
- privacy (for themselves and their belongings)
- make decisions (unless advanced directives or durable power of attorney exist)
- see visitors in private
- receive information regarding their medical care and treatments
- have social services
- leave the nursing home after giving the required amount of notice (A stay in a nursing home is normally considered voluntary; however, the facility will consider a variety of factors before discharging a resident. These factors include the resident's health, safety, and potential danger to self or others, as well as the resident's payment for services. The contract will state how much notice is required before a resident may transfer to another facility, return home, or move in with a family member.)

Family involvement

In some cases, a nursing home is chosen after the family has only a short time to prepare for the change. For example, when a patient is unable to care for himself or herself due to a sudden illness or injury, the family must turn to nursing home care without having the luxury of researching this option over time. The nursing home's costs must be explained to the resident or family prior to admission. It is important for the nursing home staff to be willing to answer the family's questions and reassure them about the care their loved one will receive. To help with choosing a nursing home, Medicare has set up a Nursing Home Compare website at <http://www.medicare.gov/NHCompare/> that allows users to search by geography, proximity, the name of the nursing home, or special focus.

Nursing home professionals have an opportunity to continue to work closely with the resident's family and loved ones over the course of a resident's stay. In these facilities, concerned family members and friends of the resident are involved in his or her care, and may have guardianship or other decision-making responsibility. These individuals may voice their concerns through meetings between staff and family members. Those with legal guardianship are entitled to see a resident's medical records, care plans, and other related material.

Communication

As in other health care settings, communication among nursing home staff is very important. In nursing homes, the care is based on a team approach. Physicians, nurses, and allied health professionals work together to make sure the resident is able to experience the highest quality of life possible.

In many cases, physicians who have had a long-term relationship with a patient continue treatment after the patient has been admitted to a nursing home. It is important for the nursing home staff to leave blocks of time open in the schedule for physician visits. It is also the staff's duty to keep the personal physicians apprised of a resident's medical condition.

The resident, physician, and resident's legal guardian and family must be told immediately if any of the following situations arise: an accident involving the resident, the need for a major treatment change, and a decision regarding discharge or transfer. Unless an emergency arises, the nursing home must give 30 days written notice of discharge or transfer. The family may appeal the decision.

Culture change

Culture change refers to a movement to transform nursing homes into more homelike and less hospital-like communities. Spearheaded by groups like LIFESPAN, the Eden Alternative, and the Green House Project, people involved in changing nursing homes formed the Pioneer Network in 2000. The network advocates giving elders as much choice and self-determination as possible, including more opportunities for human companionship and keeping pets. As of 2004, nine states (Colorado, Florida, Illinois, Michigan, New Jersey, North Carolina, Pennsylvania, South Carolina, and Washington) had formed culture change coalitions.

The Pioneer Network drew up a list of values and principles that has been adopted by the NCCNHR (formerly the National Citizens' Coalition for Nursing Home Reform and other groups:

- Know each person.
- Each person can and does make a difference.
- Relationship is the fundamental building block of a transformed culture.
- Respond to spirit, as well as mind and body.
- Risk taking is a normal part of life.
- Put person before task.
- All elders are entitled to self-determination wherever they live.
- Community is the antidote to institutionalization.
- Do unto others as you would have them do unto you—yes, the Golden Rule.
- Promote the growth and development of all.
- Shape and use the potential of the environment in all its aspects: physical, organizational, psycho/social/spiritual.
- Practice self-examination, searching for new creativity and opportunities for doing better.
- Recognize that culture change and transformation are not destinations but a journey, always a work in progress.

Results

The quality of care in nursing homes is an important issue. Quality issues include:

- Ratios of staff to patients. Advocacy groups are pushing for increased staff-to-patient ratios in nursing homes.) The NCCNHR recommends one direct care staff member (R.N., L.V.N., or C.N.A.) per five residents during the day shift, per 10 residents during the evening shift, and per 15 residents during the night shift.
- Elder abuse. It is important for nursing home personnel to look for signs of abuse or neglect when a

---

WHO PERFORMS THE PROCEDURE AND WHERE IS IT PERFORMED?

The nursing home staff may include an administrator, medical director, director of nursing, and directors for other allied health services. It is important for nursing home staff to understand the policies regarding care in these types of facilities.

The following professionals may provide care and treatments in nursing homes:

- physicians, including psychiatrists
- nurses
- nursing assistants
- dietitians
- physical, occupational, and speech therapists
- pharmacists
- social activities staff
- dentists
- social workers or psychological counselors
- chaplains
- such other staff as custodians and office personnel

---

resident checks in and during a resident's stay. Signs of abuse include bodily injuries that appear suspicious, visible harm to the wrist or ankles that may indicate the use of restraints, skin ulcers that seem neglected, poor hygiene, inadequate nutrition, unexplained dehydration, untreated medical problems, or such personality disorders as excessive nervousness or withdrawal. The nurse or allied health professional is to report any signs of abuse to the supervisor or physician.

- Reimbursement. Nursing home administrators report that reimbursements do not cover the expenses, while nursing home advocates would like a higher portion of revenues to be allocated for direct patient care.

Resources

BOOKS

Baker, Beth. *Old Age in a New Age: The Promise of Transformative Nursing Homes.* Nashville, TN: Vanderbilt University Press, 2007.

Birkett, D. Peter, M.D., ed. *Psychiatry in the Nursing Home.* 2nd Edition. Binghamton, NY: Haworth Press Inc, 2001.

Chapman, Reynolds C. *Nursing Homes from A to Z: A Guide Designed to Educate Residents and Family*

Members in Navigating the Complex Environment of a Nursing Home. New York: iUniverse, 2007.

Frolik, Lawrence A. Residence Options for Older and Disabled Clients. Chicago: American Bar Association, 2008.

Weiner, Audrey S., and Judah L. Ronch, eds. Culture Change in Long-Term Care. New York: Haworth Social Work Practice Press, 2003.

PERIODICALS

Feng, Z., D. C. Grabowski, O. Intrator, et al. "Medicaid Payment Rates, Case-Mix Reimbursement, and Nursing Home Staffing-1996-2004." Medical Care 46 (January 2008): 33–40.

Labossiere, R., and M. A. Bernard. "Nutritional Considerations in Institutionalized Elders." Current Opinion in Clinical Nutrition and Metabolic Care 11 (January 2008): 1–6.

Marx, T. L. "Partnering with Hospice to Improve Pain Management in the Nursing Home Setting." Journal of the American Osteopathic Association 105 (March 2005): S22–S26.

Reuben, D. B. "Better Care for Older People with Chronic Diseases: An Emerging Vision." Journal of the American Medical Association 298 (December 12, 2007): 2673–2674.

Robinson, S. B., and R. B. Rosher. "Tangling with the Barriers to Culture Change: Creating a Resident-Centered Nursing Home Environment." Journal of Gerontological Nursing 32 (October 2006): 19–25.

Winningham, R. G., and N. L. Pike. "A Cognitive Intervention to Enhance Institutionalized Older Adults' Social Support Networks and Decrease Loneliness." Aging and Mental Health 11 (November 2007): 716–721.

ORGANIZATIONS

American Nurses Association. 8515 Georgia Avenue, Suite 400, Silver Spring, MD 20910-3492. (800) 274-4ANA or (301) 628-5000. http://www.nursingworld.org.

Centers for Medicare & Medicaid Services (CMS). 7500 Security Boulevard, Baltimore, MD 21244-1850. (800) 633-4227. < http://www.cms.hhs.gov/>.

e-Healthcare Solutions, Inc., 953 Route 202 North, Branchburg, N.J. 08876. (908) 203-1350. Fax: (908) 203-1307. info@e-healthcaresolutions.com. http://www.digitalhealthcare.com/.

Joint Commission. One Renaissance Blvd., Oakbrook Terrace, IL 60181. (630) 792-5000. http://www.jointcommission.org.

National Center for Health Statistics (NCHS). 3311 Toledo Road, Hyattsville, MD 20782. (800) 232-4636. < http://www.cdc.gov/nchs/.

NCCNHR (formerly the National Citizens' Coalition for Nursing Home Reform). 1828 L Street, NW, Suite 801, Washington, DC 20036. (202) 332-2275. <www.nccnhr.org>.

Pioneer Network. P.O. Box 18648, Rochester, NY 14618. (585) 271-7570. < http://www.pioneernetwork.net/>.

U.S. Department of Health and Human Services. 200 Independence Avenue, S.W., Washington, DC 20201. (202) 619-0257. (877) 696-6775. < http://www.dhhs.gov/>.

OTHER

Coates, Karen J. Senior Class. May 2002 [cited March 1, 2003]. http://www.nurseweek.com/news/features/02-05/senior.asp.

NCCNHR. A Consumer Guide to Choosing a Nursing Home. Washington, DC: NCCNHR, 2007. Available online in PDF format at < http://nccnhr.newc.com/uploads/NhConsumerGuide.pdf>.

Rhonda Cloos, R.N.
Crystal H. Kaczkowski, M.Sc.
Rebecca Frey, Ph.D.

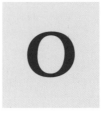

O

Obstetric and gynecologic surgery

Definition

Obstetric and gynecologic surgery refers to procedures that are performed to treat a variety of conditions affecting the female reproductive organs. The main structures of the reproductive system are the vagina, the uterus, the ovaries, and the fallopian tubes.

Description

Obstetrics is the branch of medicine that focuses on women during pregnancy, childbirth, and the postpartum period. Gynecology is a broader field, focusing on the general health care of women and treating conditions that affect the female reproductive organs. Medical doctors who choose to specialize in obstetrics and gynecology must undergo at least four years of post-medical school training (called a residency) in the areas of women's general health, pregnancy, labor and delivery, preconceptional and postpartum care, prenatal testing, and genetics. Obstetrician-gynecologists (also called OB-GYNs) may also subspecialize in the areas of gynecologic oncology (the treatment of cancers that affect the reproductive system), maternal-fetal medicine (the care of high-risk pregnancies), reproductive endocrinology and infertility (the study and treatment of the reproductive glands and hormones and the causes of infertility), and urogynecology (treatment of urinary tract and pelvic disorders).

Surgical procedures

There are a wide range of surgical procedures that have been developed to treat the various conditions that affect the female reproductive organs.

THE VAGINA. The vagina is the muscular canal that extends from the opening of the vulva (the external female genitals) to the cervix, the lower part of the uterus. The vagina is the outlet for menstrual blood and is also where the penis is inserted during sexual intercourse.

Some common surgical procedures that are performed on the vagina include:

- Episiotomy. A surgical incision made in the perineum (the area between the vagina and anus) to expand the opening of the vagina to prevent tearing during delivery.

- Colporrhaphy. Surgical repair of the vagina may be necessary after childbirth, sexual assault, or other injuries.

- Colpotomy. This incision into the wall of the vagina may be used to excise ovarian cysts, perform tubal ligation, or remove uterine fibroids.

- Egg Retrieval. This is a procedure used to extract the eggs from the ovaries prior to in vitro fertilization. A needle is placed through the vaginal wall to extract the eggs from the ovaries under ultrasound guidance.

- Colposcopy. A colposcope is a specialized instrument used to visualize the vagina and cervix, to diagnose abnormalities, or to test for the presence of precancerous or cancerous cells.

THE UTERUS. The uterus is the hollow, muscular organ at the top of the vagina. The cervix is the neck-shaped opening at the lower part of the uterus, while the fundus is the rounded upper portion. The endometrium is the inner lining of the uterus; it is where a fertilized egg will implant during the early days of pregnancy. The endometrium normally sheds during each menstrual cycle if the egg released during ovulation has not been fertilized. The myometrium is the middle muscular layer of the uterus; it is the myometrium that rhythmically contracts during labor contractions.

Some common surgical procedures that are performed on the uterus include:

KEY TERMS

Ectopic pregnancy—A pregnancy that occurs outside of the uterus, most often in the fallopian tubes.

Endometriosis—A condition in which the endometrium (lining of the uterus) grows outside of the uterus.

Ovarian cysts—Fluid-filled cavities on the surface of the ovary that may cause pain and bleeding if they become too large.

Uterine fibroids—Also called leiomyomas; benign growths in the smooth muscle of the uterus.

Uterine prolapse—A condition which the uterus descends into or beyond the vagina.

- Myomectomy. A procedure in which myomas (uterine fibroids) are surgically removed from the uterus.

- **Cesarean section**. A surgical procedure in which incisions are made through the woman's abdomen and uterus to deliver her baby.

- Cervical cerclage. The cervix is stitched closed to prevent a miscarriage or premature birth.

- Cervical cryosurgery. Cryosurgery freezes and destroys an area of the cervix in which precancerous cells have been found.

- Induced abortion. The intentional termination of a pregnancy before the fetus can live independently.

- Hysterectomy. The removal of part or all of the uterus may be done to treat uterine cancer, fibroid tumors, endometriosis, uterine prolapse, or other conditions of the uterus.

- Hysterotomy. This incision into the uterus is done during a cesarean section, open fetal surgery, and some second-trimester abortions.

- Dilatation and curettage. D&C is a gynecological procedure in which the cervix is dilated (expanded) and the lining of the uterus (endometrium) is scraped away.

THE OVARIES. The ovaries are egg-shaped structures located to each side of the uterus. It is within the ovaries that the female egg develops. A mature egg is released from one of the ovaries approximately every 28 days during a process called ovulation.

The surgical procedures that are performed on the ovaries include:

- Oophorectomy. One or both ovaries may be removed during this procedure to prevent or treat ovarian or other cancers, to remove large ovarian cysts, or to treat endometriosis.

- Cystectomy. An ovarian cystectomy may be used to remove part of an ovary to treat ovarian tumors or cysts.

THE FALLOPIAN TUBES. The fallopian tubes are the structures that carry a mature egg from the ovaries to the uterus. These tubes, which are about 4 in (10 cm) long and 0.2 in (0.5 cm) in diameter, are found on the upper outer sides of the uterus, and open into the uterus through small channels. It is within a fallopian tube that fertilization, the joining of the egg and the sperm, takes place.

Some common surgical procedures that are performed on the fallopian tubes include:

- Salpingostomy. An incision is made in the fallopian tube, often to excise an ectopic pregnancy.

- Salpingectomy. One or both fallopian tubes are removed in this procedure. It may be used to treat ruptured or bleeding fallopian tubes (as a result of ectopic pregnancy), infection, or cancer.

- **Tubal ligation**. A permanent form of birth control in which a woman's fallopian tubes are surgically cut or blocked off to prevent pregnancy.

THE VULVA. The external female genital organs (or vulva) include the labia majora, two lips or folds that enclose the labia minora. The labia minora, in turn, are two lips or folds that enclose the clitoris, a small sensitive organ with a high number of nerve endings.

Some examples of surgeries that affect the vulva are:

- Vulvectomy. The vulva may be partially or completely removed, as in the case of vulvar cancer.

- Laceration or hematoma repair. Vulvar hematoma (a localized collection of blood) or laceration may result from a "straddle" injury, sexual assault, or childbirth. Severe hematomas may need surgical drainage.

Obstetric and gynecologic anesthesia

There are a number of options available to women for pain relief during obstetric or gynecologic surgery. Pain medications given intravenously (into a vein) or intramuscularly (into a muscle) help to decrease the amount of pain during childbirth or certain procedures, although they will generally not completely eliminate pain.

Regional anesthesia, either a spinal or an epidural, is the preferred method of pain relief during childbirth and certain surgical procedures such as cesarean section, tubal ligation, **cervical cerclage**, and others that do not require the patient to be unconscious. The benefits of regional anesthesia include allowing the patient to be awake during the surgery, avoiding the risks of **general anesthesia**, and allowing early contact between mother and child in the case of a cesarean section. Spinal anesthesia involves inserting a needle into a region between the vertebrae of the lower back and injecting numbing medications. An epidural is similar to a spinal except that a catheter is inserted so that numbing medications may be administered as needed. Some women experience a drop in blood pressure when a regional anesthetic is administered; this can be countered with fluids and/or medications.

In some instances, use of general anesthesia may be indicated. General anesthesia can be more rapidly administered in the case of an emergency (e.g. severe fetal distress). If the mother has a coagulation disorder that would be complicated by a drop in blood pressure (a risk with regional anesthesia), general anesthesia is an alternative. General anesthesia is also used for some of the more complicated and prolonged obstetric and gynecologic surgeries.

Resources

BOOKS

Hammond, Charles B. "Gynecology: The Female Reproductive Organs." In *Sabiston Textbook of Surgery*. Philadelphia: W. B. Saunders Company, 2001.

Hawkins, Joy L., David H. Chestnut, and Charles P. Gibbs. "Obstetric Anesthesia." In *Obstetrics: Normal & Problem Pregnancies*. Philadelphia: Churchill Livingstone, 2002.

ORGANIZATIONS

American Board of Obstetrics and Gynecology. 2915 Vine Street, Dallas, TX 75204. (214) 871-1619. http://www.abog.org.

American College of Obstetricians and Gynecologists. 409 12th St., SW, PO Box 96920, Washington, DC 20090-6920. (202)638-5577. http://www.acog.org.

Gynecologic Surgery Society. 2440 M Street, NW, Suite 801, Washington, DC 20037. (202) 293-2046. http://www.gynecologicsurgerysociety.org.

OTHER

"Atlas of the Body: Female Reproductive Organs." American Medical Association. January 28, 2002 [cited March 1, 2003]. http://www.ama-assn.org/ama/pub/category/7163.html.

Camaan, William, and Bhavani Shankar Kodali. "Obstetrical Anesthesia." Brigham & Women's Hospital Health and Information Services, February 10, 2008. http://www.brighamandwomens.org/painfreebirthing.

"Health Conditions and Medical Procedures." OBGYN.net [cited March 1, 2003]. http://www.obgyn.net/women/conditions/conditions.asp.

Stephanie Dionne Sherk
Renee Laux, M.S.

Obstetric sonogram *see* **Pelvic ultrasound**

Omphalocele repair

Definition

An omphalocele is a congenital defect in which internal organs such as the liver, stomach, and intestines, are on the outside of the abdomen, at the umbilical cord, instead of being located inside the body. These abdominal cavity contents are enclosed in a thin, transparent, membranous sac that is actually formed inside the umbilical cord tissue. An omphalocele repair is a surgical procedure in which the organs are returned to the inside of the body, and the opening in the abdominal wall is closed. Whenever possible, a normal-looking belly button is created.

Purpose

The internal organs need to be enclosed inside the abdomen for protection against injury, and to ensure that the tissue remains properly hydrated. The omphalocele repair is necessary to return the tissue to the inside of the body.

Demographics

Omphaloceles usually occur in full-term infants, more frequently in boys than in girls. A recent study found that the ratio is two girls to three boys.

The presence of an omphalocele often occurs with other birth defects, including:

- heart defects, such as the tetralogy of Fallot
- imperforate anus, a malformation of the anorectal area of the gastrointestinal system
- urinary problems
- genetic disorders
- Beckwith-Wiedemann syndrome, with enlarged tongue, gigantism, and enlarged internal organs
- pentalogy of Cantrell, with malformations in the chest and abdominal area, including heart defects, and high mortality rate

To check for other congenital defects, x rays are usually taken of the heart, lungs, and diaphragm once the infant's condition has been stablized after birth.

Description

An omphalocele is a defect that can be viewed on sonogram during an **ultrasound** performed while the mother is pregnant. At about six to eight weeks of fetal development, the abdominal contents come out of the fetus's abdomen at the base of the umbilical cord. They return to the inside as development continues.

KEY TERMS

Congenital—Present at the time of birth.

Edema—Swelling, or filling with fluid.

Gigantism—A condition in which the individual grows to an abnormally large size. Mental development may or may not be normal.

Intravenous—The use of a special tube, or catheter, inserted into a vein. Through the catheter, the infant may receive medications, as well as feedings, until taking food directly into the stomach is possible.

Sonogram—Image, or picture, obtained when using a machine called an ultrasound to look inside the uterus when the mother is pregnant. It is a painless procedure that sends out sound waves to the baby, and as the sound waves bounce off the object—the baby—an image is created on a monitor.

If this process is interrupted in some way during the seventh to tenth week of fetal development, the contents remain on the outside, and an omphalocele develops. Because the abdominal contents are now on the outside of the body, the inside cavity may not develop properly. For this reason, a large omphalocele cannot simply be placed back inside because the cavity may be too small. The internal organs will need to be protected and kept hydrated while the inside is gradually stretched. Small amounts of the omphalocele are returned at any one time to allow the cavity to gradually stretch to accommodate them. If the sac surrounding the tissue has ruptured, or broken, there is a greater risk of infection, tissue damage, loss of **body temperature**, and dehydration.

The repair may be performed in stages. If the omphalocele is very small, it may be possible to return all of the contents to the inside, and surgically close the opening. If the omphalocele is too large to do this all at once, some contents will remain on the outside while a sterile pouch is created to protect the tissue that remains on the outside. To be sure that the tissue does not dry out, it will be covered with warm and moist sterile **dressings**. The infant can lose considerable body heat through the large amount of exposed surface area, so keeping him or her warm, and closely monitoring body temperature is a high priority. An antibacterial solution may be used to decrease the risk of infection. The infant will have a tube that goes in through the nose or mouth and down into the stomach, called a nasogastric tube. Suction is used to keep the stomach empty, avoiding the chance of vomiting, or of the fluid moving from the stomach up into the lungs. The contents of the sac will be carefully examined to make sure that none of the tissue is damaged or dead, and to check for signs of intestinal birth defects before being inserted into the body.

The omphalocele repair is a surgical procedure performed under **general anesthesia**. The infant will receive medication to relax his or her muscles, and to help the surgery move forward without causing any pain. A large omphalocele repair may be done in stages over several weeks. The contents of the sac are often swollen, which makes it impossible to return them into the small cavity all at once. The return of the sac contents into the abdominal cavity creates intra-abdominal pressure, which may cause the infant to have difficulty breathing. To help the infant breathe, a special breathing tube may be inserted. The tube is attached to a machine that regulates the length and frequency of the breaths. When the necessary surgeries have been completed, the suturing will be done in such a way as to leave, if possible, a somewhat normal-looking belly button. A large omphalocele repair can leave a large, unsightly scar. For cosmetic purposes, the scar may be operated on at a later date to make it less noticeable. Gastroesophageal reflux, which may require additional surgery, is common in patients with a repaired omphalocele.

Diagnosis/Preparation

The diagnosis of an omphalocele may take place during an ultrasound while the mother is still pregnant. A recent study found that 75% of omphaloceles were diagnosed by ultrasound, most commonly around week 18 of pregnancy. To avoid any injury to the omphalocele sac, a cesarean birth may be performed so that the infant does not travel through the birth canal. If the omphalocele has not been detected prior to birth, it is immediately noticeable upon birth.

Aftercare

The infant will need to spend some time after the surgery in the **intensive care unit**. Because infants are unable to properly regulate their temperature, they are placed in special beds that are kept warm. They will usually need oxygen and a breathing tube to help them breathe for a while. The breathing machine is referred to as **mechanical ventilation**, or a ventilator. This machine helps the baby breathe at the right depth and frequency for his or her age, allowing the infant to conserve energy for other functions. An infant that is struggling for air spends much energy on breathing, which slows the healing process.

WHO PERFORMS THE PROCEDURE AND WHERE IS IT PERFORMED?

This procedure is performed by a surgeon, preferably board certified, who specializes in pediatric surgery and has experience with such conditions. The repair needs to be done in a hospital, preferably one with a neonatal intensive care unit, with specially-trained pediatric intensive care nurses and staff.

Once the bowels are moving normally, feedings will be slowly started. Feedings are usually first done through a nasogastric tube so the infant does not need to use energy for sucking and swallowing. Sucking on a pacifier is avoided because this could cause the bowel to expand with air and slow down the healing process. Until the nasogastric tube is used, the infant will be fed intravenously. The intravenous line provides the infant with needed **antibiotics**, pain medication, and fluids.

Infants with an omphalocele may spend quite some time, perhaps several months, in the hospital before being discharged home. It may take them some time to learn to feed through normal infant sucking and swallowing. Their development may be delayed, and they may require help for months as they catch up to the physical and mental development that is normal for their age. If the parents do not live near the hospital, they should be encouraged to spend as much time with their infant as possible to ensure infant-parent bonding. When the repair is done in stages, it can be difficult for the parents to remain patient. The birth of a child with a birth defect can be quite emotionally difficult for the parents. Individuals trained to assist parents through this time should meet with them to provide information and support.

Risks

All surgery has risks, from the procedure itself as well as the anesthesia. Infection and bleeding are the two primary risks of surgery. Breathing problems and reactions to the anesthetics are the main risks from anesthesia. In addition to these standard surgical risks, an omphalocele repair has the associated risks of damage to the organs on the outside of the body, additional breathing problems from the added pressure inside the abdominal cavity when the contents are returned, infection of the abdominal cavity (peritonitis), and a slowing or paralysis of the bowels (paralytic ileus).

QUESTIONS TO ASK THE DOCTOR

- In addition to the omphalocele, what other medical conditions does the child have?
- What is the chance of surviving the procedures needed to correct these problems?
- What quality of life can the child have if all the procedures are successfully performed?
- How many of these procedures has the surgeon performed?
- What outcomes has the surgeon's patients had?
- How long will the child need to stay in the hospital?
- What about breastfeeding?
- What is the likelihood of a similar condition being present in future children for this couple?

Normal results

The expected results depend on many factors, including:

- size of the omphalocele
- degree of development of the abdominal cavity
- presence and extent of other congenital defects
- damage to or loss of intestinal tissue
- whether the infant was full-term or premature at birth

Many omphaloceles can be completely corrected with excellent results.

Morbidity and mortality rates

An omphalocele occurs in about one in 5,000 live births. Other congenital defects are common. In one recent study, 50% of infants with omphalocele had other birth defects, primarily heart-related. On average, the infants spent three days on a ventilator, with about 45 total days spent in the hospital. The mortality rate was 8%, mostly due to heart problems.

Alternatives

There are no non-surgical alternatives to omphalocele repair. The abdominal contents need to be returned to the abdominal cavity, and the opening closed. While awaiting surgical repair, a sterile elastic bandage may be placed on the omphalocele to decrease edema (fluid accumulation).

Resources

BOOKS

Ashcraft, Keith W. *Pediatric surgery*. W. B. Saunders Company, 2000.

Pillitteri, Adele. *Maternal & Child Nursing: Care of the childbearing & childrearing family*. 3rd edition. Lippincott, 1999.

PERIODICALS

Barisic, I. et al. "Evaluation of Prenatal Ultrasound Diagnosis of Fetal Abdominal Wall Defects by 19 European Registries."*Ultrasound Obstet Gynecol* 18 (October 2001): 309–16.

Saxena, A. and G.H. Willital. "Omphalocele: Clinical Review and Surgical Experience Using Dura Patch Grafts."*Hernia* 6 (July 2002): 73–8

ORGANIZATIONS

National Library of Medicine: Medline Plus Health Information. [cited July 7, 2003]. http://www.nlm.nih.gov

Esther Csapo Rastegari, R.N., B.S.N., Ed.M.

Onocology surgery *see* **Surgical oncology**

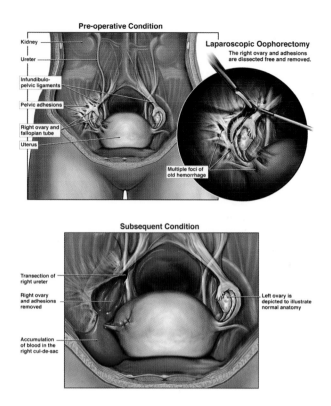

Ovarian surgery. *(Nucleus Medical Art, Inc. / Alamy)*

Oophorectomy

Definition

Unilateral oophorectomy (also called an ovariectomy) is the surgical removal of an ovary. If one ovary is removed, a woman may continue to menstruate and have children. If both ovaries are removed, a procedure called a bilateral oophorectomy, menstruation stops and a woman loses the ability to have children.

Purpose

Oophorectomy is performed to:

• remove cancerous ovaries
• remove the source of estrogen that stimulates some cancers
• remove a large ovarian cyst
• excise an abscess
• treat endometriosis

In an oophorectomy, one or a portion of one ovary may be removed or both ovaries may be removed. When an oophorectomy is done to treat ovarian cancer or other spreading cancers, both ovaries are removed (called a bilateral oophorectomy). Removal of the ovaries and fallopian tubes is performed in about one-third of hysterectomies (surgical removal of the uterus), often to reduce the risk of ovarian cancer.

Oophorectomies are sometimes performed on premenopausal women who have estrogen-sensitive breast cancer in an effort to remove the main source of estrogen from their bodies. This procedure has become less common than it was in the 1990s. Today, chemotherapy drugs are available that alter the production of estrogen and tamoxifen blocks any of the effects any remaining estrogen may have on cancer cells.

Until the 1980s, women over age 40 having hysterectomies routinely had healthy ovaries and fallopian tubes removed at the same time. This operation is called a bilateral **salpingo-oophorectomy**. Many physicians reasoned that a woman over 40 was approaching menopause and soon her ovaries would stop secreting estrogen and releasing eggs. Removing the ovaries would eliminate the risk of ovarian cancer and only accelerate menopause by a few years.

In the 1990s, the thinking about routine oophorectomy began to change. The risk of ovarian cancer in women who have no family history of the disease is less than 1%. Meanwhile, removing the ovaries increases the risk of cardiovascular disease and accelerates osteoporosis unless a woman takes prescribed hormone replacements.

Under certain circumstances, oophorectomy may still be the treatment of choice to prevent breast and

KEY TERMS

Cyst—An abnormal sac containing fluid or semi-solid material.

Endometriosis—A benign condition that occurs when cells from the lining of the uterus begin growing outside the uterus.

Fallopian tubes—Slender tubes that carry ova from the ovaries to the uterus.

Hysterectomy—Surgical removal of the uterus.

Osteoporosis—The excessive loss of calcium from the bones, causing the bones to become fragile and break easily.

ovarian cancer in certain high-risk women. A study done at the University of Pennsylvania and released in 2000 showed that healthy women who carried the BRCA1 or BRCA2 genetic mutations that predisposed them to breast cancer had their risk of breast cancer drop from 80% to 19% when their ovaries were removed before age 40. Women between the ages of 40 and 50 showed less risk reduction, and there was no significant reduction of breast cancer risk in women over age 50. A 2002 study showed that five years after being identified as carrying BRCA1 or BRCA2 genetic mutations, 94% of women who had received a bilateral salpingo-oophorectomy were cancer-free, compared to 79% of women who had not received surgery.

The value of ovary removal in preventing both breast and ovarian cancer has been documented. However, there are disagreements within the medical community about when and at what age this treatment should be offered. Preventative oophorectomy, also called prophylactic oophorectomy, is not always covered by insurance. One study conducted in 2000 at the University of California at San Francisco found that only 20% of insurers paid for preventive bilateral oophorectomy (PBO). Another 25% had a policy against paying for the operation, and the remaining 55% said that they would decide about payment on an individual basis.

Demographics

Overall, ovarian cancer accounts for only 4% of all cancers in women. But the lifetime risk for developing ovarian cancer in women who have mutations in BRCA1 is significantly increased over the general population and may cause an ovarian cancer risk of 30% by age 60. For women at increased risk,

oophorectomy may be considered after the age of 35 if childbearing is complete.

Other factors that increase a woman's risk of developing ovarian cancer include age (most ovarian cancers occur after menopause), the number of menstrual periods a woman has had (affected by age of onset, pregnancy, breastfeeding, and oral contraceptive use), history of breast cancer, diet, and family history. The incidence of ovarian cancer is highest among Native Americans (17.5 cases per 100,000 population), white (15.8 per 100,000), Vietnamese (13.8 per 100,000), white Hispanic (12.1 per 100,000), and Hawaiian (11.8 per 100,000) women; it is lowest among Korean (7.0 per 100,000) and Chinese (9.3 per 100,000) women. African American women have an ovarian cancer incidence of 10.2 per 100,000 population.

Description

Oophorectomy is done under general or regional anesthesia. It is often performed through the same type of incision, either vertical or horizontal, as an abdominal **hysterectomy**. Horizontal incisions leave a less noticeable scar, but vertical incisions give the surgeon a better view of the abdominal cavity. After the incision is made, the abdominal muscles are stretched apart, not cut, so that the surgeon can see the ovaries. Then the ovaries, and often the fallopian tubes, are removed.

Oophorectomy can sometimes be done with a laparoscopic procedure. With this surgery, a tube containing a tiny lens and light source is inserted through a small incision in the navel. A camera can be attached that allows the surgeon to see the abdominal cavity on a video monitor. When the ovaries are detached, they are removed though a small incision at the top of the vagina. The ovaries can also be cut into smaller sections and removed.

The advantages of abdominal incision are that the ovaries can be removed even if a woman has many adhesions from previous surgery. The surgeon gets a good view of the abdominal cavity and can check the surrounding tissue for disease. A vertical abdominal incision is mandatory if cancer is suspected. The disadvantages are that bleeding is more likely to be a complication of this type of operation. The operation is more painful than a laparoscopic operation and the recovery period is longer. A woman can expect to be in the hospital two to five days and will need three to six weeks to return to normal activities.

Diagnosis/Preparation

Before surgery, the doctor will order blood and urine tests, and any additional tests such as **ultrasound** or x rays to help the surgeon visualize the woman's condition. The woman may also meet with the anesthesiologist to evaluate any special conditions that might affect the administration of anesthesia. A colon preparation may be done, if extensive surgery is anticipated.

On the evening before the operation, the woman should eat a light dinner, then take nothing by mouth, including water or other liquids, after midnight.

Aftercare

After surgery a woman will feel discomfort. The degree of discomfort varies and is generally greatest with abdominal incisions, because the abdominal muscles must be stretched out of the way so that the surgeon can reach the ovaries. In order to minimize the risk of postoperative infection, **antibiotics** will be given.

When both ovaries are removed, women who do not have cancer are started on hormone replacement therapy to ease the symptoms of menopause that occur because estrogen produced by the ovaries is no longer present. If even part of one ovary remains, it will produce enough estrogen that a woman will continue to menstruate, unless her uterus was removed in a hysterectomy. To help offset the higher risks of heart and bone disease after loss of the ovaries, women should get plenty of **exercise**, maintain a low-fat diet, and ensure intake of calcium is adequate.

Return to normal activities takes anywhere from two to six weeks, depending on the type of surgery. When women have cancer, chemotherapy or radiation are often given in addition to surgery. Some women have emotional trauma following an oophorectomy, and can benefit from counseling and support groups.

Risks

Oophorectomy is a relatively safe operation, although, like all major surgery, it does carry some risks. These include unanticipated reaction to anesthesia, internal bleeding, blood clots, accidental damage to other organs, and post-surgery infection.

Complications after an oophorectomy include changes in sex drive, hot flashes, and other symptoms of menopause if both ovaries are removed. Women who have both ovaries removed and who do not take estrogen replacement therapy run an increased risk for cardiovascular disease and osteoporosis. Women with a history of psychological and emotional problems before an oophorectomy are more likely to experience psychological difficulties after the operation.

WHO PERFORMS THE PROCEDURE AND WHERE IS IT PERFORMED?

Oophorectomies are usually performed in a hospital operating room by a gynecologist, a medical doctor who has completed specialized training in the areas of women's general health, pregnancy, labor and childbirth, prenatal testing, and genetics.

Complications may arise if the surgeon finds that cancer has spread to other places in the abdomen. If the cancer cannot be removed by surgery, it must be treated with chemotherapy and radiation.

Normal results

If the surgery is successful, the ovaries will be removed without complication, and the underlying problem resolved. In the case of cancer, all the cancer will be removed. A woman will become infertile following a bilateral oophorectomy.

Morbidity and mortality rates

Studies have shown that the complication rate following oophorectomy is essentially the same as that following hysterectomy. The rate of complications associated with hysterectomy differs by the procedure performed. Abdominal hysterectomy is associated with a higher rate of complications (9.3%), while the overall complication rate for vaginal hysterectomy is 5.3%, and 3.6% for laparoscopic vaginal hysterectomy. The risk of **death** is about one in every 1,000 women having a hysterectomy. The rates of some of the more commonly reported complications are:

- excessive bleeding (hemorrhaging): 1.8–3.4%
- fever or infection: 0.8–4.0%
- accidental injury to another organ or structure: 1.5–1.8%

Because of the cessation of hormone production that occurs with a bilateral oophorectomy, women who lose both ovaries also prematurely lose the protection these hormones provide against heart disease and osteoporosis. Women who have undergone bilateral oophorectomy are seven times more likely to develop coronary heart disease and much more likely to develop bone problems at an early age than are premenopausal women whose ovaries are intact.

QUESTIONS TO ASK THE DOCTOR

- Why is a oophorectomy being recommended?
- How will the procedure be performed?
- Will I have a remaining ovary (or portion of ovary)?
- What alternatives to oophorectomy are available to me?

Alternatives

Depending on the specific condition that warrants an oophorectomy, it may be possible to modify the surgery so at least a portion of one ovary remains, allowing the woman to avoid early menopause. In the case of prophylactic oophorectomy, drugs such as tamoxifen may be administered to block the effects that estrogen may have on cancer cells.

Resources

PERIODICALS

Kauff, N. D., J. M. Satagopan, M. E. Robson, et al. "Risk-Reducing Salpingo-oophorectomy in Women With a BRC1 or BRC2 Mutation." *New England Journal of Medicine* 346 (May 23, 2002): 1609–15.

ORGANIZATIONS

American Cancer Society. 1599 Clifton Road NE, Atlanta, GA 30329. (800) ACS-2345. http://www.cancer.org.

American College of Obstetricians and Gynecologists. 409 12th St., SW, PO Box 96920, Washington, DC 20090-6920. http://www.acog.org.

Cancer Information Service, National Cancer Institute. Building 31, Room 10A19, 9000 Rockville Pike, Bethesda, MD 20892. (800) 4-CANCER. http://www.nci.nih.gov/cancerinfo/index.html.

OTHER

"Ovarian Cancer: Detailed Guide." *American Cancer Society.* October 20, 2000 [cited March 14, 2003]. http://www.cancer.org/downloads/CRI/CRC_-_OVARIAN_CANCER.pdf.

"Prophylactic Oophorectomy." *American College of Obstetricians and Gynecologists.* September 7, 1999 [cited March 14, 2003]. http://www.medem.com/MedLB/article_detaillb.cfm?article_ID=ZZZONIHKUJC&sub_cat=9.

"Removing Ovaries Lowers Risk for Women at High Risk of Breast, Ovarian Cancer." *ACS News Today* November 8, 2000. [cited May 13, 2003]. http://www.cancer.org.

Surveillance, Epidemiology, and End Results. "Racial/Ethnic Patterns of Cancer in the United States: Ovary." *National Cancer Institute.* 1996 [cited March 14, 2003]. <http://seer.cancer.gov/publications/ethnicity/ovary.pdf>.

Tish Davidson, A.M.
Stephanie Dionne Sherk

Open decompression *see* **Laminectomy**
Open fracture reduction *see* **Fracture repair**

Open prostatectomy

Definition

Open prostatectomy is a procedure for removal of an enlarged prostate gland.

Purpose

The prostate gland is located at the base of the male urethra. The primary indication for open prostatectomy is benign prostatic hyperplasia (BPH), a condition whereby benign or noncancerous nodules grow in the prostate gland. The prostate gland is composed of smooth muscle cells, glandular cells, and cells that give the gland structure (stromal cells). A dense fibrous capsule surrounds the prostate gland. The glandular cells produce a milky fluid that mixes with seminal fluid and sperm to make semen. The prostate gland also produces a hormone called dihydrotestosterone (DHT) that has a major impact on the gland's development.

Description

The prostate gland undergoes several changes as a man ages. The pea-size gland at birth grows only slightly during puberty and reaches its normal adult shape and size (similar to a walnut) when a male is in his early twenties. The prostate gland remains stable until the mid-forties. At that time in most men, the number of cells begins to multiply, and the gland starts to enlarge. The enlargement, called hyperplasia, is due to an increase in the number of cells. Cell proliferation in the prostates of older men can cause symptoms (referred to as lower urinary tract symptoms, LUTS), which often include:

- straining when urinating
- hesitation before urine flow starts
- dribbling at the end of urination or leakage afterward
- weak or intermittent urinary strain
- painful urination

Open prostatectomy

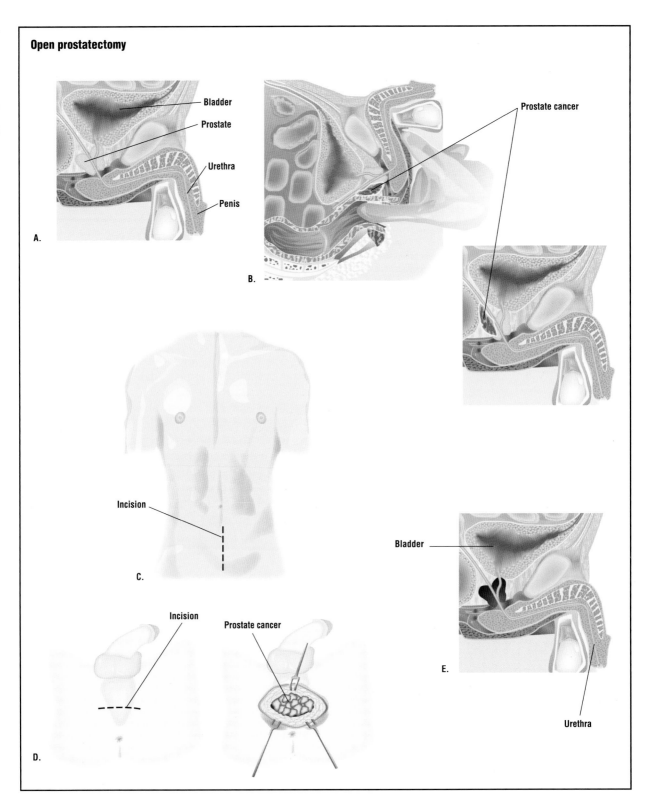

During a digital rectal exam (B), the doctor may feel an enlargement of the prostate that can be benign or cancerous. If an open prostatectomy is needed, an incision may made the lower abdomen (C) or the perineal area (D). In either case, the prostate and any cancer is removed (E). *(Illustration by GGS Information Services. Cengage Learning, Gale.)*

KEY TERMS

Bladder mucosa—Mucous coat of the bladder.

Cerebrovascular accident—Brain hemorrhage, also known as a stroke.

Cystoscopy—Examination of the bladder using a special instrument to visualize the organ.

Cystotomy—An incision in the bladder.

Pulmonary embolus—A thrombus that typically detaches from a deep vein of a lower extremity.

Trendelenburg—Position in which the head is low and the body and legs are on an inclined plane.

Other symptoms (called storage symptoms) sometime appear, and may include:

- urgent need to urinate
- bladder pain when urinating
- increased frequency of urination, especially at night
- bladder irritation during urination

The cause of BPH is not fully understood. Currently, it is thought to be caused by a hormone that the prostate gland synthesizes, called dihydrotestosterone (DHT). The hormone is synthesized from testosterone.

Surgery is generally indicated for persons with moderate to severe symptoms, particularly if urinary retention is very poor or if the enlarged prostate (BPH) contributes to urinary tract infections, blood in the urine, bladder stones, or kidney problems.

Open prostatectomy is the treatment of choice for approximately 2–3% of BPH patients who have a very large prostate, a damaged bladder, or another serious related problem. Open prostatectomy is used when the prostate is so large (2.8–3.5 oz [80–100 g]) that **transurethral resection of the prostate** (TURP, a less invasive surgical procedure to remove a smaller prostate) cannot be performed. Additionally, open prostatectomy is indicated for males with:

- recurrent or persistent urinary tract infections.
- acute urinary distention.
- bladder outlet obstructions.
- recurrent blood in urine of prostate origin.
- pathological changes in the bladder, ureters, or kidneys due to prostate obstruction.

Contraindications to open prostatectomy (reasons not to do the procedure) include previous prostatectomy, prostate cancer, a small fibrous prostate gland, and previous pelvic surgery that may obstruct access to the prostate gland.

Demographics

The cause of BPH is not entirely known; however, the incidence increases with advancing age. Before 40 years of age, approximately 10% of males have BPH. A small amount of hyperplasia is present in 80% of males over 40 years old. Approximately 8–31% of males experience moderate to severe lower urinary tract symptoms (LUTS) in their fifties. By age 80, about 80% of men have LUTS. A risk factor is the presence of normally functioning testicles; research indicates that castration can minimize prostatic enlargement. It appears that the glandular tissues that multiply abnormally use male hormones produced in the testicles differently than the normal tissues do.

Approximately 10 million American men and 30 million men worldwide have symptoms of BPH. It is more prevalent in the United States and Europe, and less common among Asians. BPH is more common in men who are married rather than single, and there is a strong genetic correlation. A man's chance for developing BPH is greater if three of more family members have the condition.

Description

Open prostatectomy can be performed by either the retropubic or suprapubic approach. The preferred anesthesia for open prostatectomy is a spinal or epidural nerve block. Regional anesthesia can help reduce blood loss during surgery, and lowers the risk of complications such as pulmonary embolus and postoperative deep vein thrombosis. **General anesthesia** may be used if the patient has an anatomic or medical contraindication for regional anesthesia.

Retropubic prostatectomy

The retropubic prostatectomy is accomplished through a direct incision of the anterior (front) prostatic capsule. The overgrowth of glandular cells (hyperplastic prostatic adenoma) is removed. These are the cells forming a mass in the prostate because of their abnormal multiplication.

A **cystoscopy** is performed before the open prostatectomy. The patient lies on his back on the operating table, and is prepared and draped for this procedure. Following the cystoscopy, the patient is changed to a Trendelenburg (feet higher than head) position. The surgical area is shaved, draped, and prepared. A catheter is placed in the urethra to drain urine. An incision is made from the umbilicus to the pubic area. The abdominal muscle (rectus abdominis) is separated, and a retractor is placed at the incision site to widen the surgical field. Further maneuvering is essential to clearly locate the veins (dorsal vein complex) and the bladder neck. Visualization of the bladder neck exposes the patient's main arterial blood supply to the prostate gland. Once the structures have been identified and the blood supply controlled, an incision is made deep into the level of the tumor. Scissors are used to dissect the prostatic tissue (prostatic capsule) from the underlying tissue of the prostatic tumor. The wound is closed after complete removal of the tumor and hemostasis (stoppage of bleeding) occurs.

The advantages of the retropubic prostatectomy include:

• direct visualization of the prostatic tumor.

• accurate incisions in the urethra, which will minimize the complication of urinary continence.

• excellent anatomic exposure and visualization of the prostate.

• clear visualization to control bleeding after tumor removal.

• little or no surgical trauma to the urinary bladder.

Suprapubic prostatectomy

Suprapubic prostatectomy (also called transvesical prostatectomy) is a procedure to remove the prostatic overgrowth via a different surgical route. The suprapubic approach utilizes an incision of the lower anterior (front) bladder wall. The primary advantage over the retropubic approach is that the suprapubic route allows for direct visualization of the bladder neck and bladder mucosa. Because of this, the procedure is ideally suited for persons who have bladder complications, as well as obese men. The major disadvantage is that visualization of the top part of the tumor is reduced. Additionally, with the subrapubic approach, hemostasis (stoppage of bleeding during surgery) may be more difficult due to poor visualization after removal of the tumor.

Using a scalpel, a lower midline incision is made from the umbilicus to the pubic area. A cystotomy (incision into the bladder) is made, and the bladder inspected. Using electrocautery (a special tool that produces heat at the tip, useful for hemostasis or tissue excision) and scissors, dissection proceeds until the prostatic tumor is identified and removed. After maintaining hemostasis and arterial blood supply to the prostate, the incisions to the bladder and abdominal wall are closed.

WHO PERFORMS THE PROCEDURE AND WHERE IS IT PERFORMED?

The procedure is performed by a urological surgeon who typically completes one year of general surgery training, and four to five years of urology training. The procedure is usually performed in a large hospital.

Diagnosis/Preparation

The presence of symptoms is indicative of the disease. Age also has an associated risk for an enlarged prostate, and can help establish diagnostic criteria.

Men must have a special blood test called the prostate specific antigen (PSA) test and routine digital rectal examination (DRE) before surgery. If the PSA levels and DRE are suspiciously indicative of prostate cancer, a transrectal **ultrasound** guided needle biopsy of the prostate must be performed before open prostatectomy, to detect the presence of prostate cancer.

Additionally, preoperative patients should have lower urinary tract studies, including urinary flow rate and post void residual urine in the bladder. Because most patients are age 60 or older, preoperative evaluation should also include a detailed history and **physical examination**; standard blood tests; chest x-ray; and **electrocardiogram** (EKG) to detect any possible preexisting conditions.

Aftercare

Open prostatectomy is a major surgical operation requiring an inpatient hospital stay of four to seven days. Blood transfusions are generally not required due to improvements in surgical technique. Immediately after the operation, the surgeon must closely monitor urinary output and fluid status. On the first day after surgery, most patients are given a clear liquid diet and asked to sit up four times. Morphine sulfate, given via a patient controlled analgesic pump (IV), is used to control pain.

On the second postoperative day, the urethral catheter is removed if the urine does not contain blood. Oral pain medications are begun if the patient can tolerate a regular diet.

On the third postoperative day, the pelvic drain is removed if drainage is less than 75 ml in 24 hours. The patient should gradually increase activity. Follow-up with the surgeon is necessary following **discharge**

QUESTIONS TO ASK THE DOCTOR

- Why is an open prostatectomy recommended?
- What form of open prostatectomy—retropubic or suprapubic—will be used?
- What forms of anesthesia and pain relief will be given?
- Where will the incision be located?
- What are the risks of the procedure?
- Is the surgeon a board certified urologist?
- Is there an alternative to open prostatectomy?
- What are the chances of after effects, including erectile problems?

from the hospital. Full activity is expected to resume within four to six weeks after surgery.

Risks

Improvements in surgical technique have lowered blood loss to a minimal level. For several weeks after open prostatectomy, patients may have urgency and urge incontinence. The severity of bladder problems depends on the patient's preoperative bladder status. Erectile dysfunction occurs in 3–5% of patients undergoing this procedure. Retrograde (backward flow) ejaculation occurs in approximately 50–80% of patients after open prostatectomy. The most common non-urologic risks include pulmonary embolism, myocardial infarction (heart attack), deep vein thrombosis, and cerebrovascular accident (stroke). The incidence of any one of these potentially adverse effects is less than 1%.

Normal results

Normally, patients will not have the adverse effects of bleeding. Hematuria (blood in the urine) is typically resolved within two days after surgery. The patient should begin a regular diet and moderate increases in activity soon after surgery. His presurgical activity level should be restored within four to six weeks after surgery.

Morbidity and mortality rates

The overall rate of morbidity and mortality is extremely low. The overall mortality (**death**) rate for open prostatectomy is approximately zero.

Alternatives

For smaller prostates, treatment using medication may help to control abnormal prostatic growth. When the prostate gland is large (75 grams and bigger), surgery is indicated.

Resources

BOOKS

Kirby, Roger S., Francesco Montorsi, Joseph Smith, and Paolo Gontero, eds. Radical Prostatectomy: From Open to Robotic. New York: Informa Healthcare, 2007.

OTHER

Miles, B. and Khera. M. "Simple Prostatectomy." eMedicine.com January 29, 2007 [cited January 5, 2008]. http://www.emedicine.com/med/topic3041.htm
"Prostatectomy" Medline Plus. date. November 15, 2006. [cited January 5, 2008]. http://www.nlm.nih.gov/medlineplus/ency/article/002996.htm.

Laith Farid Gulli, M.D., M.S.
Alfredo Mori, M.B.B.S.
Abraham F. Ettaher, M.D.
Bilal Nasser, M.D.,M.S.
Tish Davidson, A. M.

Operating room

Definition

An operating room (OR), also called surgery center, is the unit of a hospital where surgical procedures are performed.

Purpose

An operating room may be designed and equipped to provide care to patients with a range of conditions, or it may be designed and equipped to provide specialized care to patients with specific conditions.

Description

OR environment

Operating rooms are sterile environments. All personnel wear protective clothing called scrubs, as well as shoe covers, masks, caps, eye shields, and other coverings to prevent the spread of germs. The operating room is brightly lit and the temperature is very cool; operating rooms are air-conditioned to help prevent infection.

Advance directives—Legal documents that increase a patient's control over medical decisions. A patient may select medical treatment in advance, in the event that he or she becomes physically or mentally unable to communicate his or her wishes. Advance directives either state what kind of treatment the patient wants to receive (living will), or authorize another person to make medical decisions for the patient when he or she is unable to do so (durable power of attorney).

Anesthesiologist—A specially trained physician who administers anesthesia.

Arterial line—A catheter inserted into an artery and connected to a physiologic monitoring system to allow direct measurement of oxygen, carbon dioxide, and invasive blood pressure.

Catheter—A small, flexible tube used to deliver fluids or medications. A catheter may also be used to drain fluid or urine from the body.

Central venous line—A catheter inserted into a vein and connected to a physiologic monitoring system to directly measure venous blood pressure.

Chest tube—A tube inserted into the chest to drain fluid and air from around the lungs.

Critical care—The multidisciplinary healthcare specialty that provides care to patients with acute, life-threatening illness or injury.

Edema—An abnormal accumulation of fluids in intercellular spaces in the body; causes swelling.

Endotracheal tube—A tube inserted through the patient's nose or mouth that functions as an airway and is connected to a ventilator.

Foley catheter—A tube inserted into the bladder to drain urine into an external bag.

Gastrointestinal tube—A tube surgically inserted into the stomach for feeding a patient who is unable to eat by mouth.

Infectious disease team—A team of physicians and hospital staff who help control the hospital environment to protect patients against harmful sources of infection.

Inpatient surgery—Surgery that requires an overnight stay of one or more days in the hospital. The number of days spent in the hospital after surgery depends on the type of procedure performed.

Life support—Methods of replacing or supporting a failing bodily function, such as using mechanical ventilation to support breathing. In treatable or curable conditions, life support is used temporarily to aid healing until the body can resume normal functioning.

Nasogastric tube—A tube inserted through the nose and throat and into the stomach for directly feeding the patient.

Nothing by mouth (NPO)—NPO refers to the time after which the patient is not allowed to eat or drink prior to a procedure or treatment.

Outpatient surgery—Also called same-day or ambulatory surgery. The patient arrives for surgery and returns home on the same day. Outpatient surgery can take place in a hospital, surgical center, or outpatient clinic.

Swan-Ganz catheter—Also called a pulmonary artery catheter, this is a type of tubing inserted into a large vessel in the neck or chest. It is used to measure the amount of fluid in the heart, and to determine how well the heart is functioning.

The patient is brought to the operating room in a wheelchair or a bed with wheels called a gurney. The patient is transferred to the operating table, which is narrow and has safety straps to keep him or her positioned correctly.

The monitoring equipment and anesthesia used during surgery are usually kept at the head of the operating table. The anesthesiologist sits here to monitor the patient's condition during surgery.

Depending on the nature of the surgery, various forms of anesthesia or sedation are administered. The surgical site is cleansed and surrounded by a sterile drape.

The instruments used during a surgical procedure are different for external and internal treatment; different tools are used on the outside and on the inside of the body. Once internal surgery is started, the surgeon uses smaller, more delicate devices.

OR equipment

An operating room has special equipment such as respiratory and cardiac support, emergency resuscitative devices, patient monitors, and diagnostic tools.

Life support and emergency resuscitative equipment

Equipment for life support and emergency resuscitation includes:

- Heart-lung bypass machine, also called a cardiopulmonary bypass pump, which takes over for the heart and lungs during some surgeries, especially heart or lung procedures. The heart-lung machine removes carbon dioxide from the blood and replaces it with oxygen. A tube is inserted into the aorta to carry the oxygenated blood from the bypass machine to the aorta for circulation to the body. The heart-lung machine allows the heart's beating to be stopped during surgery.

- Ventilator, also called a respirator, which assists with or controls pulmonary ventilation. Ventilators consist of a flexible breathing circuit, gas supply, heating/humidification mechanism, monitors, and alarms. They are microprocessor-controlled and programmable, and regulate the volume, pressure, and flow of respiration.

- Infusion pump is a device that delivers fluids intravenously or epidurally through a catheter. Infusion pumps employ automatic, programmable pumping mechanisms to deliver continuous anesthesia, drugs, and blood infusions to the patient.

- Crash cart, also called resuscitation cart or code cart, is a portable cart containing emergency resuscitation equipment for patients who are "coding" (i.e., vital signs are in a dangerous range). The emergency equipment includes a defibrillator, airway intubation devices, resuscitation bag/mask, and medication box. Crash carts are strategically located in the operating room for immediate accessibility if a patient experiences cardiorespiratory failure.

- Intra-aortic balloon pump is a device that helps reduce the heart's workload and helps blood flow to the coronary arteries for patients with unstable angina, myocardial infarction, or those awaiting organ transplants. Intra-aortic balloon pumps use a balloon placed in the patient's aorta. The balloon is on the end of a catheter that is connected to the pump's console, which displays heart rate, pressure, and electrocardiogram (ECG) readings. The patient's ECG is used to time the inflation and deflation of the balloon.

Patient monitoring equipment

Patient monitoring equipment includes:

- Acute care physiologic monitoring system is a comprehensive patient monitoring system that can be configured to continuously measure and display various parameters via electrodes and sensors connected to the patient. Parameters monitored may include the electrical activity of the heart via an ECG, respiratory (breathing) rate, blood pressure (noninvasive and invasive), body temperature, cardiac output, arterial hemoglobin oxygen saturation (blood oxygen level), mixed venous oxygenation, and end-tidal carbon dioxide.

- Pulse oximeter monitors the arterial hemoglobin oxygen saturation (oxygen level) of the patient's blood with a sensor clipped over the finger or toe.

- Intracranial pressure monitor measures the pressure of fluid in the brain in patients with head trauma or other conditions affecting the brain (such as tumors, edema, or hemorrhage). Intracranial pressure monitors are connected to sensors inserted into the brain through a cannula (tube) or bur hole. These devices signal elevated pressure and record or display pressure trends. Intracranial pressure monitoring may be a capability included in a physiologic monitor.

Diagnostic equipment

The use of diagnostic equipment may be required in the operating room. Mobile x-ray units are used for bedside radiography, particularly of the chest. These portable units use a battery-operated generator that powers an x-ray tube. Handheld portable clinical laboratory devices, called point-of-care analyzers, are used for blood analysis at the bedside. A small amount of whole blood is required, and blood chemistry parameters can be provided much faster than if samples were sent to the central laboratory.

Other OR equipment

Disposable OR equipment includes urinary (Foley) catheters to drain urine during surgery, catheters used for arterial and central venous lines to monitor blood pressure during surgery or to withdraw blood samples, Swan-Ganz catheters to measure the amount of fluid in the heart and to determine how well the heart is functioning, chest and endotracheal tubes, and monitoring electrodes.

New surgical techniques

Minimally invasive surgery, also called laparoscopic surgery, is an operative technique performed through a few small incisions, rather than one large incision. Through these small incisions, surgeons insert a laparoscope (viewing instrument that displays the site on a computer screen for easier viewing) and endoscopic instruments to perform the surgery.

Robot-assisted surgery allows surgeons to perform certain procedures through small incisions. In robotic surgery, a surgeon sits at a console several feet from the operating table and uses a joystick, similar to that used for video games, to guide the movement of robotic arms that hold endoscopic instruments, as well as an endoscope (small camera). The surgeon uses the robotic arms to perform precise, fine hand movements and to provide access to parts of the body that are difficult to reach manually. In addition, robotic surgery provides a three-dimensional image, and the surgical field can be magnified to a greater extent than traditional or minimally invasive surgery. The goal of robotic surgery is to decrease incision size and **length of hospital stay**, while improving patient comfort and lessening recovery time.

Lasers are "scalpels of light" that offer new alternatives for some surgical procedures. Lasers can be used to cut, burn, or destroy abnormal or diseased tissue; shrink or destroy lesions or tumors; sculpt tissue; and seal blood vessels. Lasers may help surgeons perform some procedures more effectively than other traditional methods. Because lasers cause minimal bleeding, the operative area may be more clearly viewed by the surgeon. Lasers may also provide access to parts of the body that may not have been as easily reached manually.

Surgery centers

Freestanding surgery centers are available in many communities, primarily for the purpose of providing outpatient surgical procedures. The patient should make sure that the surgery center has been accredited by the Joint Commission on Accreditation of Healthcare Organizations (JCAHO), a professionally sponsored program that stimulates a high quality of patient care in healthcare facilities. There is also an accreditation option that is available for **ambulatory surgery centers**.

Choosing a surgery center with experienced staff is important. Here are some questions to consider when choosing a surgery center:

- How many surgeries are performed annually and what are the outcomes and survival rates for those procedures?
- How does the surgery center's outcomes compare with the national average?
- Does the surgery center offer procedures to treat a particular disease?
- Does the surgery center have experience treating patients in certain age groups?
- How much does surgery cost at this facility?
- Is financial assistance available?
- If the surgery center is far from the patient's home, will accommodations be provided for caregivers?

Resources

BOOKS

Deardoff, PhD, William, and John Reeves, PhD. *Preparing for Surgery: A Mind-Body Approach to Enhance Healing and Recovery*. Oakland, CA: New Harbinger Publications, 1997.

Furlong, Monica Winefryck. *Going Under: Preparing Yourself for Anesthesia: Your Guide to Pain Control and Healing Techniques Before, During and After Surgery*. Albuquerque, NM: Autonomy Publishing Company, 1993.

Goldman, Maxine A. *Pocket Guide to the Operating Room*, 2nd Edition. Philadelphia, PA: F.A. Davis Co., 1996.

PERIODICALS

"Recommended practices for managing the patient receiving anesthesia." *AORN Journal* 75, no.4 (April 2002): 849.

ORGANIZATIONS

American Board of Surgery. 1617 John F. Kennedy Boulevard, Suite 860, Philadelphia, PA 19103. (215) 568-4000. http://www.absurgery.org/ (accessed April 3, 2008).

American College of Surgeons. 633 N. Saint Clair Street, Chicago, IL 60611-3211. (312) 202-5000. http://www.facs.org/ (accessed April 2, 2008).

American Society of Anesthesiologists. 520 N. Northwest Highway, Park Ridge, IL 60068-2573. (847) 825-5586. E-mail: mail@asahq.org http://www.asahq.org/ (accessed April 2, 2008).

Association of Perioperative Registered Nurses (AORN, Inc.). 2170 South Parker Road. Suite 300, Denver, CO 80231. (800) 755-2676 or (303) 755-6304. http://www.aorn.org/ (accessed April 2, 2008).

National Heart, Lung and Blood Institute. Information Center. P.O. Box 30105, Bethesda, MD 20824-0105. (301) 251-2222. http://www.nhlbi.nih.gov (accessed April 2, 2008).

National Institutes of Health. U.S. Department of Health and Human Services, 9000 Rockville Pike, Bethesda, MD 20892. (301) 496-4000. http://www.nih.gov (accessed April 2, 2008).

OTHER

preSurgery.com. http://www.presurgery.com (accessed April 2, 2008).

Reports of the Surgeon General, National Library of Medicine. http://sgreports.nlm.nih.gov/NN (accessed April 2, 2008).

SurgeryLinx (surgery medical news and newsletters from top medical journals). MDLinx, Inc. 1025 Vermont Avenue, NW, Suite 810, Washington, DC 20005. (202) 543-6544.

Surgical Procedures, Operative, (collection of links). http://www.mic.ki.se/Diseases/e4.html (accessed April 2, 2008).

Angela M. Costello
Fran Hodgkins

Ophthalmologic surgery

Definition

Ophthalmologic surgery is a surgical procedure performed on the eye or any part of the eye.

Purpose

Surgery on the eye is routinely performed to repair retinal defects, remove cataracts or cancer, or to repair eye muscles. The most common purpose of ophthalmologic surgery is to restore or improve vision.

Demographics

Patients from the very young to very old have ocular conditions that warrant eye surgery. Two of the most common procedures are **phacoemulsification for cataracts** and elective refractive surgeries.

Cataract surgery is the most common ophthalmic procedure. More than 1.5 million cataract surgeries are performed in the United States each year. According to the National Eye Institute (NEI), more than half of all Americans age 80 or older have a cataract or have had cataract surgery.

Elective refractive surgeries, especially **laser in-situ keratomileusis (LASIK)**, attract younger patients in their 30s and 40s. Recently, the American Academy of Ophthalmology (AAO) estimated that 95% of the 1.8 million refractive surgery procedures performed in a year were **LASIK**.

Description

The surgeon, **operating room** nurses, and an anesthesiologist are present for ophthalmologic surgery. For many eye surgeries, only a local anesthetic is used, and the patient is awake. The patient's eye area is scrubbed prior to surgery, and sterile drapes are placed over the shoulders and head. Heart rate and blood pressure are monitored throughout the procedure. The patient is required to lie still and, for some surgery, especially refractive surgery, he or she is asked to focus on the light of the operating microscope. A speculum is placed in the eye to hold it open throughout surgery.

Common ophthalmologic surgery tools include scalpels, blades, forceps, speculums, and scissors. Many ophthalmologic surgeries now use lasers, which decrease the operating time as well as recovery time.

Surgeries requiring suturing can take as long as two or three hours. These intricate surgeries sometimes require the skill of a corneal or vitreo-retinal

KEY TERMS

Ablation—During LASIK, the vaporization of eye tissue.

Cataract—A clouding of the eye's lens that affects vision.

Cornea—The clear, curved tissue layer in front of the eye. It lies in front of the colored part of the eye (iris) and the black hole in the center of the iris (pupil).

Glaucoma—Disease of the eye characterized by increased pressure of the fluid inside the eye. Untreated, glaucoma can lead to blindness.

Macular degeneration—A condition usually associated with age in which the area of the retina called the macula is impaired due to hardening of the arteries (arteriosclerosis). This condition interferes with vision.

Retina—The inner, light-sensitive layer of the eye containing rods and cones; transforms the images it receives into electrical messages sent to the brain via the optic nerve.

specialist, and require the patient to be put under **general anesthesia**.

Refractive surgeries

Refractive surgeries use an excimer laser to reshape the cornea. The surgeon creates a flap of tissue across the cornea with an instrument called a microkeratome, ablates the cornea for about 30 seconds, and then replaces the flap. The laser allows this surgery to take only minutes, without the use of **stitches**.

Trabeculectomy

Trabeculectomy surgery uses a laser to open the drainage canals or make an opening in the iris to increase outflow of aqueous humor. The purpose is to lower intraocular pressure in the treatment of glaucoma.

Laser photocoagulation

Laser photocoagulation is used to treat some forms of wet age-related macular degeneration. The procedure stops leakage of abnormal blood vessels by burning them to slow the progress of the disease.

Diagnosis/Preparation

Patients complaining of any ocular problem that requires surgery will receive a similar initial examination. A complete patient history is taken, including the chief complaint. The patient needs to disclose any allergies, medication usage, family eye and medical histories, and vocational and recreational vision requirements.

The diagnostic exam should include measurement of visual acuity under both low and high illumination, biomicroscopy with pupillary dilation, stereoscopic fundus examination with pupillary dilation, assessment of ocular motility and binocularity, visual fields, evaluation of pupillary responses to rule out afferent pupillary defects, refraction, and measurement of intraocular pressure (IOP).

Other examination procedures include corneal mapping, a keratometer reading to determine the curvature of the central part of the cornea, and a slit lamp exam to determine any damage to the cornea and evidence of glaucoma and cataracts. A fundus exam also will be performed to check for retinal holes, and macular degeneration and disease.

The patient's overall health must also be considered. Poor general health will affect the ophthalmologic-surgery outcome. Surgeons may request a complete **physical examination**, in addition to the eye examination, prior to surgery.

Presurgery preparation

Patients having ophthalmologic surgery usually must stop taking **aspirin**, or aspirin-like products, 10 days before surgery unless directed otherwise by the surgeon. Patients taking blood thinners also must check with their physician to find out when they should stop taking the medication before surgery. A number of pain relievers may affect outcomes, making it important for the patient to disclose all medication. Some prescription medicines have been known to cause postsurgical scarring or flecks under the corneal flap after LASIK.

To reduce the chance of infection, the surgeon may request that the patient begin using antibiotic drops before surgery. Depending on the procedure, the patient may also be advised to discontinue contact lens wear and stop using creams, lotions, make-up, or perfume. Patients may also be asked to scrub their eyelashes for a period of time to remove any debris.

Patients are advised not to drink alcoholic beverages at least 24 hours before and after the ophthalmic procedure.

Patients must usually avoid eating or drinking anything after midnight on the day before the surgery; however, some patients may be allowed to have clear liquids in the morning. It is important for patients to ask their physician for a list of foods and medications permitted on the morning of surgery. Some patients may take morning medications (with physician approval) with the exclusion of **diuretics**, insulin, or diabetes pills. Patients are advised to dress comfortably for the surgery, and wear shirts that will not have to pass over the head.

Pre-surgical tests sometimes are administered when the patient arrives for surgery. For refractive surgeries, this ensures the laser is set for the correct refractive error. Before cataract surgery, measurements help determine the refractive power of the intraocular lens (IOL). Other tests, such as a **chest x ray**, blood work, or **urinalysis**, may also be requested depending on the patient's overall health.

Most ophthalmic surgeries are done on an outpatient basis, and patients must arrange for someone to take them home after the procedure.

Before surgery, doctors will review the pre-surgical tests and instill any dilating eye drops, antibiotic drops, and a corticosteroid or nonsteroidal anti-inflammatory drops as needed. Anesthetic eye drops also will be administered. Many ophthalmologic surgeries are performed under a local anesthetic, and patients remain in an awake but relaxed state.

Aftercare

After surgery, the patient is monitored in a recovery area. For most outpatient procedures, the patient is advised to rest for at least 24 hours until he or she returns to the surgeon's office for follow-up care. Over-the-counter (OTC) medications are usually advised for pain relief, but patients should check with their doctor to see what is recommended. Some pain relievers interfere with surgical outcomes. Patients may also use ice packs to help ease pain.

Some patients may experience slight drooping or bruising of the eye. This condition improves as the eye heals. Severe pain, nausea, or vomiting should be reported to the surgeon immediately.

After surgery, patients may be advised not to stoop, lift heavy objects, **exercise** vigorously, or swim. Patients may also be required to wear an eye shield while sleeping, and sunglasses or some type of protective lens during the day to avoid injury. Wearing make-up may be prohibited for weeks after surgery. The patient may be restricted from driving and air travel.

WHO PERFORMS THE PROCEDURE AND WHERE IS IT PERFORMED?

Ophthalmologists and optometrists may detect ophthalmic problems; however, only an ophthalmologist can perform surgery. An ophthalmologist has received specialized training in diseases of the eye and their surgical treatment. Some ophthalmologists further specialize in certain areas of the eye, such as corneal or vitreo-retinal specialists. Depending on the severity of the disease, the general ophthalmologist may refer the patient to a specialist for treatment.

An anesthesiologist may be on hand during surgery to administer the local anesthetic. Surgical nurses will assist the ophthalmologist in the operating room, and assist the patient preoperatively and postoperatively.

Most ophthalmic surgery is performed on an outpatient basis. Ambulatory surgery centers designed for ophthalmologic surgery are commonly used. Surgery may also be performed in hospital operating rooms designed for outpatient surgeries.

Patients usually have their first postoperative visit the day after the eye surgery. Subsequent exams are commonly scheduled at one, three, and six to eight weeks following surgery. This schedule depends on the patient's healing, and any complications he or she might experience.

Some patients will be required to instill eye drops for a number of weeks after surgery to prevent infection, pain, and to lessen inflammation. Eye drops also are used to lower intraocular pressure. In some cases, correct eye drop usage is critical to a successful surgery outcome.

Risks

Complications may occur during any surgery. Ophthalmologic surgery, however, is usually very safe.

Some risks include:

- Undercorrection or overcorrection in refractive surgery. Undercorrected refractive surgery patients usually can be treated with an enhancement, but overcorrected patients will need to use eyeglasses or contact lenses.
- Debilitating symptoms. These include glare, halos, double vision, and poor nighttime vision. Some

- If both eyes are diseased, will they be treated simultaneously?
- Will the eyes need to rest after surgery? Will protective lenses be required following the procedure?
- Will eyeglasses be needed?
- How many times has the surgeon performed this specific procedure?
- Should the physician be contacted if pain develops after the surgery?
- When can normal activities, such as driving, be resumed?

patients may also lose contrast sensitivity. These symptoms may be temporary or permanent.

- Dry eye. Some patients are treated with artificial tears or punctal plugs.
- Retinal detachment. The retina can become detached by the surgery if this part of the eye has any weakness when the procedure is performed. This may not occur for weeks or months.
- Endophthalmitis. An infection in the eyeball is a complication that is less common today because of newer surgery techniques and antibiotics.

Other serious complications that may occur are blindness, glaucoma, or hemorrhage.

Normal results

Normal results include restored or improved vision, and a much improved quality of life. Specific improvements depend on the type of ophthalmologic surgery performed, and the type of ocular ailment being treated.

Morbidity and mortality rates

Death from ophthalmologic surgery is rare. However, complications can still arise from the use of general anesthesia. With most ophthalmic surgeries requiring only local anesthetic, that risk has been widely eliminated.

Blindness, which was sometimes caused by serious infection, has also been reduced because of more effective **antibiotics**.

Alternatives

Some medications can be used to treat certain ophthalmic conditions. For example, surgery for glaucoma is performed only in patients who do not respond to medication. Patients with myopia (nearsightedness), hyperopia (farsightedness), or presbyopia (difficulty focusing up close) can wear contact lenses or eyeglasses instead of having refractive surgery to improve their refractive errors.

Resources

BOOKS

Berkow, Robert, ed. *The Merck Manual of Medical Information.* Whitehouse Station, NJ: 1997.

Columbia University College of Physicians & Surgeons Complete Home Medical Guide, 3rd Edition. New York: Crown Publishers, 1995.

Daly, Stephen, ed. *Everything You Need to Know About Medical Treatments.* Springhouse, PA: Springhouse Corp., 1996.

ORGANIZATIONS

American Academy of Ophthalmology. PO Box 7424, San Francisco, CA 94120-7424. (415) 561-8500. http://www.aao.org (accessed April 2, 2008).

American Optometric Association. 243 North Lindbergh Blvd., St. Louis, MO 63141. (314) 991-4100. http://www.aoanet.org (accessed April 2, 2008).

American Society of Cataract and Refractive Surgery. 4000 Legato Road, Suite 850, Fairfax, VA 22033-4055. (703) 591-2220. E-mail: ascrs@ascrs.org; http://www.ascrs.org (accessed April 2, 2008).

National Eye Institute. 2020 Vision Place Bethesda, MD 20892-3655. (301) 496-5248. http://www.nei.nih.gov (accessed April 2, 2008).

University of Michigan Kellogg Eye Center Department of Ophthalmology and Visual Sciences. 1000 Wall Street, Ann Arbor, MI 48105. (734) 763-1415. http://www.kellogg.umich.edu (accessed April 2, 2008).

OTHER

Vision Channel. http://www.visionchannel.net (accessed April 2, 2008).

Mary Bekker
Fran Hodgkins

Ophthalmoscopy

Definition

Ophthalmoscopy involves the use of a lighted scope (ophthalmoscope) that has a very bright light and a number of magnifying lenses. The scope used may be a handheld scope that provides both light source and magnifying lenses (direct ophthalmoscope). Alternatively, the examiner may wear a binocular device and hold a lens to perform this examination (indirect ophthalmoscope). The ophthalmoscope is used to examine the back of the eye (called the fundus). The fundus is lined by the light-sensitive tissue of the retina, and also contains the optic disc, choroids, and blood vessels.

Purpose

Ophthalmoscopy is performed during the course of all routine physical examinations. Additionally, ophthalmoscopy can be performed when symptoms suggest the possible presence of a condition that could affect the eyes. For example, eye diseases such as macular degeneration, glaucoma, retinal detachment, or tumors on the optic nerve can be diagnosed or monitored through ophthalmoscopy. Optalmoscopy may also be used to evaluate and monitor the deleterious effects of diseases of other body systems that may also affect the health of the eye, including such conditions as high blood pressure, atherosclerosis, vascular disease, diabetes, and brain tumors.

Description

Ophthalmosocopy is performed in a dark room. The bright light from the opthalmoscope will be shined into each of the patient's eyes, and the examiner will change the internal lens of the scope to the power that provides the clearest image. The scope will be moved so that all quadrants of the eye can be examined. The individual undergoing the examination may be asked to move his or her eyes in various directions. An instrument to measure pressure in the eyeball may be briefly applied to each eyeball to test for glaucoma. The entire examination is usually completed in under five to ten minutes.

Preparation

There is no advance preparation required for opthalmoscopy. In some cases, such as indirect opthalmoscopy, drops which can dilate the pupils may be put into the patient's eyes several minutes prior to the examination. When the pupils are dilated, it can make the examination easier to perform, and the structures within the eye can be more clearly visualized by the examiner.

Aftercare

When patients have received dilating eyedrops prior to opthalmoscopy, they should wear sunglasses

KEY TERMS

Atherosclerosis—A disease in which plaques of material along the arterial walls cause the arteries to become abnormally hard and stiff. This disease puts people at higher risk for heart attack and stroke.

Choroid—Blood vessels which run between the white of the eye (sclera) and the retina, carrying nutrients and oxygen to the retina.

Glaucoma—A disease in which there is excessive fluid pressure within the eyeball.

Macular degeneration—A progressive disease in which the central portion of the retina (the macula) is gradually destroyed.

Optic disc—A visually inactive portion of the retina from which the optic nerve and blood vessels emerge.

Retina—The light-sensing tissue within the eye that sends signals to the brain in order to generate a visual image.

while outside for the next several hours to protect their eyes from sunlight. Some people find that their vision is affected by the dilatation of their pupils. In this case, they should be advised not to drive until they feel that their vision has returned to normal. Other than these precautions, there is no aftercare necessary following ophthalmoscopy. The patient can immediately return to a normal diet and normal activities.

Risks

Ophthalmoscopy poses no risk to the patient. Under rare circumstances, patients may have a reaction to the dilating eyedrops, such as nausea, vomiting, dry mouth, flushing, dizziness, or a glaucoma episode.

Normal results

Normal results of ophthalmoscope reveal normal anatomy of the back of the eye.

Abnormal results

Abnormalities in the opthalmoscopic examination may indicate a variety of eye disease, trauma to the eye, or other systemic diseases that have effects on the structure or functioning of structures within the eye.

Resources

BOOKS

Yanoff, M., et al. *Ophthalmology*. 2nd ed. St. Louis: Mosby, 2004.

Rosalyn Carson-DeWitt, MD

Opioid analgesics *see* **Analgesics, opioid**
Optional surgery *see* **Elective surgery**

Oral glucose tolerance test

Definition

The oral glucose tolerance test (OGTT) is a series of blood tests that are used to evaluate an individual's response to drinking a standard quantity of a specific glucose-containing solution. The patient drinks the solution, and then the blood is drawn at specific intervals over the next several hours. Each blood test measures the amount of glucose (a particular form of simple sugar) in the blood. The tests are used to evaluate patients for the possibility that they have diabetes.

When carbohydrates are ingested, they are broken down in the intestines into component parts, including sugars such as glucose. Glucose is absorbed from the small intestine into the bloodstream. It circulates throughout the body and is used by all of the body's tissues and organs to generate the energy necessary for their normal functioning. In order for glucose to enter the body's cells, insulin must be present. Insulin is a hormone produced in and excreted by the pancreas. Insulin functions to allow the transport of glucose into the cells of the body, as well as being involved in the body's storage of excess glucose in the form of glycogen or triglycerides.

The blood levels of glucose and insulin are intimately related. When carbohydrates are metabolized after a meal, the blood glucose begins to rise. Under normal circumstances, the pancreas then secretes insulin, in an amount relative to the blood glucose elevation. Between meals, or after heavy exertion, glucose levels may begin to drop below a safe threshold for the body's cells (particular cells of the brain and nervous system). In response to this lowering of blood glucose, the pancreas secretes a different hormone, called glucagon. Glucagon prompts the liver to convert glycogen into glucose, thereby elevating the blood glucose back into a safe range.

Abnormal levels of blood glucose can be life-threatening. High blood glucose is termed hyperglycemia; low blood glucose is termed hypoglycemia. Either of these conditions can result in organ failure, severe brain damage, coma, or **death**. Diabetes occurs when the pancreas fails to produce normal amounts of insulin, or when it completely stops producing any insulin at all (this is often referred to as insulin-dependent or type I diabetes). Diabetes can also occur when cells of the body become less responsive to the effects of insulin (this is often referred to as insulin-resistance, or type II diabetes). Diabetes causes abnormal perturbations of the **serum glucose level**. Over time, chronic high levels of serum glucose (which may occur in poorly controlled diabetes) can result in severe damage to the heart, the eyes, the kidneys, the circulatory system, and the nervous system. In diabetics, sudden, acute increases in the serum glucose level can result in the condition called diabetic ketoacidosis, in which the extremely high levels of blood glucose lead a life-threatening illness. Diabetics can also suffer from sudden drops in serum glucose levels; if untreated, glucose deprivation affecting the organs and tissues of the body can also be life-threatening.

Women are at risk of developing gestational diabetes during pregnancy. While this condition usually resolves after the birth of the baby, and rarely leads to a permanent diagnosis of diabetes, untreated gestational diabetes can result in problems for the baby as well as the mother. Gestational diabetes in early pregnancy can cause birth defects (particularly of the brain and/or heart) and increase the chance of miscarriage. Gestational diabetes in the second and third trimesters can cause the baby to grow very large (termed macrosomia). The baby's size can result in problems for the mother during labor and delivery. Additionally, once the baby is born, it can suffer sudden hypoglycemia. In utero, the baby will have acclimated to its mother's high serum glucose levels by producing high levels of insulin. After birth, suddenly deprived of that glucose, the baby's relatively high insulin levels can result in severe hypoglycemia. If the mother is known to have gestational diabetes, then the baby will be monitored more carefully for potential drops in its blood glucose, and, if necessary, treatment with an IV solution containing glucose can be instituted rapidly.

Purpose

An oral glucose tolerance test is usually performed when there is a suspicion that an individual has Type II diabetes, for example when a serum glucose level has revealed an abnormality, when there is a strong family history of diabetes, when an individual has specific risk factors for diabetes (such as being overweight), or when an individual is experiencing symptoms suggestive of diabetes (excessive thirst and/or hunger, urinary frequency, unintentional weight loss, severe fatigue and weakness, and poor healing). Additionally, an oral glucose tolerance test is almost always ordered as a routine part of prenatal care during the second trimester of pregnancy, usually between 24 and 28 weeks of pregnancy.

Precautions

Serum glucose levels can be affected by a number of medications. Patients who are on these medications should inform their doctor, so that test results can be interpreted appropriately. Medications that may affect serum glucose levels include birth control pills, high blood pressure medications, phenytoin, furosemide, triamterene, hydrochlorothiazide, niacin, propranolol, and steroid medications. Additionally, the use of alcohol, caffeine, or recent illness, infection or emotional distress may affect test results.

Patients who are taking anticoagulant medications should inform their healthcare practitioner, since this may increase their chance of bleeding or bruising after a blood test.

Description

This test requires blood to be drawn from a vein (usually one in the forearm), generally by a nurse or phlebotomist (an individual who has been trained to draw serum). The initial blood draw is performed prior to the patient drinking the glucose solution. The other blood draws are performed at set intervals over the three or so hours after the solution has been ingested.

A tourniquet is applied to the arm above the area where the needle stick will be performed. The site of the needle stick is cleaned with antiseptic, and the needle is inserted. The serum is collected in vacuum tubes. After collection, the needle is withdrawn, and pressure is kept on the serum draw site to stop any bleeding and decrease bruising. A bandage is then applied.

Preparation

The oral glucose tolerance test should only be performed when the individual is in perfectly good health and normally ambulatory/active. For the 72 hours prior to undergoing the OGTT, the individual should be instructed to eat a high-carbohydrate diet (150-200 grams of carbohydrate per day). The test is done on a fasting basis, meaning that nothing should be eaten or drunk after midnight prior to the test (the

KEY TERMS

Gestational diabetes—A type of diabetes that occurs during pregnancy. Untreated, it can cause severe complications for the mother and the baby. However, it usually does not lead to long-term diabetes in either the mother or the child.

Glucose—A simple sugar that is the product of carbohydrate metabolism. It is the major source of energy for all of the organs and tissues of the body.

Glucagon—A hormone produced in the pancreas that is responsible for elevating blood glucose when it falls below a safe level for the body's organs and tissues.

Glycogen—The form in which glucose is stored in the body.

Hyperglycemia—Elevated blood glucose levels.

Hypoglycemia—Low blood glucose levels.

Insulin—A hormone produced by the pancreas that is responsible for allowing the body's cells to utilize glucose. The deficiency or absence of insulin is one of the causes of the disease diabetes.

Ketoacidosis—A potentially life-threatening condition in which abnormally high blood glucose levels result in the blood become too acidic.

Macrosomia—The term used to describe a new-born baby with an abnormally high birth weight.

Pancreas—An organ located near the liver and stomach, responsible for various digestive functions. The pancreas produces insulin and glucagon, hormones that are responsible for maintaining safe blood levels of glucose.

fast should last a minimum of eight and a maximum of sixteen hours). The morning of the exam, the individual should be instructed not to smoke or drink any caffeinated beverages.

Upon arrival at the laboratory, a baseline fasting serum blood glucose will be drawn. Following this, the individual will be asked to drink a solution that contains 75 grams of glucose (pregnant women will drink a 100-gram solution). The solution must be ingested in no more than five minutes. Serum blood glucose levels will be drawn at 30- to 60-minute intervals over the next several hours. A classic oral glucose tolerance test involves five blood draws over the course of the three hour testing period. An abbreviated oral glucose tolerance involves a baseline serum glucose determination, a two-hour wait, and then a second serum glucose level.

Aftercare

As with any blood tests, discomfort, bruising, and/or a very small amount of bleeding is common at the puncture site. Immediately after the needle is withdrawn, it is helpful to put pressure on the puncture site until the bleeding has stopped. This decreases the chance of significant bruising. Warm packs may relieve minor discomfort. Some individuals may feel briefly woozy after a serum test, and they should be encouraged to lie down and rest until they feel better.

Risks

Basic blood tests, such as serum glucose levels, do not carry any significant risks, other than slight bruising and the chance of brief dizziness.

Results

Normal results of a random serum glucose test range from 70-125 milligrams per deciliter (mg/dL). A normal serum glucose level at the two-hour point (two hours after ingesting the glucose solution) is less than 140 mg/dL. During the course of the two hours, any serum glucose levels should be less than 200 mg/dL.

High levels

High serum glucose levels suggest the possibility of diabetes. However, a single high, random serum glucose level is not sufficient for definitively diagnosing diabetes. The American Diabetes Association has specific criteria that must be met in order to diagnose diabetes. They require that results are verified through testing on a minimum of two different days. The oral glucose tolerance is considered to be positive for diabetes when the blood draw at the two-hour point measures 200 mg/dL or higher.

Some individuals don't meet the criteria for an actual diagnosis of diabetes, but have a higher-than-normal fasting serum glucose level, also known as an impaired fasting glucose (ranging from 100 mg/dL to 125 mg/dL), and an elevated 2-hour serum glucose level (ranging between 140 and 199 mg/dL). These individuals are thought to have an increased risk of eventually developing diabetes, and should be followed closely. Some practitioners believe that these serum glucose levels are indicative of "prediabetes."

When an oral glucose tolerance test is performed on a pregnant woman, gestational diabetes is diagnosed if the test reveals any two of the following criteria:

- A fasting serum glucose level greater than 95 mg/dL
- A serum glucose level greater than 180 mg/dL, one hour after ingesting the standardized glucose solution

- A serum glucose level greater than 155 mg/dL, two hours after ingesting the standardized glucose solution
- A serum glucose level greater than 140 mg/dL, three hours after ingesting the standardized glucose solution

A number of conditions other than diabetes can cause high serum glucose levels, including:

- Severe stress
- Heart attack
- Stroke
- Cushing's syndrome
- Steroid medications
- Pheochromocytoma
- Polycystic ovarian disease
- Acromegaly (elevated growth hormone)

Low levels

Low serum glucose levels may be due to:

- The presence of an insulinoma (a tumor that secretes insulin)
- Addison's disease
- Hypothyroidism (underactive thyroid)
- Pituitary gland tumor
- Liver disease, including cirrhosis
- Kidney disease
- Malnutrition
- Eating disorders, including anorexia nervosa
- Inappropriate doses of medicines used to treat diabetes, such as insulin or oral hypoglycemic agents

Resources

BOOKS

Goldman L, Ausiello D., eds. Cecil Textbook of Internal Medicine. 23rd ed. Philadelphia: Saunders, 2008.

Kronenberg HM, Melmed S, Polonsy KS, Larsen PR.Williams Textbook of Endocrinology. 11th ed. Philadelphia: Saunders Elsevier, 2008.

McPherson RA et al. Henry's Clinical Diagnosis and Management By Laboratory Methods. 21st ed. Philadelphia: Saunders, 2007.

ORGANIZATIONS

American Association of Clinical Chemistry. 1850 K St., N.WSuite 625, Washington, DC 20006. http://www.aacc.org.

OTHER

National Institutes of Health. [cited February 10, 2008]. http://www.nlm.nih.gov/medlineplus/encyclopedia.html.

American Diabetes Association. [cited February 10, 2008]. http://www.diabetes.org/home.jsp.

Rosalyn Carson-DeWitt, MD

Orchiectomy

Definition

Orchiectomy is the surgical removal of one or both testicles, or testes, in the human male. It is also called an orchidectomy, particularly in British publications. The removal of both testicles is known as a bilateral orchiectomy, or castration, because the person is no longer able to reproduce. Emasculation is another word that is sometimes used for castration of a male. Castration in women is the surgical removal of both ovaries (bilateral **oophorectomy**).

Purpose

An orchiectomy is done to treat cancer or, for other reasons, to lower the level of testosterone, the primary male sex hormone, in the body. Surgical removal of a testicle is the usual treatment if a tumor is found within the gland itself, but an orchiectomy may also be performed to treat prostate cancer or cancer of the male breast, as testosterone causes these cancers to grow and metastasize (spread to other parts of the body). An orchiectomy is sometimes done to prevent cancer when an undescended testicle is found in a patient who is beyond the age of puberty.

A bilateral orchiectomy is commonly performed as one stage in male-to-female (MTF) gender reassignment surgery. It is done both to lower the levels of male hormones in the patient's body and to prepare the genital area for later operations to construct a vagina and external female genitalia.

Some European countries and four states in the United States (California, Florida, Montana, and Texas) allow convicted sex offenders to request surgical castration to help control their sexual urges. This option is considered controversial in some parts of the legal system. A small number of men with very strong sex drives request an orchiectomy for religious reasons; it should be noted, however, that official Roman Catholic teaching is opposed to the performance of castration for spiritual purity.

Demographics

Cancer

Cancers in men vary widely in terms of both the numbers of men affected and the age groups most likely to be involved. Prostate cancer is the single most common malignancy affecting American men over the age of 50; about 220,000 cases are reported each year. According to the Centers for Disease Control and Prevention

Orchiectomy

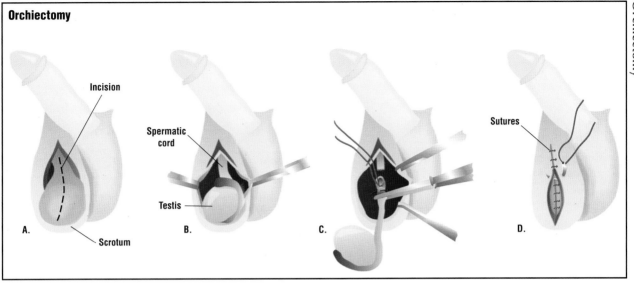

In an orchiectomy, the scrotum is cut open (A). Testicle covering is cut to expose the testis and spermatic cord (B). The cord is tied and cut, removing the testis (C), and the wound is repaired (D). *(Illustration by GGS Information Services. Cengage Learning, Gale.)*

(CDC), 31,000 men in the United States die every year from prostate cancer. African-American men are almost 70% more likely to develop prostate cancer than either Caucasian or Asian-American men; the reasons for this difference are not yet known. Other factors that increase a man's risk of developing prostate cancer include a diet high in red meat, fat, and dairy products, and a family history of the disease. Men whose father or brother(s) had prostate cancer are twice as likely as other men to develop the disease themselves. Today, however, there are still no genetic tests available for prostate cancer.

Testicular cancer, on the other hand, frequently occurs in younger men; in fact, it is the most common cancer diagnosed in males between the ages of 15 and 34. The rate of new cases in the United States each year is about 3.7 per 100,000 people. The incidence of testicular cancer has been rising in the developed countries at a rate of about 2% per year since 1970. It is not yet known whether this increase is a simple reflection of improved diagnostic techniques or whether there are other causes. There is some variation among racial and ethnic groups, with men of Scandinavian background having higher than average rates of testicular cancer, and African-American men having a lower than average incidence. Testicular cancer occurs most often in males in one of three age groups: boys 10 years old or younger; adult males between the ages of 20 and 40; and men over 60.

Other risk factors for testicular cancer include:

- Cryptorchidism, which is a condition in which a boy's testicles do not move down from the abdomen into the scrotum at the usual point in fetal development. It is also called undescended testicle(s). Ordinarily, the testicles descend before the baby is born; however, if the baby is born prematurely, the scrotal sac may be empty at the time of delivery. About 3–4% of full-term male infants are born with undescended testicles. Men with a history of childhood cryptorchidism are three to 14 times more likely to develop testicular cancer.

- Family history of testicular cancer.

- A mother who took diethylstilbestrol (DES) during pregnancy. DES is a synthetic hormone that was prescribed for many women between 1938 and 1971 to prevent miscarriage. It has since been found to increase the risk of certain types of cancer in the offspring of these women.

- Occupational and environmental factors. Separate groups of researchers in Germany and New Zealand reported in 2003 that firefighters have an elevated risk of testicular cancer compared to control subjects. The specific environmental trigger is not yet known.

Gender reassignment

Statistics for orchiectomies in connection with gender reassignment surgery are difficult to establish

KEY TERMS

Androgen—Any substance that promotes the development of masculine characteristics in a person. Testosterone is one type of androgen; others are produced in the adrenal glands located above the kidneys.

Bilateral—On both sides. A bilateral orchiectomy is the removal of both testicles.

Capsule—A general medical term for a structure that encloses another structure or body part. The capsule of the testicle is the membrane that surrounds the glandular tissue.

Castration—Removal or destruction by radiation of both testicles (in a male) or both ovaries (in a female), making the individual incapable of reproducing.

Cryptorchidism—A developmental disorder in which one or both testes fail to descend from the abdomen into the scrotum before birth.

Emasculation—Another term for castration of a male.

Epidural—A type of regional anesthetic delivered by injection into the area around the patient's lower spine. An epidural numbs the body below the waist but allows the patient to remain conscious throughout the procedure.

Gender identity disorder (GID)—A mental disorder in which a person strongly identifies with the other sex and feels uncomfortable with his or her biological sex. It occurs more often in males than in females.

Gender reassignment surgery—The surgical alteration and reconstruction of a person's sex organs to resemble those of the other sex as closely as possible; it is sometimes called sex reassignment surgery.

Inguinal—Referring to the groin area.

Metastasis—A process in which a malignant tumor transfers cells to a part of the body not directly connected to its primary site. A cancer that has spread from its original site to other parts of the body is said to be metastatic.

Oophorectomy—Removal of one or both ovaries in a woman.

Orchiectomy—Surgical removal of one or both testicles in a male. It is also called an orchidectomy.

Scrotum—The pouch of skin on the outside of the male body that holds the testes.

Spermatic cord—A tube-like structure that extends from the testicle to the groin area. It contains blood vessels, nerves, and a duct to carry spermatic fluid.

Subcapsular—Inside the outer tissue covering of the testicle. A subcapsular orchiectomy is a procedure in which the surgeon removes the inner glandular tissue of the testicle while leaving the outer capsule intact.

Testis (plural, testes)—The medical term for a testicle.

Testosterone—The major male sex hormone, produced in the testes.

Tumor marker—A circulating biochemical compound that indicates the presence of cancer. Tumor markers can be used in diagnosis and in monitoring the effectiveness of treatment.

Urology—The branch of medicine that deals with disorders of the urinary tract in both males and females, and with the genital organs in males.

---

because most patients who have had this type of surgery prefer to keep it confidential. Persons undergoing the hormonal treatments and periods of real-life experience as members of the other sex that are required prior to genital surgery frequently report social rejection, job discrimination, and other negative consequences of their decision. Because of widespread social disapproval of surgical gender reassignment, researchers do not know the true prevalence of gender identity disorders in the general population. Early estimates were 1:37,000 males and 1:107,000 females. A recent study in the Netherlands, however, maintains that a more accurate estimation is 1:11,900 males and 1:30,400 females. In any case, the number of surgical procedures is lower than the number of patients diagnosed with gender identity disorders.

Description

There are three basic types of orchiectomy: simple, subcapsular, and inguinal (or radical). The first two types are usually done under local or epidural anesthesia, and take about 30 minutes to perform. An inguinal orchiectomy is sometimes done under **general anesthesia**, and takes between 30 minutes and an hour to complete.

Simple orchiectomy

A simple orchiectomy is performed as part of gender reassignment surgery or as palliative treatment for advanced cancer of the prostate. The patient lies flat on an operating table with the penis taped against the abdomen. After the anesthetic has been given, the surgeon makes an incision in the midpoint of the scrotum and cuts through the underlying tissue. The surgeon removes the testicles and parts of the spermatic cord through the incision. The incision is closed with two layers of sutures and covered with a surgical dressing. If the patient desires, a prosthetic testicle can be inserted before the incision is closed to give the appearance of a normal scrotum from the outside.

Subcapsular orchiectomy

A subcapsular orchiectomy is also performed for treatment of prostate cancer. The operation is similar to a simple orchiectomy, with the exception that the glandular tissue is removed from the lining of each testicle rather than the entire gland being removed. This type of orchiectomy is done primarily to keep the appearance of a normal scrotum.

Inguinal orchiectomy

An inguinal orchiectomy, which is sometimes called a radical orchiectomy, is done when testicular cancer is suspected. It may be either unilateral, involving only one testicle, or bilateral. This procedure is called an inguinal orchiectomy because the surgeon makes the incision, which is about 3 in (7.6 cm) long, in the patient's groin area rather than directly into the scrotum. It is called a radical orchiectomy because the surgeon removes the entire spermatic cord as well as the testicle itself. The reason for this complete removal is that testicular cancers frequently spread from the spermatic cord into the lymph nodes near the kidneys. A long non-absorbable suture is left in the stump of the spermatic cord in case later surgery is necessary.

After the cord and testicle have been removed, the surgeon washes the area with saline solution and closes the various layers of tissues and skin with various types of sutures. The wound is then covered with sterile gauze and bandaged.

Diagnosis/Preparation

Diagnosis

CANCER. The doctor may suspect that a patient has prostate cancer from feeling a mass in the prostate in the course of a rectal examination, from the results of a transrectal **ultrasound** (TRUS), or from elevated levels of prostate-specific antigen (PSA) in the patient's blood. PSA is a tumor marker, or chemical, in the blood that can be used to detect cancer and monitor the results of therapy. A definite diagnosis of prostate cancer, however, requires a tissue biopsy. The tissue sample can usually be obtained with the needle technique. Testicular cancer is suspected when the doctor feels a mass in the

patient's scrotum, which may or may not be painful. In order to perform a biopsy for definitive diagnosis, however, the doctor must remove the affected testicle by radical orchiectomy.

GENDER REASSIGNMENT. Patients requesting gender reassignment surgery must undergo a lengthy process of physical and psychological evaluation before receiving approval for surgery. The Harry Benjamin International Gender Dysphoria Association (HBIGDA), which is presently the largest worldwide professional association dealing with the treatment of gender identity disorders, has published standards of care that are followed by most surgeons who perform genital surgery for gender reassignment. HBIGDA stipulates that a patient must meet the diagnostic criteria for gender identity disorders as defined by either the *Diagnostic and Statistical Manual of Mental Disorders,* fourth edition (*DSM-IV*) or the *International Classification of Diseases–10 (ICD-10)*.

Preparation

All patients preparing for an orchiectomy will have standard blood and urine tests before the procedure. They are asked to discontinue aspirin-based medications for a week before surgery and all non-steroidal anti-inflammatory drugs (NSAIDs) two days before the procedure. Patients should not eat or drink anything for the eight hours before the scheduled time of surgery.

Most surgeons ask patients to shower or bathe on the morning of surgery using a special antibacterial soap. They should take extra time to lather, scrub, and rinse their genitals and groin area.

Patients who are anxious or nervous before the procedure are usually given a sedative to help them relax.

CANCER. Patients who are having an orchiectomy as treatment for testicular cancer should consider banking sperm if they plan to have children following surgery. Although it is possible to father a child if only one testicle is removed, some surgeons recommend banking sperm as a precaution in case the other testicle should develop a tumor at a later date.

GENDER REASSIGNMENT. Most males who have requested an orchiectomy as part of male-to-female gender reassignment have been taking hormones for a period of several months to several years prior to surgery, and have had some real-life experience dressing and functioning as women. The surgery is not performed as an immediate response to the patient's request.

Because the standards of care for gender reassignment require a psychiatric diagnosis as well as a **physical examination**, the surgeon who is performing the orchiectomy should receive two letters of evaluation and recommendation by mental health professionals, preferably one from a psychiatrist and one from a clinical psychologist.

Aftercare

Patients who are having an orchiectomy in an ambulatory surgery center or other outpatient facility must have a friend or family member to drive them home after the procedure. Most patients can go to work the following day, although some may need an additional day of rest at home. Even though it is normal for patients to feel nauseated after the anesthetic wears off, they should start eating regularly when they get home. Some pain and swelling is also normal; the doctor will usually prescribe a pain-killing medication to be taken for a few days.

Other recommendations for aftercare include:

- Drinking extra fluids for the next several days, except for caffeinated and alcoholic beverages.

- Avoiding sexual activity, heavy lifting, and vigorous exercise until the follow-up appointment with the doctor.

- Taking a shower rather than a tub bath for a week following surgery to minimize the risk of absorbable stitches dissolving prematurely.

- Applying an ice pack to the groin area for the first 24–48 hours.

- Wearing a jock strap or snug briefs to support the scrotum for two weeks after surgery.

Some patients may require psychological counseling following an orchiectomy as part of their long-term aftercare. Many men have very strong feelings about any procedure involving their genitals, and may feel depressed or anxious about their bodies or their relationships after genital surgery. In addition to individual psychotherapy, support groups are often helpful. There are active networks of prostate cancer support groups in Canada and the United States as well as support groups for men's issues in general.

Long-term aftercare for patients with testicular cancer includes frequent checkups in addition to radiation treatment or chemotherapy. Patients with prostate cancer may be given various hormonal therapies or radiation treatment.

Risks

Some of the risks for an orchiectomy done under general anesthesia are the same as for other procedures. They include deep venous thrombosis, heart or breathing problems, bleeding, infection, or reaction to the anesthesia. If the patient is having epidural anesthesia, the risks include bleeding into the spinal canal, nerve damage, or a spinal headache.

Specific risks associated with an orchiectomy include:

- loss of sexual desire (This side effect can be treated with hormone injections or gel preparations.)
- impotence
- hot flashes similar to those in menopausal women, controllable by medication
- weight gain of 10–15 lb (4.5–6.8 kg)
- mood swings or depression
- enlargement and tenderness in the breasts
- fatigue
- loss of sensation in the groin or the genitals
- osteoporosis (Men who are taking hormone treatments for prostate cancer are at greater risk of osteoporosis.)

An additional risk specific to cancer patients is recurrence of the cancer.

Normal results

Cancer

Normal results depend on the location and stage of the patient's cancer at the time of surgery. Most prostate cancer patients, however, report rapid relief from cancer symptoms after an orchiectomy. Patients with testicular cancer have a 95% survival rate five years after surgery if the cancer had not spread beyond the testicle. Metastatic testicular cancer, however, has a poorer prognosis.

Gender reassignment

Normal results following orchiectomy as part of a sex change from male to female are a drop in testosterone levels with corresponding decrease in sex drive and gradual reduction of such masculine characteristics as beard growth. The patient may choose to have further operations at a later date.

Morbidity and mortality rates

Orchiectomy by itself has a very low rate of morbidity and mortality. Patients who are having an orchiectomy as part of cancer therapy have a higher risk of **dying** from the cancer than from testicular surgery.

WHO PERFORMS THE PROCEDURE AND WHERE IS IT PERFORMED?

Orchiectomy performed as part of cancer therapy may be done in a hospital under general anesthesia, but is most often done as an outpatient procedure in a urology clinic or similar facility. Most surgeons who perform orchiectomies to treat cancer are board-certified urologists or general surgeons.

Orchiectomies performed as part of gender reassignment surgery are usually done in clinics that specialize in genital surgery. The standards of care defined by the Harry Benjamin International Gender Dysphoria Association stipulate that the surgeon should be a board-certified urologist, gynecologist, plastic surgeon, or general surgeon, and that he or she must have undergone supervised training in genital reconstruction.

The morbidity and mortality rates for persons having an orchiectomy as part of gender reassignment surgery are about the same as those for any procedure involving general or epidural anesthesia.

Alternatives

Cancer

There is no effective alternative to radical orchiectomy in the treatment of testicular cancer; radiation and chemotherapy are considered follow-up treatments rather than alternatives.

There are, however, several alternatives to orchiectomy in the treatment of prostate cancer:

- watchful waiting
- hormonal therapy (The drugs that are usually given for prostate cancer are either medications that oppose the action of male sex hormones [anti-androgens, usually flutamide or nilutamide] or medications that prevent the production of testosterone [goserelin or leuprolide acetate].)
- radiation treatment
- chemotherapy

Gender reassignment

The primary alternative to an orchiectomy for gender reassignment is hormonal therapy. Most patients seeking MTF gender reassignment begin taking female

QUESTIONS TO ASK THE DOCTOR

- How effective is an orchiectomy in preventing a recurrence of my cancer?
- What side effects of this procedure am I most likely to experience?
- How many orchiectomies have you performed?
- Can you recommend a local men's network or support group?

hormones (estrogens) for three to five months minimum before requesting genital surgery. Some persons postpone surgery for a longer period of time, often for financial reasons; others choose to continue on estrogen therapy indefinitely without surgery.

Resources

BOOKS

"Congenital Anomalies: Renal and Genitourinary Defects." Section 19, Chapter 261 in *The Merck Manual of Diagnosis and Therapy,* edited by Mark H. Beers and Robert Berkow. Whitehouse Station, NJ: Merck Research Laboratories, 1999.

Morris, Jan. *Conundrum.* New York: Harcourt Brace Jovanovich, Inc., 1974.

"Principles of Cancer Therapy: Other Modalities." Section 11, Chapter 144 in *The Merck Manual of Diagnosis and Therapy,* edited by Mark H. Beers and Robert Berkow. Whitehouse Station, NJ: Merck Research Laboratories, 1999.

"Sexual and Gender Identity Disorders." In *Diagnostic and Statistical Manual of Mental Disorders,* 4th edition, text revision. Washington, DC: American Psychiatric Association, 2000.

PERIODICALS

Berruti, A., et al. "Background to and Management of Treatment-Related Bone Loss in Prostate Cancer." *Drugs and Aging* 19 (2002): 899–910.

Dawson, C. "Testicular Cancer: Seek Advice Early." *Journal of Family Health Care,* 12 (2002): 3.

Elert, A., K. Jahn, A. Heidenreich, and R. Hofmann. "The Familial Undescended Testis." [in German] *Klinische Padiatrie* 215 (January–February 2003): 40–45.

Geldart, T. R., P. D. Simmonds, and G. M. Mead. "Orchidectomy after Chemotherapy for Patients with Metastatic Testicular Germ Cell Cancer." *BJU International* 90 (September 2002): 451–455.

Incrocci, L., W. C. Hop, A. Wijnmaalen, and A. K. Slob. "Treatment Outcome, Body Image, and Sexual Functioning After Orchiectomy and Radiotherapy for Stage I-II Testicular Seminoma." *International Journal of*

Radiation Oncology, Biology, Physics 53 (August 1, 2002): 1165–1173.

Landen, M., et al. "Done Is Done—and Gone Is Gone. Sex Reassignment is Presently the Best Cure for Transsexuals." [in Swedish] *Lakartidningen* 98 (July 25, 2001): 3322–3326.

Papanikolaou, Frank, and Laurence Klotz. "Orchiectomy, Radical." *eMedicine* October 3, 2001 [March 30, 2003]. http://www.emedicine.com/med/topic3063.htm.

Roberts, L. W., M. Hollifield, and T. McCarty. "Psychiatric Evaluation of a 'Monk' Requesting Castration: A Patient's Fable, with Morals." *American Journal of Psychiatry* 155 (March 1998): 415–420.

Smith, M. R. "Osteoporosis and Other Adverse Body Composition Changes During Androgen Deprivation Therapy for Prostate Cancer." *Cancer and Metastasis Reviews* 21 (2002): 159–166.

Stang, A., K. H. Jockel, C. Baumgardt-Elms, and W. Ahrens. "Firefighting and Risk of Testicular Cancer: Results from a German Population-Based Case-Control Study." *American Journal of Industrial Medicine* 43 (March 2003): 291–294.

Stone, T. H., W. J. Winslade, and C. M. Klugman. "Sex Offenders, Sentencing Laws and Pharmaceutical Treatment: A Prescription for Failure." *Behavioral Sciences and the Law* 18 (2000): 83–110.

ORGANIZATIONS

American Board of Urology (ABU). 2216 Ivy Road, Suite 210, Charlottesville, VA 22903. (434) 979-0059. http://www.abu.org.

American Cancer Society (ACS). (800) ACS-2345. http://www.cancer.org.

American Prostate Society. P. O. Box 870, Hanover, MD 21076. (800) 308-1106. http://www.ameripros.org.

Canadian Prostate Cancer Network. P. O. Box 1253, Lakefield, ON K0L 2H0 Canada. (705) 652-9200. http://www.cpcn.org.

Centers for Disease Control and Prevention (CDC) Cancer Prevention and Control Program. 4770 Buford Highway, NE, MS K64, Atlanta, GA 30341. (888) 842-6355. http://www.cdc.gov/cancer/comments.htm.

Harry Benjamin International Gender Dysphoria Association, Inc. (HBIGDA). 1300 South Second Street, Suite 180, Minneapolis, MN 55454. (612) 625-1500. http://www.hbigda.org.

National Cancer Institute (NCI). NCI Public Inquiries Office. Suite 3036A, 6116 Executive Boulevard, MSC8332, Bethesda, MD 20892-8322. (800) 4-CANCER or (800) 332-8615 (TTY). http://www.nci.nih.gov.

OTHER

Harry Benjamin International Gender Dysphoria Association (HBIGDA). *Standards of Care for Gender Identity Disorders,* 6th version, February, 2001 [April 1, 2003]. http://www.hbigda.org/socv6.html.

National Cancer Institute (NCI) Physician Data Query (PDQ). *Male Breast Cancer: Treatment,* December 9, 2002 [March 29, 2003]. http://www.nci.nih.gov/cancer-info/pdq/treatment/malebreast/healthprofessional.

NCI PDQ. *Testicular Cancer: Treatment,* February 20, 2003 [March 29, 2003]. http://www.nci.nih.gov/cancerinfo/pdq/treatment/testicular/healthprofessional.

Rebecca Frey, PhD

Orchiopexy

Definition

Orchiopexy is a procedure in which a surgeon fastens an undescended testicle inside the scrotum, usually with absorbable sutures. It is done most often in male infants or very young children to correct cryptorchidism, which is the medical term for undescended testicles. Orchiopexy is also occasionally performed in adolescents or adults, and may involve one or both testicles. In adults, orchiopexy is most often done to treat testicular torsion, which is a urologic emergency resulting from the testicle's twisting around the spermatic cord and losing its blood supply.

Other names for orchiopexy include orchidopexy, inguinal orchiopexy, repair of undescended testicle, cryptorchidism repair, and testicular torsion repair.

Purpose

To understand the reasons for performing an orchiopexy in children, it is helpful to have an outline of the normal pattern of development of the testes in a male infant. The gubernaculum is an embryonic cord-like ligament that attaches the testes within the inguinal (groin) region of a male fetus up through the seventh month of pregnancy. Between the 28th and the 35th week of pregnancy, the gubernaculum migrates into the scrotum and creates space for the testes to descend. In normal development, the testes have followed the gubernaculum downward into the scrotum by the time the baby is born. The normal pattern may be interrupted by several possible factors, including inadequate androgen (male sex hormone) secretion, structural abnormalities in the boy's genitals, and defective nerves in the genital region.

Orchiopexy is performed in children for several reasons:

• To minimize the risk of infertility. Adult males with cryptorchidism typically have lower sperm counts and produce sperm of poorer quality than men with normal testicles. The risk of infertility rises

Orchiopexy

An orchiopexy is used to repair an undescended testicle in childhood. An incision is made into the abdomen, the site of the undescended testicle, and another is made in the scrotum (A). The testis is detached from surrounding tissues (B) and pulled out of the abdominal incision attached to the spermatic cord (C). The testis is then pulled down into the scrotum (D) and stitched into place (E). *(Illustration by GGS Information Services. Cengage Learning, Gale.)*

with increasing age at the time of orchiopexy and whether both testicles are affected. Men with one undescended testicle have a 40% chance of being infertile; this figure rises to 70% in men with bilateral cryptorchidism.

• To lower the risk of testicular cancer. The incidence of malignant tumors in undescended testes has been estimated to be 48 times the incidence in normal testes. Men with cryptorchidism have a 10% chance of eventually developing testicular cancer.

KEY TERMS

Cremasteric reflex—A reflex in which the cremaster muscle, which covers the testes and the spermatic cord, pulls the testicles back into the scrotum. It is important for a doctor to distinguish between an undescended testicle and a hyperactive cremasteric reflex in small children.

Cryptorchidism—A developmental disorder in which one or both testes fail to descend from the abdomen into the scrotum before birth. It is the most common structural abnormality in the male genital tract.

Ectopic—Located in an abnormal site or tissue. An ectopic testicle is one that is located in an unusual position outside its normal line of descent into the scrotum.

Gonadotropins—Hormones that stimulate the activity of the ovaries in females and testes in males.

Hernia—The protrusion of a loop or piece of tissue through an incision or abnormal opening in other tissues.

Inguinal—Referring to the groin area.

Laparoscope—An instrument that allows a surgeon to look inside the abdominal cavity.

Non-palpable—Unable to be detected through the sense of touch. A non-palpable testicle is one that is located in the abdomen or other site where the doctor cannot feel it by pressing gently on the child's body.

Orchiectomy—Surgical removal of one or both testicles in a male; also called an orchidectomy.

Perineum—The area between the scrotum and the anus.

Peritoneum—The smooth, colorless membrane that lines the inner surface of the abdomen.

Prune belly syndrome (PBS)—A genetic disorder associated with abnormalities of human chromosomes 18 and 21. Male infants with PBS often have cryptorchidism along with other defects of the genitals and urinary tract. PBS is also known as triad syndrome and Eagle-Barrett syndrome.

Scrotum—The pouch of skin on the outside of the male body that holds the testes.

Spermatic cord—A tube-like structure that extends from the testicle to the groin area. It contains blood vessels, nerves, and a duct to carry spermatic fluid.

Testicular torsion—Twisting of the testicle around the spermatic cord, cutting off the blood supply to the testicle. It is considered a urologic emergency.

Testis (plural, testes)—The medical term for a testicle.

Urology—The branch of medicine that deals with disorders of the urinary tract in both males and females, and with the genital organs in males.

• To lower the risk of traumatic injury to the testicle. Undescended testicles that remain in the patient's groin area are vulnerable to sports injuries and pressure from car seat belts.

• To prevent the development of an inguinal hernia. An inguinal hernia is a disorder that occurs when a portion of the contents of the abdomen pushes through an abnormal opening in the abdominal wall. It is likely to occur in a male infant with cryptorchidism because a sac known as the processus vaginalis, which connects the scrotum and the abdominal cavity, remains open after birth. In normal development, the processus vaginalis closes shortly after the testes descend into the scrotum. If the sac remains open, a section of the child's intestine can extend into the sac. It may become trapped (incarcerated) in the sac, forming what is called a strangulated hernia. The portion of the intestine that is trapped in the sac may die, which is a medical emergency.

• To prevent testicular torsion in adolescence.

• To maintain the appearance of a normal scrotum. Orchiopexy is considered a necessary procedure for psychological reasons, as boys with only one visible testicle are frequently subjected to teasing and ridicule after they start school.

The primary reason for performing an orchiopexy in an adolescent or adult male is treatment of testicular torsion, rather than cryptorchidism. Testicles that have not descended by the time a boy reaches puberty are usually removed by a complete **orchiectomy**.

Demographics

Cryptorchidism

Cryptorchidism is the most common abnormality of the male genital tract, affecting 3–5% of full-term male infants and 30–32% of premature male infants. In most cases, the condition resolves during the first few months after delivery; only 0.8% of infants over three months of age still have undescended testicles.

Because of the potentially serious consequences of cryptorchidism, however, doctors do not advise watchful waiting once the child is over six months old. Undescended testicles rarely come down into the scrotum of their own accord after that age.

Cryptorchidism is a frequent occurrence in prune belly syndrome (PBS) and a few other genetic disorders characterized by structural abnormalities of the genitourinary tract.

No variation in the incidence of cryptorchidism among different racial and ethnic groups has been reported.

Testicular torsion

Most American males suffering from testicular torsion are below age 30, with the majority between the ages of 12 and 18. The peak ages for an acute episode of testicular torsion are the first year of life and age 14. Testicular torsion occurs on the left side of the body slightly more often than on the right side, about 52% versus 48% of cases.

Description

Cryptorchidism

Some orchiopexies in children are relatively simple procedures; however, others are complicated by the location of the undescended testicle. In general, an orchiopexy for an undescended testicle that lies in front of the scrotum or just above it is a less complicated operation than one done to treat a non-palpable testicle. The procedure is usually done under **general anesthesia**.

If the undescended testis is in the groin area, the surgeon will make a small incision in the groin and a second small incision in the scrotum. The testis is moved downward from the groin without complete separation from the gubernaculum. It is then placed inside a small pouch created by the surgeon between the skin of the scrotum and a layer of muscle in the scrotum called the dartos muscle. The testicle is held in place with sutures that are eventually absorbed by the body.

The Fowler-Stephens technique is often used when the undescended testicle is located high above the scrotum or in the abdomen. It may be done in two stages scheduled several months apart. In the first stage, the surgeon moves the testicle downward and attaches it temporarily to the inside of the thigh. In the second stage, the testicle is transferred into the scrotum itself and sutured into place.

A third type of orchiopexy is called testicular autotransplantation. The surgeon removes the undescended testicle completely from its present location and re-implants it in the scrotum by reattaching its surrounding tissues and blood vessels to nearby blood vessels. This technique minimizes the risk of an inadequate blood supply to the re-implanted testicle.

Testicular torsion

An orchiopexy done to treat testicular torsion is usually done under general or epidural anesthesia. The surgeon makes an incision in the patient's scrotum and untwists the spermatic cord. The affected testicle is inspected for signs of necrosis, or tissue **death**. If too much tissue has died due to loss of blood supply, the surgeon will remove the entire testicle. If the tissue appears to be healthy, the surgeon sutures the testicle to the wall of the scrotum and then closes the incision. In most cases, the surgeon will also attach the unaffected testicle to the scrotal wall as a preventive measure.

Diagnosis/Preparation

Cryptorchidism

The diagnosis of cryptorchidism is usually made when a pediatrician examines the newborn baby, although the condition can occur at any time before the boy reaches puberty. The first stage in diagnosis is an external **physical examination** of the child's genitals. If either testicle does not appear to be in the scrotum, the doctor will palpate, or touch, the groin area and abdomen to determine whether a testicle can be felt in any of those locations. If the testicle can be felt, the doctor will decide on the basis of its location whether it is an undescended testicle, a so-called ectopic testicle, or a retractile testicle. An ectopic testicle is one that has developed in a location outside the normal path of development in the inguinal canal. Ectopic testicles are most often discovered along the inner part of the thigh near the groin, at the base of the penis, or below the scrotum in the perineum (the area between the scrotum and the rectum). A retractile testicle is one that is readily pulled back out of the scrotum by an overly sensitive reflex called the cremasteric reflex; it is not a genuinely undescended testicle. It is important for the doctor to distinguish a retractile testicle from genuine cryptorchidism because retractile testicles do not need surgical treatment. At this point in the diagnostic workup, a general pediatrician will often consult a specialist in pediatric urology.

In about 20% of male infants with cryptorchidism, the missing testicle cannot be felt at all. It is known as a non-palpable testicle. The child may be given a hormone challenge test to help determine whether the testicle is located in the abdomen or whether it has failed to develop fully. If the testosterone level in the blood rises in response to the test, the doctor knows that there is a testis present somewhere in the child's body. In other cases, the testis has atrophied, or shriveled up due to an inadequate blood supply before birth. If neither testicle can be felt, the child should be examined further for evidence of intersexuality. The doctor may order an **ultrasound** to check for the presence of a uterus, particularly if the child's external genitals are ambiguous in appearance.

Surgery is the next step in searching for a non-palpable testicle. The surgeon may perform either an open inguinal procedure or a laparoscopic approach. In an open inguinal exploration, the surgeon makes an incision in the child's groin; if nothing is found, the incision may be extended into the lower abdomen. In a laparoscopic approach, the surgeon uses an instrument that looks like a small telescope with a light attached in order to see inside the groin or the abdominal cavity through a much smaller incision. If the surgeon is able to find the testicle, he or she may then proceed directly to perform an orchiopexy.

Testicular torsion

Testicular torsion is usually diagnosed in the emergency room. The doctor will usually suspect testicular torsion on the basis of sudden onset of severe pain on one side of the scrotum; it is unusual for pain to develop gradually in this disorder. The patient's history often indicates recent hard physical work, vigorous **exercise**, or trauma to the genital area; however, testicular torsion can also occur without any apparent reason. Other symptoms may include swelling of the scrotum, blood in the semen, nausea and vomiting, pain in the abdomen, and fever. A few patients feel the need to urinate frequently. When the doctor examines the patient's scrotum, the affected testicle is usually enlarged and is painful when the doctor touches it. It usually lies higher in the scrotum than the unaffected testicle and may be lying in a horizontal position.

Since testicular torsion is a medical emergency, most doctors will not risk permanent damage to the testicle by taking the time to perform imaging studies. If the diagnosis is unclear, however, the doctor may order a radionuclide scan or a color Doppler ultrasound to determine whether the blood flow to the testicle has been cut off. The patient will be given a mild pain medication and referred to a urologist for surgery as soon as possible.

Aftercare

Cryptorchidism

Aftercare in children depends partly on the complexity of the procedure. If the child has an uncomplicated orchiopexy, he can usually go home the same day. If the surgeon had to make an incision in the abdomen to find a non-palpable testicle before performing the orchiopexy, the child may remain in the hospital for two to three days. The doctor will usually prescribe a pain medication for the first few days after the procedure.

After the child returns home, he should not bathe until the day after surgery. In addition, he should not ride a bicycle, climb trees, or do anything else that requires straddling for two to three weeks. An older boy should avoid sports or rough games that might result in injury to the genitals until he has a post-surgical checkup.

Most surgeons will schedule the child for a checkup one or two weeks after the orchiopexy, with a second checkup three months later.

Testicular torsion

Aftercare is similar to that for orchiopexy in a child. The area around the incision should be washed very gently the next day and a clean dressing applied. Medication will be prescribed for postoperative pain. The patient is advised to rest at home for several days after surgery, to remain in bed as much as possible, to drink extra fluids, and to elevate the scrotum on a small pillow to ease the discomfort. Vigorous physical and sexual activity should be avoided until the pain and swelling go away.

Risks

Cryptorchidism

The risks of orchiopexy in treating cryptorchidism include:

- infection of the incision
- bleeding
- damage to the blood vessels and other structures in the spermatic cord, leading to eventual loss of the testicle
- failure of the testicle to remain in the scrotum (This problem can be repaired by a second operation.)
- difficulty urinating for a few days after surgery

WHO PERFORMS THE PROCEDURE AND WHERE IS IT PERFORMED?

A pediatric surgeon or pediatric urologist is the specialist most likely to perform an orchiopexy in an infant or small child. In an adult patient, the procedure is usually performed by a urologist after referral from the patient's primary physician or the emergency care physician.

An orchiopexy can be performed in the surgical unit of a children's hospital or an ambulatory surgical center. Most orchiopexies in adults are performed as outpatient procedures.

Testicular torsion

The risks of orchiopexy as a treatment for testicular torsion include:

- infection of the incision
- bleeding
- loss of blood circulation in the testicle leading to loss of the testicle
- reaction to anesthesia

Normal results

In a normal orchiopexy, the testicle remains in the scrotum without re-ascending. If the procedure has been successful, there is no damage to the blood vessels supplying the testicle, no loss of fertility, and no recurrence of torsion.

Morbidity and mortality rates

Cryptorchidism

Orchiopexy is most likely to be successful in children when the undescended testicle is relatively close to the scrotum. The rate of failure for orchiopexy performed as a treatment for cryptorchidism is 8% if the testicle lies just above the scrotum; 10–20% if the testicle is located in the inguinal canal; and 25% if the testicle lies within the abdomen.

Testicular torsion

The mortality rate for orchiopexy in adults is very low because almost all patients are young males in good health. The procedure has a 99% rate of success in saving the testicle when the diagnosis is made promptly and treated within six hours. After 12 hours, however,

QUESTIONS TO ASK THE DOCTOR

- How often have you treated a child for cryptorchidism?
- What are the chances that the treatment will be successful?
- What should I tell my son about the operation?
- Are there likely to be any long-term aftereffects?

the rate of success in saving the testicle drops to 2%. The average rate of testicular atrophy following orchiopexy for testicular torsion is about 27%.

Alternatives

Cryptorchidism

Hormonal therapy using gonadotropins to stimulate the production of more testosterone is effective in some children in causing the testes to descend into the scrotum without surgery. This approach, however, is usually successful only with undescended testes that are already close to the scrotum; its rate of success ranges from 10–50%. Undescended testes that are located higher almost never respond to hormonal therapy. In addition, treatment with hormones has several undesirable side effects, including aggressive behavior.

Some surgeons will, however, prescribe hormonal treatment before an orchiopexy in order to increase the size of the undescended testis and make it easier to identify during surgery.

Testicular torsion

Pain caused by testicular torsion can be relieved temporarily by manual detorsion. To perform this maneuver, the doctor stands at the patient's feet and gently rotates the affected testicle toward the outside of the patient's body in a sidewise direction. Manual detorsion is effective in relieving pain in 30–70% of patients; however, it is not considered an alternative to orchiopexy in preventing a recurrence of the torsion or loss of the testicle.

Resources

BOOKS

"Congenital Anomalies: Renal and Genitourinary Defects." Section 19, Chapter 261 in *The Merck Manual of*

Diagnosis and Therapy, edited by Mark H. Beers and Robert Berkow. Whitehouse Station, NJ: Merck Research Laboratories, 1999.

PERIODICALS

Baker, L. A., et al. "A Multi-Institutional Analysis of Laparoscopic Orchidopexy." *BJU International,* 87 (April 2001): 484–489.

Chang, B., L. S. Palmer, and I. Franco. "Laparoscopic Orchidopexy: A Review of a Large Clinical Series." *BJU International,* 87 (April 2001): 490–493.

Docimo, S. G., R. I. Silver, and W. Cromie. "The Undescended Testicle: Diagnosis and Management." *American Family Physician,* 62 (November 1, 2000): 2037–2044, 2047–2048.

Dogra, Vikram S., and Hamid Mojibian. "Cryptorchidism." *eMedicine,* June 21, 2002 [April 4, 2003]. www.emedicine.com/radio/topic201.htm.

Franco, Israel. "Prune Belly Syndrome." *eMedicine,* August 24, 2001 [April 4, 2003]. www.emedicine.com/med/topic3055.htm.

Jawdeh, Bassam Abu, and Samir Akel. "Cryptorchidism: An Update." *American University of Beirut Surgery,* (Summer 2002) [April 3, 2003]. www.staff.aub.edu.lb/~websurgp/sc0a.html.

Nair, S. G., and B. Rajan. "Seminoma Arising in Cryptorchid Testis 25 Years After Orchiopexy: Case Report." *American Journal of Clinical Oncology,* 25 (June 2002): 287–288.

Rupp, Timothy J., and Mark Zwanger. "Testicular Torsion." *eMedicine,* March 25, 2003 [April 4, 2003]. www.emedicine.com/EMERG/topic573.htm.

Sessions, A. E., et al. "Testicular Torsion: Direction, Degree, Duration, and Disinformation." *Journal of Urology,* 169 (February 2003): 663–665.

Shekarriz, B., and M. L. Stoller. "The Use of Fibrin Sealant in Urology." *Journal of Urology,* 167 (March 2002): 1218–1225.

Tsujihata, M., et al. "Laparoscopic Diagnosis and Treatment of Nonpalpable Testis." *International Journal of Urology,* 8 (December 2001): 692–696.

ORGANIZATIONS

American Academy of Pediatrics (AAP). 141 Northwest Point Boulevard, Elk Grove Village, IL 60007. (847) 434-4000. http://www.aap.org.

American Board of Urology (ABU). 2216 Ivy Road, Suite 210, Charlottesville, VA 22903. (434) 979-0059. http://www.abu.org.

National Organization for Rare Disorders (NORD). 55 Kenosia Avenue, P. O. Box 1968, Danbury, CT 06813-1968. (203) 744-0100. http://www.rarediseases.org.

Prune Belly Syndrome Network. P. O. Box 2125, Evansville, IN 47728-0125. http://www.prunebelly.org.

Rebecca Frey, PhD

Orthopedic surgery

Definition

Orthopedic (sometimes spelled orthopaedic) surgery is an operation performed by a medical specialist such as an orthopedist or orthopedic surgeon, who is trained to assess and treat problems that develop in the bones, joints, and ligaments of the human body.

Purpose

Orthopedic surgery addresses and attempts to correct problems that arise in the skeleton and its attachments, the ligaments and tendons. It may also include some problems of the nervous system, such as those that arise from injury of the spine. These problems can occur at birth, through injury, or as the result of aging. They may be acute, as in an accident or injury, or chronic, as in many problems related to aging.

Orthopedics comes from two Greek words, *ortho,* meaning straight, and *pais,* meaning child. Originally, orthopedic surgeons treated skeletal deformities in children, using braces to straighten the child's bones. With the development of anesthesia and an understanding of the importance of **aseptic technique** in surgery, orthopedic surgeons extended their role to include surgery involving the bones and related nerves and connective tissue.

The terms orthopedic surgeon and orthopedist are used interchangeably today to indicate a medical doctor with special training and certification in orthopedics.

Many orthopedic surgeons maintain a general practice, while some specialize in one particular aspect of orthopedics such as **hand surgery**, joint replacements, or disorders of the spine. Orthopedists treat both acute and chronic disorders. Some orthopedic surgeons specialize in trauma medicine and can be found in emergency rooms and trauma centers, treating injuries. Others find their work overlapping with plastic surgeons, geriatric specialists, pediatricians, or podiatrists (foot care specialists). A rapidly growing area of orthopedics is sports medicine, and many sports medicine doctors are board certified in orthopedic surgery.

Demographics

The American Academy of Orthopedic Surgeons reports that in January 2008, there are 31,309 members within all categories of orthopedic surgeons in the United States.

KEY TERMS

Arthroplasty—The surgical reconstruction or replacement of a joint.

Prosthesis—A synthetic replacement for a missing part of the body such as a knee or a hip.

Range of motion—The normal extent of movement (flexion and extension) of a joint.

Description

The range of treatments provided by orthopedists is extensive. They include procedures such as **traction, amputation,** hand reconstruction, **spinal fusion,** and joint replacements. They also treat strains and sprains, broken bones, and dislocations. Some specific procedures performed by orthopedic surgeons are listed as separate entries in this book, including **arthroplasty, arthroscopic surgery, bone grafting, fasciotomy, fracture repair, kneecap removal,** and traction.

In general, orthopedists are employed by hospitals, medical centers, trauma centers, or free-standing surgical centers where they work closely with a **surgical team,** including an anesthesiologist and surgical nurse. Orthopedic surgery can be performed under general, regional, or **local anesthesia.**

Much of the work of an orthopedic surgeon involves adding foreign material to the body in the form of screws, wires, pins, tongs, and prosthetics to hold damaged bones in their proper alignment or to replace damaged bone or connective tissue. Great improvements have been made in the development of artificial limbs and joints, and in the materials available to repair damage to bones and connective tissue. As developments occur in the fields of metallurgy and plastics, changes will take place in orthopedic surgery that will allow surgeons to more nearly duplicate the natural functions of bones, joints, and ligaments, and to more accurately restore damaged parts to their original ranges of motion.

Diagnosis/Preparation

Persons are usually referred to an orthopedic surgeon by a primary care physician, emergency room physician, or other doctor. Prior to any surgery, candidates undergo extensive testing to determine appropriate corrective procedures. Tests may include x rays, computed tomography (CT) scans, **magnetic resonance imaging** (MRI), myelograms, diagnostic arthroplasty, and blood tests. The orthopedist will determine the

WHO PERFORMS THE PROCEDURE AND WHERE IS IT PERFORMED?

Orthopedic surgery is performed by a physician with specialized training in orthopedic surgery. It is most commonly performed in operating room of a hospital. Very minor procedures such as setting a broken bone may be performed in a professional office or an emergency room of a hospital.

history of the disorder and any treatments that were previously tried. A period of rest to the injured part may be recommended before surgery is undertaken.

Surgical candidates undergo standard blood and urine tests before surgery and, for major procedures, may be given an **electrocardiogram** or other diagnostic tests prior to the operation. Individuals may choose to donate some of their own blood to be held in reserve for their use in major surgery such as **knee replacement,** during which heavy bleeding is common.

Aftercare

Rehabilitation from orthopedic injuries can require long periods of time. Rehabilitation is usually physically and mentally taxing. Orthopedic surgeons will work closely with physical therapists to ensure that patients receive treatment that will enhance the range of motion and return function to all affected body parts.

Risks

As with any surgery, there is always the risk of excessive bleeding, infection, and allergic reaction to anesthesia. Risks specifically associated with orthopedic surgery include inflammation at the site where foreign materials (pins, prostheses, or wires) are introduced into the body, infection as the result of surgery, and damage to nerves or to the spinal cord.

Normal results

Thousands of people have successful orthopedic surgery each year to recover from injuries or to restore lost function. The degree of success in individual recoveries depends on an individual's age and general health, the medical problem being treated, and a person's willingness to comply with rehabilitative therapy after the surgery.

QUESTIONS TO ASK THE DOCTOR

- What tests will be performed prior to surgery?
- How will the procedure affect daily activities after recovery?
- Where will the surgery be performed?
- What form of anesthesia will be used?
- What will be the resulting appearance and level of function after surgery?
- Is the surgeon board certified by the American Academy of Orthopedic Surgeons?
- How many similar procedures has the surgeon performed?
- What is the surgeon's complication rate?

Abnormal results from orthopedic surgery include persistent pain, swelling, redness, drainage or bleeding in the surgical area, surgical wound infection resulting in slow healing, and incomplete restoration of pre-surgical function.

Morbidity and mortality rates

Mortality from orthopedic surgical procedures is not common. The most common causes for mortality are adverse reactions to anesthetic agents or drugs used to control pain, post-surgical clot formation in the veins, and post-surgical heart attacks or strokes.

Alternatives

For the removal of diseased, non-functional, or non-vital tissue, there is no alternative to orthopedic surgery. Alternatives to orthopedic surgery depend on the condition being treated. Medications, acupuncture, or hypnosis are used to relieve pain. Radiation is an occasional alternative for shrinking growths. Chemotherapy may be used to treat bone cancer. Some foreign bodies may remain in the body without harm.

Resources

BOOKS

Browner BD et al. Skeletal Trauma: Basic science, management, and reconstruction. 3rd ed. Philadelphia: Elsevier, 2003.

Canale, ST, ed. Campbell's Operative Orthopaedics. 10th ed. St. Louis: Mosby, 2003.

DeLee, JC and D. Drez.DeLee and Drez's Orthopaedic Sports Medicine. 2nd ed. Philadelphia: Saunders, 2005.

PERIODICALS

O'Brien, J. G. "Orthopedic Surgery: A New Frontier." Mayo Clinic Proceedings 78, no.3 (2003): 275–277.

Ribbans, W. J. "Orthopaedic Care in Haemophilia." Hospital Medicine 64, no.2 (2003): 68–69.

Showstack, J. "Improving Quality of Care in Orthopedic Surgery." Arthritis and Rheumatism 48, no.2 (2003): 289–290.

ORGANIZATIONS

American Academy of Orthopedic Surgeons. 6300 North River Road Rosemont, IL 60018-4262. (847) 823-7186 or (800) 346-2267. http://www.aaos.org/wordhtml/home2.htm.

American College of Sports Medicine. 401 West Michigan Street, Indianapolis, IN 46202-3233 (Mailing Address: P.O. Box 1440, Indianapolis, IN 46206-1440). (317) 637-9200, Fax: (317) 634-7817. http://www.acsm.org.

American College of Surgeons. 633 North Saint Claire Street, Chicago, IL 60611. (312) 202-5000. http://www.facs.org/.

American Society for Bone and Mineral Research 2025 M Street, NW, Suite 800, Washington, DC 20036-3309. (202) 367-1161. http://www.asbmr.org/.

Orthopedic Trauma Association. 6300 N. River Road, Suite 727, Rosemont, IL 60018-4226. (847) 698-1631. http://www.ota.org/links.htm.

OTHER

American Osteopathic Association. [cited April 7, 2003]. http://www.aoa-net.org/Certification/orthopedsurg.htm.

Brigham and Woman's Hospital (Harvard University School of Medicine). [cited April 7, 2003]. <http://splweb.bwh.harvard.edu:8000/pages/projects/ortho/ortho.html>.

Martindale's Health Science Guide, 2003. [cited April 7, 2003]. <http://www-sci.lib.uci.edu/HSG/Medical Surgery.html>.

Thomas Jefferson University Hospital. [cited April 7, 2003]. http://www.jeffersonhospital.org/e3front.dll?durki=4529.

University of Maryland College of Medicine. [cited April 7, 2003]. http://www.umm.edu/surg-ortho/.

L. Fleming Fallon, Jr, MD, DrPH

Orthopedic x rays *see* **Bone x rays**

Orthotopic transplantation *see* **Liver transplantation**

Osteotomy, hip *see* **Hip osteotomy**

Osteotomy, knee *see* **Knee osteotomy**

Otolaryngologic surgery *see* **Ear, nose, and throat surgery**

Otoplasty

Definition

Otoplasty refers to a group of **plastic surgery** procedures done to correct deformities of or disfiguring injuries to the external ear. It is the only type of plastic surgery that is performed more often in children than adults.

Purpose

Otoplastic surgery may done for the following reasons:

• To reconstruct an external ear in children who are born with a partially or completely missing auricle (the visible part of the external ear). This type of birth defect is called microtia; it occurs in such disorders as hemifacial microsomia and Treacher Collins syndrome. Most cases of microtia, however, involve only one ear.

• To correct the appearance of protruding or prominent ears. This procedure is also known as setback otoplasty or pinback otoplasty.

• To correct major disparities in the size or shape of a patient's ears.

• To reshape deformed ears. One congenital type of deformity is known as Stahl's ear, which is characterized by a pointed upper edge produced by the flattening of the ear rim and folding of the cartilage. Stahl's deformity is also known as Vulcan ear or Spock ear because it resembles the ears of the well-known *Star Trek* character.

• To repair or reconstruct the auricle after traumatic injuries or cancer surgery.

Otoplasty is considered reconstructive rather than **cosmetic surgery**. Consequently, it is often covered by health insurance. People who are considering

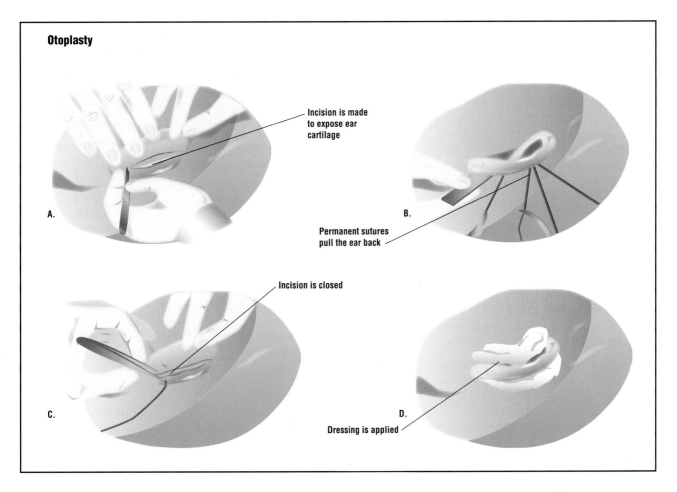

Otoplasty

Incision is made to expose ear cartilage

A.

Permanent sutures pull the ear back

B.

Incision is closed

C.

Dressing is applied

D.

During an otoplasty, an incision is made in the back of the ear, exposing cartilage (A). Permanent sutures in the cartilage pull the ear back closer to the skull (B). The incision is closed (C), and dressings are applied (D). *(Illustration by GGS Information Services. Cengage Learning, Gale.)*

otoplasty for themselves or their children should check with their insurance carrier about coverage. The average surgeon's fee for an otoplasty in the United States in 2001 was $3,114.

Otoplasty is not done to correct hearing difficulties related to the structures of the middle and inner ear. Hearing problems are treated surgically by otolaryngologists (physicians who specialize in ear, nose, and throat procedures).

Demographics

Statistics for congenital deformities of the external ear are difficult to obtain because the causes are so diverse. Such genetic disorders as Treacher Collins syndrome and hemifacial microsomia affect between one in 3,500 and one in 10,000 children. In addition, microtia has been associated with certain medications taken during pregnancy—particularly anticonvulsants, which are drugs given to treat epilepsy, and isotretinoin, a drug prescribed for severe acne.

Stahl's deformity is found more often among Asian Americans than among Caucasian or African Americans. As of 2003, it is thought to be a hereditary disorder.

Setback or pinback otoplasty is the most frequently performed procedure for reconstruction of prominent or protruding ears. According to the American Society of Plastic Surgeons, 30,137 setback otoplasties were performed in the United States in 2006. There are no exact statistics on the incidence of protruding ears in the general population, although about 8% of patients treated for this deformity have a family history of it. Large or protruding ears appear to be equally common in males and females; however, it is easier for girls and women to avoid social discomfort by styling their hair to cover their ears. This factor may explain why a slight majority (53%) of setback otoplasties is done on boys. Although most setback otoplasties are performed in children between the ages of four and 14, the second largest group of patients in this category is women in their 20s and 30s.

The most common cause of trauma requiring otoplasty is human and animal bites. Although exact figures are not known because many bite cases are not reported, a large percentage of dog and human bites cause wounds on the head and neck. With regard to human bites, the single most common injury requiring medical treatment is auricular avulsion, or tearing of the external ear. In the United States, 93% of patients treated for ear injuries caused by human bites are males between the ages of 15 and 25. Most cases of auricular avulsion in children, however, are

KEY TERMS

Auricle—The portion of the external ear that is not contained inside the head. It is also called the pinna.

Avulsion—A type of injury caused by ripping or tearing. Most ear injuries requiring otoplasty are avulsion injuries.

Concha—The hollow shell-shaped portion of the external ear.

Congenital—Present at the time of birth.

Ear molding—A non-surgical method for treating ear deformities shortly after birth with the application of a mold held in place by tape and surgical glue.

Hematoma—A localized collection of blood in an organ or tissue due to broken blood vessels.

Hemifacial microsomia (HFM)—A term used to describe a group of complex birth defects characterized by underdevelopment of one side of the face.

Microtia—The partial or complete absence of the auricle of the ear.

Pinna—Another name for the auricle; the visible portion of the external ear.

Setback otoplasty—A surgical procedure done to reduce the size or improve the appearance of large or protruding ears; it is also known as pinback otoplasty.

Stahl's deformity—A congenital deformity of the ear characterized by a flattened rim and pointed upper edge caused by a fold in the cartilage; it is also known as Vulcan ear or Spock ear.

Treacher Collins syndrome—A disorder that affects facial development and hearing, thought to be caused by a gene mutation on human chromosome 5. Treacher Collins syndrome is sometimes called mandibulofacial dysostosis.

caused by dog bites, which are likely to cause crushing as well as tearing of the tissues.

Description

Otoplasty in children is performed under **general anesthesia**; in adults, it may be done under either general anesthesia or **local anesthesia** with sedation. Most otoplasties take about two to three hours to complete. Many plastic surgeons prefer to use absorbable sutures when performing an otoplasty in order to minimize the risk of disturbing the shape of the ear by removing **stitches** later.

Otoplasty for microtia

Otoplasty for microtia requires a series of three or four separate operations. In the first operation, a piece of cartilage is removed from the child's rib cage on the side opposite the affected ear, so that the surgeon can use the natural curve of the cartilage in fashioning the new ear. The surgeon works from a template derived from photographs and computer models when he or she carves the cartilage into the desired shape. The cartilage is then carefully positioned under the skin on the side of the face. The skin will shape itself to fit the cartilage framework of the new ear. The second and third operations are done to shape the ear lobe and to raise the new ear into its final position.

Otoplasty for protruding ears

There is no universally accepted single technique for performing a setback otoplasty. Variations in the procedure are due partly to the different causes of ear protrusion. The patient's ear may have a large concha (the shell-like hollow of the external ear); the angle of the fold in the ear cartilage may cause the ear to protrude; or the ear lobe may be unusually large.

After the patient has been anesthetized, the surgeon makes an incision behind the ear in the fold of skin where the ear meets the head. In one technique, the surgeon exposes the ear cartilage beneath the skin and reshapes it or removes a small piece. The cartilage is bent back toward the head and secured in place with non-removable sutures. Removal of cartilage is sometimes referred to as a conchal resection.

Another procedure for protruding ears involves the removal of skin and suturing the cartilage back on itself. This technique reshapes the ear without the need to remove cartilage; it is sometimes called a cartilage-sparing otoplasty.

After the surgeon has finished reshaping the ear and carefully drying the area, the incision is closed. The surgeon covers the ear with a cotton dressing moistened with mineral oil or other soft dressing.

Diagnosis/Preparation

Congenital abnormalities of the ear

Diagnosis of microtia is made by the obstetrician or pediatrician at the time of the child's birth. The diagnosis of prominent or protruding ears, however, is somewhat more complex because the deformity is a matter of shape and proportion rather than the absence or major malformation of a body part. The head of a newborn infant is larger in proportion to its body than is the case in adults, and as a result, the shape of the ears may not concern the parents until the child is two to three years old.

Otoplasty to correct microtia is usually started when the child is at least five years old. The surgeon must remove a portion of rib cartilage in order to construct a framework for the missing ear, and children younger than five may not have enough cartilage. In addition, it is easier for the surgeon to use the child's normal ear as a model for the size and shape of the reconstructed ear when the child is five to seven years old. Otoplasty for microtia is preceded by consultations between the surgeon and the child's parents. Following the diagnosis, a comprehensive treatment plan is made that includes long-term psychosocial as well as surgical follow-up. The reconstruction of a missing ear must be done in several stages because the surgeon must allow for changes in the proportions of the child's face and skull as he or she matures as well as attempt to make the new ear look as normal as possible.

There continues to be some debate among plastic surgeons concerning the best age for performing a setback otoplasty. Many recommend the operation when the child is between five and seven years old. One reason is that the human ear has attained 85–90% of its adult size by this age, and therefore the surgeon can estimate the final size and shape of the ear with considerable accuracy. In addition, the cartilage in the ear is still relatively soft and easier for the surgeon to reshape. Another reason for performing an otoplasty in children in the early elementary school years is psychological; name-calling and teasing by peers can be emotionally destructive for children in this age bracket. On the other hand, some surgeons have reported performing setback otoplasties on children as young as nine months with no disturbances in the growth of the ear or recurrence of the problem.

Preparation for otoplasty in children should include an assessment of the child's feelings about the procedure. Some surgeons consider opposition on the child's part to be a contraindication for surgery, as well as unrealistic expectations on the part of the parents. In general, a positive attitude is associated with faster recovery and better overall results.

Preparation for otoplasty in adults includes a **physical examination** and standard blood tests. Patients are usually advised to discontinue taking **aspirin** and any other medications that thin the blood for two weeks prior to surgery. Plastic surgeons strongly urge adult patients to quit smoking before the surgery, because smoking delays and complicates the healing process. Adult patients are also asked to shower and shampoo their hair thoroughly on the morning of the procedure. Men should have a haircut or trim a day or two before surgery; women should braid or pin their hair close to the head.

Trauma

Avulsion injuries caused by bites, thermal or chemical burns resulting from industrial accidents, and other traumatic injuries of the auricle are diagnosed by emergency physicians.

Plastic surgery for traumatic injuries of the auricle is preceded by thorough cleansing of the wound and **debridement** of damaged tissue. It is important to treat ear injuries promptly because the ears are not well supplied with blood vessels. This characteristic makes it easier for infection to develop in parts of the auricle where the skin has been torn open or crushed. In some cases, plastic surgery is postponed for a few days and the patient is given oral penicillin to prevent infection.

Aftercare

After an otoplasty, the patient's head is wrapped with a turban-type bandage that is worn for four to five days following surgery. The patient is instructed to wear a ski-type headband over the ears continuously for about a month after the turban is removed, and then at night for an additional two months. Warm compresses should be applied to the ears two to three times a day for two weeks after the turban is removed.

Patients should follow the surgeon's instructions about washing their hair, and avoid holding hot-air blow dryers too close to the ear.

Patients should also avoid contact sports for at least three months after otoplasty. An anti-inflammatory medication (Kenalog) can be applied to the ear in the event of abnormal scar formation.

Risks

Some risks associated with otoplasties are common to all operations performed under general anesthesia. They include bleeding or infection of the incision; numbness or loss of feeling in the area around the incision; and a reaction to the anesthesia.

Specific risks associated with otoplasties include the following:

- Formation of abnormal scar tissue. This complication can usually be corrected later; plastic surgeons advise waiting at least six months for revision surgery.
- Hematoma, which is a collection of blood within a body organ or tissue caused by leakage from broken

WHO PERFORMS THE PROCEDURE AND WHERE IS IT PERFORMED?

Otoplasties for microtia and prominent or deformed ears are specialized procedures performed only by qualified plastic surgeons. Plastic surgeons are doctors who have completed three years of general surgical training, followed by two to three years of specialized training in plastic surgery. There are, however, relatively few plastic surgeons who perform otoplasties for microtia.

Ear molding as an alternative to surgery is performed by a plastic surgeon as an outpatient or office procedure.

Traumatic injuries of the external ear are treated initially by an emergency physician, trauma surgeon, or plastic surgeon; in most cases, an otolaryngologist is consulted to determine whether the inner structures of the ear have also been injured. Revision plastic surgery may be performed later to remove scar tissue.

blood vessels. In the case of the ear, a hematoma can damage the results of plastic surgery because it creates tension and pressure that distort the final shape of the ear. Careful drying of the ear at the end of the procedure and application of a pressure bandage can reduce the risk of a hematoma. In the event that one develops, it is treated by reopening the incision and draining the collected blood.

- Distortion of the shape of the ear caused by overcorrection of deformed features.
- Reappearance of ear protrusion (in setback otoplasty). This complication is most likely to occur in the first six months after surgery.

Normal results

The normal result of an otoplasty is a reconstructed or reshaped ear that resembles a normal ear (or the patient's other ear) more closely. In a setback otoplasty, the normal result is an ear that lies closer to the patient's head without an overcorrected, "pinned-back" look.

Morbidity and mortality rates

The mortality rate in otoplasty is extremely low and is almost always associated with anesthesia reactions. The most common complication reported is

QUESTIONS TO ASK THE DOCTOR

- How long will it take for the ear to assume its final shape?
- How much change in the shape of the ear can be reasonably expected?
- Would my child benefit from ear molding rather than surgery?
- How many otoplasties have you performed?

asymmetrical ears (18.4%), followed by skin irritation (9.8%); increased sensitivity to cold (7.5%); soreness when the ear is touched (5.7%); abnormal shape to the ear (4.4%); loss of feeling in the ear (3.9%); bleeding (2.6%); and hematoma (0.4%).

Alternatives

Some ear deformities in children, including protruding ears and Stahl's deformity, can be treated with ear molding in the early weeks of life, when the cartilage in the ear can be reshaped by the application of splints and Steri-Strips. One technique involves making a mold in the shape desired for the child's ear from dental compound and attaching it to the ear with methylmethacrylate **glue**. The ear and the mold are held in place with surgical tape and covered with a tubular bandage or ear wrap for reinforcement. The mold and tape must be worn constantly for six weeks, with a change of dressing every two weeks. Ear molding is reported to be about 85% effective when it is started within six weeks after the baby's birth. It costs less than surgery—about $600—and is considerably less painful. The chief disadvantage of ear molding is its ineffectiveness in treating ear deformities characterized by the absence of skin and cartilage rather than distorted shape.

There are no effective alternatives to otoplasty in treating ear deformities or injuries in adults; however, some plastic surgeons use custom-made silicone molds to help maintain the position of the ears in adult patients for several weeks after surgery.

Resources

BOOKS

Cummings, CW, et al.Otolayrngology: Head and Neck Surgery. 4th ed. St. Louis: Mosby, 2005.

PERIODICALS

Adamson PA "Otoplasty technique." Otolaryngology Clinics of North America 40 (April 2007): 305–18.

Aygit, A. C. "Molding the Ears After Anterior Scoring and Concha Repositioning: A Combined Approach for Protruding Ear Correction." Aesthetic Plastic Surgery 27 (March 14, 2003) [e-publication ahead of print].

Bauer, B. S., D. H. Song, and M. E. Aitken. "Combined Otoplasty Technique: Chondrocutaneous Conchal Resection as the Cornerstone to Correction of the Prominent Ear." Plastic and Reconstructive Surgery 110 (September 15, 2002): 1033–1040.

Furnas, D. W. "Otoplasty for Prominent Ears." Clinics in Plastic Surgery 29 (April 2002): 273–288.

Gosain, A. K., and R. F. Recinos. "Otoplasty in Children Less than Four Years of Age: Surgical Technique." Journal of Craniofacial Surgery 13 (July 2002): 505–509.

Manstein, Carl H. "Ear, Congenital Deformities." eMedicine, May 31, 2005 [accessed April 22, 2008]. www.emedicine.com/plastic/topic207.htm.

Peker, F., and B. Celikoz. "Otoplasty: Anterior Scoring and Posterior Rolling Technique in Adults." Aesthetic Plastic Surgery 26 (July–August 2002): 267–273.

Vital, V., and A. Printza. "Cartilage-Sparing Otoplasty: Our Experience." Journal of Laryngology and Otology 116 (September 2002): 682–685.

Yugueros, P., and J. A. Friedland. "Otoplasty: The Experience of 100 Consecutive Patients." Plastic and Reconstructive Surgery 108 (September 15, 2001): 1045–1051.

ORGANIZATIONS

American Academy of Facial Plastic and Reconstructive Surgery (AAFPRS). 310 South Henry Street, Alexandria, VA 22314. (703) 299-9291. www.facemd.org.

American Society of Plastic Surgeons (ASPS). 444 East Algonquin Road, Arlington Heights, IL 60005. (847) 228-9900. www.plasticsurgery.org.

FACES: The National Craniofacial Association. P. O. Box 11082, Chattanooga, TN 37401. (800) 332-2373. www.faces-cranio.org.

National Organization for Rare Disorders (NORD). 55 Kenosia Avenue, P. O. Box 1968, Danbury, CT 06813-1968. (203) 744-0100.

OTHER

American Academy of Facial Plastic and Reconstructive Surgery. 2001 Membership Survey: Trends in Facial Plastic Surgery. Alexandria, VA: AAFPRS, 2002.

American Academy of Facial Plastic and Reconstructive Surgery. Procedures: Understanding Otoplasty Surgery, [April 6, 2003]. www.facial-plastic-surgery.org/patient/procedures/otoplasty.html.

American Society of Plastic Surgeons. Procedures: Otoplasty, [April 5, 2003]. www.plasticsurgery.org/public_education/procedures/Otoplasty.cfm.

Rebecca Frey, PhD

Otosclerosis surgery *see* **Stapedectomy**

Outpatient surgery

Definition

Outpatient surgery, also referred to as ambulatory surgery, is defined by the American Hospital Association (AHA) as "a surgical operation, whether major or minor, performed on patients who do not remain in the hospital overnight." Outpatient surgery may be performed in inpatient operating suites, outpatient surgery suites, or procedure rooms within an outpatient care facility. Patients may go home after being released following the procedure and time spent in the **recovery room**.

Purpose

Mounting pressure to keep hospitalization costs down and improved technology have increased the frequency of outpatient surgery, with shorter medical procedure duration, fewer complications, and lower cost. As of 2006, about 53% of all surgical procedures in the United States are performed on an outpatient basis.

According to the Agency for Healthcare Research and Quality, about 90% of outpatient surgeries in the United States are performed to treat an illness or disorder; the remaining 10% are diagnostic procedures.

Description

Due to improved pain control, advanced medical techniques—including those that reduce recovery time—and cost-cutting considerations, more and more surgeries are being performed on an outpatient basis. Surgeries suited to a nonhospital setting generally are those with a low percentage of postoperative complications, which would require serious attention by a physician or nurse. Outpatient surgery continues to mushroom: in 1984, roughly 400,000 outpatient surgeries were performed; by 2000, the number had risen to 8.3 million; and from 1993 to 2001, the number of freestanding **ambulatory surgery centers** in the United States increased by 150%. A 2002 study reported that 65% of all surgical procedures did not involve a hospital stay; this proportion is expected to increase to 75% by 2015. These statistics also reflect the fact that many patients (especially children) prefer to recover at home or in a familiar setting.

With increased technological advances in instruments such as the arthroscope and laparoscope, more physicians are performing surgery in their offices or in other outpatient settings, primarily ambulatory clinics and surgical centers, or surgicenters. Among the most frequently performed outpatient surgeries are tonsillectomies, arthroscopy, **cosmetic surgery**, removal of cataracts, gynecological, urological and orthopedic procedures, wound and hernia repairs, and gallbladder removals. Even such procedures as microscopically controlled surgery under **local anesthesia** for skin cancer have been recommended on an outpatient basis.

Preparation

While many outpatient surgeries are covered by insurance plans, many are not. Candidates for such surgeries should check in advance with their insurance carrier concerning whether their procedures are covered on an outpatient basis. **Medicare** and **Medicaid** patients should also check whether these programs will cover the cost of their surgeries.

Preparing for outpatient surgery varies, of course, with the surgical procedure to be performed. There are, however, guidelines common to most outpatient surgeries. Patients should be in good health before undergoing ambulatory surgery. Colds, fever, chills, or flu symptoms are all reasons to postpone a procedure, and surgical candidates should notify their primary health care physicians if such conditions exist.

Patients should check with their physician for all information covering preparation for outpatient procedures. A near-universal requirement is to have a family member or friend take charge of delivering the patient to surgery, either to wait there or to arrive in time to pick up the patient on release from recovery. The evening before, a light meal is recommended to preoperative patients, with no alcohol taken for a full day before surgery. Nothing is to be taken by mouth after midnight of the day preceding surgery. Smokers should stop or cut back on smoking prior to surgery. Loose-fitting clothing is recommended, and patients should bring along enough money to cover postoperative prescription drugs.

KEY TERMS

Ambulatory surgery—Surgery done on an outpatient basis; the patient goes home the same day.

Ambulatory surgery center—An outpatient facility with at least two operating rooms, either connected or not connected to a hospital.

Outpatient procedures—Surgeries that are performed on an outpatient basis, involving less recovery time and fewer expected complications.

This same information applies if the outpatient is a child. If children are permitted clear liquids on the day of outpatient surgery, parents will be told when the child must stop taking them. Surgery will be cancelled or delayed if these requirements are not met.

Results

The benefits of outpatient surgery include lower medical costs, tighter scheduling—because patients are not subject to the potential delays encountered in hospital operating rooms—and what many patients would consider a less stressful environment than a hospital setting. Recovery time spent in one's own home, either with familiar caregivers or home nurses, is a choice many postoperative patients prefer to recuperation in a hospital.

Complications related to surgery occur less than 1% of the time in outpatient settings. However, in terms of patient safety, nonhospital settings are not as closely regulated as are hospitals, so patients should inquire about potential risks concerning outpatient surgery that arise in ambulatory clinics, surgical centers, and physicians' offices. There are guidelines for surgery in outpatient settings, but oversight and enforcement may vary. Patients may wish to find out whether their outpatient center is licensed or certified as a medical facility or is accredited in the states that require this. The latter may be accomplished by contacting the Joint Commission (formerly the Joint Commission for Accreditation of Healthcare Organizations).

Among problems encountered during outpatient surgery are those concerning anesthesia administration, infection, bleeding that calls for a **transfusion**, and respiratory and resuscitation events. Some patients are at higher risk than others of requiring inpatient admission after an outpatient procedure. These include patients over the age of 65; operations lasting longer than 120 minutes; the need for **general anesthesia**; and patients with heart problems, cancer, or vascular disease.

Resources

BOOKS

Fiebach, Nicholas H., ed. *Principles of Ambulatory Medicine*, 7th ed. Philadelphia: Lippincott Williams and Wilkins, 2007.

Joint Commission on Accreditation of Healthcare Organizations. *Standards for Ambulatory Surgical Centers*. Oakbrook Terrace, IL: JCAHO, 2007.

PERIODICALS

Bian, J., and M. A. Morrisey. "Free-standing Ambulatory Surgery Centers and Hospital Surgery Volume." *Inquiry* 44 (Summer 2007): 200–210.

Eggertson, L. "Ten-Year Trend: Surgeries Up, Hospitalizations Down." *Canadian Medical Association Journal* 176 (March 13, 2007): 756.

Fleisher, L. A., L. R. Pasternak, and A. Lyles. "A Novel Index of Elevated Risk of Inpatient Hospital Admission Immediately Following Outpatient Surgery." *Archives of Surgery* 142 (March 2007): 263–268.

ORGANIZATIONS

American Hospital Association (AHA). One North Franklin, Chicago, IL 60606-3421. (312) 422-3000. http://www.aha.org/aha_app/index.jsp (accessed April 2, 2008).

Joint Commission. One Renaissance Blvd. Oakbrook Terrace, IL 60181. (630) 792-5000. http://www.jointcommission.org/ (accessed April 2, 2008).

OTHER

Questions To Ask Your Doctor Before You Have Surgery, Agency for Health Care Research and Quality. http://www.ahcpr.gov/consumer/surgery.htm#head2/ (accessed April 2, 2008).

Russo, C. Allison, et al. *Ambulatory Surgery in U.S. Hospitals, 2003*. Rockville, MD: Agency for Healthcare Research and Quality, 2007.

Wax, C. M. *Preparation for Surgery*. http://healthisnumberone.com/libsurgprep.htm (accessed April 2, 2008).

Nancy McKenzie, PhD
Rebecca Frey, PhD

Ovary and fallopian tube removal *see* **Salpingo-oophorectomy**

Ovary removal *see* **Oophorectomy**

Oxygen therapy

Definition

Oxygen may be classified as an element, a gas, and a drug. Oxygen therapy is the administration of oxygen at concentrations greater than that in room air to treat or prevent hypoxemia (not enough oxygen in the blood). Oxygen delivery systems are classified as stationary, portable, or ambulatory. Oxygen can be administered by nasal cannula, mask, and tent. Hyperbaric oxygen therapy involves placing the patient in an airtight chamber with oxygen under pressure.

Purpose

The body is constantly taking in oxygen and releasing carbon dioxide. If this process is inadequate, oxygen levels in the blood decrease, and the patient may need supplemental oxygen. Oxygen therapy is a

KEY TERMS

Arterial blood gas test—A blood test that measures oxygen and carbon dioxide in the blood.

Atelectasis—Partial or complete collapse of the lung, usually due to a blockage of the air passages with fluid, mucus or infection.

Breathing rate—The number of breaths per minute.

Cannula—Also called nasal cannula. A small, lightweight plastic tube with two hollow prongs that fit just inside the nose. Nasal cannulas are used to supply supplemental oxygen through the nose.

Cyanosis—Blue, gray, or dark purple discoloration of the skin caused by a deficiency of oxygen.

Ductus arteriosis—A fetal blood vessel that connects the aorta and pulmonary artery.

Flow meter—Device for measuring the rate of a gas (especially oxygen) or liquid.

Hypoxemia—Oxygen deficiency, defined as an oxygen level less than 60 mm Hg or arterial oxygen saturation of less than 90%. Different values are used for infants and patients with certain lung diseases.

Oxygenation—Saturation with oxygen.

Peak expiratory flow rate—A test used to measure how fast air can be exhaled from the lungs.

Pulmonary function tests—A series of tests that measure how well air is moving in and out of the lungs and carrying oxygen to the bloodstream.

Pulmonary rehabilitation—A program that helps patients learn how to breathe easier and improve their quality of life. Pulmonary rehabilitation includes treatment, exercise training, education, and counseling.

Pulmonologist—A physician who specializes in caring for people with lung diseases and breathing problems.

Pulse oximetry—A non-invasive test in which a device that clips onto the finger measures the oxygen level in the blood.

Residual volume—The volume of air remaining in the lungs, measured after a maximum expiration.

Respiratory failure—The sudden inability of the lungs to provide normal oxygen delivery or normal carbon dioxide removal.

Respiratory therapist—A health care professional who specializes in assessing, treating, and educating people with lung diseases.

Total lung capacity test—A test that measures the amount of air in the lungs after a person has breathed in as much as possible.

Vital capacity—Maximal breathing capacity; the amount of air that can be expired after a maximum inspiration.

key treatment in respiratory care. The purpose is to increase oxygen saturation in tissues where the saturation levels are too low due to illness or injury. Breathing prescribed oxygen increases the amount of oxygen in the blood, reduces the extra work of the heart, and decreases shortness of breath. Oxygen therapy is frequently ordered in the **home care** setting, as well as in acute (urgent) care facilities.

Some of the conditions oxygen therapy is used to treat include:

- documented hypoxemia
- severe respiratory distress (e.g., acute asthma or pneumonia)
- severe trauma
- chronic obstructive pulmonary disease (COPD, including chronic bronchitis, emphysema, and chronic asthma)
- pulmonary hypertension
- cor pulmonale

- acute myocardial infarction (heart attack)
- short-term therapy, such as postanesthesia recovery

Oxygen may also be used to treat chronic lung disease patients during **exercise**.

Hyperbaric oxygen therapy is used to treat the following conditions:

- gas gangrene
- decompression sickness
- air embolism
- smoke inhalation
- carbon monoxide poisoning
- cerebral hypoxic event

Helium-oxygen therapy is a treatment that may be used for patients with severe airway obstruction. The combination of helium and oxygen, known as heliox, reduces the density of the delivered gas, and has been shown to reduce the effort of breathing and improve ventilation when an airway obstruction is present.

This type of treatment may be used in an emergency room for patients with acute, severe asthma.

Description

Oxygen delivery (other than mechanical ventilators and hyperbaric chambers)

In the hospital, oxygen is supplied to each patient room via an outlet in the wall. Oxygen is delivered from a central source through a pipeline in the facility. A flow meter attached to the wall outlet accesses the oxygen. A valve regulates the oxygen flow, and attachments may be connected to provide moisture. In the home, the oxygen source is usually a canister or air compressor. Whether in home or hospital, plastic tubing connects the oxygen source to the patient.

Oxygen is most commonly delivered to the patient via a nasal cannula or mask attached to the tubing. The nasal cannula is usually the delivery device of choice since it is well tolerated and doesn't interfere with the patient's ability to communicate, eat, or drink. The concentration of oxygen inhaled depends upon the prescribed flow rate and the ventilatory minute volume (MV).

Another delivery option is transtracheal oxygen therapy, which involves a small flexible catheter inserted in the trachea or windpipe through a tracheostomy tube. In this method, the oxygen bypasses the mouth, nose, and throat, and a humidifier is required at flow rates of 1 liter (2.1 pt) per minute and above. Other oxygen delivery methods include tents and specialized infant oxygen delivery systems.

TYPES OF OXYGEN DELIVERY SYSTEMS. The types of oxygen delivery systems include:

- Compressed oxygen—oxygen that is stored as a gas in a tank. A flow meter and regulator are attached to the oxygen tank to adjust oxygen flow. Tanks vary in size from very large to smaller, portable tanks. This system is generally prescribed when oxygen is not needed constantly (e.g., when it is only needed when performing physical activity).
- Liquid oxygen—oxygen that is stored in a large stationary tank that stays in the home. A portable tank is available that can be filled from the stationary tank for trips outside the home. Oxygen is liquid at very cold temperatures. When warmed, liquid oxygen changes to a gas for delivery to the patient.
- Oxygen concentrator—electric oxygen delivery system approximately the size of a large suitcase. The concentrator extracts some of the air from the room, separates the oxygen, and delivers it to the patient via a nasal cannula. A cylinder of oxygen is provided as a

backup in the event of a power failure, and a portable tank is available for trips outside the home. This system is generally prescribed for patients who require constant supplemental oxygen or who must use it when sleeping.
- Oxygen conserving device, such as a demand inspiratory flow system or pulsed-dose oxygen delivery system—uses a sensor to detect when inspiration (inhalation) begins. Oxygen is delivered only upon inspiration, thereby conserving oxygen during exhalation. These systems can be used with either compressed or liquid oxygen systems, but are not appropriate for all patients.

Preparation

A physician's order is required for oxygen therapy, except in emergency use. The need for supplemental oxygen is determined by inadequate oxygen saturation, indicated in blood gas measurements, pulse oximetry, or clinical observations. The physician will prescribe the specific amount of oxygen needed by the patient. Some patients require supplemental oxygen 24 hours a day, while others may only need treatments during exercise or sleep. No special patient preparation is required to administer oxygen therapy.

Patient education

SELECTING AN OXYGEN SYSTEM. A health care provider will meet with the patient to discuss the oxygen systems available. A system recommendation will be made, based on the patient's overall condition and personal needs, as well as the system's ease of use, reliability, cost, range of oxygen delivery, and features. The health care provider can give the patient a list of medical supply companies that stock home oxygen equipment and supplies. The patient can meet with home care representatives from these companies to evaluate the product lines that best fit his or her needs. Patients in the home setting are directed to notify the vendors when replacement oxygen supplies are needed.

OXYGEN SAFETY. Patients will receive instructions about the safe use of oxygen in the home. Patients must be advised not to change the flow rate of oxygen unless directed to do so by the physician.

Oxygen supports combustion, therefore no open flame or combustible products should be permitted when oxygen is in use. These include petroleum jelly, oils, and aerosol sprays. A spark from a cigarette, electric razor, or other electrical device could easily ignite oxygen-saturated hair or bedclothes around the patient. Explosion-proof plugs should be used for vaporizers and humidifier attachments. The patient should be sure to have a functioning smoke detector and fire extinguisher in the home at all times.

Care must be taken with oxygen equipment used in the home or hospital. The oxygen system should be kept clean and dust-free. Cylinders should be kept in carts, or have collars for safe storage. If not stored in a cart, smaller canisters may be lain on the floor. Knocking cylinders together can cause sparks, so bumping them should be avoided. In the home, the oxygen source must be placed at least 6 ft (1.8 m) away from flames or other sources of ignition, such as a lit cigarette. Oxygen tanks should be kept in a well–ventilated area. Oxygen tanks should not be kept in the trunk of a car. "No Smoking—Oxygen in Use" signs should be used to warn visitors not to smoke near the patient.

Special care must be given when administering oxygen to premature infants because of the danger of high oxygen levels causing retinopathy of prematurity, or contributing to the construction of ductus arteriosis. PaO_2 (partial pressure of oxygen) levels greater than 80 mm Hg should be avoided.

Patients who are undergoing a laser **bronchoscopy** should receive concurrent administration of supplemental oxygen to avoid burns to the trachea.

Insurance clearance

The patient should check with his or her insurance provider to determine if the treatment is covered and what out-of-pocket expenses may be incurred. Oxygen therapy is usually fully or partially covered by most insurance plans, including **Medicare**, when prescribed according to specific guidelines. Usually test results indicating the medical necessity of the supplemental oxygen are needed before insurance clearance is granted.

Travel guidelines

Traveling with oxygen requires advanced planning. The patient needs to obtain a letter from his or her health care provider that verifies all medications, including oxygen. In addition, a copy of the patient's oxygen prescription must be shown to travel personnel. Home health care companies can help the patient make travel plans, and can arrange for oxygen when the patient arrives at his or her destination. Patients cannot bring or use their own oxygen tanks on an airplane; therefore the patient must leave his or her portable oxygen tank at the airport before boarding. Oxygen suppliers can pick up the oxygen unit from the airport if necessary, or a family member can take it home.

Aftercare

Once oxygen therapy is initiated, periodic assessment and documentation of oxygen saturation levels is required. Follow-up monitoring includes blood gas measurements and pulse oximetry tests. If the patient is using a mask or a cannula, gauze can be tucked under the tubing to prevent irritation of the cheeks or the skin behind the ears. Water-based lubricants can be used to relieve dryness of the lips and nostrils.

Risks

Oxygen is not addictive and causes no side effects when used as prescribed. Complications from oxygen therapy used in appropriate situations are infrequent. Respiratory depression, oxygen toxicity, and absorption atelectasis are the most serious complications of oxygen overuse.

A physician should be notified and emergency services may be required if the following symptoms develop:

- frequent headaches
- anxiety
- cyanotic (blue) lips or fingernails
- drowsiness
- confusion
- restlessness
- slow, shallow, difficult, or irregular breathing

Oxygen delivery equipment may present other problems. Perforation of the nasal septum as a result of using a nasal cannula and non–humidified oxygen has been reported. In addition, bacterial contamination of nebulizer and humidification systems can occur, possibly leading to the spread of pneumonia. High-flow systems that employ heated humidifiers and aerosol generators, especially when used by patients with artificial airways, also pose a risk of infection.

Normal results

A normal result is a patient that demonstrates adequate oxygenation through pulse oximetry, blood gas tests, and clinical observation. Signs and symptoms of inadequate oxygenation include cyanosis, drowsiness, confusion, restlessness, anxiety, or slow, shallow, difficult, or irregular breathing. Patients with obstructive airway disease may exhibit "aerophagia" (air hunger) as they work to pull air into the lungs. In cases of carbon monoxide inhalation, the oxygen saturation can be falsely elevated.

Resources

BOOKS

Mason, RJ et al. Murray & Nadel's Textbook of Respiratory Medicine. 4th ed. Philadelphia: Saunders, 2007.

Hyatt, Robert E., Paul D. Scanlon, Masao Nakamura,. Interpretation of Pulmonary Function Tests: A Practical Guide, 2nd ed. Philadelphia: Lippincott Williams and Wilkins Publishers, 2003.

Wilkins, Robert, et al. Egan's Fundamentals of Respiratory Care, 8th ed. St. Louis: Mosby, 2003.

Yutsis, Pavel I. Oxygen to the Rescue: Oxygen Therapies and How They Help Overcome Disease, Promote Repair, and Improve Overall Function. Basic Health Publications, Inc., 2003.

ORGANIZATIONS

American Association for Cardiovascular and Pulmonary Rehabilitation (AACVPR). 7600 Terrace Avenue, Suite 203, Middleton, Wisconsin 53562. (608) 831-6989. E-mail: aacvpr@tmahq.com. http://www.aacvpr.org.

American Association for Respiratory Care. 11030 Ables Lane, Dallas, Texas 75229. (972) 243-2272. E-mail: info@aarc.org. http://www.aarc.org.

American College of Chest Physicians. 3300 Dundee Road, Northbrook, Illinois 60062-2348. (847) 498-1400. http://www.chestnet.org.

American Lung Association and American Thoracic Society. 1740 Broadway, New York, NY 10019-4374. (800) LUNG-USA or (800) 586-4872. http://www.lungusa.org.

National Heart, Lung and Blood Institute. Information Center. P.O. Box 30105, Bethesda, Maryland 20824. (301) 251-2222. http://www.nhlbi.nih.gov/nhlbi/.

National Jewish Medical and Research Center. Lung-Line. 14090 Jackson Street, Denver, Colorado 80206. http://www.nationaljewish.org.

OTHER

Daily Lung. http://www.dailylung.com. A full-feature magazine covering lung disease and related health topics.

National Lung Health Education Program. http://www.nlhep.org.

Pulmonary Paper. P.O. Box 877, Ormond Beach, Florida 32175. (800) 950-3698. http://www.pulmonarypaper.org. Not-for-profit newsletter supporting people with chronic lung problems.

Maggie Boleyn, R.N., B.S.N.
Angela M. Costello
Rosalyn Carson-DeWitt, MD

Oxytocin *see* Uterine stimulants

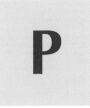

Pacemaker implantation *see* **Pacemakers**

Pacemakers

Definition

A pacemaker is a surgically implanted electronic device that regulates a cardiac arrhythmia.

Pacemakers are most frequently prescribed when the heartbeat decreases under 60 beats per minute at rest (severe symptomatic bradycardia). They are also used in some cases to slow a fast heart rate over 120 beats per minute at rest (tachycardia).

Demographics

The population for pacemaker implant is not limited by age, sex, or race. Over 100,000 pacemakers are implanted per year in the United States. The occurrence is more frequent in the elderly with over 85% of implants received by those over age 65. A history of myocardial infarction (heart attack), congenital defect, or cardiac transplant also increases the likelihood of pacemaker implant.

Description

Approximately 500,000 Americans have an implantable permanent pacemaker device. A pacemaker implantation is performed under **local anesthesia** in a hospital by a surgeon assisted by a cardiologist. An insulated wire called a lead is inserted into an incision above the collarbone and guided through a large vein into the chambers of the heart. Depending on the configuration of the pacemaker and the clinical needs of the patient, as many as three leads may be used in a pacing system. Current pacemakers have a double, or bipolar, electrode attached to the end of each lead. The electrodes deliver an electrical charge to the heart to regulate

heartbeat. They are positioned on the areas of the heart that require stimulation. The leads are then attached to the pacemaker device, which is implanted under the skin of the patient's chest.

Patients undergoing surgical pacemaker implantation usually stay in the hospital overnight. Once the procedure is complete, the patient's **vital signs** are monitored and a **chest x ray** is taken to ensure that the pacemaker and leads are properly positioned.

Modern pacemakers have sophisticated programming capabilities and are extremely compact. The smallest weigh less than 13 grams (under half an ounce) and are the size of two stacked silver dollars. The actual pacing device contains a pulse generator, circuitry programmed to monitor heart rate and deliver stimulation, and a lithium iodide battery. Battery life typically ranges from seven to 15 years, depending on the number of leads the pacemaker is configured with and how much energy the pacemaker uses. When a new battery is required, the unit can be exchanged in a simple outpatient procedure.

A temporary pacing system is sometimes recommended for patients who are experiencing irregular heartbeats as a result of a recent heart attack or other acute medical condition. The implantation procedure for the pacemaker leads is similar to that for a permanent pacing system, but the actual pacemaker unit housing the pulse generator remains outside the patient's body. Temporary pacing systems may be replaced with a permanent device at a later date.

Diagnosis/Preparation

Patients being considered for pacemaker implantation will undergo a full battery of cardiac tests, including an **electrocardiogram** (ECG), electrophysiological study, or both, to fully evaluate the bradycardia or tachycardia.

The symptoms of fatigue and lightheadedness that are characteristic of bradycardia can also be caused by

KEY TERMS

Electrocardiogram (ECG)—A recording of the electrical activity of the heart. An ECG uses externally attached electrodes to detect the electrical signals of the heart.

Electrophysiological study—A test that monitors the electrical activity of the heart in order to diagnose arrhythmia. An electrophysiological study measures electrical signals through a cardiac catheter that is inserted into an artery in the leg and guided up into the atrium and ventricle of the heart.

Embolism—A blood clot, air bubble, or clot of foreign material that blocks the flow of blood in an artery. When an embolism blocks the blood supply to a tissue or organ, the tissue the artery feeds dies (infarction). Without immediate and appropriate treatment, an embolism can be fatal.

Magnetic resonance imaging (MRI)—An imaging technique that uses a large circular magnet and radio waves to generate signals from atoms in the body. These signals are used to construct images of internal structures.

a number of other medical conditions, including anemia. Certain prescription medications can also slow the heart rate. A doctor should take a complete medical history and perform a full physical work-up to rule out all non-cardiac causes of bradycardia.

Patients are advised to abstain from eating six to eight hours before the surgical procedure. The patient is usually given a sedative to help him or her relax for the procedure. An intravenous (IV) line will also be inserted into a vein in the patient's arm before the procedure begins in case medication or blood products are required during the insertion.

Aftercare

After an implant without complications the patient can expect a hospital stay of one to five postprocedure days. Pacemaker patients should schedule a follow-up visit with their cardiologist approximately six weeks after the surgery. During this visit, the doctor will make any necessary adjustments to the settings of the pacemaker. Pacemakers are programmed externally with a handheld electromagnetic device. Pacemaker batteries must be checked regularly. Some pacing systems allow patients to monitor battery life through a special telephone monitoring service that can read pacemaker signals.

WHO PERFORMS THIS PROCEDURE AND WHERE IS IT PERFORMED?

Pacemaker implants are performed by a cardiologist who has completed medical school and an additional internship and residency program. Additional training as an electrophysiologist may be acquired by the physician during the residency program. Specific training by the pacemaker manufacturer may also be acquired. Hospitals performing these procedures have access to cardiac catheterization facilities or operating rooms equipped with portable fluoroscopy units.

Patients with cardiac pacemakers should not undergo a **magnetic resonance imaging** (MRI) procedure. Devices that emit electromagnetic waves (including magnets) may alter pacemaker programming or functioning. A 1997 study found that cellular phones often interfere with pacemaker programming and cause irregular heart rhythm. However, advances in pacemaker design and materials have greatly reduced the risk of pacemaker interference from electromagnetic fields.

Risks

Because pacemaker implantation is an invasive surgical procedure, internal bleeding, infection, hemorrhage, and embolism are all possible complications. Infection is more common in patients with temporary pacing systems. Antibiotic therapy given as a precautionary measure can reduce the risk of pacemaker infection. If infection does occur, the entire pacing system may have to be removed.

The placing of the leads and electrodes during the implantation procedure also presents certain risks for the patient. The lead or electrode could perforate the heart or cause scarring or other damage. The electrodes can also cause involuntary stimulation of nearby skeletal muscles.

A complication known as pacemaker syndrome develops in approximately 7% of pacemaker patients with single-chamber pacing systems. The syndrome is characterized by the low blood pressure and dizziness that are symptomatic of bradycardia. It can usually be corrected by the implantation of a dual-chamber pacing system.

QUESTIONS TO ASK THE DOCTOR

- How many pacemaker implants has the physician performed?
- What type of pacemaker will be implanted, univentricular or biventricular, and how many of the specific procedure has the physician performed?
- How long will the expected hospital stay be?
- What precautions should be taken in the weeks following discharge from the hospital?
- What precautions will need to taken in day to day activities following pacemaker implant?
- When can normal daily, such as driving, exercise and work, activities be initiated?
- What will indicate that the pacemaker is failing and when should emergency care be sought?
- How long will the battery function and when should treatment to replace the device be sought?
- Is there special documentation I will need for air travel during security screenings?
- Will there be notification of manufacturer recalls?

Normal results

Pacemakers that are properly implanted and programmed can correct a patient's arrhythmia and resolve related symptoms.

Morbidity and mortality rates

In the United States, patients experience complications in 3.3% and 3.8% of cases, with those over 65 years of age demonstrating a slightly higher complication rate of 6.1%. The most common complications include lead dislodgement, pneumothorax (collapsed lung), and cardiac perforation. The risk of **death** is less then 0.5% throughout the course of the hospital stay.

Resources

BOOKS

Libby, P. et al. Braunwald's Heart Disease. 8th ed. Philadelphia: Saunders, 2007.

PERIODICALS

Gregoratas, Gabriel, et al. "ACC/AHA Guideline Update for Implantation of Pacemakers and Antiarrhythmia Devices." Circulation 106(2002): 1175–209.

ORGANIZATIONS

American Heart Association. 7320 Greenville Ave. Dallas, TX 75231. (214) 373-6300. http://www.american heart. org.

Paula Anne Ford-Martin
Allison J. Spiwak, MSBME

Packed cell volume *see* **Hematocrit**

Packed red blood cell volume *see* **Hematocrit**

Pain management

Definition

Pain itself is defined by the International Association for the Study of Pain (IASP) as "an unpleasant sensory and emotional experience associated with actual or potential tissue damage or described in terms of such damage." Thus, pain management encompasses all interventions used to understand and ease pain, and if possible to alleviate the cause of the pain.

Purpose

Pain serves to alert a person to potential or actual damage to the body. The definition of damage is quite broad: pain can arise from injury as well as disease. After the message is received and interpreted, further pain can be counterproductive. Pain can have a negative impact on a person's quality of life and impede recovery from illness or injury, thus contributing to escalating health care costs. Unrelieved pain can become a syndrome in its own right and cause a downward spiral in a person's health and emotional outlook. Managing pain properly facilitates recovery, prevents additional health complications, and improves an individual's quality of life.

Yet the experiencing of pain is a completely unique occurrence for each person, a complex combination of several factors other than the pain itself. It is influenced by:

- Ethnic and cultural values. In some cultures, tolerating pain is related to showing strength and endurance. In others, pain is considered punishment for misdeeds.
- Age. Many people have been taught that grownups never cry. On the other hand, in some cultures, the

elderly are allowed to complain freely about pain and discomfort.

- Anxiety and stress. This factor is related to being in a strange or unfamiliar place such as a hospital, and the fear of the unknown consequences of the pain and the condition causing it, which can all combined to make pain feel more severe. For patients being treated for pain, knowing the duration of activity of an analgesic leads to anxiety about the return of pain when the drug wears off. This anxiety can make the pain more severe. In addition, patients who interpret their pain as meaning that their disease is recurring or getting worse often experience pain as more severe.

- Fatigue and depression. It is known that pain in itself can actually cause emotional depression. Fatigue from lack of sleep or the illness itself also contributes to depressed feelings.

Precautions

The perception of pain is an individual experience. Healthcare providers play an important role in understanding their patients' pain. All too often, both physicians and nurses have been found to incorrectly assess the severity of pain. A study reported in the *Journal of Advanced Nursing* evaluated nurses' perceptions of a select group of white American and Mexican-American women patients' pain following gallbladder surgery. Objective assessments of each patient's pain showed little difference between the perceived severities for each group. Yet, the nurses involved in the study consistently rated all patients' pain as less than the patients reported, and with equal consistency, believed that better-educated women born in the United States were suffering more than less-educated Mexican-American women. Nurses from a northern European background were more apt to minimize the severity of pain than nurses from eastern and southern Europe or Africa. The study indicated how healthcare staff, and especially nursing staff, need to be aware of how their own background and experience contributes to how they perceive a person's pain.

Some patient populations are particularly susceptible to inadequate pain management. These include cancer patients; children; trauma victims receiving treatment in hospital emergency departments; and the elderly in **nursing homes**.

Description

Before considering pain management, a review of pain definitions and mechanisms may be useful. Pain is the means by which the peripheral nervous system

KEY TERMS

Acute—Referring to pain in response to injury or other stimulus that resolves when the injury heals or the stimulus is removed.

Central nervous system (CNS)—The part of the nervous system that includes the brain and the spinal cord.

Chronic—Referring to pain that endures beyond the term of an injury or painful stimulus. Can also refer to cancer pain, pain from a chronic or degenerative disease, and pain from an unidentified cause.

Iatrogenic—Resulting from the activity of the physician.

Neuropathy—Nerve damage.

Neurotransmitter—Chemicals within the nervous system that transmit information from or between nerve cells.

Nociceptor—A nerve cell that is capable of sensing pain and transmitting a pain signal.

Nonpharmacological—Referring to therapy that does not involve drugs.

Parasympathetic nervous system—That part of the autonomic nervous system consisting of nerves that arise from the cranial and sacral regions and function in opposition to the sympathetic nervous system.

Peripheral nervous system (PNS)—Nerves that are outside of the brain and spinal cord.

Pharmacological—Referring to therapy that relies on drugs.

Stimulus—A factor capable of eliciting a response in a nerve.

Sympathetic nervous system—That portion of the autonomic nervous system consisting of nerves that originate in the thoracic and lumbar spinal cord and function in opposition to the parasympathetic nervous system.

(PNS) warns the central nervous system (CNS) of injury or potential injury to the body. The CNS comprises the brain and spinal cord, and the PNS is composed of the nerves that stem from and lead into the CNS. PNS includes all nerves throughout the body, except the brain and spinal cord. Pain is sometimes categorized by its site of origin, either cutaneous (originating in the skin, or subcutaneous tissue, such as a shaving nick or paper cut), deep somatic pain (arising from bone, ligaments and tendons, nerves, or veins and arteries), or visceral (appearing as a result of stimulation of pain receptor nerves around such organs as the brain, lungs, or stomach and intestines).

A pain message is transmitted to the CNS by special PNS nerve cells called nociceptors, which are distributed throughout the body and respond to different stimuli depending on their location. For example, nociceptors that extend from the skin are stimulated by such sensations as pressure, temperature, and chemical changes.

When a nociceptor is stimulated, neurotransmitters are released within the cell. Neurotransmitters are chemicals found within the nervous system that facilitate nerve cell communication. The nociceptor transmits its signal to nerve cells within the spinal cord, which conveys the pain message to the thalamus, a specific region in the brain.

Once the brain has received and processed the pain message and coordinated an appropriate response, pain has served its purpose. The body uses natural pain-killers called endorphins to derail further pain messages from the same source. However, these natural pain-killers may not adequately dampen a continuing pain message. Also, depending on how the brain has processed the pain information, certain hormones such as prostaglandins may be released. These hormones enhance the pain message and play a role in immune system responses to injury, such as inflammation. Certain neurotransmitters, especially substance P and calcitonin gene-related peptide, actively enhance the pain message at the injury site and within the spinal cord.

Pain is generally divided into two additional categories: acute and chronic. Nociceptive pain, or the pain that is transmitted by nociceptors, is typically called acute pain. This kind of pain is associated with injury, headaches, disease, and many other conditions. Response to acute pain is made by the sympathetic nervous system (the nerves responsible for the fight-or-flight response of the body). It normally resolves once the condition that precipitated it is resolved.

There are some disorders that produce pain that does not resolve following the disorder. Even after healing or a cure has been achieved, the brain continues to perceive pain. In this situation, the pain may be considered chronic. Chronic pain is within the province of the parasympathetic nervous system, and the changeover occurs as the body attempts to adapt to the pain. The time limit used to define chronic pain typically ranges from three to six months, although some healthcare professionals prefer a more flexible definition and consider chronic pain as pain that

endures beyond a normal healing time. The pain associated with cancer, persistent and degenerative conditions, and neuropathy, or nerve damage, is included in the chronic category. Also, unremitting pain that lacks an identifiable physical cause such as the majority of cases of low back pain may be considered chronic. The underlying biochemistry of chronic pain appears to be different from that of acute nociceptive pain.

It has been hypothesized that uninterrupted and unrelenting pain can induce changes in the spinal cord. In the past, severing a nerve's connection to the CNS has treated intractable pain. However, the lack of any sensory information being relayed by that nerve can cause pain transmission in the spinal cord to go into overdrive, as evidenced by the phantom limb pain experienced by amputees. Evidence is accumulating that unrelenting pain or the complete lack of nerve signals increases the number of pain receptors in the spinal cord. Nerve cells in the spinal cord may also begin secreting pain-amplifying neurotransmitters independent of actual pain signals from the body. Immune chemicals, primarily cytokines, may play a prominent role in such changes.

Managing pain

Considering the different causes and types of pain, as well as its nature and intensity, management usually requires a multidisciplinary approach. The elements of this approach include treating the underlying cause of pain, pharmacological and non-pharmacological therapies, and some invasive (surgical) procedures.

Treating the cause of pain underlies the basic strategy of pain management. Injuries are repaired, diseases are diagnosed, and certain encounters with pain can be anticipated and treated prophylactically (by prevention). However, there are no guarantees of immediate relief from pain. Recovery can be impeded by pain and quality of life can be damaged. Therefore, pharmacological and other therapies have developed over time to address these aspects of disease and injury.

PHARMACOLOGICAL OPTIONS. General guidelines developed by the World Health Organization (WHO) have been developed for pain management. These guidelines operate upon the three-step ladder approach, including:

- Mild pain is alleviated with acetaminophen or a non-steroidal anti-inflammatory drug (NSAID). NSAIDs and acetaminophen are available as over-the-counter (OTC) and prescription medications, and are frequently the initial pharmacological treatment for pain. These drugs can also be used as adjuncts to the other drug therapies that might require a doctor's prescription. NSAIDs include aspirin, ibuprofen (Motrin, Advil, Nuprin), naproxen sodium (Aleve), and ketoprofen (Orudis KT). These drugs are used to treat pain from inflammation and work by blocking production of pain-enhancing neurotransmitters. Acetaminophen is also effective against pain, but its ability to reduce inflammation is limited. NSAIDs and acetaminophen are effective for most forms of acute (sharp, but of a short duration) pain.

- Mild to moderate pain is eased with a milder opioid medication, plus acetaminophen or NSAIDs. Opioids include both drugs derived from the opium poppy, such as morphine and codeine, and synthetic drugs based on the structure of opium. This drug class includes drugs such as oxycodone, methadone, and meperidine (Demerol). They provide pain relief by binding to specific opioid receptors in the brain and spinal cord. One drawback of opioids, however, is that they frequently cause constipation because they slow down the rhythmic muscular contractions of the intestines that push food along during the process of digestion.

- Moderate to severe pain is treated with stronger opioid drugs, plus acetaminophen or NSAIDs. Morphine is sometimes referred to as the gold standard of palliative care as it is not expensive; can be given by starting with smaller doses and gradually increased; and is highly effective over a long period of time. It can also be given by a number of different routes, including by mouth, rectally, or by injection.

Although antidepressant drugs were developed to treat depression, it has been discovered that they are also effective in combating chronic headaches, cancer pain, and pain associated with nerve damage. Antidepressants that have been shown to have analgesic (pain-reducing) properties include amitriptyline (Elavil), trazodone (Desyrel), and imipramine (Tofranil). Anticonvulsant drugs share a similar background with antidepressants. Developed to treat epilepsy, anticonvulsants were found to relieve pain as well. Drugs such as phenytoin (Dilantin) and carbamazepine (Tegretol) are prescribed to treat the pain associated with nerve damage.

In some cases, chronic pain caused by complications of diabetes or cancer can be eased by administering local anesthetics. The most commonly used are mexiletine (Mexitil) and a lidocaine patch.

Corticosteroids are another class of drugs commonly given to manage chronic pain caused by arthritis or other diseases affecting the muscles and joints; they may also be given to control nausea. Dexamethasone (Decadron) and prednisone are the most commonly used corticosteroids in pain management. They work by reducing inflammation and suppressing the immune system.

Close monitoring of the effects of pain medications is required in order to assure that adequate amounts of medication are given to produce the desired pain relief. When a person is comfortable with a certain dosage of medication, oncologists typically convert to a long-acting version of that medication. Transdermal fentanyl patches (Duragesic) are a common example of a long-acting opioid drug often used for cancer pain management. A patch containing the drug is applied to the skin and continues to deliver the drug to the person for an average of three days. Pumps are also available that provide an opioid medication upon demand when the person is experiencing pain. By pressing a button, they can release a set dose of medication into an intravenous solution or an implanted catheter. Another mode of administration involves implanted catheters that deliver pain medication directly to the spinal cord. Because these pumps offer the patient some degree of control over the amount of analgesic administered, the system, commonly called **patient-controlled analgesia** (PCA), reduces the level of anxiety about availability of pain medication. Delivering drugs in this way can reduce side effects and increase the effectiveness of the drug. Research is underway to develop toxic substances that act selectively on nerve cells that carry pain messages to the brain. These substances would kill the selected cells and stop transmission of the pain message.

NONPHARMACOLOGICAL OPTIONS. Pain treatment options that do not use drugs are often used as adjuncts to, rather than replacements for, drug therapy. One of the benefits of nondrug therapies is that an individual can take a more active role in pain management. Such relaxation techniques as yoga and meditation are used to focus the brain elsewhere than on the pain, decrease muscle tension, and reduce stress. Tension and stress can also be reduced through **biofeedback**, in which an individual consciously attempts to modify skin temperature, muscle tension, blood pressure, and heart rate.

Hypnosis is another nonpharmacological option for pain relief. Although doctors do not yet fully understand how hypnosis works, it is used successfully in some patients to manage pain related to childbirth, oral surgery, burn treatment, and other procedures that require the patient to remain conscious.

Participating in normal activities and exercising can also help control pain levels. Through physical therapy, an individual learns beneficial exercises for reducing stress, strengthening muscles, and staying fit. Regular **exercise** has been linked to production of endorphins, the body's natural painkillers.

Acupuncture involves the insertion of small needles into the skin at key points. Acupressure uses these same key points, but involves applying pressure rather than inserting needles. Both of these methods may work by prompting the body to release endorphins. Applying heat or being massaged are very relaxing and help reduce stress. Transcutaneous electrical nerve stimulation (TENS) applies a small electric current to certain parts of nerves, potentially interrupting pain signals and inducing release of endorphins. To be effective, use of TENS should be medically supervised.

INVASIVE PROCEDURES. There are three types of invasive procedures that may be used to manage or treat pain: anatomic, augmentative, and ablative. These procedures involve surgery, and certain guidelines should be followed before carrying out a procedure with permanent effects. First, the cause of the pain must be clearly identified. Next, surgery should be done only if noninvasive procedures are ineffective. Third, any psychological issues should be addressed. Finally, there should be a reasonable expectation of success.

Anatomic procedures involve correcting the injury or removing the cause of pain. Relatively common anatomic procedures are decompression surgeries such as repairing a herniated disk in the lower back or relieving the nerve compression related to carpal tunnel syndrome. Another anatomic procedure is neurolysis, also called a nerve block, which involves destroying a portion of a peripheral nerve.

Augmentative procedures include electrical stimulation or direct application of drugs to the nerves that are transmitting the pain signals. Electrical stimulation works on the same principle as TENS. In this procedure, instead of applying the current across the skin, electrodes are implanted to stimulate peripheral nerves or nerves in the spinal cord. Augmentative procedures also include implanted drug-delivery systems. In these systems, catheters are implanted in the spine to allow direct delivery of drugs to the CNS.

Ablative procedures are characterized by severing a nerve and disconnecting it from the CNS. However, this method may not address potential alterations within the spinal cord. These changes perpetuate pain messages and do not cease, even when the connection between the sensory nerve and the CNS is severed. With growing understanding of neuropathic pain and development of less invasive procedures, ablative procedures are used less frequently. However,

they do have applications in select cases of peripheral neuropathy, cancer pain, and other disorders.

Preparation

Prior to beginning management, the patient's pain should be thoroughly evaluated, including a psychosocial as well as a physical assessment. Pain scales or questionnaires can be administered by a member of the healthcare team, although there is no single questionnaire that is universally accepted as of 2007. Some questionnaires are verbal, while others use pictures or drawings to help the patient describe the pain. Some questionnaires are filled out by the patient, while others may be given to relatives or friends to complete. It is often necessary to ask other family members to complete a pain questionnaire if the patient is cognitively impaired.

In spite of their limitations, questionnaires and self-report forms do allow healthcare workers to better understand the pain being suffered by the patient. Evaluation also includes physical examinations and diagnostic tests to determine the underlying physical causes of the pain. Some evaluations require assessments from several viewpoints, including neurology, psychiatry and psychology, and physical therapy. If the pain is caused by a medical procedure, management consists of anticipating the type and intensity of associated pain and managing it preemptively.

Nurses or physicians often take what is called a pain history. This history will help to provide important information that can help health care providers to better manage the patient's pain. A typical pain history includes the following questions:

• Where is the pain located?

• On a scale of 1 to 10, with 1 indicating the least pain, how would the person rate the pain being experienced?

• What does the pain feel like?

• When did (or does) the pain start?

• How long has the person had it?

• Is the person sometimes free of pain?

• Is the pain constant, or is it episodic?

• Does the person know of anything that triggers the pain or makes it worse?

• Does the person have other symptoms (nausea, dizziness, blurred vision, etc.) during or after the pain?

• What pain medications or other measures has the person found to help in easing the pain?

• How does the pain affect the person's ability to carry on normal activities?

• What does it mean to the person that he or she is experiencing pain?

Aftercare

An assessment by nursing staff as well as other healthcare providers should be made to determine the effectiveness of the pain management interventions employed. There are objective, measurable signs and symptoms of pain that can be looked for. The goal of good pain management is the absence of these signs. Signs of acute pain include:

- rise in pulse and blood pressure
- more rapid breathing
- perspiring profusely, clammy skin
- taut muscles
- more tense appearance, fast speech, very alert
- unusually pale skin
- dilated pupils of the eye

  Signs of chronic pain include:

- lower pulse and blood pressure
- changeable breathing pattern
- warm, dry skin
- nausea and vomiting
- slow or monotone speech
- inability or difficulty in getting out of bed and performing activities of daily living (ADLs)
- constricted pupils of the eye

When these signs are absent and the patient appears to be comfortable, healthcare providers can consider their interventions to have been successful. It is also important to document interventions used, and which ones were successful.

Risks

Owing to toxicity over the long term, some drugs can only be used for acute pain or as adjuncts in chronic pain management. NSAIDs have the well-known side effect of causing gastrointestinal bleeding, and long-term use of **acetaminophen** has been linked to kidney and liver damage. Other drugs, especially narcotics, have such serious side effects as constipation, drowsiness, and nausea. Serious side effects can also accompany pharmacological therapies; mood swings, confusion, bone thinning, cataract formation, increased blood pressure, and other problems may discourage or prevent use of some **analgesics**.

Nonpharmacological therapies carry little or no risks. However, individuals recovering from serious illness or injury should consult with the health care providers or physical therapists before making use of adjunct therapies. Invasive procedures carry risks similar to other surgical procedures, such as infection,

reaction to anesthesia, and iatrogenic (injury as a result of treatment) injury.

A traditional concern about narcotics use has been the risk of promoting addiction. As narcotic use continues over time, the body becomes accustomed to the drug and adjusts normal functions to accommodate to its presence. Therefore, to elicit the same level of action, it is necessary to increase dosage over time. As dosage increases, an individual may become physically dependent on narcotic drugs.

However, physical dependence is different from psychological addiction. Physical dependence is characterized by discomfort if drug administration suddenly stops, while psychological addiction is characterized by an overpowering craving for the drug for reasons other than pain relief. Psychological addiction is a very real and necessary concern in some instances, but it should not interfere with a genuine need for narcotic pain relief. However, caution must be taken with people who have a history of addictive behavior.

Normal results

Effective application of pain management techniques reduces or eliminates acute or chronic pain. This treatment can improve an individual's quality of life and aid in recovery from injury and disease.

Resources

BOOKS

Gould, Harry J., III. *Understanding Pain: What It Is, Why It Happens, and How It's Managed.* St. Paul, MN: American Academy of Neurology Press, 2007.

Hughes, John, ed. *Pain Management: From Basics to Clinical Practice.* New York: Churchill Livingstone/Elsevier, 2008.

Main, Chris J., Michael J. L. Sullivan, and Paul J. Watson. *Pain Management: Practical Applications of the Biopsychosocial Perspective in Clinical and Occupational Settings.* Edinburgh and New York: Churchill Livingstone, 2008.

PERIODICALS

Cleary, J. F. "The Pharmacologic Management of Cancer Pain." *Journal of Palliative Medicine* 10 (December 2007): 1369–1394.

Coyle, N. "Assessing Cancer Pain in the Adult Patient." *Oncology (Williston Park)* 20 (September 2006): 41–49.

Curtis, K. M., H. F. Henriques, G. Fanciullo, et al. "A Fentanyl-based Pain Management Protocol Provides Early Analgesia for Adult Trauma Patients." *Journal of Trauma* 63 (October 2007): 819–826.

D'Arcy, Yvonne. "Keep Your Patient Safe during PCA." *Nursing* 38 (January 2008): 50–55.

Marx, T. L. "Partnering with Hospice to Improve Pain Management in the Nursing Home Setting." *Journal of the American Osteopathic Association* 105 (March 2005): S22–S26.

McPherson, M. L., C. D. Ponte, and R. M. Respond (eds.). "Profiles in Pain Management." *Journal of the American Pharmacists Association* (June 2003).

Schwartz, S. R. "Perioperative Pain Management." *Oral and Maxillofacial Surgery Clinics of North America* 18 (May 2006): 139–150.

ORGANIZATIONS

American Chronic Pain Association (ACPA). P.O. Box 850, Rocklin, CA 95677-0850. (800) 533-3231. http://www.theacpa.org/index.asp (accessed April 2, 2008).

American Pain Society. 4700 West Lake Ave., Glenview, IL 60025. (847) 375-4715. http://www.ampainsoc.org (accessed April 2, 2008).

International Association for the Study of Pain (IASP). 111 Queen Anne Avenue North, Suite 501, Seattle, WA 98109-4955. (206) 283-0311. http://www.iasp-pain.org//AM/Template.cfm?Section = Home (accessed April 2, 2008).

OTHER

National Cancer Institute (NCI). Pain, health professional version. Bethesda, MD: NCI, 2007. http://www.cancer.gov/cancertopics/pdq/supportivecare/pain/HealthProfessional (accessed April 2, 2008).

National Institute of Neurological Disorders and Stroke (NINDS). *Pain: Hope through Research.* NIH Publication 01-2406. Bethesda, MD: NINDS, 2007.

Joan M. Schonbeck
Sam Uretsky, PharmD
Rebecca Frey, PhD

Pain relievers *see* **Analgesics**

Pallidotomy

Definition

Pallidotomy is the destruction of a small region of the brain, the globus pallidus internus, in order to treat some of the symptoms of Parkinson's disease.

Purpose

The symptoms of Parkinson's disease (PD) include rigidity, slowed movements, and tremor, along with postural instability and a variety of non-motor symptoms (i.e., symptoms not involving movement). These symptoms are due to degeneration of a small portion of the brain called the substantia nigra, the cells of which secrete the chemical dopamine that influences cells in another brain region called the globus pallidus internus

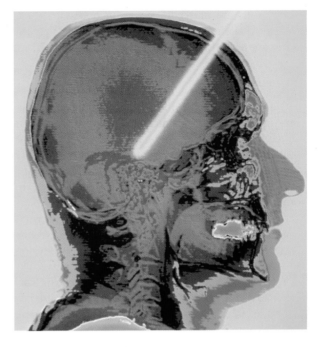

A CT scan of a surgical probe entering a patient's brain. *(John Greim / Photo Researchers, Inc.)*

(GPi). Together with other brain regions, these two structures take part in complex control loops that govern certain aspects of movement and, when substantia nigra cells degenerate, these loops are disrupted and movements become unregulated, producing the symptoms of Parkinson's disease.

The effects of dopamine on the brain can be mimicked by the drug levodopa; levodopa therapy is the mainstay of PD treatment in its early stages. Unfortunately, levodopa becomes less effective over time, and also produces unwanted and uncontrolled movements called dyskinesias. This may occur after five to 10 years or more of successful levodopa treatment. Once a patient can no longer be treated effectively with levodopa, surgery is considered as a management option. Pallidotomy is one of the main surgical options for treatment of advanced PD.

The effect of dopamine on the cells of the GPi is to suppress them by preventing them from firing. Pallidotomy mimics this action by permanently destroying the GPi cells. It may seem odd that the treatment for degeneration of one brain area is to destroy another, but in the absence of dopamine, the GPi cells are overactive, and therefore, eliminating them is an appropriate treatment.

The GPi has two halves that control movements on opposites sides: right controls left, left controls right. Unilateral (one-sided) pallidotomy may be used if symptoms are markedly worse on one side or the other, or if the risks from bilateral (two-sided) pallidotomy are judged to be too great.

Demographics

Parkinson's disease affects approximately one million Americans. The peak incidence is approximately at age 62, but young-onset PD can occur as early as age 40. Because young-onset patients live with their disease for so many more years, they are more likely to become candidates for surgery than older-onset patients. In addition, younger patients tend to do better with surgery and suffer fewer adverse effects from the surgery. Approximately 5% of older PD patients receive one form or another of PD surgery; many more develop the symptoms for which surgery may be effective, but either develop them at an advanced age, making surgery inadvisable, or decide the risks of surgery are not worth the potential benefit, or do not choose surgery for some other reason.

Description

Pallidotomy requires the insertion of a long needle-like probe deep into the brain through a hole in the top of the skull. In order to precisely locate the GPi target, and to ensure the probe is precisely placed in the target, a "stereotactic frame" is used. This device is a rigid frame attached to the patient's head, providing an immobile three-dimensional coordinate system, which can be used to precisely track the location of the GPi and the movement of the probe.

For unilateral pallidotomy, a single "burr hole" is made in the top of the skull; bilateral pallidotomy requires two holes. A strong topical anesthetic is used to numb the shaved area before this hole is drilled. Since there are no pain receptors in the brain, there is no need for deeper anesthetic. In addition, the patient must remain awake in order to report any sensory changes during the surgery. The lesion made in the GPi is very close to the optic tract that carries visual information from the eyes to the rear of the brain. Visual changes may indicate the probe is too close to this region.

Once the burr hole is made, the surgeon inserts a microelectrode probe, which is used to more precisely locate the GPi. Electrical stimulation of the brain through the electrode can help determine exactly which structure is being stimulated. This is harmless, but may cause twitching, light flashes, or other sensations. A contrast dye may also be injected into the spinal fluid, which allows the surgeon to visualize the brain's structure using one or more imaging techniques. During the procedure, the patient will be asked to make

various movements to assist in determining the location of the electrode.

When the proper target is located, the electrode tip is briefly heated, carefully destroying the surrounding tissue to about the size of a pearl. If bilateral pallidotomy is being performed, the localizing and lesioning will be repeated on the other side.

Diagnosis/Preparation

Pallidotomy is performed in patients with Parkinson's disease who are still responsive to levodopa, but who have developed disabling drug treatment complications known as motor fluctuations, including rapid wearing off of drug effect, unpredictable "off states" (times of low levodopa levels in the blood), and disabling dyskinesias. Those who are very elderly, demented, or with other significant medical conditions that would be compromised by surgery are usually not candidates for pallidotomy.

The surgical candidate should discuss all the surgical options with the neurologist before deciding on pallidotomy. A full understanding of the risks and potential benefits must be understood before consenting to the surgery.

The patient will undergo a variety of medical tests, and one or more types of neuroimaging procedures, including **magnetic resonance imaging** (MRI), computed tomagraphy (CT) scanning, **angiography** (imaging the brain's blood vessels), and ventriculography (imaging the brain's ventricles). On the day of the surgery, the stereotactic frame will be fixed to the patient's head. First, a local anesthetic is applied at the four sites where the frame's pins contact the head; there may nonetheless be some initial discomfort. A final MRI is done with the frame in place to help set the coordinates of the GPi in relation to the frame.

The patient will receive a mild sedative to ease the anxiety of the procedure.

Aftercare

The procedure requires several hours. Some centers perform pallidotomy as an outpatient procedure, sending the patient home the same day. Most centers keep the patient overnight or longer for observation. Patients will feel improved movement immediately. Medications may be adjusted somewhat to accommodate the changes in symptoms.

Risks

The key to successful outcome in pallidotomy is extremely precise placement of the electrode. While

WHO PERFORMS THE
PROCEDURE AND WHERE IS IT
PERFORMED?

Pallidotomy is performed in the hospital by a neurosurgeon, in coordination with the patient's neurologist.

QUESTIONS TO ASK THE
DOCTOR

• How many pallidotomies has the neurosurgeon performed?
• What is the surgeon's own rate of serious complications?
• Would deep brain stimulation of the subthalamic nucleus be appropriate for me?
• How will my medications change after the operation?

there are several controversies in the field of PD surgery, all experts agree that risks are reduced in procedures performed by the most experienced neurosurgeons.

Hemorrhage in the brain is a possible complication, as is infection. There are small but significant risks of damage to the optic tract, which can cause visual deficits. Speech impairments may also occur, including difficulty retrieving words and slurred speech. Some cognitively fragile patients may become even more impaired after surgery.

Normal results

Pallidotomy improves the motor ability of patients, especially during "off" periods. Studies show the procedure generally improves tremor, rigidity, and slowed movements by 25–60%. Dyskinesias typically improve by 75% or more. Improvements from unilateral pallidotomy are primarily on the side opposite the surgery. Balance does not improve, nor do non-motor symptoms such as drooling, constipation, and orthostatic hypotension (lightheadness on standing).

Morbidity and mortality rates

Among the best surgeons, the risk of serious morbidity or mortality is 1–2%. Hemorrhage may occur in 2–6%, visual field deficits in 0–6%, and weakness in 2–8%. Most patients gain weight after surgery.

Alternatives

Patients whose symptoms are well managed by drugs are not recommended for surgery, and significant effort will usually be made to adjust medications to control symptoms before surgery is considered.

Thalamotomy, surgery to the thalamus, was recommended in the past to control tremor. It is rarely performed today, and few centers would consider thalamotomy for any patient unless tremor was the only troubling and uncontrolled symptom.

Deep-brain stimulation (DBS) of the GPi is an alternative treatment in widespread use, as is DBS of another brain region, the subthalamic nucleus. Both

procedures use permanemtly implanted, programmable electrodes to deliver a very small, continuous electric current to the target region. This has the same effect as a lesion, but is adjustable. DBS of the subthalamic nucleus typically produces better symtomatic results that either DBS to the GPi or pallidotomy. However, both forms of DBS carry the risk of long-term complications from the implanted hardware, as well as other risks.

Resources

BOOKS

Goetz, CG. Goetz's Textbook of Clinical Neurology. 3rd ed. Philadelphia: Saunders, 2007.

ORGANIZATIONS

National Parkinson's Disease Foundation. http://www.npf.org.
WE MOVE. http://www.wemove.org.

Richard Robinson

Pancreas removal *see* **Pancreatectomy**

Pancreas transplantation

Definition

Pancreas transplantation is a surgical procedure in which a diseased pancreas is replaced with a healthy pancreas that has been obtained from an immunologically compatible cadavear or living donor.

Purpose

The pancreas secretes insulin that regulates glucose (blood sugar) metabolism. Patients with type I

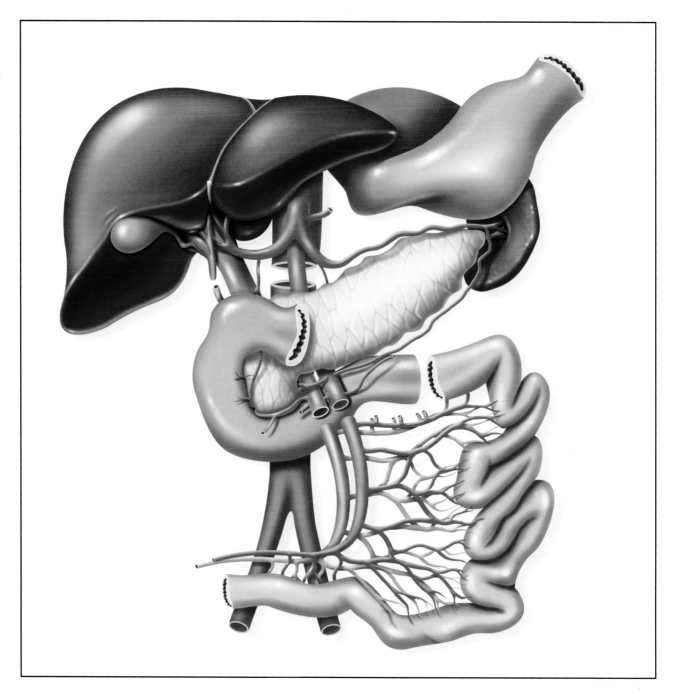

The pancreas transplantation procedure. *(BSIP/Phototake. Reproduced by permission.)*

diabetes have experienced partial or complete damage to the insulin-producing beta cells of the pancreas. Consequently, they are unable to generate sufficient insulin to control blood glucose levels. Long-term uncontrolled high blood glucose levels can cause damage to every system of the body, so type I patients must inject insulin to do the work of the beta cells. Pancreas transplantation allows the body to once again make

and secrete its own insulin, and establishes insulin independence for these individuals.

Demographics

It is estimated that over one million people in the United States have type 1 diabetes mellitus (also called insulin-dependant diabetes or juvenile diabetes). Among these individuals, the best candidates for pancreas transplantation are typically:

- between the ages of 20 and 40
- those who have extreme difficulty regulating their glucose levels with insulin therapy (a condition called brittle diabetes)
- those who have few secondary complications of diabetes
- those who are in good cardiovascular health

A pancreas-only transplant is an uncommon procedure, with only 163 procedures occurring in the United States in 2001. More common is the combined kidney-pancreas transplant, which was performed on 885 patients the same year. An additional 305 patients received a PAK, or pancreas after kidney transplant, according to the United Network for Organ Sharing (UNOS).

Description

Once a donor pancreas is located and tissue typing deems it compatible, the patient is contacted and prepared for surgery. Blood tests, a **chest x ray**, and an **electrocardiogram** (ECG) are performed and an intravenous (IV) line is started for fluid and medication administration. Once the transplant procedure is ready to start, **general anesthesia** is administered.

The surgeon makes an incision under the ribs and locates the pancreas and duodenum. The pancreas and duodenum (part of the small intestine) are removed. The new pancreas and duodenum are then connected to the patient's duodenum, and the blood vessels are sutured together to restore blood flow to the new pancreas. The patient's original pancreas is left in place.

Replacing the duodenum allows the pancreas to drain into the gastrointestinal system. The transplant can also be done creating bladder drainage. Bladder drainage makes it easier to monitor organ rejection because pancreatic secretions can be measured in the patient's urine. Once the new pancreas is in place, the abdomen and skin are sutured closed. This surgery is often done at the same time as kidney **transplant surgery**.

Diagnosis/Preparation

After the patient and doctor have decided on a pancreas transplant, a complete immunological study is performed to match the patient to a donor. An extensive medical history and **physical examination** is performed, including radiological exams, blood and urine tests, and psychological evaluation. Once the patient is approved for transplant, he or she will be placed on the United Network for Organ Sharing

---

KEY TERMS

Cadaver organ—A pancreas, kidney, or other organ from a brain-dead organ donor.

Duodenum—The section of the small intestine immediately after the stomach.

(UNOS) Organ Center waiting list. The timing of surgery depends on the availability of a donated living or cadaver organ.

Aftercare

Patients receiving a pancreas transplantation are monitored closely for organ rejection. The average hospital stay is three weeks, and it takes about six months to recover from surgery. Patients will take **immunosuppressant drugs** for the rest of their lives.

Risks

Diabetes and poor kidney function greatly increase the risk of complications from anesthesia during surgery. Organ rejection, excessive bleeding, and infection are other major risks associated with this surgery.

The reason simultaneous kidney-pancreas transplants and pancreas after kidney transplants are performed more frequently than pancreas only transplants is the relative risk of immunosuppressant drugs in people with diabetes. People with type I diabetes are already at risk for autoimmune problems, are more prone to infections, and have a complicated medical history that makes suppressing the immune system unadvisable.

On the other hand, diabetes is also the number one cause of chronic kidney failure, or end-stage renal disease (ESRD), which makes this group more likely to eventually require a kidney transplant for survival. In those patients with diabetes who will receive or are already receiving immunosuppressive treatment for a life-saving kidney transplant, a pancreas transplant can return their ability to self-produce insulin.

Patients with type I diabetes considering pancreas transplantation alone must weigh the risks and benefits of the procedure and decide with their doctors whether life-long treatment with immunosuppressive drugs is preferable to life-long insulin dependence.

Normal results

In a successful transplant, the pancreas begins producing insulin, bringing the regulation of glucose

WHO PERFORMS THE PROCEDURE AND WHERE IS IT PERFORMED?

A pancreas transplant is performed by a transplant surgeon in one of over 200 UNOS-approved hospitals nationwide. The patient must go through an evaluation procedure at his or her hospital of choice to get on the UNOS national waiting list and the UNOS Organ Center's UNet database.

back under control. Natural availability of insulin prevents the development of additional complications associated with diabetes, including kidney damage, vision loss, and nerve damage. Many patients report an improved quality of life.

Morbidity and mortality rates

In their 2002 Annual Report, the Organ Procurement and Transplant Network (OPTN) reported that the patient survival rate for pancreas transplant alone was 98.6% after one year and 86% after three years. Survival rates for pancreas-kidney transplant recipients were 95.1% after one year and 89.2% after three years.

Alternatives

Innovations in islet cell transplants, a procedure that involves transplanting a culture of the insulin-producing islet cells of a healthy pancreas to a patient with type I diabetes, have increased the frequency of this procedure. The Edmonton Protocol, a type of islet cell transplant developed in 1999 by Dr. James Shapiro at the University of Alberta (Canada), uses a unique immunosuppresant drug regimen that has dramatically improved success rates of the islet transplant procedure. As of early 2003, the Edmonton Protocol was still considered investigational in the United States, and a number of clinical trials were ongoing.

Resources

PERIODICALS

Norton, Patrice. "Pancreatic Human Islet Cells Offer Alternative to Pancreas Transplant." *Family Practice News.* 33 (January 2003): 14.

Reddy, K.S. et al. "Long-term survival following simultaneous kidney-pancreas transplantation versus kidney transplantation alone in patients with type 1 diabetes mellitus and renal failure." *American Journal of Kidney Disease* 41 (February 2003): 464–70.

QUESTIONS TO ASK THE DOCTOR

- How many pancreas or pancreas-kidney transplants have both you and the hospital performed?
- What are your success rates? How about those of the hospital?
- Who will be on my transplant team?
- Can I get on the waiting list at more than one hospital?
- What type of immunosuppressive drugs will I be on post-transplant?
- How long will my recovery period be?

ORGANIZATIONS

American Diabetes Association. 1701 North Beauregard Street, Alexandria, VA 22311. (800) 342-2383. http://www.diabetes.org.

United Network for Organ Sharing (UNOS). 700 North 4th St., Richmond, VA 23219. (888) 894-6361. http://www.transplantliving.org.

Tish Davidson, A.M.
Paula Anne Ford-Martin

Pancreatectomy

Definition

A pancreatectomy is the surgical removal of the pancreas. A pancreatectomy may be total, in which case the entire organ is removed, usually along with the spleen, gallbladder, common bile duct, and portions of the small intestine and stomach. A pancreatectomy may also be distal, meaning that only the body and tail of the pancreas are removed, leaving the head of the organ attached. When the duodenum is removed along with all or part of the pancreas, the procedure is called a pancreaticoduodenectomy, which surgeons sometimes refer to as "Whipple's procedure." Pancreaticoduodenectomies are increasingly used to treat a variety of malignant and benign diseases of the pancreas. This procedure often involves removal of the regional lymph nodes as well.

Purpose

A pancreatectomy is the most effective treatment for cancer of the pancreas, an abdominal organ that

KEY TERMS

Chemotherapy—A cancer treatment that uses synthetic drugs to destroy the tumor either by inhibiting the growth of the cancerous cells or by killing the cancer cells.

Computed tomography (CT) scan—An imaging technique that creates a series of pictures of areas inside the body, taken from different angles. The pictures are created by a computer linked to an x-ray machine.

Endoscopic retrograde cholangiopancreatography (ERCP)—A procedure to x-ray the ducts (tubes) that carry bile from the liver to the gallbladder and from the gallbladder to the small intestine.

Laparoscopy—In this procedure, a laparoscope (a thin, lighted tube) is inserted through an incision in the abdominal wall to determine if the cancer is within the pancreas only or has spread to nearby tissues and if it can be removed by surgery later. Tissue samples may be removed for biopsy.

Magnetic resonance imaging (MRI)—A procedure in which a magnet linked to a computer is used to create detailed pictures of areas inside the body.

Pancreas—A large gland located on the back wall of the abdomen, extending from the duodenum (first part of the small intestine) to the spleen. The pancreas produces enzymes essential for digestion, and

the hormones insulin and glucagon, which play a role in diabetes.

Pancreaticoduodenectomy—Removal of all or part of the pancreas along with the duodenum. Also known as "Whipple's procedure" or "Whipple's operation."

Pancreatitis—Inflammation of the pancreas, either acute (sudden and episodic) or chronic, usually caused by excessive alcohol intake or gallbladder disease.

Positron emission tomography (PET) scan—An imaging system that creates a picture showing the location of tumor cells in the body. A substance called radionuclide dye is injected into a vein, and the PET scanner rotates around the body to create the picture. Malignant tumor cells show up brighter in the picture because they are more active and take up more dye than normal cells.

Radiation therapy—A treatment using high energy radiation from x-ray machines, cobalt, radium, or other sources.

Ultrasonogram—A procedure where high-frequency sound waves that cannot be heard by human ears are bounced off internal organs and tissues. These sound waves produce a pattern of echoes which are then used by the computer to create sonograms, or pictures of areas inside the body.

secretes digestive enzymes, insulin, and other hormones. The thickest part of the pancreas near the duodenum (a part of the small intestine) is called the head, the middle part is called the body, and the thinnest part adjacent to the spleen is called the tail.

While surgical removal of tumors in the pancreas is the preferred treatment, it is only possible in the 10–15% of patients who are diagnosed early enough for a potential cure. Patients who are considered suitable for surgery usually have small tumors in the head of the pancreas (close to the duodenum, or first part of the small intestine), have jaundice as their initial symptom, and have no evidence of metastatic disease (spread of cancer to other sites). The stage of the cancer will determine whether the pancreatectomy to be performed should be total or distal.

A partial pancreatectomy may be indicated when the pancreas has been severely injured by trauma, especially injury to the body and tail of the pancreas. While such surgery removes normal pancreatic tissue as well, the long-term consequences of this surgery are

minimal, with virtually no effects on the production of insulin, digestive enzymes, and other hormones.

Chronic pancreatitis is another condition for which a pancreatectomy is occasionally performed. Chronic pancreatitis—or continuing inflammation of the pancreas that results in permanent damage to this organ—can develop from long-standing, recurring episodes of acute (periodic) pancreatitis. This painful condition usually results from alcohol abuse or the presence of gallstones. In most patients with the alcohol-induced disease, the pancreas is widely involved, therefore, surgical correction is almost impossible.

Description

A pancreatectomy can be performed through an open surgery technique, in which case one large incision is made, or it can be performed laparoscopically, in which case the surgeon makes four small incisions to insert tube-like **surgical instruments**. The abdomen is filled with gas, usually carbon dioxide, to help the surgeon view the abdominal cavity. A camera is inserted through one of the tubes and displays images on a monitor in the **operating room**. Other instruments are placed through the additional tubes. The laparoscopic approach allows the surgeon to work inside the patient's abdomen without making a large incision.

If the pancreatectomy is partial, the surgeon clamps and cuts the blood vessels, and the pancreas is stapled and divided for removal. If the disease affects the splenic artery or vein, the spleen is also removed.

If the pancreatectomy is total, the surgeon removes the entire pancreas and attached organs. He or she starts by dividing and detaching the end of the stomach. This part of the stomach leads to the small intestine, where the pancreas and bile duct both attach. In the next step, he removes the pancreas along with the connected section of the small intestine. The common bile duct and the gallbladder are also removed. To reconnect the intestinal tract, the stomach and the bile duct are then connected to the small intestine.

During a pancreatectomy procedure, several tubes are also inserted for **postoperative care**. To prevent tissue fluid from accumulating in the operated site, a temporary drain leading out of the body is inserted, as well as a **gastrostomy** or g-tube leading out of the stomach in order to help prevent nausea and vomiting. A jejunostomy or j-tube may also be inserted into the small intestine as a pathway for supplementary feeding.

Diagnosis/Preparation

Patients with symptoms of a pancreatic disorder undergo a number of tests before surgery is even considered. These can include ultrasonography, x-ray examinations, computed tomography scans (CT scan), and **endoscopic retrograde cholangiopancreatography** (ERCP), a specialized imaging technique to visualize the ducts that carry bile from the liver to the gallbladder. Tests may also include **angiography**, another imaging technique used to visualize the arteries feeding the pancreas, and needle aspiration cytology, in which cells are drawn from areas suspected to contain cancer. Such tests are required to establish a correct diagnosis for the pancreatic disorder and in the planning the surgery.

Since many patients with pancreatic cancer are undernourished, appropriate nutritional support, sometimes by tube feedings, may be required prior to surgery.

Some patients with pancreatic cancer deemed suitable for a pancreatectomy will also undergo chemotherapy and/or radiation therapy. This treatment is aimed at shrinking the tumor, which will improve the chances for successful surgical removal. Sometimes,

patients who are not initially considered surgical candidates may respond so well to chemoradiation that surgical treatment becomes possible. Radiation therapy may also be applied during the surgery (intraoperatively) to improve the patient's chances of survival, but this treatment is not yet in routine use. Some studies have shown that intraoperative radiation therapy extends survival by several months.

Patients undergoing distal pancreatectomy that involves removal of the spleen may receive preoperative medication to decrease the risk of infection.

Aftercare

Pancreatectomy is major surgery. Therefore, extended hospitalization is usually required with an average hospital stay of two to three weeks.

Some pancreatic cancer patients may also receive combined chemotherapy and radiation therapy after surgery. This additional treatment has been clearly shown to enhance survival rates.

After surgery, patients experience pain in the abdomen and are prescribed pain medication. Follow-up exams are required to monitor the patient's recovery and remove implanted tubes.

A total pancreatectomy leads to a condition called pancreatic insufficiency, because food can no longer be normally processed with the enzymes normally produced by the pancreas. Insulin secretion is likewise no longer possible. These conditions are treated with pancreatic enzyme replacement therapy, which supplies digestive enzymes; and with insulin injections. In some case, distal pancreatectomies may also lead to pancreatic insufficiency, depending on the patient's general health condition before surgery and on the extent of pancreatic tissue removal.

Risks

There is a fairly high risk of complications associated with any pancreatectomy procedure. A recent Johns Hopkins study documented complications in 41% of cases. The most devastating complication is postoperative bleeding, which increases the mortality risk to 20–50%. In cases of postoperative bleeding, the patient may be returned to surgery to find the source of hemorrhage, or may undergo other procedures to stop the bleeding.

One of the most common complications from a pancreaticoduodenectomy is delayed gastric emptying, a condition in which food and liquids are slow to leave the stomach. This complication occurred in 19% of patients in the Johns Hopkins study. To manage

WHO PERFORMS THE PROCEDURE AND WHERE IS IT PERFORMED?

A pancreatectomy is performed by a surgeon trained in gastroenterology, the branch of medicine that deals with the diseases of the digestive tract. An anesthesiologist is responsible for administering anesthesia and the operation is performed in a hospital setting, with an oncologist on the treatment team if pancreatic cancer motivated the procedure.

this problem, many surgeons insert feeding tubes at the original operation site, through which nutrients can be fed directly into the patient's intestines. This procedure, called enteral nutrition, maintains the patient's nutrition if the stomach is slow to recover normal function. Certain medications, called promotility agents, can help move the nutritional contents through the gastrointestinal tract.

The other most common complication is pancreatic anastomotic leak. This is a leak in the connection that the surgeon makes between the remainder of the pancreas and the other structures in the abdomen. Most surgeons handle the potential for this problem by checking the connection during surgery.

Normal results

After a total pancreatectomy, the body loses the ability to secrete insulin, enzymes, and other substances; therefore, the patient has to take supplements for the rest of his or her life.

Patients usually resume normal activities within a month after surgery, although they are asked to avoid heavy lifting for six to eight weeks and not to drive as long as they take narcotic medication.

When a pancreatectomy is performed for chronic pancreatitis, the majority of patients obtain some relief from pain. Some studies report that one-half to three-quarters of patients become free of pain.

Morbidity and mortality rates

The mortality rate for pancreatectomy has decreased in recent years to 5–10%, depending on the extent of the surgery and the experience of the surgeon. A study of 650 patients at Johns Hopkins Medical Institution, Baltimore, found that only nine patients, or 1.4%, died from complications related to surgery.

QUESTIONS TO ASK THE DOCTOR

- What do I need to do before surgery?
- What type of anesthesia will be used?
- How long will it take to recover from the surgery?
- When can I expect to return to work and/or resume normal activities?
- What are the risks associated with a pancreatectomy?
- How many pancreatectomies do you perform in a year?
- Will there be a scar?

Unfortunately, pancreatic cancer is the most lethal form of gastrointestinal malignancy. However, for a highly selective group of patients, a pancreatectomy offers a chance for cure, especially when performed by experienced surgeons. The overall five-year survival rate for patients who undergo pancreatectomy for pancreatic cancer is about 10%; patients who undergo pancreaticoduodenectomy have a 4–5% survival at five years. The risk for tumor recurrence is thought to be unaffected by whether the patient undergoes a total pancreatectomy or a pancreaticoduodenectomy, but is increased when the tumor is larger than 1.2 in (3 cm) and the cancer has spread to the lymph nodes or surrounding tissue.

Alternatives

Depending on the medical condition, a **pancreas transplantation** may be considered as an alternative for some patients.

Resources

BOOKS

Bastidas, J. Augusto, and John E. Niederhuber. "The Pancreas." In *Fundamentals of Surgery*. Edited by John E. Niederhuber. Stamford: Appleton & Lange, 1998.

Mayer, Robert J. "Pancreatic Cancer." In *Harrison's Principles of Internal Medicine*. Edited by Anthony S. Fauci, et al. New York: McGraw-Hill, 1997.

PERIODICALS

Cretolle, C., C. N. Fekete, D. Jan, et al. "Partial elective pancreatectomy is curative in focal form of permanent hyperinsulinemic hypoglycaemia in infancy: A report of 45 cases from 1983 to 2000." *Journal of Pediatric Surgery* 37 (February 2002): 155–158.

Lillemoe, K. D., S. Kaushal, J. L. Cameron, et al. "Distal pancreatectomy: indications and outcomes in 235 patients." *Annals of Surgery* 229 (May 1999): 698–700.

McAndrew, H. F., V. Smith, and L. Spitz. "Surgical complications of pancreatectomy for persistent hyperinsulinaemic hypoglycaemia of infancy." *Journal of Pediatric Surgery* 38 (January 2003): 13–16.

Patterson, E. J., M. Gagner, B. Salky, et al. "Laparoscopic pancreatic resection: single-institution experience of 19 patients." *Journal of the American College of Surgeons* 193 (September 2001): 281–287.

ORGANIZATIONS

American College of Gastroenterology. 4900 B South 31st St., Arlington, VA 22206. (703) 820-7400. http://www.acg.gi.org.

American Gastroenterological Association (AGA). 4930 Del Ray Avenue, Bethesda, MD 20814. (301) 654-2055. http://www.gastro.org.

National Cancer Institute (NCI). NCI Public Inquiries Office, Suite 3036A, 6116 Executive Boulevard, MSC8322 Bethesda, MD 20892-8322. (800) 422-6237. http://www.cancer.gov.

OTHER

NIH CancerNet: Pancreatic Cancer Homepage. [cited July 1, 2003]. http://www.cancer.gov/cancerinfo/types/pancreatic.

Caroline A. Helwick
Monique Laberge, Ph.D.

Paracentesis

Definition

Paracentesis is a minimally invasive procedure that uses a needle to remove fluid from the abdomen.

Purpose

There are two reasons to take fluid out of the abdomen. One is to analyze it for diagnostic purposes; the other is to relieve pressure. Liquid that accumulates in the abdomen is called ascites. Ascites seeps out of organs for several reasons related either to disease in the organ or fluid pressures that are changing.

Liver disease

All the blood flowing through the intestines passes through the liver on its way back to the heart. When progressive disease such as alcohol damage or hepatitis destroys enough liver tissue, the scarring that results shrinks the liver and constricts blood flow. Such scarring of the liver is called cirrhosis. Pressure builds in the intestinal blood circulation, slowing flow and pushing fluid into surrounding tissues. Slowly the

> **KEY TERMS**
>
> **Ascites**—Fluid in the abdomen.
>
> **Ectopic pregnancy**—A pregnancy occurring outside the womb that often ruptures and requires surgical removal.
>
> **Hepatitis**—An inflammation of the liver.

fluid accumulates in areas with the lowest pressure and greatest capacity. The free space around abdominal organs receives the greatest amount. This space is called the peritoneal space because it is enclosed by a thin membrane called the peritoneum. The peritoneum wraps around nearly every organ in the abdomen, providing many folds and spaces for the fluid to gather.

Infections

Peritonitis is an infection of the peritoneum that can develop in several ways. Many abdominal organs contain germs that do not occur elsewhere in the body. If they spill their contents into the peritoneum, infection is the result. Infection changes the dynamics of body fluids, causing them to seep into tissues and spaces. The gall bladder, the stomach, any part of the intestine, and most especially the appendix—all cause peritonitis when they leak or rupture. Tuberculosis can infect many organs in the body; it is not confined to the lungs. Tuberculous peritonitis causes ascites.

Other inflammations

Peritoneal fluid is not just produced by infections. An inflamed pancreas, called pancreatitis, can cause a massive sterile peritonitis when it leaks its digestive enzymes into the abdomen.

Cancer

Any cancer that begins in or spreads to the abdomen can leak fluid. One particular tumor of the ovary that leaks fluid and results in fluid accumulation is called Meigs' syndrome.

Kidney disease

Since the kidneys are intimately involved with the body's fluid balance, diseases of the kidney often cause excessive fluid to accumulate. Nephrosis and nephrotic syndrome are the general terms for diseases that cause the kidneys to retain water and promote its movement into body tissues and spaces.

Heart failure

The ultimate source of fluid pressure in the body is the heart, whose pumping generates blood pressure. All other pressures in the body are related to blood pressure. As the heart starts to fail, blood backs up, waiting to be pumped. This increases pressure in the veins leading to the heart, particularly below the it where gravity is also pulling blood down. The extra fluid from heart failure is first noticed in the feet and ankles, where gravitational effects are most evident. In the abdomen, the liver swells first, then it and other abdominal organs start to leak.

Pleural fluid

The other major body cavity (besides the abdomen) is the chest. The tissue in the chest corresponding to the peritoneum is called the pleura, and the space contained within the pleura, between the ribs and the lungs, is called the pleural space. Fluid is often found in both cavities, and fluid from one cavity can find its way into the other.

Fluid that accumulates in the abdomen creates abnormal pressures on organs in the abdomen. Digestion is hindered; blood flow is slowed. Pressure upward on the chest from fluid-filled organs compromises breathing. The kidneys function poorly in the presence of such external pressures and may even fail.

Description

During paracentesis, special needles puncture the abdominal wall, being careful not to hit internal organs. If fluid is needed only for analysis, less than 7 oz (200 ml) are removed. If pressure relief is an additional goal, many quarts may be removed. Rapid removal of large amounts of fluid can cause blood pressure to drop suddenly. For this reason, the physician will often leave a tube in place so that fluid can be removed slowly, giving the system time to adapt.

A related procedure called culpocentesis removes ascitic fluid from the very bottom of the abdominal cavity through the back of the vagina. This is used most often to diagnose female genital disorders like ectopic pregnancy, which may bleed or exude fluid into the peritoneal space.

Fluid is sent to the laboratory for testing, where cancer and blood cells can be detected, infections identified, and chemical analysis can direct further investigations.

Aftercare

An adhesive bandage and perhaps a single stitch close the insertion site. Nothing more is required.

Risks

Risks are negligible. It is remotely possible that an organ could be punctured and bleed or that an infection could be introduced.

Normal results

A diagnosis of the cause and/or relief from accumulated fluid pressure are the expected results. Fluid will continue to accumulate until the cause is corrected. Repeated procedures may be needed.

Resources

BOOKS

Chung, Raymond T. and Daniel K. Podolsky. "Cirrhosis and its Complications." In *Harrison's Principles of Internal Medicine*, edited by Eugene Braunwald, et al. New York: McGraw-Hill, 2001.

Henry, J. B. *Clinical Diagnosis and Management by Laboratory Methods*. 20th ed. Philadelphia, PA: W. B. Saunders Company, 2001.

OTHER

Lehrer, Jennifer K. *Abdominal tap—paracentesis*. National Institutes of Health. January 1, 2003 [cited April 4, 2003]. http://www.nlm.nih.gov/medlineplus/encyclopedia.html.

"Paracentesis." American Thoracic Society. April, 2003 [cited April 4, 2003]. http://www.thoracic.org/assemblies/cc/ccprimer/infosheet10.html.

J. Ricker Polsdorfer, MD
Mark A. Best, MD

Paralytic ileus *see* **Intestinal obstruction repair**

Parathyroid gland removal *see* **Parathyroidectomy**

Parathyroidectomy

Definition

Parathyroidectomy is the removal of one or more parathyroid glands. A person usually has four parathyroid glands, although the exact number may vary from three to seven. The glands are located in the neck, in front of the Adam's apple, and are closely linked to

Parathyroidectomy

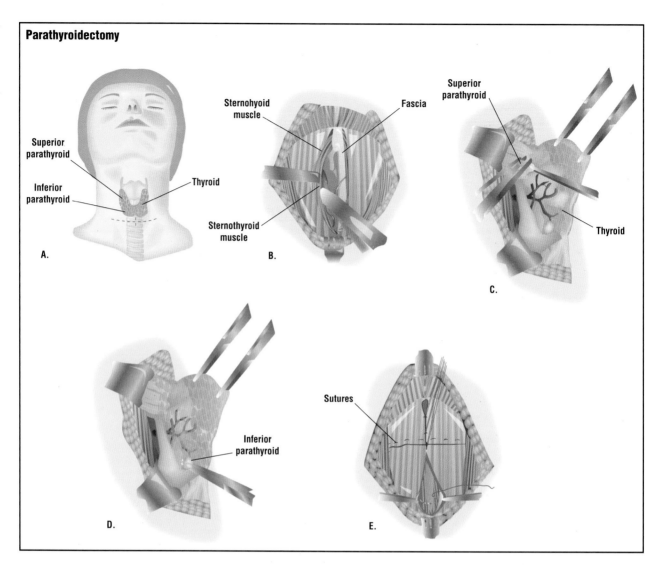

The parathyroid gland is accessed through an incision in the neck (A). Muscles and connecting tissues, or fascia, are cut open (B). The thyroid gland is exposed, and the superior (C) and inferior parathyroid glands are removed (D). The muscle layers are stitched, and the wound closed (E). *(Illustration by GGS Information Services. Cengage Learning, Gale.)*

the thyroid gland. The parathyroid glands regulate the balance of calcium in the body.

Purpose

Parathyroidectomy is usually performed to treat hyperparathyroidism (abnormal over-functioning of the parathyroid glands).

Demographics

The number of parathyroidectomy procedures has risen due to routine measurement of calcium in the blood. Incidence rates vary between 25 and 50 per 100,000 persons. The number of procedures in females is approximately twice that of males. The incidence of parathyroidectomy rises after age 40.

Description

The operation begins when an anesthesiologist administers **general anesthesia**. The surgeon makes an incision in the front of the neck where a tight-fitting necklace would rest. All of the parathyroid glands are identified. The surgeon then identifies the diseased gland or glands, and confirms the diagnosis by sending a piece of the gland(s) to the pathology department for immediate microscopic examination. The diseased glands are then removed, and the incision is closed and covered with a dressing.

KEY TERMS

Anesthesiologist—A physician who specializes in anesthetizing persons for operations or other medical procedures.

Ectopic parathyroid tissue—Parathyroid tissue located in an abnormal place.

Hyperparathyroidism—Abnormal over-functioning of the parathyroid glands.

Hypoparathyroidism—Abnormal under-functioning of the parathyroid glands.

Otolaryngologist—A surgeon who treats people with abnormalities in the head and neck regions of the body.

Recurrent laryngeal nerve—A nerve that lies very near the parathyroid glands, and serves the larynx or voice box.

Parathyroidectomy patients usually stay overnight in the hospital after the operation. Some patients remain hospitalized for one or two additional days.

Diagnosis/Preparation

Prior to the operation, the diagnosis of hyperparathyroidism should be confirmed using lab tests. Occasionally, physicians order computed tomography scans (**CT scans**), **ultrasound** exams, or **magnetic resonance imaging** (MRI) tests to determine the total number of parathyroid glands, and their location prior to the procedure.

Parathyroidectomy should only be performed when other non-operative methods have failed to control a person's hyperparathyroidism.

Preparation is similar to other surgical procedures requiring general anesthetic. The patient is not allowed any food or drink by mouth after midnight the night before surgery. He or she should ask the physician for specific directions regarding preparation for surgery, including food, drink, and medication intake.

Aftercare

The incision should be watched for signs of infection. In general, no special **wound care** is required.

The calcium level is monitored during the first 48 hours after the operation by obtaining frequent blood samples for laboratory analysis.

Most individuals require only two or three days of hospitalization to recover from the operation. They

WHO PERFORMS THE PROCEDURE AND WHERE IS IT PERFORMED?

Parathyroidectomy is an operation performed most commonly by a general surgeon, or occasionally by an otolaryngologist, in the operating room of a hospital.

can usually resume most of their normal activities within one to two weeks.

Risks

The major risk of parathyroidectomy is injury to the recurrent laryngeal nerve (a nerve that lies very near the parathyroid glands and serves the larynx or voice box). If this nerve is injured, the voice may become hoarse or weak.

Occasionally, too much parathyroid tissue is removed, and a person may develop hypoparathyroidism (under-functioning of the parathyroid glands). If this occurs, he or she will require daily calcium supplements.

In some cases, the surgeon is unable to locate all of the parathyroid glands, and cannot remove them in one procedure. A fifth or sixth gland may be located in an aberrant place such as the chest (ectopic parathyroid). If this occurs, the hyperparathyroidism may not be corrected with one operation, and a second procedure may be required to find all of the patient's remaining parathyroid gland tissue.

Normal results

The surgery progresses normally if the diseased parathyroid glands are located and removed from the neck region.

Morbidity and mortality rates

Hematoma formation (collection of blood under the incision) is a possible complication of any operative procedure. However, in procedures that involve the neck it is of particular concern because a rapidly enlarging hematoma can obstruct the airway.

Infection of the surgical incision may occur, as it may in any operative procedure, but this is uncommon in parathyroidectomy.

Before the function of the parathyroid gland was understood, people undergoing a **thyroidectomy** often

QUESTIONS TO ASK THE DOCTOR

- What type of physician performs the surgery?
- Is the surgeon board certified in head and neck surgery?
- How many parathyroidectomy procedures has the surgeon performed?
- What is the surgeon's complication rate?
- Is there an alternative to surgery?
- What is the risk of complication?
- How will the body's function change after the surgery?

died due to the lack of calcium in their blood caused by removal of the parathyroid glands. This is not a problem today.

Alternatives

There is no safe or reliable alternative to removal of the parathyroid glands for the treatment of hyperparathyroidism. Oral phosphates can lower serum calcium levels, but the long-term use of this approach is not well understood.

Resources

BOOKS

Bilezikan, J.P., R. Marcus, M. Levine. *The Parathyroids* 2nd Edition. St. Louis: Academic Press, 2001.

Bland, K.I, W.G. Cioffi, M.G. Sarr. *Practice of General Surgery*. Philadelphia: Saunders, 2001.

Randolph, G. *Surgery of Thyroid and Parathyroid Glands*. St. Louis: Elsevier, 2002.

Schwartz, S.I., J.E. Fischer, F.C. Spencer, G.T. Shires, J.M. Daly. *Principles of Surgery* 7th edition. New York: McGraw Hill, 1998.

Townsend C., K.L. Mattox, R.D. Beauchamp, B.M. Evers, D.C. Sabiston *Sabiston Review of Surgery* 3rd Edition. Philadelphia: Saunders, 2001.

PERIODICALS

Awad, S.S., J. Miskulin, N. Thompson. "Parathyroid Adenomas versus Four-gland Hyperplasia as the Cause of Primary Hyperparathyroidism in Patients with Prolonged Lithium Therapy." *World Journal of Surgery* 27, no.4 (2003): 486-8.

Genc, H., E. Morita, N.D. Perrier, D. Miura, P. Ituarte, Q.Y. Duh, O.H. Clark. "Differing Histologic Findings after Bilateral and Focused Parathyroidectomy." *Journal of the American College of Surgery* 196, no.4 (2003): 535-40.

Goldstein, R.E., D. Billheimer, W.H. Martin, K. Richards. "Sestamibi Scanning and Minimally Invasive Radio-guided Parathyroidectomy without Intraoperative Parathyroid Hormone Measurement." *Annals of Surgery* 237, no.5 (2003): 722-31.

Miccoli, P., P. Berti, G. Materazzi, G. Donatini. "Minimally Invasive Video Assisted Parathyroidectomy (MIVAP)." *European Journal of Surgical Oncology* 29, no.2 (2003): 188-90.

ORGANIZATIONS

American College of Surgeons. 633 North St. Clair Street, Chicago, IL 60611-32311. (312) 202-5000, fax: (312) 202-5001. http://www.facs.org, E-mail: postmaster@facs.org.

American Medical Association. 515 N. State Street, Chicago, IL 60610. (312) 464-5000. http://www.ama-assn.org.

American Academy of Otolaryngology-Head and Neck Surgery. One Prince St., Alexandria, VA 22314-3357. (703) 836-4444. http://www.entnet.org/index2.cfm.

American Osteopathic College of Otolaryngology-Head and Neck Surgery. 405 W. Grand Avenue, Dayton, OH 45405. (937) 222-8820 or (800) 455-9404, fax (937) 222-8840. Email: info@aocoohns.org.

Association of Thyroid Surgeons. 717 Buena Vista St., Ventura, CA 93001. Fax: (509) 479-8678. info@thyroidsurgery.org.

OTHER

Columbia University Medical Center. [cited May 5, 2003] http://cpmcnet.columbia.edu/dept/thyroid/parasurgHP.html.

Mayo Clinic. [cited May 5, 2003] http://www.mayoclinic.org/checkup/02mar-parathyroid.html.

Ohio State University. [cited May 5, 2003] http://www.acs.ohio-state.edu/units/osuhosp/patedu/ Materials/PDFDocs/surgery/thyroid.pdf.

University of California-San Diego. [cited May 5, 2003] http://www-surgery.ucsd.edu/ent/PatientInfo/th_parathyroid.html.

University of Wisconsin. [cited May 5, 2003] http://www.surgery.wisc.edu/general/patients/endocrine.shtml.

L. Fleming Fallon, Jr., M.D., Dr.PH.

Paravaginal surgery *see* **Needle bladder neck suspension**

Parentage testing

Definition

Parentage testing (previously called paternity testing) refers to a variety of DNA tests used in an attempt to verify whether someone could possibly be the mother or the father of a particular child. Parentage testing has two possible results: an individual can be definitively excluded as the parent, or an individual can be defined as having some degree of probability of being the parent.

In fact, neither paternity nor maternity can actually be definitively demonstrated through current tests. Instead, these tests provide information that a particular individual cannot be excluded as the child's parent. A mathematical model is then utilized to determine an estimate of the probability that, based on the results of the testing, a particular individual IS that child's parent. The probability is called the parentage index, and it uses DNA results, as well as situational information (where the alleged parent was at the time of the child's conception, comparison of the alleged parent's and the child's physical appearance) to generate a percent chance of parentage.

The first step in parentage testing involves collecting some type of DNA sample from the child in question, the known parent, and the alleged parent. Any type of biological tissue can be used for this testing. Most commonly, a testing sample is obtained either through a buccal (inside of the cheek) swab, or through blood testing. DNA is the genetic material stored inside the nucleus of every cell within the human body. The DNA can be extracted from the nucleus of the cells which have been procured in the testing sample for each individual. Laboratory testing then evaluates the known parent's DNA, and compares this to the child's DNA. The DNA of each individual is sequenced, and DNA sequences that match the known relationship are excluded. The remaining DNA sequences are then compared to DNA sequences of the alleged parent. This gives the examiners information on the probability that this individual is or is not capable of having parented the child, up to a probability of over 99.9%.

Purpose

This test is performed to exclude the possibility that a particular individual could be the biological mother or father of a baby or child, or to provide evidence of probability that the individual might be the biological mother or father of a baby or child. These tests are often run when a mother is uncertain of her baby's paternity, to clarify child support issues, to clarify issues that may come up relative to an adoption, or in forensic medicine (medicine pertaining to a crime).

Precautions

Parentage testing is not effected by illness, medications, activity level or diet. However, the test results can be affected by a recent blood transfusion. Therefore, if

KEY TERMS

Buccal—The interior surface of the cheek.

DNA—Deoxyribonucleic acid; the substance within the nucleus of all human cells in which the genetic information is stored.

Maternity—Refers to the mother.

Paternity—Refers to the father.

blood is being used for the DNA testing, 90 days should elapse between a blood transfusion and parentage testing.

Patients who are taking anticoagulant medications should inform their healthcare practitioner prior to a blood draw, since this may increase their chance of bleeding or bruising after a blood test.

Description

While blood testing is frequently performed for parentage testing, other types of tissue may be used to provide DNA samples appropriate for testing. This includes a buccal (inside of the cheek) swab, in which a cotton-swab like instrument is used to scrape a few of the cells from the inside of the cheek. In some cases, other types of biological tissue, bone, or teeth may be used for testing.

This test may be performed using blood drawn from a vein (usually one in the forearm), generally by a nurse or phlebotomist (an individual who has been trained to draw blood). A tourniquet is applied to the arm above the area where the needle stick will be performed. The site of the needle stick is cleaned with antiseptic, and the needle is inserted. The blood is collected in vacuum tubes. After collection, the needle is withdrawn, and pressure is kept on the blood draw site to stop any bleeding and decrease bruising. A bandage is then applied. Alternatively, a finger stick can be used to draw just a few drops of blood from a finger tip.

Because the results of parentage testing are frequently utilized in court or as evidence in legal decisions, there are very careful regulations on the way the samples are drawn, labeled, stored, and transported. It is crucial that the chain-of-custody of all samples is clearly delineated, and that all packaging is tamper-free and appropriately labeled. Individuals who are involved in the actual parentage case are restrained from being involved in the actual acts of either collecting or transporting the DNA-containing samples.

Preparation

There are no restrictions on diet or physical activity, either before or after the testing.

Aftercare

There is no aftercare necessary following a buccal swab.

As with any blood tests, discomfort, bruising, and/or a very small amount of bleeding is common at the puncture site. Immediately after the needle is withdrawn, it is helpful to put pressure on the puncture site until the bleeding has stopped. This decreases the chance of significant bruising. Warm packs may relieve minor discomfort. Some individuals may feel briefly woozy after a blood test, and they should be encouraged to lie down and rest until they feel better.

Risks

Neither a buccal swab nor basic blood tests carry any significant risk.

Results

One possible outcome of parentage testing is exclusion of the possibility that an individual has any chance whatsoever of being able to be genetically related as a parent to the child in question—this is referred to as a zero-percent probability. Positive proof of parentage can approach 99.9% probability that a particular individual could be a particular child's parent.

Resources

BOOKS

McPherson, R. A., et al. *Henry's Clinical Diagnosis and Management By Laboratory Methods,* 21st ed. Philadelphia: Saunders, 2007.

ORGANIZATIONS

American Association of Clinical Chemistry. 1850 K St., N.WSuite 625, Washington, DC 20006. http://www.aacc.org.

Rosalyn Carson-DeWitt, MD

Parkinson's surgery *see* **Deep brain stimulation**

Parotid gland removal *see* **Parotidectomy**

Parotidectomy

Definition

Parotidectomy is the removal of the parotid gland, a salivary gland near the ear.

Purpose

The parotid gland is the largest of the salivary glands. There are two parotid glands, one on each side of the face, just below and to the front of the ear. A duct through which saliva is secreted runs from each gland to the inside of the cheek.

The main purpose of parotidectomy is to remove abnormal growths (neoplasms) that occur in the parotid gland. Parotid gland neoplasms may be benign (approximately 80%) or malignant. Tumors may spread from other areas of the body, entering the parotid gland by way of the lymphatic system.

Demographics

Benign parotid gland growths usually appear after the age of 40. Malignant growths most often affect women over the age of 60, while benign tumors affect both sexes equally. Cancer of the salivary glands accounts for only 1% of all cancers, and 7% of all head and neck cancers.

Description

During surgery, two different areas of the parotid gland are identified: the superficial lobe and the deep lobe. Superficial parotidectomy removes just the superficial lobe, while total parotidectomy removes both lobes.

The patient is first placed under **general anesthesia** to ensure that no pain is experienced and that all muscles remain relaxed. An incision is made directly to the front or back of the ear and down the jaw line. The skin is folded back to expose the parotid gland. The various facial nerves are identified and protected during the surgery so as to avoid permanent facial paralysis or numbness. A superficial or total parotidectomy is then performed, depending on the type and location of the tumor. If the tumor has spread to involve the facial nerve, the operation is expanded to include parts of the bone behind the ear (mastoid) to remove as much tumor as possible. Before the incision is closed, a drain is inserted into the area to collect any leaking saliva, if a superficial parotidectomy was performed. The procedure typically takes from two to five hours to complete, depending on the extent of surgery and the skill of the surgeon.

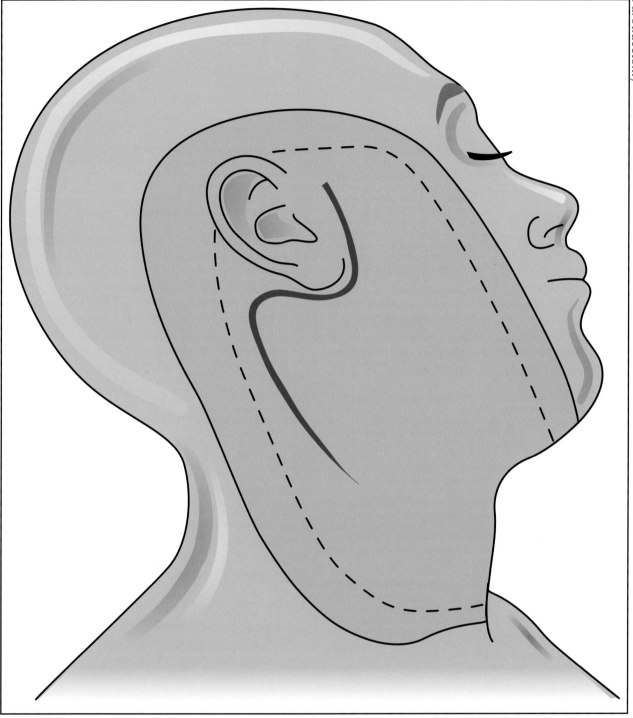

Parotidectomy is a surgical procedure performed to remove cancerous tumors in the parotid gland, a salivary gland near the ear. Among the tumors seen in the parotid gland are lymphoma, melanoma, and squamous cell carcinoma. The illustration above shows the facial incision sites for this procedure. *(Illustration by Electronic Illustrators Group. Cengage Learning, Gale.)*

Diagnosis/Preparation

A complete **physical examination** and medical history is performed, as are diagnostic tests to help the surgeon better plan for the surgery. Some tests that may be performed include computed tomography (CT) scan, **magnetic resonance imaging** (MRI),

KEY TERMS

Fistula—An abnormal opening or duct through tissue that results from injury, disease, or other trauma.

Salivary glands—Three pairs of glands that secrete into the mouth and aid digestion.

and fine-needle aspiration biopsy (using a thin needle to withdraw fluid and cells from the growth).

Aftercare

After surgery, the patient will remain in the hospital for one to three days. The incision site will be watched closely for signs of infection and heavy bleeding (hemorrhage). The incision site should be kept clean and dry until it is completely healed. If the patient has difficulty smiling, winking, or drinking fluids, the physician should be contacted immediately. These are signs of facial nerve damage.

Risks

There are a number of complications that are associated with parotidectomy. Facial nerve paralysis after minor surgery should be minimal. After major surgery, a graft is attempted to restore nerve function to facial muscles. Salivary fistulas can occur when saliva collects in the incision site or drains through the incision. Recurrence of cancer is the single most important consideration for patients who have undergone parotidectomy. Long-term survival rates are largely dependent on the tumor type and the stage of tumor development at the time of the operation.

Other risks include hematoma (collection of blood under the skin) and infection. The most common long-term complication of parotidectomy is redness and sweating in the cheek, known as Frey's syndrome. Rarely, paralysis may extend throughout all the branches of the facial nervous system.

Normal results

Although some facial numbness or weakness is normal immediately following parotidectomy, these symptoms usually subside within a few months, with most patients regaining full function within one year. Return of a benign tumor is very rare.

WHO PERFORMS THE PROCEDURE AND WHERE IS IT PERFORMED?

Parotidectomy is performed in a hospital operating room, usually by an otolaryngologist, a medical doctor who specializes in the treatment of diseases that affect the ear, nose, throat, and other structures of the head and neck.

Morbidity and mortality rates

There is a 25–50% risk of temporary facial weakness following parotidectomy, and a 1–2% risk of permanent weakness. Frey's syndrome may be experienced by up to 90% of patients to some extent and causes perspiration on that side of the face with eating. There is very little or no risk of mortality associated with the surgery. The survival rate of malignant parotid gland tumors depends on their size, location, extension, and if metastasis has occurred. The 10-year survival rate ranges from 32% to 83%.

Alternatives

A benign parotid neoplasm may be managed expectantly (i.e., adhering to a period of watchful waiting) so that the growth is of a larger size before it is removed (the risk of facial nerve damage increases with each subsequent parotidectomy). There is generally no alternative to surgical treatment of parotid gland neoplasms, although radiation therapy may be recommended after the procedure in the case of malignant tumors.

Resources

PERIODICALS

Califano, Joseph, and David W. Eisele. "Benign Salivary Gland Neoplasms." *Otolaryngology Clinics of North America* 32, no. 5 (October 1, 1999): 861–73.

Carlson, Grant W. "The Salivary Glands: Embryology, Anatomy, and Surgical Applications." *Surgical Clinics of North America* 80, no. 1 (February 1, 2000): 261–73.

Sinha, Uttam, and Matthew Ng. "Surgery of the Salivary Glands." *Otolaryngology Clinics of North America* 32, no. 5 (October 1, 1999): 887–906.

ORGANIZATIONS

American Academy of Otolaryngology. One Prince St., Alexandria, VA 22314-3357. (703) 836-4444. http://www.entnet.org.

QUESTIONS TO ASK THE DOCTOR

- Why is a parotidectomy being recommended?
- How many parotidectomies do you perform each year?
- What is your rate of complications?
- What diagnostic tests will be performed prior to surgery?
- Will a superficial or total parotidectomy be performed?

OTHER

Gordon, Ashley D. "Parotid Tumors, Benign." *eMedicine,* December 27, 2001 [cited April 7, 2003] http://www. emedicine.com/plastic/topic371.htm.

Johns, Michael M. "Salivary Gland Neoplasms." *eMedicine,* May 17, 2002 [cited April 7, 2003] http://www.emedicine. com/ent/topic679.htm.

Shelato, Dwight. *The Patient's Forum on Tumors of the Parotid Gland,* [cited April 7, 2003] <http://patientsforum. com>.

Mary K. Fyke
Stephanie Dionne Sherk

Partial thromboplastin time

Definition

The partial thromboplastin time (PTT) test is a blood test that is done to investigate bleeding disorders and to monitor patients taking an anticlotting drug (heparin).

Purpose

Diagnosis

Blood clotting (coagulation) depends on the action of substances in the blood called clotting factors. Measuring the partial thromboplastin time helps to assess which specific clotting factors may be missing or defective.

Monitoring

Certain surgical procedures and diseases cause blood clots to form within blood vessels. Heparin is used to treat these clots. The PTT test can be used to monitor the effect of heparin on a patient's coagulation system.

Precautions

Certain medications besides heparin can affect the results of the PPT test. These include antihistamines, vitamin C (ascorbic acid), **aspirin**, and chlorpromazine (Thorazine).

Description

When a body tissue is injured and begins to bleed, it starts a sequence of clotting factor activities called the coagulation cascade, which leads to the formation of a blood clot. The cascade has three pathways: extrinsic, intrinsic, and common. Many of the thirteen known clotting factors in human blood are shared by both pathways; several are found in only one. The PTT test evaluates the factors found in the intrinsic and common pathways. It is usually done in combination with other tests, such as the prothrombin test, which evaluate the factors of the extrinsic pathway. The combination of tests narrows the list of possible missing or defective factors.

Heparin prevents clotting by blocking certain factors in the intrinsic pathway. The PTT test allows a doctor to check that there is enough heparin in the blood to prevent clotting, but not so much as to cause bleeding. The test is done before the first dose of heparin or whenever the dosage level is changed; and again when the heparin has reached a constant level in the blood. The PTT test is repeated at scheduled intervals.

The PTT test uses blood to which a chemical has been added to prevent clotting before the test begins. About 5 mL of blood are drawn from a vein in the patient's inner elbow region. Collection of the sample takes only a few minutes. The blood is spun in a centrifuge, which separates the pale yellow liquid part of blood (plasma) from the cells. Calcium and activating substances are added to the plasma to start the intrinsic pathway of the coagulation cascade. The partial thromboplastin time is the time it takes for a clot to form, measured in seconds.

The test can be done without activators, but they are usually added to shorten the clotting time, making the test more useful for monitoring heparin levels. When activators are used, the test is called activated partial thromboplastin time or APTT.

Test results can be obtained in less than one hour. The test is usually covered by insurance.

Preparation

The doctor should check to see if the patient is taking any of the medications that may influence the test results. If the patient is on heparin therapy, the blood sample is drawn one hour before the next dose of heparin.

Aftercare

Aftercare includes routine care of the puncture site. In addition, patients on heparin therapy must be watched for signs of spontaneous bleeding. The patient should not be left alone until the doctor or nurse is sure that bleeding has stopped. Patients should also be advised to watch for bleeding gums, bruising easily, and other signs of clotting problems; to avoid activities that might cause minor cuts or bruises; and to avoid using aspirin.

Risks

The patient may develop a bruise or swelling around the puncture site, which can be treated with moist warm compresses. People with coagulation problems may bleed for a longer period than normal.

Normal results

Normal results vary based on the method and activators used. Normal APTT results are usually between 25–40 seconds; PTT results are between 60–70 seconds. APTT results for a patient on heparin should be 1.5–2.5 times normal values. An APTT longer than 100 seconds indicates spontaneous bleeding.

Abnormal results

Increased levels in a person with a bleeding disorder indicate a clotting factor may be missing or defective. Further tests are done to identify the factor involved. Liver disease decreases production of factors, increasing the PTT.

Low levels in a patient on heparin indicate too little heparin is in the blood to prevent clots. High levels indicate too much heparin is present, placing the person at risk of excessive bleeding.

Morbidity and mortality rates

Morbidity rates are excessively miniscule. The most common problems are minor bleeding and bruising. Since neither are reportable events, morbidity can only be estimated. Mortality is essentially zero.

KEY TERMS

Activated partial thromboplastin time—Partial thromboplastin time test that uses activators to shorten the clotting time, making it more useful for heparin monitoring.

Clotting factors—Substances in the blood that act in sequence to stop bleeding by forming a clot.

Coagulation—The process of blood clotting.

Coagulation cascade—The sequence of biochemical activities, involving clotting factors, that stop bleeding by forming a clot.

Common pathway—The pathway that results from the merging of the extrinsic and intrinsic pathways. The common pathway includes the final steps before a clot is formed.

Extrinsic pathway—One of three pathways in the coagulation cascade.

Heparin—A medication that prevents blood clots.

Intrinsic pathway—One of three pathways in the coagulation cascade.

Partial thromboplastin time—A test that checks the clotting factors of the intrinsic pathway.

Plasma—The fluid part of blood, as distinguished from blood cells.

Alternatives Resources

There are no alternatives to a partial thromboplastin time.

Precautions

The only precaution needed is to clean the venipuncture site with alcohol.

Side effects

The most common side effects of a partial thromboplastin time test are minor bleeding and bruising.

Resources

BOOKS

Fischbach, F. T. and M. B. Dunning. A Manual of Laboratory and Diagnostic Tests. 8th ed. Philadelphia: Lippincott Williams & Wilkins, 2008.

McGhee, M. A Guide to Laboratory Investigations. 5th ed. Oxford, UK: Radcliffe Publishing Ltd, 2008.

Price, C. P. Evidence-Based Laboratory Medicine: Principles, Practice, and Outcomes. 2nd ed. Washington, DC: AACC Press, 2007.

Scott, M.G., A. M. Gronowski, and C. S. Eby. Tietz's Applied Laboratory Medicine. 2nd ed. New York: Wiley-Liss, 2007.

Springhouse, A. M.. Diagnostic Tests Made Incredibly Easy!. 2nd ed. Philadelphia: Lippincott Williams & Wilkins, 2008.

PERIODICALS

Aksungar, F. B., A. E. Topkaya, Z. Yildiz, S. Sahin, and U. Turk. "Coagulation status and biochemical and inflammatory markers in multiple sclerosis." Journal of Clinical Neuroscience 15, no. 4 (2008): 393–397.

Awan, M. S., M. Iqbal, and S. Z. Imam. "Epistaxis: when are coagulation studies justified?" Emergency Medicine Journal 25, no. 3 (2008): 156–157.

Mueck, W., B. I. Eriksson, K. A. Bauer et al. "Population pharmacokinetics and pharmacodynamics of rivaroxaban - an oral, direct factor Xa inhibitor - in patients undergoing major orthopaedic surgery." Clinical Pharmacokinetics 47, no. 3 (2008): 203–216.

Rosenkrantz, A., M. Hinden, B. Leschmik, et al. "Calibrated automated thrombin generation in normal uncomplicated pregnancy." Thrombosis and Hemostasis 99, no. 2 (2008): 331–337.

ORGANIZATIONS

American Association for Clinical Chemistry. http://www.aacc.org/AACC/.

American Society for Clinical Laboratory Science. http://www.ascls.org/.

American Society of Clinical Pathologists. http://www.ascp.org/.

College of American Pathologists. http://www.cap.org/apps/cap.portal.

OTHER

American Clinical Laboratory Association. Information about clinical chemistry. 2008 [cited February 24, 2008]. http://www.clinical-labs.org/.

Clinical Laboratory Management Association. Information about clinical chemistry. 2008 [cited February 22, 2008]. http://www.clma.org/.

Lab Tests On Line. Information about lab tests. 2008 [cited February 24, 2008]. http://www.labtestsonline.org/.

National Accreditation Agency for Clinical Laboratory Sciences. Information about laboratory tests. 2008 [cited February 25, 2008]. http://www.naacls.org/.

L. Fleming Fallon, Jr, MD, DrPH

Patella removal *see* **Kneecap removal**

Patent ductus arteriosis repair *see* **Heart surgery for congenital defects**

Patent urachus repair

Definition

Patent urachus repair is surgery to correct a urachus (a tube that connects the fetal bladder to the umbilical cord) that fails to close after birth.

Purpose

A patent urachus is an anomaly, and repair is recommended for these defects occurring at birth.

Demographics

The condition occurs three times more often in male infants than in females.

Description

As fetal development progresses, the urachus, a tube that can measure from 1.2–3.9 in (3–10 cm) long and 0.3–0.4 in (8–10 mm) in diameter, forms, extending from the front dome of the bladder to the umbilicus. Following birth, the tube, adjacent to the umbilical ligaments, closes and itself becomes ligament. Should this closure fail, it may result in several types of urachal remnants. If the urachus remains completely open, it is known as a patent urachus. This type of abnormality makes up 50% of all urachal anomalies.

If the urachus remains open all the way to the bladder, there is the danger that bacteria will enter the bladder through the open tube and cause infection. For this reason, the patent urachus of the infant must be removed.

Diagnosis/Preparation

This anomaly occurs as an isolated event or in association with prune-belly syndrome, in which there is continuous drainage of urine from the umbilicus. If urine freely discharges through the umbilicus, the patent urachus is rarely found. It should be suspected, however, if a local cord is enlarged and affected with edema, or is slow to slough normally. The condition customarily is diagnosed in infants.

The child is given a general anesthetic, after which an incision is made in the lower abdomen.

Patent urachus repair

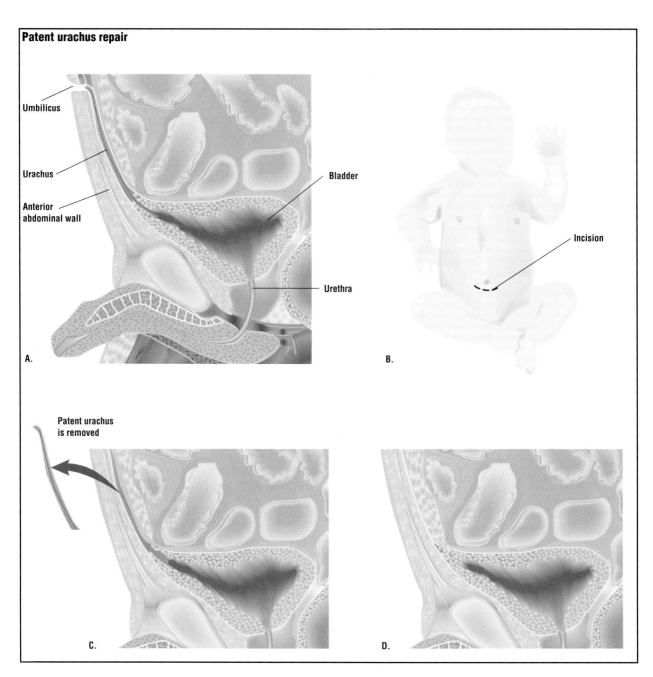

A patent urachus is an abnormal opening from the bladder to the umbilicus, which is retained from fetal life (A). To repair it, an incision is made in the baby's abdomen (B). The patent urachus is removed (C), and the opening to the bladder is closed (D). *(Illustration by GGS Information Services. Cengage Learning, Gale.)*

Aftercare

Surgery for patent urachus repair may require several days' hospitalization, during which infants can be fed as normal.

Risks

Risks are the same as for those patients receiving any anesthesia: a reaction to medication and/or breathing problems. There is also the risk of bladder infection or bladder leaks. In the latter case, a catheter is put in place until the bladder heals.

Normal results

The outcomes of patent urachus repair in infants are excellent, as a rule, and most children recover rapidly.

KEY TERMS

Adenocarcinoma—A malignant tumor that originates in the membranous tissue that serves as the covering of a gland.

Antereolateral—Situated in front and to the side.

Patency—The state of being open or unblocked.

WHO PERFORMS THE PROCEDURE AND WHERE IS IT PERFORMED?

Patent urachus repair is performed by the pediatric surgeon in a hospital setting.

Morbidity and mortality rates

Patent urachal anomalies do not usually cause significant morbidity or mortality. However, adenocarcinoma has been reported in adults with urachal remnants, presumably from chronic inflammation and infection. Patency is noted in only 2% of adults.

Alternatives

Sometimes more conservative treatment than surgery is advised, with radical excision reserved for persistent or recurring cases. Because the urachus may not completely close at birth, but may close within the first few months of the infant's life, observation may be advised before moving forward with surgery.

Resources

BOOKS

Campbell, Meredith F. and Patrick C. Walsh, eds. *Campbell's Urology*, 8th ed. Philadephia: W.B. Saunders Company, 2002.

PERIODICALS

Razvi, S., R. Murphy, E. Shlasko, and C. Cunningham-Rundles. "Delayed Separation of the Umbilical Cord Attributable to Urachal Anomalies." *NIH/NLM MEDLINE* 108, no.2 (August 1, 2001): 493–494.

Nancy McKenzie, PhD

QUESTIONS TO ASK THE DOCTOR

- Is it advisable to put off surgery during the first few months of the child's life and see if the urachus will close on its own?
- What effects will surgery have on a newborn?

Patient-controlled analgesia

Definition

Patient-controlled analgesia (PCA) is a means for the patient to self-administer **analgesics** (pain medications) intravenously by using a computerized pump, which introduces specific doses into an intravenous line.

Purpose

The purpose of PCA is improved pain control. The patient receives immediate delivery of pain medication without the need for a nurse to administer it. The patient controls when the medication is given. More importantly, PCA uses more frequent but smaller doses of medication, and thus provides more even levels of medication within the patient's body. Syringe-injected **pain management** by a nurse requires larger doses of medication given less frequently. Larger doses peak shortly after administration, often causing undesirable side effects such as nausea and difficulty in breathing. Their pain-suppressing effects also often wear off before the next dose is scheduled.

Description

PCA uses a computerized pump, which is controlled by the patient through a hand-held button that is connected to the machine. The pump usually delivers medications in small regular doses, and it can be programmed to issue a large initial dose and then a steady, even flow. The PCA pump can deliver medicine into a vein (intravenously, the most common method), under the skin (subcutaneously), or between the dura mater and the skull (epidurally).

When the patient feels the need for medication, the patient presses a button similar to a nurse call button. When this button is pressed, some sound (usually a beep) is heard, indicating that the pump is working properly and that the button was pressed correctly. The pump delivers the medication through an intravenous line, a plastic tube connected to a needle

KEY TERMS

Analgesia—A medicine that relieves pain.

Epidural—Between the vertebrae and the dura mater of the spinal cord. Analgesia is introduced into this space anywhere along the spinal column.

Intravenous—Within a vein, usually meaning something introduced into a vein such as an injection.

Lockout time—The minimum amount of time (usually expressed in minutes) after one dose of pain medication on demand is given before the patient is allowed to receive the next dose on demand.

Opioid—A synthetic drug resembling opium or alkaloids of opium.

Respiratory depression—Decreased rate (number of breaths per minute) and depth (how much air is inhaled with each breath) of breathing.

Subcutaneous—Under the skin, as in an injection under the skin.

inserted into a vein. Glucose and other medications can also be administered through intravenous lines, along with analgesics.

The medications most commonly used in PCA pumps are synthetic, opium-like pain-relievers (opioids), usually morphine and meperidine (Demerol).

The pump may be set to deliver a larger initial dose of the prescribed drug. The health-care provider sets the pump to deliver a specified dose, determined by the physician, on demand with a lockout time (for example, 1 mg of morphine on demand, but not more frequently than one dose every six minutes). If the patient presses the button before six minutes have elapsed, the pump will not dispense the medication. The pump also generates a record that the health personnel can access. An around-the-clock, even dose may also be set. The practitioner sets a total limit for an hour (or any other period) that takes into account the initial dose, the demand doses, and the around-the-clock doses. The pump's internal computer calculates all these amounts, makes a record of the requests it received and those it refused, and also keeps inventory of the medication being administered, which warns the staff when the supply is getting low.

An example of how a nurse might program the pump might be for a patient who has a prescription for a maximum of 11 mg of morphine an hour. The nurse sets the machine to deliver 1 mg at the beginning of the hour, and 1 mg on demand with a six-minute lockout. There are 10 six-minute periods in an hour, so the patient can request and receive 10 mg over that hour.

Using a PCA pump requires that the patient understand how the system works and has the physical strength to press the button. Therefore, PCA should not be offered to patients who are confused, unresponsive, or paralyzed. Patients with neurologic disease or head injuries in whom narcotics would mask neurologic changes are not eligible for PCA. Patients with poor kidney or lung function are usually not good candidates for PCA, unless they are monitored very closely.

PCA may be used by children as young as seven years old. It has proven safe and successful in such children in the control of postoperative pain, sickle-cell pain, and pain associated with bone-marrow transplantation. In all cases, the child should manage the PCA pump himself or herself. As morphine can slow breathing in young patients, the blood oxygen levels of children must be closely monitored.

In addition, PCA has been found safe for nursing mothers after a **cesarean section**. Very small amounts of morphine do pass into the milk of breastfeeding mothers, but it has not proved harmful to infants.

Preparation

When preparing for PCA, the nurse must assess the patient to determine whether PCA is appropriate and then must set the total dose and the timing of the doses as prescribed by the physician. Since there is only a small amount of drug administered (3,000 doses at 10 mg each weigh less than 1 oz total), it is not sufficient fluid to keep the tubing and the needle from clogging and the contents from coagulating. Therefore, the drug must be put in a solution (flush solution) that will flow through the tube and needle easily, and permit rapid administration. The flush solution also keeps the line open for administration of other medications or in case the patient has a reaction to the pain medications. For example, a patient may have a reaction to morphine and would need counteractive medication immediately. The flush solution can also keep the patient from becoming dehydrated. In addition, many painkillers that are prescribed (such as morphine sulfate) are solid crystals at room temperature and need to be dissolved in some fluid to be absorbed by the body.

When entering the settings into the PCA system, the nurse must pay close attention to the physician's orders to ensure that the correct medication is used, that the concentration of the drug in the flushing solution is correct, that the dose of the drug itself is correct, that the lockout time is appropriate, and that the total hourly limit is properly entered into the pump's computerized controls. To eliminate the risk of incorrect programming, many institutions have adopted policies that require verification by a registered nurse (RN) for all programming. That is, everything must be checked by two nurses, and both must sign the written record.

Another important aspect of PCA is patient education. The settings on the PCA pump must be explained to patients so that they understand how and when medications will be available. The nurse should observe patients as they first start using the button, should ensure that the equipment is functioning properly, and be clear that the patients understand their role in the process and are carrying it out correctly.

Whenever opium-like painkillers are administered to the elderly patient, it must be remembered that older adults may be more susceptible to the side effects of narcotics because the heart, liver, and kidneys of the elderly function less efficiently than those of younger patients. The elderly may also clear the narcotic out of their system at a slower pace. If the pump's timing device is calibrated for a younger person's rate of elimination, the elderly patient could accidentally receive an overdose. Doses for such elderly patients should be calculated more conservatively.

Normal results

The goal of patient-controlled analgesia is managed pain control, enhanced by a stable and constant level of the pain medication in the body. The patient is able to rest better and breathe more deeply. Since the patient is comfortable, he or she is more able to participate in activities that would enhance recovery. PCA also gives the patient in the hospital some control in an unfamiliar and uncomfortable situation. When administered properly, and with watchful assessment by health-care providers, PCA can be a safe alternative to traditional methods of relieving pain.

Interestingly enough, studies have shown that when patients control their pain medication, most use less medication overall than patients who have nurse-administered painkillers.

Risks

Problems that may occur with PCA include allergic reactions to the medications and adverse side effects such as nausea, a dangerous drop in the rate and effectiveness of breathing, and excessive sedation. The PCA device must be monitored frequently to prevent tampering. Even sophisticated devices that monitor themselves and sound an alarm should be checked often, since no machine is perfect. Ineffective pain control must be assessed to determine whether the problem stems from inadequate dosage or from inability, or unwillingness, of the patient to carry out his or her own pain management.

Resources

BOOKS

Miller RD. Miller's Anesthesia. 6th ed. Philadelphia: Elsevier 2005.

PERIODICALS

Baka, Nour-Eddine. "Colostrum Morphine Concentrations during Postcesarean Intravenous Patient-controlled Analgesia." Journal of the American Medical Association 287, no. 12 (March 27, 2002): 1508.

ORGANIZATIONS

American Association of Nurse Anesthetists/AANA. 222 South Prospect Avenue, Park Ridge, IL 60068-4001. (847) 692-7050; Fax: (847) 692-6968. E-mail: info@aana.com. http://www.aana.com.

American Association of Nurse Anesthetists/AANA, Federal Government Affairs Office. 412 1st Street, SE, Suite 12, Washington, DC 20003. (202) 484-8400; Fax: (202) 484-8408. E-mail: info@aanadc.com.

American Society of PeriAnesthesia Nurses/ASPAN. 10 Melrose Avenue, Suite 110, Cherry Hill, NJ 08003-3696. (877) 737-9696; Fax: (856) 616-9601. E-mail: aspan@aspan.org. http://www.aspan.org.

American Society of Anesthesiologists/ASA. 520 North Northwest Highway, Park Ridge, IL 60068-2573. (847) 825-5586; Fax: (847) 825-1692. E-mail: mail@asahq.org.

The National Hospice and Palliative Care Organization/ NHPCO. 1700 Diagonal Road, Suite 300, Alexandria, VA 22314. (703) 837-1500. E-mail: info@nhpco.org.

Janie F. Franz
Jennifer Lee Losey, RN
Rosalyn Carson-DeWitt, MD

Patient charts *see* **Medical charts**

Patient confidentiality

Definition

Confidentiality is the right of an individual to have personal, identifiable medical information kept private. Such information should be available only to the physician of record and other health care and insurance personnel as necessary. As of 2003, patient confidentiality was protected by federal statute.

Purpose

The passage of federal regulations (the Health Insurance Portability and Accountability Act of 1996) was prompted by the need to ensure privacy and protection of personal records and data in an environment of electronic medical records and third-party insurance payers.

Description

Patient confidentiality means that personal and medical information given to a health care provider will not be disclosed to others unless the individual has given specific permission for such release.

Because the disclosure of personal information could cause professional or personal problems, patients rely on physicians to keep their medical information private. It is rare for medical records to remain completely sealed, however. The most benign breach of confidentiality takes place when clinicians share medical information as case studies. When this data is published in professional journals the identity of the patient is never divulged, and all identifying data is either eliminated or changed. If this confidentiality is breached in any way, patients may have the right to sue.

The greatest threat to medical privacy, however, occurs because most medical bills are paid by some form of health insurance, either private or public. This makes it difficult, if not impossible, to keep information truly confidential. Health records are routinely viewed not only by physicians and their staffs, but by the employees of insurance companies, medical laboratories, public health departments, researchers, and many others. If an employer provides health insurance, the employer and designated employees may have access to employee files.

The Health Insurance Portability and Accountability Act (HIPAA) of 1996 requires all professionals and organizations to guard the privacy of their patients and customers. Individuals must provide written consent for any and all releases of medical or

KEY TERMS

HIPAA—Health Insurance Portability and Accountability Act of 1996.

Joint Commission on Accreditation of Healthcare Organizations (JCAHO)—The accrediting organization that evaluates virtually all U.S. health care organizations and programs. Accreditation is maintained with onsite surveys every three years; laboratories are surveyed every two years.

health-related information. Employees at all levels are required to maintain confidentiality. Similar policies have been in place for some time. This was a requirement of the Joint Commission on Accreditation of Healthcare Organizations (JCAHO) to maintain accreditation. All confidentiality releases must identify the types of information that can be released, the people or groups that have been permitted access to the information, and limit the length of time for which the release is valid.

Before the enactment of HIPAA, despite having voluntary safeguards, patient confidentiality had eroded with the almost-complete dominance of health-maintenance organizations and other types of third-party payers. Confidentiality is essential for a good relationship between patient and practitioner, whose duty to keep information private stems from the Hippocratic Oath. If personal information is disseminated without the patient's permission, it can erode confidence in the medical profession and expose health care professionals to legal action.

Physicians are increasingly being sued by patients whose information has been released without their permission. Even though the plaintiffs do not always prevail, the costs of legal action are burdensome to both sides.

Each state and the federal government have enacted laws to protect the confidentiality of health care information generally, with particular attention paid to information about communicable diseases and mental health. For example, through the 1960s substance and alcohol abuse were treated as mental illnesses, with patient confidentiality determined by the laws in each state, since at the time the state was responsible for mental health care and treatment.

In the early 1970s, however, the rising numbers of those needing substance abuse treatment came to the attention of the federal government, because drug-related activity, including the treatment for substance abuse, could be the basis for criminal prosecution on a federal level. Congress concluded that this might stop individuals needing treatment from seeking it. HIPAA was enacted to provide a strict confidentiality law and limit disclosure of information that could reveal a patient's identity.

Confusion ensued when practitioners who were treating substance abusers were required to follow two practices for patient confidentiality. One set of requirements was mandated by the state. The federal government dictated the other. With the varying degrees of protection provided by state mental health laws, the confusion increased. While all states specify exceptions to confidentiality, few have spelled out the necessary elements of valid consent for disclosure of mental health information. Some states presently allow disclosure of the following types of mental health information without patient consent:

- to other treatment providers
- to health care services payers or other sources of financial assistance to the patient
- to third parties that the mental health professional feels might be endangered by the patient
- to researchers
- to agencies charged with oversight of the health care system or the system's practitioners
- to families under certain circumstances
- to law enforcement officials under certain circumstances aa
- to public health officials

Prior to 2003, providers had become increasingly concerned that these exceptions are not addressed uniformly, particularly when providers and payers conducted business across state lines. This resulted in open-ended disclosures that specify neither the parties to whom disclosure is to be made nor the specific information allowed to be revealed. Since 2003, implementation of HIPPA requirements have rectified this problem.

Both the ethical and the legal principles of confidentiality are rooted in a set of values regarding the relationship between caregiver and patient. It is essential that a patient trust a caregiver so that a warm and accepting relationship may develop. This is particularly true in a mental health treatment.

Normal results

The Health Insurance Portability and Accountability Act of 1996 was enacted to address the issue of patient confidentiality. Full implementation of HIPAA regulations began in April 2003. If individuals and organizations having patient data adhere to the requirements of HIPAA, patient confidentiality will be enhanced.

HIPAA provides a uniform set of guidelines that apply to all providers and organizations. HIPAA requirements are not affected by state boundaries.

Resources

BOOKS

Carter, P. I. HIPAA Compliance Handbook 2008. Gaithersburg, Maryland: Aspen, 2007.

Clarke, S., and J. Oakley. Informed Consent and Clinician Accountability: The Ethics of Report Cards on Surgeon Performance. New York: Cambridge University Press, 2007.

Fix, R. M. Informed Consent. Florence, KY: Frontline Publishing Company, 2007.

Getz, K., and D. Borfitz. Informed Consent: The Consumer's Guide to the Risks and Benefits of Volunteering for Clinical Trials. Boston, MA: CenterWatch, 2002.

Glahn, S. Informed Consent. Paris, Ontario, Canada: David C. Cook, 2007.

Hubbard, M. W., K. E. Glover, and C. P. Hartley. HIPAA Policies and Procedures Desk Reference. Chicago: American Medical Association, 2003.

Manson, N.C., and O. O'Neill. Rethinking Informed Consent in Bioethics. New York: Cambridge University Press, 2007.

Pabrai, U. A. Getting Started with HIPAA Boston: Premier Press, 2003.

PERIODICALS

Ackerman, M. J. "The personal health record." Journal of Medical Practice Management 23, no. 2 (2007): 84–85.

Barash, C. I. "Threats to privacy protection." Science 317, no. 5838 (2007): 600–602.

Butler, D. "Data sharing threatens privacy." Nature 449, no. 7163 (2007): 644–645.

Recupero, P. R. "Ethics of medical records and professional communications." Child and Adolescent Psychiatric Clinics of North America 55, no. 7 (2008): 37–51.

Reilley, P. R., and R. M. Debusk. "Ethical and legal issues in nutritional genomics." Journal of the American Dietetic Association 108, no. 1 (2008): 36–40.

ORGANIZATIONS

American Academy of Family Physicians. 11400 Tomahawk Creek Parkway, Leawood, KS 66211-2672. (913) 906-6000. http://www.aafp.org. <fp@aafp.org>.

American College of Physicians. 190 N Independence Mall West, Philadelphia, PA 19106-1572. (800) 523-1546, ext. 2600. (215) 351-2600. http://www.acponline.org.

American Medical Association. 515 N. State Street, Chicago, IL 60610. (312) 464-5000. http://www.ama-assn.org.

National Patient Advocate Foundation. 725 15th St. NW, 10th Floor, Washington, DC 20005, Phone: (202) 347-8009, Fax: (202) 347-5579. http://www.npaf.org. <action@npaf.org>.

OTHER

American Psychological Association. Information about Patent Confidentiality. 2007 [cited December 28, 2007]. http://www.apa.org/practice/senate_compromises.html.

American Society of Cosmetic Breast Surgery. Information about Patent Confidentiality. 2007 [cited December 28, 2007]. http://www.hipaa.org/.

National Academy of Sciences. Information about Patent Confidentiality. 2007 [cited December 28, 2007]. http://www.nap.edu/readingroom/books/for/index.html.

Persons United Limiting Substandards and Errors in Health Care (P.U.L.S.E.). Information about Patent Confidentiality. 2007 [cited December 28, 2007]. http://www.pulseamerica.org/.

Stanford University. *Information about Patent Confidentiality.* 2007 [cited December 28, 2007]. http://www.stanford.edu/class/siw198q/websites/HearingMar01/bill.html.

L. Fleming Fallon, Jr., MD, DrPH

Patient rights

Definition

Patient rights encompass legal and ethical issues in the provider-patient relationship, including a person's right to privacy, the right to quality medical care without prejudice, the right to make informed decisions about care and treatment options, and the right to refuse treatment.

Purpose

The purpose of delineating patient rights is to ensure the ethical treatment of persons receiving medical or other professional health care services. Without exception, all persons in all settings are entitled to receive ethical treatment.

Description

Many issues comprise the rights of patients in the medical system, including a person's ability to sue a health plan provider; access to emergency and specialty care, diagnostic testing, and prescription medication without prejudice; confidentiality and protection of patient medical information; and continuity of care.

Health care reform led to an emergence of health maintenance organizations (HMOs) and other managed health care plans. The rapid change in medical care moved health care decision making from medical professionals to business entities, a move many consider to be detrimental to the health care industry in general.

Establishing a patient's bill of rights has been the response to this concern. The Bipartisan Patient Protection Act of 2001 has been signed into law.

At issue, besides basic rights of care and privacy, is the education of patients concerning what to expect of their health care facility and its providers. These basic rights include the right to:

- participate in the development and implementation in the plan of care
- be treated with respect and dignity
- be informed about condition, treatment options, and the possible results and side effects of treatment
- refuse treatment in accordance with the law, and receive information about the consequences of refusal
- quality health care without discrimination because of race, creed, gender, religion, national origin, or source of payment
- privacy and confidentiality, which includes access to medical records upon request
- personal safety
- know the identity of the person treating the patient, as well as any relationship between professionals and agencies involved in the treatment
- informed consent for all procedures
- information, including the medical records by the patient or by the patient's legally authorized representative and hospital charges, except for Medicaid and general assistance
- consultation and communication
- complain or compliment without the fear of retaliation or compromise of access or quality of care

Patients are expected to meet a fair share of responsibility by following the plan of care, providing complete and accurate health information, and communicating comprehension of instructions on procedures and treatment. The patient is further responsible for consequences of refusal of treatment, of not following the rules and regulations of a hospital, and of not being considerate of others' rights. The patient is also responsible for providing assurance that financial obligations of care are met.

The American Hospital Association provides an informal bill of rights for patients who are hospitalized, which informs patients that they have the right to refuse any procedure or medication that is prescribed, and that states that full information should be provided by the attending physician if the patient has expressed doubts or concerns.

Persons United Limiting Substandards and Errors in Health Care (PULSE), a non-profit organization concerned with patient education and improving communication within the health care system, encourages the partnership of health care professionals and patients. A patient who is educated about his or her own medical condition can work together with health care providers regarding treatment decisions.

New federal privacy rules, beyond the proposed patient bill of rights, give patients additional control over private medical information. Patients have the right to examine their own medical records and to amend them if necessary. In practice, medical personnel have often been reluctant to part with patient records, even when requested by the patients themselves. While health care providers and patients assume that medical records are private, the widespread use of computer transmissions opens the potential for seriously compromising **patient confidentiality**. Regulations recently imposed by the federal government are aimed at protecting patient records by creating limits on the methods in which medical information is shared. Direct authorization from a patient must be gained before information may be released. Criminal and civil penalties may be imposed for a privacy violation. Intentional disclosure of private information can bring a $50,000 fine and a one-year prison term. Penalties for selling medical information are higher. These rules became enforceable in 2003.

Alternatives

Not all individuals or organizations agree with the new regulations. Some complain that they are too restrictive, while others maintain that they are not restrictive enough. The Joint Commission on Accreditation of Healthcare Organizations (JCAHO) cites complexity and cost factors as major problems, and that the full extent of the impact caused by the ruling was not adequately considered when it passed in 2003. The government estimated that it will cost taxpayers $17.6 billion over 10 years to comply with the privacy regulations. Critics of the regulations imply that the cost will be more than triple the estimate, and that billable hours for attorneys specializing in the complexities of the regulations will skyrocket, thus resulting in even higher costs of patient care.

Resources

BOOKS

Annas, G. The Rights of Patients: The Authoritative ACLU Guide to the Rights of Patients. 3rd ed. New York: New York University Press, 2004.

Biegbeder, Y. International Public Health: Patients' Rights Vs. the Protection of Patents. 3rd ed. London: Ashgate Publishing, 2004.

Bondeson, W., and J. Jones. The Ethics of Managed Care: Professional Integrity and Patient Rights. New York: Springer, 2002.

Colby, W. Unplugged: Reclaiming Our Right to Die in America. Chicago: AMACOM/American Management Association, 2007.

PERIODICALS

Ackerman, M. J. "The personal health record." Journal of Medical Practice Management 23, no. 2 (2007): 84–85.

Applebaum, P. S. "Clinical practice. Assessment of patients' competence to consent to treatment." New England Journal of Medicine 357, no. 18 (2007): 1834–1840.

Barash, C. I. "Threats to privacy protection." Science 318, no. 5838 (2007): 913–914.

Campbell, B., H. Thompson, J. Slater, C. Coward, K. Wyatt, and K. Sweeney. "Extracting information from hospital records: what patients think about consent." Quality and Safety in Health Care 16, no. 6 (2007): 404–408.

Haque, O. S., and H. Bursztajn. "Decision-making capacity, memory and informed consent, and judgment at the boundaries of the self." Journal of Clinical Ethics 18, no. 3 (2007): 256–261.

Mitka, M. "Aiding emergency research aim of report on exceptions to informed consent." Journal of the American Medical Association 298, no. 22 (2007): 2608–2609.

ORGANIZATIONS

American Academy of Family Physicians. 11400 Tomahawk Creek Parkway, Leawood, KS 66211-2672. (913) 906-6000. E-mail: <fp@aafp.org>. http://www.aafp.org.

American College of Physicians. 190 N Independence Mall West, Philadelphia, PA 19106-1572. (800) 523-1546, x2600, or (215) 351-2600. http://www.acponline.org.

American Medical Association. 515 N. State Street, Chicago, IL 60610. (312) 464-5000. http://www.ama-assn.org.

National Patient Advocate Foundation, 725 15th St. NW, 10th Floor, Washington, DC 20005. Phone: (202) 347-8009, Fax: (202) 347-5579. http://www.npaf.org .

OTHER

American Cancer Society. Information about Patient Rights. 2007 [cited December 28, 2007]. http://www.cancer.org/docroot/MIT/content/MIT_3_2_Patients_Bill_Of_Rights.asp.

American Psychological Association. Information about Patient Rights. 2007 [cited December 28, 2007]. http://www.apa.org/practice/senate_compromises.html .

National Association for Home Care. Information about Patient Rights. 2007 [cited December 28, 2007]. http://www.nahc.org/Consumer/wamraap.html.

National Institute of Health. Information about Patient Rights. 2007 [cited December 28, 2007]. http://clinicalcenter.nih.gov/participate/patientinfo/legal/bill_of_rights.shtml.

National Library of Medicine. Information about Patient Rights. 2007 [cited December 28, 2007]. http://www.nlm.nih.gov/medlineplus/patientrights.html.

Persons United Limiting Substandards and Errors in Health Care (P.U.L.S.E.). Information about Patent Confidentiality. 2007 [cited December 28, 2007]. http://www.pulseamerica.org/.

Stanford University. Information about Patent Confidentiality. 2007 [cited December 28, 2007]. http://www.stanford.edu/class/siw198q/websites/Hearing Mar01/bill.html.

L. Fleming Fallon, Jr, MD, DrPH

PCA *see* **Patient-controlled analgesia**
PCNL *see* **Nephrolithotomy, percutaneous**
PCV *see* **Hematocrit**

KEY TERMS

Marfan syndrome—A condition occasionally associated with chest wall deformities, in which the patients have a characteristic tall, thin appearance, and cardiac and great vessel abnormalities.

Pectus carinatum—A chest wall deformity characterized by a protrusion of the sternum.

Pectus excavatum—A chest wall deformity in which the chest wall takes on a sunken appearance.

Poland syndrome—A condition associated with chest wall deformities in which varying degrees of underdevelopment of one side of the chest and arm may occur.

Sternum—The breastbone. It connects to ribs one through seven on either side of the chest.

Pectus excavatum repair

Definition

Pectus excavatum repair, also called "funnel chest repair" or "chest deformity repair," is a type of surgery performed to correct pectus excavatum, a deformity of the front of the chest wall with depression of the breastbone (sternum) and rib (costal) cartilages. It is sometimes associated with Marfan or Poland syndrome.

Purpose

The chest consists of the rib cage and sternum, which protect the upper-abdominal cavity and its contents. Pectus excavatum, also called "funnel chest" or "depressed sternum" is a deformity that is usually diagnosed shortly after birth. In some people, it is not visible until they are older. The exact cause is not known, but it is believed to be due to overgrowth of the rib cartilage connected to the sternum, which connects to the sternum being pushed backward toward the spine. Most people have no symptoms, but if the breastbone is pushed back far enough, heart and lung function may be affected. The purpose of pectus excavatum repair surgery is to correct the deformity to improve physical appearance, posture, and breathing.

Demographics

In the United States, pectus excavatum is the most common chest wall deformity observed in children, occurring more commonly in boys than in girls. Pectus excavatum tends to run in families. The funnel chest usually progresses as the child grows, often showing a dramatic deterioration during the puberty growth spurt.

Pectus excavatum repair is technically easiest to perform in preadolescent children, and the recovery is faster. However, almost half of the patients undergoing the operation are teenagers. Repair is rarely performed on children under eight years of age. In recent years, a large number of adults over the age of 21 years have undergone repair with equally good results as those observed with children.

Description

Pectus excavatum repair is always performed with the patient under **general anesthesia**. An epidural catheter is inserted for the management of pain after the operation. The surgeon makes two incisions over the sternum, on either side of the chest, for insertion of a curved steel bar or strut under the sternum. He or she proceeds to remove the deformed cartilages. The rib lining is left in place to allow renewed cartilage growth. The sternum is then repositioned, and the metal strut is placed behind it and brought out through the muscles and skin for future attachment to a brace, which will stay in place six to 12 weeks. The metal strut is fixed to the ribs on either side, and the incisions are closed and dressed. A small steel grooved plate may be used at the end of the bar to help stabilize and fix the bar to the rib. A blood **transfusion** is not required during surgery. The surgeon may insert a temporary chest tube to re-expand the lung if the lining of the lung is entered.

A variety of surgical procedures are available to repair pectus excavatum.

Nuss procedure

A common technique is the Nuss procedure, developed in 1987 by Dr. Donald Nuss, a pediatric surgeon at Children's Hospital of the The King's Daughters and Eastern Virginia Medical School in Norfolk, Virginia. The procedure is minimally invasive, and results in very little blood loss and short recovery times.

Leonard procedure

Another surgical approach that drastically reduces the time required for surgery is the Leonard procedure, developed by Dr. Alfred Leonard, a Minneapolis thoracic and pediatric surgeon. This operation does not violate the chest, and is combined with a bracing technique.

Diagnosis/Preparation

A pediatrician diagnoses pectus excavatum after observing a child when he or she inhales, exhales, and rests. The pediatrician also calculates the depth of the chest from front to back using x rays of the chest to determine whether the diameter is shorter than average, as is the case with funnel chest. The heart is usually larger and displaced to the left. The pediatrician also evaluates lung capacity using **exercise** tests and lung scans that can reveal mismatched lungs.

Other diagnostic tests may include:

- Electrocardiogram (ECG or EKG). This test records the electrical activity of the heart, and shows abnormal rhythms (arrhythmias or dysrhythmias).
- Echocardiogram (echo). This test evaluates the structure and function of the heart by using sound waves recorded on an electronic sensor that yields a moving picture of the heart and its valves.

Before surgery, a bone density test is performed to ensure that the patient does not have soft bones that would deform again right after the surgery. After a complete **health history** is taken, a patient whose condition is considered severe enough to warrant surgery is sent for a CT scan and further evaluation of his or her pulmonary function.

Because of the great variablity of pectus excavatum among those who have it, custom-made bars (or braces) must be used. The brace is a light vest to which the deformity-correcting wire will be attached at surgery. Patients are fitted with the brace prior to surgery.

WHO PERFORMS THE PROCEDURE AND WHERE IS IT PERFORMED?

Pectus excavatum repair is performed in a hospital by experienced thoracic surgeons who specialize in pectus excavatum repair.

Aftercare

Usual recovery time in the hospital is four to five days. Attention is paid to post-operative **pain management**. The patient is encouraged to breathe deeply, and receives assistance with movement (to avoid dislodging the bar). After discharge, the patient slowly resumes a normal, but restricted, activity level. Most children are able to return to school in two to three weeks, with exercise restrictions for six weeks (no physical education classes, heavy lifting, or athletics).

The pectus excavatum support bar is removed under general anesthesia two to four years after insertion, usually on an outpatient basis. In most cases, patients are able to leave the hospital within one to two hours after bar removal.

Risks

Risks associated with pectus excavatum repair include those normally associated with the administration of anesthesia (such as adverse reactions to medications and breathing problems), and risks associated with any surgery (such as bleeding and infection). Specific pectus excavatum surgery risks may include lung collapse (pneumothorax) and the recurrence of the funnel chest. Bar displacement may occasionally require repositioning.

Normal results

Pectus excavatum repair, in almost all instances, restores the ability of patients to participate in full activities, even strenuous activities and athletics. Also, there is a marked improvement in the patient's self image.

Morbidity and mortality rates

According to the National Institutes of Health (NIH), excellent results (95–98%) are reported over a lengthy follow-up time of 25 years. Long-term follow-up (over 15 years) shows that the Nuss procedure provides excellent results with less than 5% recurrence of the deformity after the bar is removed.

QUESTIONS TO ASK THE DOCTOR

- Can exercises correct pectus excavatum?
- How is pectus excavatum surgery performed?
- Should everyone with pectus excavatum have surgery?
- What surgical procedures does the doctor use?
- How many pectus excavatum surgeries does the physician perform each year?

Alternatives

Mild cases of pectus excavatum may respond to an exercise and posture physiotherapy program. Many patients with rounded shoulders and a slouching posture have benefited from these techniques, with or without additional surgical correction. However, body-building exercises usually result in worsening of cosmetic appearance due to the enhancement of the pectoral muscles.

Resources

BOOKS

Pearson, F. G. *Thoracic Surgery*. Philadelphia: W. B. Saunders Co., 2002.

Ravitch, M. M. *Congenital Deformities of the Chest Wall and Their Operative Correction*. Philadelphia: W. B. Saunders Co., 1977.

PERIODICALS

Engum, S., F. Rescorla, K. West, T. Rouse, L.R. Scherer, and J. Grosfeld. "Is the Grass Greener? Early Results of the Nuss Procedure." *Journal of Pediatric Surgery* 35 (2000): 246-51.

Genc, A., and O. Mutaf. "Polytetrafluoroethylene Bars in Stabilizing the Reconstructed Sternum for Pectus Excavatum Operations in Children." *Chest* 110 (July 2002): 54-7.

Hebra, A., B. Swoveland, M. Egbert, E.P. Tagge, K. Georgeson, H.B. Othersen, and D. Nuss. "Outcome Analysis of Minimally Invasive Repair of Pectus Excavatum: Review of 251 Cases." *Journal of Pediatric Surgery* 35 (2000): 252-7.

Jacobs, J. P., J.A. Quintessenza, V.O. Morell, L.M. Botero, H.M. van Gelder, and C. I. Tchervenkov. "Minimally Invasive Endoscopic Repair of Pectus Excavatum." *European Journal of Cardiothoracic Surgery* 21 (2002): 869-83.

ORGANIZATIONS

American Pediatric Surgical Association (APSA). 60 Revere Drive, Suite 500, Northbrook, IL 60062. (847) 480-9576. www.eapsa.org.

Southern Thoracic Surgical Association. 633 N. Saint Clair St., Suite 2320, Chicago, IL, 60611-3658. (800) 685-7872. www.stsa.org/.

OTHER

"Pectus Excavatum Repair." *BestHealth*.www.besthealth.com/surgery/PectusExcavatumRepair_1.html.

Monique Laberge, Ph.D.

Pediatric concerns

Definition

Pediatric concerns are those issues that are unique to the care of children when surgery and hospitalization are involved.

Description

Children are not just little adults. When dealing with children medically, it is important to keep in mind the stage of their physical growth and development; their emotional development; and their maturity level. There are many different kinds of pediatric surgeries and procedures. A pediatric hospital is designed around the special needs of children and their families. All of the staff, including doctors (pediatric surgeons, pediatric anesthesiologists, pediatric radiologists), nurses, and technical support, have special training in pediatrics. Children's hospitals have specific expertise in pediatric problems and special programs for children who are ill or injured.

Helping a child prepare for surgery

When parents are helping their child prepare for surgery, it is important to realize that, no matter how mature the child may act, he or she still needs to be treated differently than adults. Some children find it comforting to know exactly what will happen, when, and how, all in great detail. Others do not want much detail. They may need just an overview of what to expect, keeping just one step ahead of what will be done to them. The particular level of a child's development will determine the specific concerns.

For example, the biggest fear for infants and toddlers is being away from their parents. Parents should stay with the child as much as possible, and ensure that basic needs (such as eating, play, or sleeping) are met, both at home and in the hospital. Preschoolers also fear being away from the parents, but, additionally, they see hospitalization as a punishment and fear

KEY TERMS

Child life specialist—A person who has had specific training in the care of children, including understanding growth and development specific to each age range and how to talk to children of different ages.

Pediatrics—The medical specialty of caring for children.

Separation anxiety—A fear of being separated from a parent or loved one; a normal developmental process, occurring at certain points in a young child's life.

bodily harm. In this case, parents should, again, stay with the child as much as possible, and start talking to them at home about the coming operation to help reassure them. For the hospital stay, parents should bring the child's favorite blanket and/or toys, pictures from home, and maybe music tapes.

For school-age children, the biggest fears are needles and pain. Parents can help by giving them information about their body and how it works, and vaguely explain that the doctor will fix them, but parents should not use language like "cut, incision, open you up, make a hole, etc." To make the hospital feel more familiar, parents can bring pictures and music tapes and/or videos from home. By adolescence, children are worried about the loss of independence, being separated from their peers, and being different (i.e., a change in their appearance). For teenagers at this stage of development, it is extremely important to explain an illness or hospitalization to them in terms that they can understand, using examples to which they can relate, and allow them to be involved in decisions, if possible. The parents should encourage them to ask questions.

What to expect at the hospital

Being in a hospital and undergoing surgery is scary and stressful for a child. Hospitalization disrupts their normal routines. If the staff behaves in a trusting, nurturing way, the child may become comfortable enough to return to some normal behaviors. Trust is important to all ages of children. If a procedure will hurt, it is important to be honest and let them know what to expect. Children can only learn to trust the staff if the staff is honest with them and treats them with respect.

Books and videos developed for children that explain about going to the hospital can be helpful. Some hospitals provide programs for children to come and visit before the hospitalization, so that children will already be familiar with the hospital environment when they are admitted. Play is a child's way of expressing emotion, especially under difficult situations. Play can serve as a distracter as well as a means by which surgery and hospitalization can be explained to children. Dolls or stuffed animals can be used to walk young children through what they will be experiencing. Hospital play areas will often have toys that represent hospital equipment, so that a procedure can be explain with the use of props. For example, there may be pretend casts and **bandages** that a child can put on a stuffed animal. How children play can also serve as an insight for parents and staff as to understand how their children are feeling about what is happening to them. As children express their concerns through play, parents and staff can then address those concerns. Play is therapeutic for children, helping them feel safer in an unfamiliar environment, and should be considered an essential element in preparing for a child's hospital stay. Play areas help to make a strange place feel comfortable, both for the child as well as for the parents. Play areas also provide a relaxed area for parents to be with their child, a friendly home-like environment where nurturing can take place.

Unfortunately, some surgeries are not planned. Emergency situations are always more stressful, both because they are unexpected and because they are often more serious. Children take their cue on how to behave from those around them. When parents are noticeably concerned, children's anxiety levels rise. Parents should remain as calm as possible to be fully present for their children.

Parents should expect to be able to be with their children most of the time. For most day surgeries, parents can stay with their child until he or she is asleep, and then can be waiting in the **recovery room** when the child is waking up after the procedure is completed. Some facilities provide pullout beds for parents to spend the night with their children, and may even have a small kitchen where they can prepare food to eat in their child's room.

Qualified staff should be available to help parents work through their concerns and anxiety. Parents with more than one child may sometimes need to leave their hospitalized child completely in the hands of hospital staff as they attend to their other children at home. Many facilities have volunteers who can stay with children when their parents need to leave the hospital.

What to look for in health care for a child

While those hospitals designed especially for children are a wonderful resource, other hospitals that care for patients of all ages will often provide comparable care. If the surgery allows for time to select a surgeon and hospital, things to look for include:

- surgeons and physicians who are board certified in pediatrics
- staff with special training in pediatrics
- equipment designed for pediatric use
- a separate wing or floor for children
- child life specialists on staff
- play rooms and toys that can be brought into a child's room

A pediatric hospital or wing will have equipment that is smaller, better suited to the child's size. Bandages may have pictures of cartoon characters on them; there may be paintings of characters from children's movies on the walls.

Staff will usually have had special training to understand what issues are important to children at different stages of development. They should use language that is adapted to explain what is happening to the child in ways that make sense to them. For example, instead of just asking a child to blow, they may ask them to imagine that they are blowing out candles on a birthday cake. All of these techniques help to make the hospital a more familiar and friendlier place, putting the child at ease and helping to lessen anxiety.

Resources

BOOKS

Behrman, R. E., et al. *Nelson's Textbook of Pediatrics.* 17th ed. Philadelphia: Saunders, 2004.

ORGANIZATIONS

The Nemours Foundation. http://kidshealth.org.

Esther Csapo Rastegari, RN, BSN, EdM

Pediatric surgery

Definition

Pediatric surgery is a specialized field of surgery for the treatment of conditions that can be surgically corrected in a baby, child, or adolescent.

Purpose

The purpose of pediatric surgery varies with the procedure. In general, the purpose is to surgically correct a congenital condition, disease, traumatic injury, or other disorder in the pediatric patient.

Demographics

Pediatric surgeons provide treatment for young patients—newborns up through late adolescence.

Description

Pediatric surgery is the surgical branch that uses operative techniques to correct certain pediatric conditions (i.e., congenital abnormalities, tumors, chronic diseases, and traumatic injuries). There are different specialties within the field that include:

- pediatric general surgery
- pediatric otolaryngology (ear, nose, and throat)
- pediatric ophthalmology (eye)
- pediatric urology (urogenital system)
- pediatric orthopedic (bone) surgery
- pediatric neurological (brain and spinal cord) surgery
- pediatric plastic (reconstructive and cosmetic) surgery

The American Academy of Pediatrics has established specific guidelines for referral to subspecialists. The pediatric patient has special considerations that differentiate him or her, both physically and psychologically, from an adult. A neonate (newborn) poses great challenge in surgical treatment since the tiny structures and immature organ systems may not cope with disease-induced stress and the physical demands of a major operative procedure. A newborn infant may still be developing key bodily functions, or may have special requirements. Key areas of concern in the newborn include:

- cardiovascular (heart) system
- thermoregulation (temperature requirements of 73°F [22.8°C]).
- pulmonary (lung) function
- renal (kidney) function
- immature immunity and liver
- special requirements for fluid, electrolyte (necessary elements such as sodium, potassium, and calcium) and nutrition

The pediatric surgeon must take into account the special requirements unique to the young surgical patient. The pediatric surgeon is trained to treat the entire spectrum of surgical illnesses. The following is an overview (with symptoms) of the more common pediatric conditions that require surgery typically performed by the pediatric surgeon.

KEY TERMS

Atresia—Thinning or narrowing of a body passageway.

Large intestine—The portion of the colon that includes the cecum; ascending, transverse, and descending sigmoid colon; rectum; and anal canal.

Oliguria—Decreased urine production.

Pediatric aged patient—The pediatric aged patient encompasses several periods during development. The first four weeks after birth are callled the neonatal period. The first year after birth is called infancy, and childhood is from 13 months until puberty (between the ages of 12 and 15 years in girls and 13 and 16 years in boys).

Polyp—A tumor mass, generally benign and capable of surgical removal.

Pylorus—The area that controls food passage from the stomach to the first part of the small intestine (duodenum).

Small intestine—The part of the intestines that consists of the duodenum, jejunum, and ileum.

Alimentary tract obstruction

Obstruction of the alimentary tract (tubes of digestion extending from the mouth to the anus) is characterized by four cardinal symptoms:

- abdominal distention (an abdomen that becomes large and appears swollen)
- bilious vomiting (due to bile in the stomach)
- maternal polyhydramnios (excess amniotic fluid in the amniotic sac, greater than 2,000 ml) before birth
- failure to pass meconium (dark green or black sticky excretion passed via the newborn's rectum) in the first 24 hours of life

ESOPHAGEAL ATRESIA AND TRACHEOESOPHAGEAL FISTULA. This is a congenital deformity of the esophagus (the tube that passes food from the mouth to the stomach) does not connect to the stomach. Symptoms include severe respiratory distress (the neonate cannot breathe) and excessive salivation. Other clinical signs include cyanosis (bluish discoloration of the skin due to oxygen deprivation), choking, and coughing.

PYLORIC ATRESIA AND RELATED CONDITIONS. Pyloric atresia is a condition that occurs when the pyloric valve, located between the stomach and duodenum, fails to open. Food cannot pass out of the stomach, resulting in vomiting clear gastric juice at attempted feedings. Maternal polyhydramnios is present before birth in more than 60% of cases.

Other areas of the colon (duodenum, jejunum, ileum) can be obstructed during development, with symptoms present at birth. Most of these disorders share the four cardinal symptoms of alimentary obstruction.

INTUSSUSCEPTION. Intussusception accounts for 50% of intestinal obstruction in patients who are three months to one year of age. Eighty percent of cases are observed by the child's second birthday. The cause of intussusception is not known, and it is more common in males who are well nourished and apparently healthy. The symptoms include a sudden onset of abdominal pain characterized by episodic screaming and drawing up of the legs. In 60% of patients, vomiting and blood in the stool are common findings (either bright red or occult [hidden] blood). Typically, the bowel movements look like currant jelly, consisting of mucus and blood mixed together. Currant jelly stool is the most common clinical observation for patients with intussusception. During **physical examination**, patients will exhibit abdominal distention, and in 65% of cases there is a sausage-shaped mass that can be felt in the upper right portion of the abdomen toward the mid-abdomen. **Ultrasound** studies are a reliable method of diagnosis.

FAILURE TO PASS MECONIUM. Failure to pass meconium (meconium ileus) is associated with cystic fibrosis (a genetic disorder), colonic obstruction (colonic atresia), meconium plug syndrome, and aganglionic megacolon (also called Hirschsprung's disease, a congenital absence of the nerves that provide gastrointestinal tract mobility).

Anorectal anomalies

There are many different types of anorectal anomalies common to male and female neonates, as well as deformities that are gender-specific since involvement of genitalia can occur. The surgery for these cases is complicated, and must be performed by an experienced pediatric surgeon. Complications of these procedures could result in permanent problems.

Necrotizing enterocolitis (NEC)

NEC affects 1–2% of patients admitted to a neonatal **intensive care unit**. It is a life-threatening illness characterized by abdominal distention, bilious vomiting, lethargy, fever, occult (not obvious) or gross (clearly seen) rectal bleeding. Additionally, affected patients may exhibit signs of hypothermia (temperature less than 96.5°F or 35.8°C), bradycardia (slow heart rate), abdominal mass (felt during palpation), oliguria, jaundice, and episodes of breathlessness (apnea). Survival of NEC surgery can be expected for 60–70% of patients.

Abdominal wall defects

Omphalocele is a defect that involves protrusion of abdominal contents into an external sac. This disorder occurs in one per 5,000 births. More than 50% of omphalocele patients have serious genetic deformities involving these body systems: cardiovascular (heart), musculoskeletal (muscle and bones), genitourinary (genital and bladder systems), and central nervous (brain and spinal cord). The overall survival rate for infants with omphalocele varies, and depends on defect size, other associated genetic abnormalities, and age of newborn. (Many infants with omphalocele are premature.) Approximately 33% of patients with omphaloceles do not survive.

GASTROSCHISIS. Gastroschisis is a defect in the abdominal wall to the side (lateral) of the umbilicus. It usually occurs to the right of an intact normal umbilical cord. The cause is unknown. The bowel protrudes to the outside of the abdomen during intrauterine life (while the embryo is developing inside the uterus). The amniotic fluid has an irritating effect on the exposed bowel, and causes infection of the bowels. The problem can be detected by ultrasound studies during pregnancy. Some pediatric surgeons and obstetricians recommend **cesarean section** (early elective delivery) to spare bowel trauma. The newborn patients typically require surgery, tube feedings for three to four weeks, and hospitalization for several weeks. The current survival rate for infants with gastroschisis is greater than 90%.

Congenital diaphragmatic hernia (CDH)

CDH can be diagnosed by the fourth month of pregnancy via ultrasound studies. Of the infants with congenital diaphragmatic hernia (CDH), 44–66% have other congenital abnormalities as a result of developmental malformations. Anatomically, patients with CDH have a defect in development that allows a communication between the chest and abdomen. Through this defect, the abdominal contents enter the lung cavity and interfere with normal lung development. The incidence is approximately one per 2,200 live births, and males are more commonly affected than females. Usually the infants are full-term, and the defect occurs on the left side in the majority—88%—of patients.

Treatment is extensive, and usually requires three major areas:

- stabilization of patient and preoperative preparation
- operative treatment
- postoperative respiratory, metabolic, circulatory and nutritional supportive measures

Postoperatively, the infant is monitored in the neonatal intensive care setting. The postoperative period is more critical if a lung is severely underdeveloped.

Pyloric stenosis (PS)

Pyloric stenosis is an obstruction in the intestine due to a larger-than-normal size of the muscle fibers of the pylorus (lower stomach opening). Pyloric stenosis is a common hereditary condition that affects males more than females, and occurs in one per 750 births. The typical symptoms include a progressive, often projectile, vomiting after attempted feedings. The gastric vomitus (bloody in 80% of patients) usually begins during the second and third week of life, and increases in force and frequency. Typically, the infant fails to gain weight, and the number of bowel movements and rate of urination decreases.

Physical examination is usually helpful in establishing a diagnosis. Palpation of the enlarged muscle fibers can be felt as an olive-shaped mass located along the midline approximately one-third to one-half of the distance from the umbilicus to the xiphoid (end of the breastbone), when the stomach is empty. Careful abdominal examination and palpation can usually identify the pyloric mass in 85% of cases.

Gastroesophageal reflux

Gastroesophageal reflux disease (GERD) is a common disorder in infancy, and usually disappears by the baby's first birthday. The largest group of patients with clinically significant GERD are those who have neurologic impairment. Symptoms often include vomiting, repeated lung infections (from aspirating gastric contents during regurgitation of foodstuffs), and delayed gastric emptying. The success rate with infants who have procedures necessary to correct GERD is over 90%.

Meckel's diverticulum

Meckel's diverticulum occurs in approximately 2% of the U.S. population. The diverticulum is an outgrowth of intestine that is located in a portion of the intestines called the ileum. Symptoms of obstruction are more often observed in infants, and bleeding is more common in patients after age four.

Intestinal polyps

Juvenile polyps are usually present between the ages of four and 14 years, and tend to be inflammatory. The most common symptom of intestinal polyps is rectal bleeding, which is commonly due to a solitary polyp (80% of cases). Diagnosis can be done by proctosigmoidoscopy, which allows visualization of 85% of polyps.

Acute appendicitis

Acute appendicitis is a relatively common surgical emergency that is misdiagnosed in 28% of patients due to a broad spectrum of symptoms that can confuse the clinician. The classic clinical symptom of acute appendicitis is the onset of pain in the middle region of the abdomen that is followed by anorexia (loss of appetite), nausea, and vomiting. The pain is persistent and radiates to the right lower abdomen, becoming more intense and localized. The physical and abdominal examinations must be carefully and accurately performed. Patients with acute appendicitis usually have an increased white blood cell (cells that fight infection) count.

Once the diagnosis is established, the child is prepared for surgery. Preoperative **antibiotics** are started at least one half-hour before the operation. If the appendix is perforated (ruptured), complications can occur as a result of kidney (renal) failure, seizures due to fever, and gram-negative sepsis (an infection that enters the bloodstream and interferes with life-saving chemical reactions). Patients who are very young, or those who were misdiagnosed and incurred long delays in treatment, are susceptible to **death**.

Inflammatory bowel diseases

Some cases (approximately 25%) of inflammatory bowel disease are found in persons younger than 20 years of age. Two types can occur, Crohn's disease and ulcerative colitis.

The diagnosis of inflammatory bowel disease is usually based on presenting clinical symptoms, laboratory analysis results, endoscopic appearance, and radiologic findings. Approximately 50–60% of patients have bloody diarrhea, severe cramping, abdominal pain, and urgency.

CROHN'S DISEASE. The symptoms of Crohn's disease includes cramping abdominal pain, diarrhea, and strictures (constriction) resulting from bowel obstruction. Removal of diseased portions in children with Crohn's disease may be temporarily beneficial, but recurrence after surgical removal occurs in about 50% of cases within four years. Chronic symptoms may remain into adult life, making long-term follow-up essential.

ULCERATIVE COLITIS. Ulcerative colitis is limited to the colon. A surgical procedure known as colectomy is curative, and indicated for intractable disease (64% of patients). Colectomy is the removal of the entire colon, or the inflamed part of it.

Biliary tract disorders

A variety of biliary tract conditions may be present at birth, some requiring surgical correction.

NEONATAL JAUNDICE. Neonatal jaundice is common, and results from an immature system not capable of some basic biochemical reactions. Food intake can help speed these reactions, which usually resolve the condition within seven to 10 days. Jaundice that persists for over two weeks is abnormal, and could be caused by over 30 possible disorders.

BILIARY ATRESIA. Biliary atresia is a disease that causes inflammation of the ducts within the biliary system, resulting in fibrosis of these ducts. The incidence of biliary atresia is one per 15,000 live births, and is more common in females. Time is critical, and most patients must have surgery by two months of life. Approximately 25–30% of patients who receive early operative intervention have long-term successful outcomes. Some patients may require **liver transplantation**, and 85–90% of these patients survive.

CHOLELITHIASIS. Gallbladder obstruction in infants and young children is usually caused by pigmented (colored) stones resulting from blood disorders. Removal of the gallbladder (laparoscopic **cholecystectomy**) is the treatment of choice.

Trauma

Accidents are the leading cause of death in children between the ages of one and 15 years, and accounts for 50% of all deaths in the pediatric age group. More than half of these deaths are due to motor vehicle accidents, followed by falls, bicycle injuries, drowning, burns, child abuse, and birth trauma. Head trauma is the single most common organ associated with traumatic death. Within recent years, the number of fatalities related to the use of firearms and violence has increased.

More than 20 million children each year sustain injuries requiring treatment. These injuries account for 100,000 cases of permanent pediatric disability. Response to trauma in pediatric patients is significantly different from older patients. Pediatric patients require special attention concerning temperature regulation, blood volume, metabolic rate and requirements, and airway

WHO PERFORMS THE PROCEDURE AND WHERE IS IT PERFORMED?

Pediatric surgery is performed by a pediatric surgeon who has had five years of general surgery training, along with further specialized instruction and experience, and is certified in pediatric general surgery or in a specific pediatric specialty.

maintenance. Other special pediatric considerations include response to stress, communication difficulties, psychological trauma, a different pediatric trauma score system, smaller airway diameter, and increased risk of aspirating gastric contents (which could cause pneumonia). Pediatric trauma patients should have access to appropriate pre-hospital transportation, and must receive medical attention in a pediatric trauma center capable of providing the complex level of care necessary for serious pediatric trauma situations.

Neck masses

Neck masses during infancy and childhood may be caused by tumors or infections, or they may be congenital. Lymphadenitis is an infection of a lymph node that becomes enlarged and tender. Most cases are resolved by treating the primary source of infection (i.e., middle ear infection and tonsillitis). Some inflamed nodes may require an incision and drainage of infection.

Hernias

INGUINAL HERNIA AND HYDROCELE. Inguinal (groin) hernia is the most frequent disorder requiring surgery in the pediatric age group. Clinically, a right-sided inguinal hernia is more common in males (60% of cases), and there is a familial tendency. The incidence is higher in full-term infants (3.5–5%). Full-term infants and older children (without underlying diseases) can receive surgical repair in an outpatient setting. An inguinal hernia may result in herniation of the scrotum, and a communicating hydrocele (hernia with a small connection to the peritoneal cavity).

UMBILICAL HERNIA. Umbilical hernia is a defect of the umbilical ring, and is more common in females and African American children. Spontaneous involution occurs in 80% of cases. Larger defects may be observed for several years without complications, and their spontaneous resolution is possible. If the umbilical hernia persists, patients may develop feeding intolerance, pain, and local skin breakdown.

QUESTIONS TO ASK THE DOCTOR

- What are the risks of surgery?
- What is the benefit of the surgery?
- What type of anesthesia will be used?
- How many surgeries of this type has the surgeon performed?
- Is there an alternative to surgery?
- Is a full recovery expected, and if not, what deficits will the child have?
- What should the parents and child do to prepare for surgery?
- What care is needed following the surgery?
- When will the child be able to return to normal activity?

Undescended testes

Undescended testes are observed in 1–2% of full-term males. Approximately 30% of preterm males may have an undescended testis. Undescended testis in premature infants may descend by the first year of life, and observation is often the treatment during that time.

Tumors

Wilm's tumor (nephroblastoma) is a tumor in the kidneys that forms during embryonic development. The tumor is due to a genetic abnormality; and approximately 80% of children are diagnosed between one and five years of age. In about 75–95% of cases, the patient has an abdominal mass that is detected by a parent during bathing. Blood in the urine (hematuria) occurs in 10–15% of cases, and high blood pressure (hypertension) is present in 20–25% of cases. Hypertension is the result of the tumor compressing the kidney in a specific area, causing it to release a chemical called renin, which elevates blood pressure. During physical examination, the Wilm's tumor is a smooth, round, hard, nontender flank mass. The treatment of Wilm's tumor depends on its stage, and may include surgery, chemotherapy, or radiotherapy.

Resources

BOOKS

Townsend, Courtney. *Sabiston Textbook of Surgery*, 16th ed. St. Louis: W. B. Saunders Company, 2001.

PERIODICALS

Coran, A. "American Academy of Pediatrics: Guidelines for Referral to Pediatric Surgical Specialists." *Pediatrics* 110, no. 1 (July 2002).

Okada P. J., B. Hicks. "Pediatric Surgical Emergencies: Neonatal Surgical Energencies." *Clinical Pediatric Emergency Medicine* 3, no.1 (March 2002:).

ORGANIZATIONS

The American Pediatric Surgical Association. 60 Revere Drive Suite 500 Northbrook, Il 60062. (847) 480-9576. Fax: (847) 480-9282 E-mail: eapsa@eapsa.org.

Laith Farid Gulli, M.D., M.S.
Nicole Mallory, M.S., PA-C
Abraham F. Ettaher, M.D.
Robert Ramirez, B.S.

PEG tube insertion *see* **Gastrostomy**

Pelvic ultrasound

Definition

Pelvic **ultrasound** is a procedure in which high-frequency sound waves create images of the pelvic organs. The sound waves are projected into the pelvis, and measure how they reflect—or echo—back from the different tissues.

Purpose

Ultrasound is a preferred method of examining the pelvis, and functions as an extension of a **physical examination**, particularly for obese patients. It is a common initial step after physical examination when a patient complains of pelvic pain or abnormal vaginal bleeding. The procedure is performed routinely during pregnancy and examinations to determine the cause of infertility. Ultrasound has the ability to detect the size and shape of pelvic organs, such as the bladder, and is useful in evaluating the cause of bladder dysfunction. In women, pelvic ultrasound is used to examine the uterus, ovaries, cervix, and vagina. In general, ultrasound can detect inflammation, free fluid, cysts (abnormal fluid-filled spaces), and tumors in the pelvic region.

A primary use of pelvic ultrasound is during pregnancy. In early pregnancy (about five to seven weeks), ultrasound may determine the size of the fetus to confirm the suspected due date, detect multiple fetuses, or confirm that the fetus is alive (viable). Ultrasound is particularly useful in distinguishing between intrauterine (within the uterus) and ectopic (outside the uterus) pregnancies. Toward the middle of the pregnancy (about 16–20 weeks), the procedure can confirm fetal growth, reveal defects in the anatomy of the fetus, and check the placenta and amniotic fluid. Toward the end of pregnancy, it may be used to evaluate fetal size, position, growth, or to check the placenta.

Doctors may use ultrasound to guide the biopsy needle during **amniocentesis** and chorionic villus sampling. The imaging allows precise placement of the long needle that is inserted into the patient's uterus to collect cells from the placenta or amniotic fluid.

Description

Depending on the goal of the procedure, a pelvic ultrasound can also be called a bladder ultrasound, pelvic gynecologic sonogram, or obstetric sonogram. Ultrasound examinations are usually done in a doctor's office, clinic, or hospital setting. Typically, the patient will lie on an examination table with the pelvis exposed. Special gel is applied to the area to make sure that there is no air between the hand-held transducer and the skin, and to facilitate transducer movement. The physician or technologist guides the transducer over the abdomen. The transducer both creates and receives the echoes of the high-frequency sound waves (usually in the range of 3.5–10.0 megahertz). An ultrasound scan reveals the shape and densities of organs and tissues. By performing repeated scans over time, much like the frames of a movie, ultrasound can also reveal movement, such as the motions of a fetus. This technique is called real-time ultrasound.

Using a computerized tool, called a caliper, the ultrasound technologist can measure various structures shown in the image. For example, the length of the upper thigh bone (femur) or the distance between the two sides of the skull can indicate the age of the fetus.

Ultrasound technology has been safely used in medical settings for over 30 years, and several significant extensions to the procedure have made it even more useful. A specially designed transducer probe can be placed in the vagina to provide better ultrasound images. This transvaginal or endovaginal scan is particularly useful in early pregnancy or in cases where ectopic pregnancy is suspected. It is also routinely used to provide better anatomic delineation of the endometrium and pelvic masses. In men, transrectal scans, where the probe is placed in the rectum, are done to check the prostate. Doppler ultrasound has the ability to follow the flow of blood through veins and arteries, and can be useful in detecting disorders such as abnormal blood flow associated with ovarian torsion (a twisted blood supply that causes pelvic pain). Color enhancement is particularly useful in Doppler imaging, where shades of red signify flow

KEY TERMS

Acoustic window—Area through which ultrasound waves move freely.

Amniocentesis—A procedure where a needle is inserted through the pregnant woman's abdomen and into the uterus to withdraw a sample of amniotic fluid surrounding the fetus.

Chorionic villus sampling—A procedure where a needle is inserted into the placenta to withdraw a sample of the placenta's inner wall cells surrounding the fetus.

Ectopic pregnancy—A pregnancy where the fertilized egg becomes implanted somewhere other than in the uterus; if in a fallopian tube it is called a tubal pregnancy.

Real-time—A type of ultrasound that takes multiple images over time in order to record movement, or the observations obtained while scanning (rather than obtained by looking at films after the procedure).

Sonographer—A technologist or physician who uses an ultrasound unit to takes ultrasound images of patients.

Transducer—The handheld part of the ultrasound unit that produces the ultrasound waves and receives the ultrasound echos.

Ultrasound—Sound above what can be heard by the human ear, generally above 20,000 Hz (cycles per second).

away from the transducer and shades of blue signify flow toward it.

Hysterosonography is another variant ultrasound procedure. It involves the injection of saline solution into the uterus during an endovaginal scan. The saline distends the uterine cavity (or endometrium) and simplifies the identification of polyps, fibroids, and tumors. The saline outlines the lesion, making it easier to find and evaluate. Hysterosonography can also be used in the testing of patency (openness) of the fallopian tubes during infertility evaluations.

Preparation

Before undergoing a pelvic ultrasound, the patient may be asked to drink several glasses of water and to avoid urinating for about one hour prior to exam time. When the bladder is full, it forms a convenient path, called an acoustic window, for the ultrasonic waves. A full bladder is not necessary for an endovaginal

examination, sometimes making it a preferred choice in emergency situations. Women usually empty their bladders completely before an endovaginal exam.

Aftercare

For a diagnostic ultrasound, the lubricating gel applied to the abdomen is wiped off at the end of the procedure and the patient can immediately resume normal activities.

Risks

Ultrasound carries with it almost no risk for complications.

Normal results

A normal scan reveals no abnormalities in the size, shape, or density of the organs scanned. During pregnancy, a normal scan reveals a viable fetus of expected size and developmental stage. Although ultrasound is an extremely useful tool, it cannot detect all problems in the pelvic region. If a tumor or other lesion is very small or if it is masked by another structure, it may not be detected. When used during pregnancy, patients should be advised that ultrasound does not reveal all fetal abnormalities. Additionally, the reliability of ultrasound readings can depend on the skill of the technologist or physician performing the scan.

An abnormal scan may show the presence of inflammation, cysts, tumors, or abnormal blood flow patterns. These results may suggest further diagnostic procedures, or surgical or pharmacological treatment. Obstetrical ultrasound examinations may alter the anticipated due date or detect abnormalities or defects in the fetus. This information may reveal that the fetus cannot survive on its own after birth, or that it will require extensive treatment or care. The technologist performing the ultrasound should consult with a radiologist or other physician if any questionable results appear.

Resources

BOOKS

Gabbe, SG et al. *Obstetrics: Normal and Problem Pregnancies.* 5th ed. London: Churchill Livingstone, 2007.

Grainger RG, et al. *Grainger & Allison's Diagnostic Radiology: A Textbook of Medical Imaging.* 4th ed. Philadelphia: Saunders, 2001.

Katz VL et al. *Comprehensive Gynecology.* 5th ed. St. Louis: Mosby, 2007.

Mettler, FA. *Essentials of Radiology.* 2nd ed. Philadelphia: Saunders, 2005.

Townsend, CM et al. *Sabiston Textbook of Surgery*. 17th ed. Philadelphia: Saunders, 2004.

Wein, AJ et al. *Campbell-Walsh Urology*. 9th ed. Philadelphia: Saunders, 2007.

ORGANIZATIONS

American Institute of Ultrasound in Medicine. 14750 Sweiter Lane, Suite 100, Laurel, MD 20707-5906. (301) 498-4100 or (800) 638-5352. http://www.aium.org.

American Registry of Diagnostic Medical Sonographers (ARDMS). 600 Jefferson Plaza, Suite 360, Rockville, MD 20852-1150. (301) 738-8401 or (800) 541-9754. http://www.ardms.org.

OTHER

Valley, Verna T. "Ultrasonography, Pelvic." Emedicine. January 17, 2001. [cited May 6, 2001] http://www.emedicine.com/emerg/topic622.htm.

Michelle L. Johnson, M.S., J.D.
Lee A. Shratter, M.D.
Rosalyn Carson-DeWitt, MD

Penile implant surgery *see* **Penile prostheses**

Penile prostheses

Definition

Penile prostheses are semi-rigid or inflatable devices that are implanted into penises to alleviate impotence.

Purpose

The penis is composed of one channel for urine and semen, and three compartments with tough, fibrous walls containing erectile tissue. With appropriate stimulation, the blood vessels that lead out of these compartments constrict, trapping blood. Blood pressure fills and hardens the compartments producing an erection of sufficient firmness to perform sexual intercourse. Additional stimulation leads to ejaculation, where semen is pumped out of the urethra. When this system fails, erectile dysfunction or impotence (failure to create and maintain an erection) occurs.

Impotence can be caused by a number of conditions, including diabetes, spinal cord injury, prolonged drug abuse, and removal of the prostate gland. If the medical condition is irreversible, a penile prosthesis may be considered. Men whose impotence is caused by psychological problems are not recommended for implant surgery.

KEY TERMS

General anesthesia—Deep sleep induced by a combination of medicines that allows surgery to be performed.

Genital—Sexual organ.

Perineum—Area between the anus and genitals.

Scrotum—The external pouch containing the male reproductive glands (testes) and part of the spermatic cord.

Demographics

Recently, it has been reported that surgeons insert approximately 20,000 penile implants into American men yearly. The most common device is a multi-component inflatable implant (approximately 45% of all implants). Semi-rigid rods account for about 35% of the implants. Self-contained devices comprise approximately 20% of implants.

Description

Penile implant surgery is conducted on persons who have exhausted all other areas of treatment. Semi-rigid devices consist of two rods that are easier and less expensive to implant than the inflatable cylinders. Once implanted, the semi-rigid device needs no follow-up adjustments; however, it produces a penis that constantly remains semi-erect. Inflatable cylinders produce a more natural effect. Men using them are able to simulate an erection via a pump located in the scrotum.

With a surgical patient under **general anesthesia**, the device is inserted into the erectile tissue of the penis through an incision in the fibrous wall. In order to insert the pump for the inflatable implant, incisions are made in the abdomen and the perineum (area between the anus and the genitals). A fluid reservoir is placed into the groin, and the pump is placed in the scrotum. The cylinders, reservoir, and pump are connected by tubes and tested before the incisions are closed.

Diagnosis/Preparation

Surgery always requires a patient who is adequately informed about the procedure's risks and benefits. The sexual partner should also be involved in the discussion. Prior to surgery, the region undergoes antibacterial cleansing and is shaved.

WHO PERFORMS THE PROCEDURE AND WHERE IS IT PERFORMED?

A penile prosthesis is usually implanted by a urologist. This is a doctor with specialty training in diseases of the urinary system and the genital organs. The procedure is performed in a hospital with the patient under general anesthesia.

Aftercare

To minimize swelling, ice packs are applied to the penis for the first 24 hours following surgery. The incision sites are cleansed daily to prevent infection. Pain relievers may be taken.

Risks

With any implant, there is a slightly greater risk of infection than with simple surgery. The implant may irritate the penis and cause continuous pain. The inflatable prosthesis may need follow-up surgery to repair leaks in the reservoir or to reconnect the tubing.

Normal results

Successful implantation of a penile prosthesis solves some problems related to impotence. After healing from the surgical procedure, men with a penile prosthesis can resume normal sexual activities.

Morbidity and mortality rates

On a purely technical basis, morbidity associated with a surgically implanted penile implants is relatively uncommon, and is usually due to a postsurgical infection or to mechanical failure of the implanted device. Experts feel that personal dissatisfaction with a penile implant procedure is more common, and is usually due to unreasonable or inappropriate expectations for the procedure. Mortality is quite rare.

Alternatives

Medication (sildenafil citrate [Viagra]) is useful for some men with erectile dysfunction. The medication must be prescribed and monitored by a physician.

Impotence caused psychological factors can usually be treated with appropriate counseling and therapy.

Creams are available for purchase. Most experts agree that these cannot reverse physiological impotence.

QUESTIONS TO ASK THE DOCTOR

- What is the cause of the erectile dysfunction or impotence?
- How will the a penile prosthesis affect daily activities after recovery?
- How will the a penile prosthesis affect sexual activities after recovery?
- What will be the resulting appearance after surgery?
- Is the surgeon board certified?
- How many penile prosthesis procedures has the surgeon performed?
- What is the surgeon's complication rate?

Most experts consider mechanical rings that prevent blood flow out of a penis to be dangerous, and advise against their use.

Resources

BOOKS

Khatri, VP and JA Asensio. Operative Surgery Manual. 1st ed. Philadelphia: Saunders, 2003.

Townsend, CM et al. Sabiston Textbook of Surgery. 17th ed. Philadelphia: Saunders, 2004.

Wein, AJ et al. Campbell-Walsh Urology. 9th ed. Philadelphia: Saunders, 2007.

PERIODICALS

Carson, C.C. "Penile Prostheses: Are They Still Relevant?" British Journal of Urology International 91, no.3 (2003): 176-7.

ORGANIZATIONS

American Board of Surgery. 1617 John F. Kennedy Boulevard, Suite 860, Philadelphia, PA 19103. (215) 568-4000. Fax: (215) 563-5718. http://www.absurgery.org.

American Board of Urology. 2216 Ivy Road, Suite 210, Chaarlottesviille, VA 22903. (434) 979-0059. http://www.abu.org.

American College of Surgeons. 633 North St. Clair Street, Chicago, IL 60611-32311. (312) 202-5000. Fax: (312) 202-5001. E-mail: postmaster@facs.org. http://www.facs.org.

American Foundation for Urologic Disease. 1128 North Charles Street, Baltimore, MD 21201. (800) 242-2383. http://www.afud.org.

American Medical Association. 515 N. State Street, Chicago, IL 60610. (312) 464-5000. http://www.ama-assn.org.

American Urological Association. 1120 North Charles Street, Baltimore, MD 21201. (410) 727-1100. http://www.auanet.org.

OTHER

Cornell University. [cited May 5, 2003] http://www.
cornellurology.com/cornell/sexualmedicine/ed/
implant.shtml.

Ohio State University Medical Center. [cited May 5, 2003]
http://www.acs.ohio-state.edu/units/osuhosp/patedu/
Materials/PDFDocs/procedure/impo-imp.pdf.

Phoenix5. [cited May 5, 2003] http://www.phoenix5.org/
sexaids/implants/surgerydiags.html.

University of California-Davis Medical Center. [cited May
5, 2003] http://www.ucdmc.ucdavis.edu/ucdhs/health/
a-z/15Impotence/doc15procedures.html.

L. Fleming Fallon, Jr., M.D., Dr.PH.

Percutaneous nephrolithotomy *see*
Nephrolithotomy, percutaneous

Percutaneous transluminal angioplasty *see*
Angioplasty

Pericardiocentesis

Definition

A procedure performed with a needle to remove fluid for diagnostic or therapeutic purposes from the tissue covering the heart (pericardial sac).

Purpose

The heart is surrounded by a membrane covering called the pericardial sac. The sac consists of two layers, the parietal (outer) and visceral (inner) layer, and normally contains a small amount of fluid to cushion and lubricate the heart as it contracts and expands. When too much fluid gathers in the pericardial cavity, the space between the pericardium and the outer layers of the heart, a condition known as pericardial effusion occurs. Abnormal amounts of fluid may result from:

- pericarditis, infection caused by inflammation of the pericardial sac
- trauma, such as an abnormal collection of blood due to an accident
- surgery or invasive heart procedures
- heart attack (myocardial infarction) or congestive heart failure, which occurs when the heart looses its pumping capability due to a heart condition
- kidney (renal) failure
- cancer (producing malignant effusions)

The rate of pericardial fluid accumulation is important. If fluid accumulation develops slowly, then problems with blood flow will not develop until fluid retention becomes massive. Blood can also enter the pericardial sac (hemopericardium) due to trauma, blood-thinning medications, or disease. When there is rapid or excessive build-up of fluid or blood in the pericardial cavity, the resulting compression on the heart impairs the pumping action of the vascular system (a condition called cardiac tamponade). Pericardiocentesis can be used in such an emergency situation to remove the excess accumulations of blood or fluid from the pericardial sac. For diagnostic purposes, pericardiocentesis may be advised in order to obtain fluid samples from the sac for laboratory analysis.

Prior to the discovery of **echocardiography**, pericardiocentesis was a risky procedure. The clinician had to insert a long needle below the breastbone into the pericardial sac without internal visualization. This blind approach was associated with damage to the lungs, coronary arteries, myocardium, and liver. However, with direct visualization using echocardiography, pericardiocentesis can now be performed with minor risk. Some risk is still associated with the procedure since it is considered an invasive measure.

Demographics

Cardiac tamponade and pericarditis are two primary complications that require intervention with pericardiocentesis. Cardiac tamponade has an incidence of two in 10,000 the general U.S. population. Approximately 2% of cases are attributed to injuries that penetrate the chest. Pericarditis is more common in males than females, with a ratio of seven to three. In young adults, pericarditis is usually caused by HIV infection or a trauma injury. Malignancy or renal (kidney) failure are the main causes of this disorder in the elderly.

Description

The patient should sit with the head elevated 30-40 degrees. This is done to maximize fluid drainage. A site close to the pericardial sac is chosen, and if time permits the patient is sedated. The puncture site is cleaned with an antiseptic iodine solution, and the area is shaved and anesthetized with lidocaine (a local anesthetic). A long cardiac needle is inserted under the xiphoid (the bottom of the breastbone) approach on the left side of the heart using guided imagery into the chest wall until the needle reaches the pericardial sac. Usually, the patient may experience a sensation of pressure when the tip of the needle penetrates the pericardial sac. When guided imagery confirms correct placement, fluid is aspirated from the sac.

KEY TERMS

Cardiac tamponade—A condition caused by pericardial effusion, that seriously constrains cardiac contraction and access of blood to the heart.

Echocardiography—Sound waves that penetrate deep anatomical structures and generates a visual image on a monitor screen.

Egobronchophony—Increased intensity of the spoken voice.

Hemodynamic—Relating to the flow of blood through the circulatory system.

Myocardial infarction—A heart attack occurs when a coronary artery is blocked and blood flow to the blocked area is impaired.

Parietal pericardium—External or outer layer of the pericardial cavity.

Pericardial friction rub—A crackly, grating, low-pitched sound and is heard in both inspiration and expiration.

Pulsus paradoxus—A variation of the systolic pressure with respiration (diminished systolic pressure with inspiration and increased pressure with expiration).

Tactile fremitus—A tremor or vibration in any part of the body detected by palpation (palpation is when the clinician gently feels or presses with hands).

Visceral pericardium—Single layer of cells that lines both the internal surface of the heart with the parietal pericardium and the external surface of the heart.

If the procedure is performed for diagnostic purposes, aspirated fluid can be collected in specimen vials and sent for pathological analysis (i.e. for cancer cell detection in cases where malignant effusion is suspected), or the fluid is just removed if the procedure was performed urgently (i.e. cardiac tamponade). For therapeutic cases, a pericardial catheter may be attached and fixed into position to allow for continuous drainage. When the needle is removed, pressure is applied for five minutes at the puncture site to stop the bleeding, and the site is then bandaged.

Diagnosis/Preparation

The typical symptom associated with patients requiring pericardiocentesis is chest pain, usually indicative of severe effusion. Patients with cardiac tamponade commonly have dyspnea (difficulty breathing)

and those with an infection may have fever. Some patients may have a hoarse voice from compression of a nerve called the recurrent laryngeal nerve; the pericardial sac may be so large that it pushes or compresses neighboring anatomical structures. Physical symptoms may vary, dependent both on size and the rate of filling of the pericardial effusion. Patients can also present with the following physical symptoms:

- tachycardia, an increased heart rate
- tachypnea, an increase in breathing rate
- jugular vein enlargement
- narrow pulse pressure (pulsus paradoxus)
- pericardial friction rub
- elevated central venous pressure
- hiccups from esophageal compression
- Ewart's sign (dull sound when the doctor taps the chest, tactile fremitus, egobronchophony)

The procedure can be performed in an emergency room, ICU, or at the bedside. Before the procedure patients should have an echocardiogram and basic blood analysis. No special dietary restrictions are required for pericardiocentesis. The patient will receive an IV line for sedation or other necessary medications and an **electrocardiogram** (ECG) to monitor cardiac activity. The patient must lie flat on the table, with the body elevated to a 60-degree angle. If the test is elective, then food and water restriction is recommended for six hours before the test. For infants and children, preparation depends on the child's age, level of trust, and previous exposure to this or similar procedures.

Aftercare

The puncture site, or if a catheter is fixed in place, the catheter site, should be inspected regularly for signs of infection such as redness or swelling. **Vital signs** such as blood pressure and pulse are monitored following the procedure.

Risks

Pericardiocentesis is an invasive procedure and therefore has associated risks. Complications are possible, but have become less common due to guided imaging techniques that improved the past blind approach. Possible risks include:

- puncture of the myocardium, the outer muscle layer of the heart
- puncture of a coronary artery, a blood vessel that supplies blood to heart muscle
- myocardial infarction (heart attack)

WHO PERFORMS THE PROCEDURE AND WHERE IS IT PERFORMED?

A cardiologist who has received three years of training in internal medicine and three years of cardiology training typically performs the procedure. A general surgeon can also perform pericardiocentesis and typically have five years of surgical training. The procedure is performed in a hospital, either in the ER (emergency room), ICU (intensive care unit), or bedside.

- needle induced arrhythmias (irregular heartbeats)
- pneumopericardium, air entry into the pericardial sac
- infection of the pericardial membranes (pericarditis)
- accidental puncture of the stomach, lung, or liver

Normal results

Normal pericardial fluid is clear to straw colored. During pathological examination normal pericardial fluid does not contain blood, cancer cells, or bacteria. In most individuals, a small amount of fluid (10–50 ml) is in the pericardial sac to cushion the heart. Pericardial fluid volumes over 50 ml suggest pericardial effusion. The presence of microorganisms (such as *Staphylococcus aureus*) in aspirated pericardial fluid indicates bacterial pericarditis. Blood in pericardial fluid can be seen in patients with cancer; cardiac rupture, which can occur with myocardial infarction (heart attack); or hemorrhage due to traumatic injury or accident.

Morbidity and mortality rates

The success of pericardiocentesis has greatly improved with the use of guided imagery during the procedure. Only about 5% of patients will experience a major complication as a result of pericardiocentesis. Cardiac tamponade is fatal in almost all cases unless the excess fluid in the pulmonary sac is removed.

Resources

BOOKS

Khatri, VP and JA Asensio. *Operative Surgery Manual*. 1st ed. Philadelphia: Saunders, 2003.

Libby, P. et al. *Braunwald's Heart Disease*. 8th ed. Philadelphia: Saunders, 2007.

Mason, RJ et al. *Murray & Nadel's Textbook of Respiratory Medicine*. 4th ed. Philadelphia: Saunders, 2007.

Marx, J. *Rosen's Emergency Medicine: Concepts and Clinical Practice*, 5th ed. St. Louis: Mosby, Inc., 2002.

Townsend, CM et al. *Sabiston Textbook of Surgery*. 17th ed. Philadelphia: Saunders, 2004.

PERIODICALS

A.D.A.M., Inc. "Pericardiocentesis." January 31, 2003 [cited June 26, 2003]. University of Pennsylvania Health System. http://www.pennhealth.com/ency/article/003872.htm.

Desai, K., et al. "Pericardiocentesis." eMedicine.com. April 25, 2002 [cited June 26, 2003]. http://www.emedicine.com/med/topic3560.htm.

Laith Farid Gulli, MD, MS
Alfredo Mori, MBBS
Abraham F. Ettaher, MD
Robert Ramirez, BS

QUESTIONS TO ASK THE DOCTOR

- Where will the procedure take place?
- What type of anesthetic will be used?
- Will this procedure be used for diagnostic purposes?
- Who will be performing the procedure?

Peripheral endarterectomy

Definition

A peripheral endarterectomy is the surgical removal of fatty deposits, called plaque, from the walls of arteries other than those of the heart and brain. The surgery is performed when plaque blocks an artery and obstructs the flow of blood and oxygen to other parts of the body, most commonly the legs but also the arms, kidneys, or intestines. The peripheral arteries most often treated with endarterectomy are those that supply the legs, especially the aortoiliac arteries in the pelvic area. Other arteries that may be treated with endarterectomy include the femoral arteries in the groin, the renal arteries that supply the kidneys, and the superior mesenteric arteries that supply the intestines.

Purpose

Endarterectomy surgeries are performed to treat advanced peripheral arterial disease (PAD). PAD most often occurs as a result of atherosclerosis, a condition characterized by the gradual build up of fats, cholesterol, cellular waste, calcium, and other substances on the inner walls of large and medium-sized arteries. Plaque, the hardened, waxy substance that results from this build up, can cause narrowing (stenosis) of an artery and block the flow of blood and oxygen. Peripheral endarterectomies are performed to reopen blocked arteries and to restore blood flow in the body (revascularization), helping to prevent heart attack, stroke, the **amputation** of a limb, organ failure, or **death**.

Demographics

People who have been diagnosed with PAD caused by atherosclerosis are at high risk of arterial blockage (occlusion) and are candidates for peripheral endarterectomy. Occlusive arterial disease is found in 15 to 20% of men and women older than age 70. When found in people younger than 70, it occurs more often in men than in women, particularly in those who have ever smoked or who have diabetes. Women with PAD live longer than men with the same condition, which accounts for the equal incidence in older Americans. African-Americans have been shown to be at greater risk for arterial occlusion than other racial groups in the United States.

Description

PAD is a progressive occlusive disease of the arteries, common in older people who have ever smoked or who have diabetes. Although there are other forms of arterial disease that affect peripheral arteries (Buerger's disease, Raynaud's disease, and acrocyanosis), PAD in most people is caused by widespread artherosclerosis, the accumulation of plaque on the inner lining (endothelium) of the artery walls. Most commonly, occlusive PAD develops in the legs, including the femoral arteries that supply the thighs with blood or in the common iliac arteries, which are branches of the lower abdominal aorta that also supply the legs. The arteries that supply the shoulders and arms are less commonly affected. Branches of the aorta that deliver blood to the kidneys, the infrarenal aorta and renal arteries, can become narrowed as a result of artherosclerosis, but are only rarely blocked suddenly and completely, a condition requiring immediate surgery. Even more rare is blockage of the branches that supply the liver and spleen.

The development of atherosclerosis and PAD is influenced by heredity and also by lifestyle factors,

KEY TERMS

Atheroma—A collection of plaque (lesion) blocking a portion of an artery.

Atherosclerosis (arteriosclerosis)—A process of thickening and hardening of large and medium-sized arteries as a result of fatty deposits on their inner linings.

Ischemia—An inadequate blood supply (circulation) in an area of the body when arteries in the area are blocked.

Peripheral arterial disease (PAD)—An occlusive disease of the arteries most often caused by progressive artherosclerosis.

Peripheral endarterectomy—The surgical removal of fatty deposits, called plaque, from the walls of arteries other than those of the heart and brain.

Plaque—A collection of wax-like fatty deposits on the insides of artery walls.

Restenosis—The repeat narrowing of blood vessels that may occur after surgical removal of plaque when preventive measures are not taken.

Revascularization—Retoring normal blood flow (circulation) in the body's vascular (veins and arteries) system.

Stenosis—The narrowing of a blood vessel.

such as dietary habits and levels of **exercise**. The risk factors for atherosclerosis include:

- high levels of blood cholesterol and triglycerides
- high blood pressure
- cigarette smoking or exposure to tobacco smoke
- diabetes, types I and II
- obesity
- inactivity, lack of exercise
- family history of early cardiovascular disease

Just as coronary artery disease (CAD) can cause a heart attack when plaque blocks the arteries of the heart, or blockage in the carotid artery leading to the brain can cause a stroke, blockage of the peripheral arteries can create life-threatening conditions. When peripheral arteries have become narrowed by plaque accumulation (atheroma), the flow of oxygen-carrying blood to the arms, legs, or body organs will be interrupted, which can cause cell death from lack of oxygen (ischemia) and nutrition. Normal growth and cell repair cannot take place, which can lead to gangrene in the limbs and subsequent amputation. When blood flow is blocked to internal organs, such as the kidneys or intestines, the result of tissue death can be the shut-down of the affected organ system and systemic (whole body) poisoning from waste accumulation. Death can result if **emergency surgery** is not performed to correct the blockage.

In some cases, the body will attempt to change the flow of blood when a portion of an artery is blocked by plaque. Smaller arteries around the blockage will begin to take some of the blood flow. This adaptation of the body (collateral circulation) is one reason for a lack of symptoms in some people who actually have PAD. Symptoms usually occur when the blockage is over 70% or when complete blockage occurs as a result of a piece of plaque breaking off and blocking the artery. Blockage in the legs, for example, will reduce or cut off circulation, causing painful cramping in the legs during walking (intermittent claudication) and pain in the feet during rest, especially during the night. When an artery gradually becomes narrowed by plaque, the symptoms are not as severe as when sudden, complete blockage occurs. Sudden blockage does not offer time for collateral vessels to develop and symptoms can be equally sudden and dramatic. Possible symptoms of reduced blood flow in the most typically affected arteries include:

- Arteries of the arms and legs: Gradual blockage creates muscle aches and pain, cramping, and sensations of tiredness or numbness; sudden blockage may cause severe pain, coldness and numbness. A leg or arm may become blue (cyanotic) from lack of oxygen. No pulse will be felt. Paralysis may occur.

- Lower aorta, femoral artery, and common iliac arteries: Gradual narrowing causes intermittent claudication affecting the buttocks and thighs. Men may become impotent. Sudden blockage will cause both legs to become painful, pale, and cold. No pulse will be felt. Legs may become numb. The feet may become painful, infected, or even gangrenous when gradual or complete blockage limits or cuts off circulation

- Renal arteries: Gradual narrowing may produce no symptoms and no change in kidney function. Sudden, complete blockage may cause sudden pain in the side and bloody urine. This is an emergency situation.

- Superior mesenteric artery: Gradual narrowing causes steady, severe pain in the middle of the abdomen about 30 to 60 minutes after a meal. Nutrients are lost and weight loss is common. Sudden, complete blockage causes severe abdominal pain, vomiting, and the urge to move the bowels. Blood pressure falls, intestinal gangrene may develop, and the patient may go into shock. This is an emergency situation.

Sudden, complete occlusion of an artery can also happen when a clot (thrombus) forms in an already narrowed artery. Clot formation (thrombosis) can occur anywhere in the body and travel to a narrowed portion of an affected artery and become lodged (embolism), blocking blood flow. Clots can sometimes be dissolved with anticoagulant drug therapy. When this therapy is not effective or a life-threatening blockage occurs suddenly, clots can be surgically removed using thromboendarterectomy, a procedure similar to peripheral endarterectomy.

Early treatment for PAD may include medical treatment to reduce the underlying causes: lowering cholesterol, lowering blood pressure, stopping smoking, increasing exercise, and reducing the likelihood of clot formation. Clot-dissolving drugs (thrombolytic drugs) may also be used to remove a clot medically rather than to perform surgery. When these measures are not effective, or an artery becomes completely blocked, peripheral endarterectomy may be performed to remove the blockage (see also **angioplasty** and **peripheral vascular bypass surgery**). Treatment of risk factors must continue, because surgery only corrects the immediate problem, not the underlying causes.

Peripheral endarterectomy works best in narrow areas like the leg where the artery can be easily accessed, or when there is complete blockage of an artery by an atheroma that is short in length. Endarterectomy does not work as well for smaller arteries lower in the leg or in the foot or arm. Drug therapy, **angiography**, stent placement, or surgical bypass may be used to treat blockages of the arteries in these areas.

Patients undergoing peripheral endarterectomy will typically be given **general anesthesia**. The surgery is an open surgical procedure in which a vascular surgeon makes a relatively large incision in the outer skin to access the obstructed artery being treated. In order to perform the surgery, the blood that normally flows through the artery must first be rerouted through a tube connecting the blood vessels below and above the surgical site. The surgeon will then cut the obstructed artery lengthwise and will use surgical tools to clean away the accumulation of plaque. The hard, waxy substance comes out fairly easily, sometimes in a single piece. The artery will then be sutured closed or patched with a piece of a vein, usually from the patient's leg, to enlarge the repaired artery and prevent later narrowing from post-operative scarring. The entire procedure will take about one hour if there are no complications.

Diagnosis/Preparation

A complete patient history is essential to diagnosis, particularly information about family members who may have had diabetes or early cardiovascular disease. Symptoms will be important diagnostic indicators, letting the physician know what areas of the body may have reduced blood flow. Blood pressure will be taken in the arms and legs. Pulses will be measured in the arms, armpits, wrists, groin, ankles, and behind the knees. This will show where blockages may exist, since the pulse below a blockage is usually absent. Additionally, a **stethoscope** will be used to listen for abnormal sounds in the arteries that may indicate narrowing. Blood flow procedures may be performed, including:

- Doppler ultrasonography—direct measurement of blood flow and rates of flow, sometimes performed in conjunction with stress testing (exercise between tests).
- Angiography—an x-ray procedure that provides clear images of the affected arteries before surgery is performed.
- Blood tests—routine tests such as cholesterol and glucose, as well as tests to help identify other causes of narrowed arteries, such as inflammation, thoracic outlet syndrome, high homocyeteine levels, or arteritis.
- Spiral computed tomography (CT angiography) or magnetic resonance angiography (MRI)—less invasive forms of angiography.

If ultrasonography or angiography procedures were not performed earlier to diagnose arterial blockage, these tests will be performed before surgery to evaluate the amount of plaque and the extent and exact location of narrowing. **Aspirin** therapy or other clot-prevention medication may be prescribed before surgery. Any underlying medical condition, such as high blood pressure, heart disease, or diabetes will be treated prior to peripheral endarterectomy to help get the best result from the surgery. Upon **admission to the hospital**, routine blood and urine tests will be performed.

Aftercare

After the peripheral endarterectomy, the patient's blood pressure, temperature, and heart rate will be monitored in a hospital **recovery room** for an hour or more, and the surgical site will be checked regularly. The patient will then be transferred to a concentrated care unit to be observed for any sign of complications. The total hospital stay may be two to three days. When the patient returns home, activities can be resumed gradually. Walking and strenuous activity may be restricted, especially if surgery was performed on the groin or leg. During recuperation, the patient may be given pain medication as needed and clot prevention (anticoagulant) medication. Patients will be advised to reduce the risk factors for artherosclerosis in order to avoid repeat narrowing or blockage of the arteries. Repeat stenosis (restenosis) has been shown to occur frequently in people who do not make the necessary changes in lifestyle, such as changes in diet, exercise, and quitting smoking. The benefits of the surgery may only be temporary if underlying disease, such as artherosclerosis, high blood pressure, or diabetes, is not also treated.

Risks

The risks associated with peripheral endarterectomy primarily involve the underlying conditions that led to blockage of arteries in the first place. Embolism is the most serious postoperative risk; a clot or piece of tissue from the endarterectomy site that may travel to the heart, brain, or lungs can cause heart attack, stroke, or death. Restenosis, the continuing build-up of plaque, can occur within months to years after surgery if risk factors are not controlled. Other complications may include:

- reactions to anesthesia
- breathing difficulties
- changes in blood pressure
- nerve injury
- postoperative bleeding

Normal results

The outcomes of peripheral endarterectomy as a treatment for arterial blockage are usually good. Blood flow can be restored quickly to relieve symptoms and help prevent heart attack, stroke, organ failure, or limb amputation.

Morbidity and mortality rates

Morbidity and mortality depend upon the artery involved, the extent of the blockage, and the patient's overall condition, which directly influences response to the surgery. Time is also a factor. In cases of sudden and complete blockage of the mesenteric arteries, for example, only immediate surgery can save the person's life. Although death does not frequently occur during peripheral endarterectomy surgery, patients with widespread atherosclerosis and PAD have been shown to have increased morbidity and mortality associated with

WHO PERFORMS THE PROCEDURE AND WHERE IS IT PERFORMED?

Peripheral endarterectomy is performed in a hospital operating room by a vascular surgeon.

coronary artery disease, because of the common risk factors, such as cigarette smoking, high blood pressure, and diabetes. PAD patients with diabetes are shown to represent 50% of all amputations. However, only a small percentage of patients undergoing peripheral endarterectomy will suffer limb loss or associated disability and reduced quality of life.

Alternatives

Peripheral endarterectomy removes plaque directly from blocked arteries; there is no alternative way to mechanically remove plaque. However, there are alternative ways to prevent plaque build-up and reduce the risk of narrowing or blocking the peripheral arteries. Certain vitamin deficiencies in older people, for example, are known to promote high levels of homocysteine, an amino acid that contributes to atherosclerosis and a higher risk for PAD. Some nutritional supplements and alternative therapies that are recommended to help promote good vascular health include:

- Folic acid can help lower homocysteine levels and increase the oxygen-carrying capacity of red blood cells.
- Vitamins B_6 and B_{12} help lower homocysteine levels.
- Antioxidant vitamins C and E work together to promote healthy blood vessels and improve circulation.
- Angelica, an herb that contains Coumadin, a recognized anticoagulant, may help prevent clot formation in the blood.
- Essential fatty acids, as found in flax seed and other oils, can help reduce blood pressure and cholesterol, and maintain elasticity of blood vessels.
- Chelation therapy may be used to break up plaque and improve circulation.

Resources

BOOKS

Cranton, Elmer MD., ed. *Bypassing Bypass Surgery: Chelation Therapy: A Non-Surgical Treatment for Reversing Arteriosclerosis, Improving Blocked Circulation, and Slowing the Aging Process.* Hampton Roads Pub. Co., 2001.

QUESTIONS TO ASK THE DOCTOR

- Why do I need this surgery?
- How will the surgery improve my condition?
- What kind of anesthesia will I be given?
- What are the risks of having this surgery?
- How many of these procedures have you performed? How many of the surgery patients had complications after surgery?
- How can I expect to feel after surgery? How long will it take me to recover?
- What are my chances of developing this problem again after the surgery?
- What can I do to help prevent developing this condition again?

McDougal, Gene. *Unclog Your Arteries: How I Beat Artherosclerosis.* 1st Books Library, Nov 2001.

ORGANIZATIONS

American Heart Association (AHA). 7272 Greenville Ave., Dallas, TX 75231. (800) 242-8721. http://www.americanheart.org.

Vascular Disease Foundation. 3333 South Wadsworth Blvd. B104-37, Lakewood, CO 80227. (303) 949-8337; (866) PADINFO (723-4636). http://www.vdf.org.

OTHER

Hirsch, Alan T. MD. "Occlusive Peripheral Arterial Disease." *The Merck Manual of Medicine.* Home Edition [cited July 7, 2003]. http://www.merck.com/pubs.

"Patient Information: Frequently Asked Questions." Peripheral Vascular Surgery Society [cited July 7, 2003]. http://www.pvss.org.

L. Lee Culvert

Peripheral vascular bypass surgery

Definition

A peripheral vascular bypass, also called a lower extremity bypass, is the surgical rerouting of blood flow around an obstructed artery that supplies blood to the legs and feet. This surgery is performed when the build-up of fatty deposits (plaque) in an artery has blocked the normal flow of blood that carries oxygen and nutrients to the lower extremities. Bypass surgery reroutes blood from above the obstructed portion of an artery to another vessel below the obstruction.

A bypass surgery is named for the artery that will be bypassed and the arteries that will receive the rerouted blood. The three common peripheral vascular bypass surgeries are:

- Aortobifemoral bypass surgery, which reroutes blood from the abdominal aorta to the two femoral arteries in the groin.
- Femoropopliteal bypass (fem-pop bypass) surgery, which reroutes blood from the femoral artery to the popliteal arteries above or below the knee.
- Femorotibial bypass surgery, which reroutes blood between the femoral artery and the tibial artery.

A substitute vessel or graft must be used in bypass surgeries to reroute the blood. The graft may be a healthy segment of the patient's own saphenous vein (autogenous graft), a vein that runs the entire length of the thigh. A synthetic graft may be used if the patient's saphenous vein is not healthy or long enough, or if the vessel to be bypassed is a larger artery that cannot be replaced by a smaller vein.

Purpose

Peripheral vascular bypass surgery is performed to restore blood flow (revascularization) in the veins and arteries of people who have peripheral arterial disease (PAD), a form of peripheral vascular disease (PVD). People with PAD develop widespread hardening and narrowing of the arteries (atherosclerosis) from the gradual build-up of plaque. In advanced PAD, plaque accumulations (atheromas) obstruct arteries in the lower abdomen, groin, and legs, blocking the flow of blood, oxygen, and nutrients to the lower extremities (legs and feet). Rerouting blood flow around the blockage is one way to restore circulation. It relieves symptoms in the legs and feet, and helps avoid serious consequences such as heart attack, stroke, limb **amputation**, or **death**.

Demographics

Approximately 8–8 million people in the United States have PAD caused by atherosclerosis. These people are at high risk of arterial occlusion, and are candidates for peripheral vascular bypass surgery. Occlusive arterial disease is found in 12–20% of men and women older than age 65. In people younger than age 70, it occurs more often in men than women, particularly in those who have ever smoked or who

KEY TERMS

Atheroma—An accumulation of plaque blocking a portion of an artery.

Atherosclerosis (arteriosclerosis)—Process of thickening and hardening of large- and medium-sized arteries as a result of fatty deposits on their inner linings.

Intermittent claudication—Pain that occurs on walking and is relieved on rest.

Ischemia—An inadequate blood supply (circulation) in a part of the body where arteries are blocked.

Peripheral arterial disease (PAD)—An occlusive disease of the arteries most often caused by progressive atherosclerosis.

Peripheral arteries—Arteries other than those of the heart and brain, especially those that supply the lower body organs and limbs.

Plaque—A collection of wax-like fatty deposits on the insides of artery walls.

Restenosis—The repeat narrowing of blood vessels that may occur after surgical removal of plaque when preventive measures are not taken.

Revascularization—Restoring normal blood flow (circulation) in the body's vascular (veins and arteries) system.

Stenosis—Narrowing of a blood vessel.

have diabetes. Women with PAD live longer than men with the same condition, accounting for the equal incidence in older Americans. African-Americans are at greater risk for arterial occlusion than other racial groups in the United States.

Description

The circulatory system delivers blood, oxygen, and vital nutrients to the limbs, organs, and tissues throughout the body. This is accomplished via arteries that deliver oxygen-rich blood from the heart to the tissues and veins that return oxygen-poor blood from organs and tissues back to the heart and lungs for re-oxygenation. In PAD, the gradual accumulation of plaque in the inner lining (endothelium) of the artery walls results in widespread atherosclerosis that can occlude the arteries and reduce or cut off the supply of blood, oxygen, and nutrients to organ systems or limbs.

Peripheral vascular bypass surgery is a treatment option when PAD affects the legs and feet. PAD is similar to coronary artery disease (CAD), which leads to heart attacks and carotid artery disease (CAD), which causes stroke. Atherosclerosis causes each of these diseases. Most often, atherosclerotic blockage or narrowing (stenosis) occurs in the femoral arteries that supply the thighs with blood or in the common iliac arteries, which are branches of the lower abdominal aorta that also supplies the legs. The popliteal arteries (a portion of the femoral arteries near the surface of the legs) or the posterior tibial and peroneal arteries below the knee (portions of the popliteal artery) can be affected.

Just as coronary artery disease can cause a heart attack when plaque blocks the arteries of the heart, or blockage in the carotid artery leading to the brain can cause a stroke, occlusion of the peripheral arteries can create life-threatening conditions. Plaque accumulation in the peripheral arteries blocks the flow of oxygen-carrying blood, causing cells and tissue in the legs and feet to die from lack of oxygen (ischemia) and nutrition. Normal growth and cell repair cannot take place, which can lead to gangrene in the limbs and subsequent amputation. If pieces of the plaque break off, they can travel from the legs to the heart or brain, causing heart attack, stroke, or death.

The development of atherosclerosis and PAD is influenced by heredity and also by lifestyle factors, such as dietary habits and levels of **exercise**. The risk factors for atherosclerosis include:

- high levels of blood cholesterol and triglycerides.
- high blood pressure (hypertension)
- cigarette smoking or exposure to tobacco smoke
- diabetes, types 1 and 2
- obesity
- inactivity, lack of exercise
- family history of early cardiovascular disease

Sometimes the body will attempt to change the flow of blood when a portion of an artery is narrowed by plaque. Smaller arteries around the blockage begin to take over some of the blood flow. This adaptation of the body (collateral circulation) is one reason for the absence of symptoms in some people who have PAD. Another reason is that plaque develops gradually as people age. Symptoms usually don't occur until a blockage is over 70%, or when a piece of plaque breaks off and blocks an artery completely. Blockage in the legs reduces or cuts off circulation, causing painful cramping during walking, which is relieved on rest (intermittent claudication). The feet may ache even when lying down at night.

When narrowing of an artery occurs gradually, symptoms are not as severe as they are when sudden, complete blockage occurs. Sudden blockage does not allow time for collateral vessels to develop, and symptoms can be severe. Gradual blockage creates muscle aches and pain, cramping, and sensations of fatigue or numbness in the limbs; sudden blockage may cause severe pain, coldness, and numbness. At times, no pulse can be felt, a leg may become blue (cyanotic) from lack of oxygen, or paralysis may occur.

When the lower aorta, femoral artery, and common iliac arteries (all in the lower abdominal and groin areas) are blocked, gradual narrowing may produce cramping pain and numbness in the buttocks and thighs, and men may become impotent. Sudden blockage will cause both legs to become painful, pale, cold, and numb, with no pulse. The feet may become painful, infected, or even gangrenous when gradual or complete blockage limits or cuts off circulation. Feet may become purple or red, a condition called rubor that indicates severe narrowing. Pain in the feet or legs during rest is viewed as an indication for bypass surgery because circulation is reduced to a degree that threatens survival of the limb.

Early treatment for PAD usually includes medical intervention to reduce the causes of atherosclerosis, such as lowering cholesterol and blood pressure, **smoking cessation**, and reducing the likelihood of clot formation. When these measures are not effective, or an artery becomes completely blocked, lower extremity bypass surgery may be performed to restore circulation, reduce foot and leg symptoms, and prevent limb amputation.

Bypass surgery is an open procedure that requires **general anesthesia**. In femoropopliteal bypass or femorotibial bypass, the surgeon makes an incision in the groin and thigh to expose the affected artery above the blockage, and another incision (behind the knee for the popliteal artery, for example) to expose the artery below the blockage. The arteries are blocked off with vascular clamps. If an autogenous graft is used, the surgeon passes a dissected (cut and removed) segment of the saphenous vein along the artery that is being bypassed. If the saphenous vein is not long enough or is not of good quality, a tubular graft of synthetic (prosthetic) material is used. The surgeon sutures the graft into an opening in the side of one artery and then into the side of the other. In a femoropopliteal bypass, for example, the graft extends from the femoral artery to the popliteal artery. The clamps are then removed and the flow of blood is observed to make sure it bypasses the blocked portion of the affected artery.

Aortobifemoral bypass surgery is conducted in much the same way, although it requires an abdominal incision to access the lower portion of the abdominal aorta and both femoral arteries in the groin. This is generally a longer and more difficult procedure. Synthetic grafts are used because the lower abdominal aorta is a large conduit, and its blood flow cannot be handled by the smaller saphenous vein. Vascular surgeons prefer the saphenous vein graft for femoropopliteal or femorotibial bypass surgery because it has proven to stay open and provide better performance for a longer period of time than synthetic grafts. Bypass surgery patients will be given heparin, a blood thinner, immediately after the surgery to prevent clotting in the new bypass graft.

Diagnosis/Preparation

Diagnosis

After obtaining a detailed history and reviewing symptoms, the physician examines the legs and feet, and orders appropriate tests or procedures to evaluate the vascular system. Diagnostic tests and procedures may include:

- Blood pressure and pulses—pressure measurements are taken in the arms and legs. Pulses are measured in the arms, armpits, wrists, groin, ankles, and behind the knees to determine where blockages may exist, since no pulse is usually felt below a blockage.
- Doppler ultrasonography—direct measurement of blood flow and rates of flow, sometimes performed in conjunction with stress testing (tests that incorporate an exercise component).
- Angiography—an x-ray procedure that provides clear images of the affected arteries before surgery is performed.
- Blood tests—routine tests such as cholesterol and glucose, as well as tests to help identify other causes of narrowed arteries, such as inflammation, thoracic outlet syndrome, high homocyceine levels, or arteritis.
- Spiral computed tomography (CT angiography) or magnetic resonance angiography (MRA)—less invasive forms of angiography.

Preparation

If not done earlier in the diagnostic process, ultrasonography or **angiography** procedures may be performed when the patient is admitted to the hospital. These tests help the physician evaluate the amount of plaque and exact location of the narrowing or obstruction. Any underlying medical condition, such as high blood pressure, heart disease, or diabetes is treated prior to bypass surgery to help obtain the best surgical result. Regular medications, such as blood pressure drugs or **diuretics**, may be discontinued in some patients. Routine pre-operative blood and urine tests are performed when the patient is admitted to the hospital.

Aftercare

After bypass surgery, the patient is moved to a recovery area where blood pressure, temperature, and heart rate are monitored for an hour or more. The surgical site is checked regularly. The patient is then transferred to a concentrated care unit to be observed for any signs of complications. The total hospital stay for femoropopliteal bypass or femorotibial bypass surgery may be two to four days. Recovery is slower with aortobifemoral bypass surgery, which involves abdominal incisions, and the hospital stay may extend up to a week. Walking will begin immediately for patients who have had femoropopliteal or femorotibial bypasses, but patients who have had aortobifemoral bypass may be kept in bed for 48 hours. When bypass patients go home, walking more each day, as tolerated, is encouraged to help maintain blood flow and muscle strength. Feet and legs can be elevated on a footstool or pillow when the patient rests. Some swelling of the leg should be expected; it does not indicate a problem and will resolve within a month or two.

During recuperation, the patient may be given pain medication if needed, and clot prevention (anticoagulant) medication. Any redness of the surgical site or other signs of infection will be treated with **antibiotics**. Patients are advised to reduce the risk factors for atherosclerosis in order to avoid repeat narrowing or blockage of the arteries. Repeat stenosis (restenosis) has been shown to occur frequently in people who do not make the necessary lifestyle modifications, such as changes in diet, exercise, and smoking cessation. The benefits of the bypass surgery may only be temporary if underlying disease, such as atherosclerosis, high blood pressure, or diabetes, is not also treated.

Risks

The risks associated with peripheral vascular bypass surgery are related to the progressive atherosclerosis that led to arterial occlusion, including a return of pre-operative symptoms. In patients with advanced PAD, heart attack or heart failure may occur. Build up of plaque has also taken place in the

WHO PERFORMS THE PROCEDURE AND WHERE IS IT PERFORMED?

Peripheral vascular bypass surgery is performed by a vascular surgeon in a hospital operating room.

patient's arteries of the heart. Restenosis, the continuing build up of plaque, can occur within months to years after surgery if risk factors are not controlled. Other complications may include:

- clot formation in a saphenous vein graft
- failed grafts or blockages in grafts
- reactions to anesthesia
- breathing difficulties
- embolism (clot from the surgical site traveling to vessels in the heart, lungs, or brain)
- changes in blood pressure
- infection of the surgical wound
- nerve injury (including sexual function impairment after aortobifemoral bypass)
- postoperative bleeding
- failure to heal properly

Normal results

A femoropopliteal or femorotibial bypass with an autogenous graft of good quality saphenous vein has been shown to have a 60–70% chance of staying open and functioning well for five to 10 years. Aortobifemoral bypass grafts have been shown to stay open and reduce symptoms in 80% of patients for up to 10 years. Pain and walking difficulties should be relieved after bypass surgery. Success rates improve when the underlying causes of atherosclerosis are monitored and managed effectively.

Morbidity and mortality rates

The risk of death or heart attack is about 3–5% in all patients undergoing peripheral vascular bypass surgery. Following bypass surgery, amputation is still an outcome in about 40% of all surgeries performed, usually due to progressive atherosclerosis or complications caused by the patient's underlying disease condition.

QUESTIONS TO ASK THE DOCTOR

- Why is this surgery necessary?
- How will the surgery improve my condition?
- What kind of anesthesia will be given?
- How many of these procedures has the surgeon performed?
- How many surgical patients had complications after the procedure?
- How can the patient expect to feel after surgery?
- How soon will the patient be able to walk?
- How long will it take to recover completely?
- What are the chances of this problem recurring after surgery?
- What can be done to help prevent this problem from developing again?

Alternatives

Peripheral vascular bypass surgery is a mechanical way to reroute blood, and there is no alternative method. Alternative ways to prevent plaque build-up and reduce the risk of narrowing or blocking the peripheral arteries include nutritional supplements and alternative therapies, such as:

- Folic acid can help lower homocysteine levels and increase the oxygen-carrying capacity of red blood cells.
- Vitamins B_6 and B_{12} help lower homocysteine levels.
- Antioxidant vitamins C and E work together to promote healthy blood vessels and improve circulation.
- Angelica, an herb that contains Coumadin, a recognized anticoagulant, which may help prevent clot formation in the blood.
- Essential fatty acids, as found in flax seed and other oils, to help reduce blood pressure and cholesterol, and maintain blood vessel elasticity.
- Chelation therapy, used to break up plaque and improve circulation.

Resources

BOOKS

Khatri, VP and JA Asensio. Operative Surgery Manual. 1st ed. Philadelphia: Saunders, 2003.

Libby, P. et al. Braunwald's Heart Disease. 8th ed. Philadelphia: Saunders, 2007.

Townsend, CM et al. Sabiston Textbook of Surgery. 17th ed. Philadelphia: Saunders, 2004.

PERIODICALS

Perera GB. "Current trends in lower extremity revascularization." *Surgical Clinics of North America* 87, no.5 (2007): 1135–1147.

Raffetto JD. "Differences in risk factors for lower extremity arterial occlusive disease." *Journal of the American College of Surgery* 201, no.6 (2005): 1135–1147.

ORGANIZATIONS

American Heart Association (AHA). 7272 Greenville Ave., Dallas, TX 75231. (800) 242-8721. www.americanheart.org.

Vascular Disease Foundation. 3333 South Wadsworth Blvd. B104-37, Lakewood, CO 80227. (303) 949-8337 or (866)PADINFO (723-4636). www.vdf.org.

OTHER

Bypass Surgery for Peripheral Arterial Disease. Patient Information, Vascular Disease Foundation, 2003. www.vdf.org.

Hirsch, M.D., Alan T. "Occlusive Peripheral Arterial Disease." *The Merck Manual of Medicine—Home Edition, Heart and Blood Vessel Disorders* 34:3. www.merck.com/pubs.

L. Lee Culvert

Peritoneal dialysis *see* **Kidney dialysis**
Peritoneal fluid analysis *see* **Paracentesis**

Peritoneovenous shunt

Definition

A peritoneovenous shunt refers to the surgical insertion of a shunting tube to achieve the continuous emptying of ascitic fluid into the venous system.

Purpose

Ascites is a serious medical disorder characterized by the pathological accumulation of fluid in the peritoneal cavity, the smooth membrane that lines the cavity of the abdomen and surrounds the organs. Ascites is usually related to acute and chronic liver disease (cirrhosis) and to a lesser degree, to malignant tumors arising in the ovary, colon, or breast. Ascites may also be associated with chronic kidney disease and congestive heart failure. The formation of ascitic fluid results from the interplay of three factors: abnormally high pressure within the liver or the veins draining into the liver (portal hypertension); abnormally low amounts of albumin in the blood (hypoalbuminemia); and changes in sodium and water excretion by the kidneys.

When medical therapy fails, peritoneovenous shunts help manage chronic ascites.

Demographics

Cirrhosis is the seventh leading cause of **death** by disease in the United States, killing over 25,000 people each year. Fifty percent of patients with cirrhosis will develop ascites over a period of 10 years. Cirrhosis—regardless of its cause—greatly increases the risk for liver cancer. Few studies have been conducted on the risk for liver cancer in patients with primary biliary cirrhosis; however, one study reported an incidence of 2.3%. Approximately 4% of patients with cirrhosis caused by hepatitis C develop liver cancer. In Asia, about 15% of people who have chronic hepatitis B develop liver cancer, but this high rate is not seen in other parts of the world. One Italian study that followed a group of hepatitis B patients for 11 years found no liver cancer over that period of time.

Description

A variety of shunts have been designed for peritoneovenous shunting, including the Hyde shunt (1966-1974), LaVeen shunt (1974-1980), and Denver shunt. The latter predates the LaVeen shunt, but is more popular as of 2003. All designs work about equally well.

For the peritoneovenous shunt insertion procedure, the patient only requires a local anesthetic and a sedative. A long needle is inserted into the jugular vein in the neck, and is passed down through the superior vena cava, the large vein that delivers blood from the head, neck, and upper limbs back to the heart. This serves to widen the vein. The surgeon makes an incision and inserts a tube traversing the subcutaneous tissue of the chest wall. The tube connects the peritoneal cavity to the neck, where it enters the widened jugular vein. There the surgeon attaches a pressure-sensitive, one-way valve to prevent backflow.

Diagnosis/Preparation

Ascites may go unnoticed for quite some time until the patient notices a slight increase in waistline. Severe ascites with marked abdominal distension becomes very disabling, especially when associated with swelling of the legs, pleural effusions (fluid around the lungs), and shortness of breath.

Diagnosis can be established by examination of the ascitic fluid, which allows the physician to differentiate between cirrhosis and tumor-induced ascites. The fluid is taken from the peritoneal cavity in a procedure called a **paracentesis**. Ascitic fluid analysis

KEY TERMS

Ascites—An effusion and accumulation of serous fluid in the abdominal cavity.

Ascitic fluid—The fluid that accumulates in the peritoneal cavity in ascites.

Coagulopathy—A defect in the blood clotting mechanism.

Edema—The presence of abnormally large amounts of fluid in the intercellular tissue spaces of the body.

Inferior vena cava—Large vein that returns blood from the lower part of the body to the heart.

Jugular vein—Major vein of the neck that returns blood from the head to the heart.

Hypoalbuminemia—An abnormally low concentration of albumin in the blood.

Paracentesis—Surgical puncture of the abdominal cavity for the aspiration of peritoneal fluid.

Peritoneal cavity—The space enclosed by the peritoneum.

Peritoneum—The smooth membrane that lines the cavity of the abdomen, and surrounds the viscera, forming a closed sac.

Portal hypertension—Abnormally high pressure within the veins draining into the liver.

Subcutaneou—Beneath the skin.

Superior vena cava—Large vein that returns blood to the heart from the head, neck, and upper limbs.

Venous system—Circulation system that carries blood that has passed through the capillaries of various tissues, except the lungs, and is found in the veins, the right chambers of the heart, and the pulmonary arteries; it is usually dark red as a result of a lower oxygen content.

includes a total polymorph count, protein and albumin concentrations, and placement of at least 10 ml of ascitic fluid each into **blood culture** bottles for processing. If a measurement called the serum-ascitic fluid albumin gradient is greater than 11 g/L, cirrhosis, not cancer, is suspected.

Aftercare

After surgery, the patient's **vital signs** are monitored in a **recovery room**. Pain medication and **antibiotics** are administered as needed. Once released from the hospital, the patient is expected to abstain

from alcohol, and follow a low-salt diet and medication regime designed to control ascites.

Patients also require training in shunt maintenance. To keep the fluid moving out of the abdomen, the shunt has to be properly pumped on a daily basis. Twice a day—once at bedtime and again prior to rising in the morning—the shunt is pumped about 20 times. This is essential to limit the accumulation of fibrin and other debris within the shunt, and to avoid the formation of an occlusive fibrin sheath at the venous tip.

Risks

Complications following peritoneovenous shunt insertion are common and include infection, leakage of ascitic fluid, accumulation of abnormally large amounts of fluid in the intercellular tissue spaces of the body (edema), deregulation of the blood clotting mechanism (coagulopathy), and shunt blockage. Clogging of the shunt with debris is the most common complication. Some patients develop further complications from the ascitic fluid entering directly into their bloodstream. Scar tissue often develops, making future liver transplants difficult.

Normal results

In spite of the complications associated with the procedure, many patients obtain useful relief from ascites following peritoneovenous shunt insertion.

Morbidity and mortality rates

The most recent guidelines from the American Association for the Study of Liver Diseases recommend peritoneovenous shunting only under these conditions:

- Patient is diuretic-resistant and not a transplant candidate.
- Patient is not a candidate for serial therapeutic paracentesis because of multiple abdominal surgical scars.
- A physician is unavailable to perform serial paracentesis.

Cirrhosis is irreversible, but the rate of progression can be very slow depending on its cause and other factors. Five-year survival rates are about 85% in the Unites States and can be lower or higher depending on severity.

Alternatives

Alternative treatments for ascites include:

- Diuretics. Diuretics are medications that promote the excretion of urine and help eliminate excess fluids. The treatment of ascites always involves restricting dietary

WHO PERFORMS THE PROCEDURE AND WHERE IS IT PERFORMED?

Peritoneovenous shunt insertion is performed in a hospital by a surgeon specialized in gastroenterology or hepatology.

salt and taking diuretic pills to increase the output of salt in the urine. This treatment is effective, at least in the short-term, in 90% of patients.

- Repeated large-volume paracentesis. This approach, also called serial paracentesis, features repeated surgical puncture of the abdominal cavity and aspiration of the ascitic fluid.
- Transjugular portosystemic shunt. A shunting procedure designed to relieve portal hypertension.
- Portocaval shunt. Another shunting procedure designed to relieve portal hypertension.
- Liver transplantation. Replacement of the patient's liver by one obtained from a donor. Liver transplantation is the only definitive treatment for ascites, and the only treatment that has been clearly shown to improve survival.

There is no satisfactory treatment for refractory ascites in patients with cirrhosis. Both peritoneovenous shunts and paracentesis have been used, but there is uncertainty about their relative merits.

Resources

BOOKS

Arroyo, V., P. Gines, J. Rodes. and R. W. Schrier, eds. *Ascites and Renal Dysfunction in Liver Disease: Pathogenesis, Diagnosis, and Treatment.* Oxford, UK: Blackwell Science Inc, 1999.

Moore, W. S. ed. *Vascular Surgery: A Comprehensive Review.* Philadelphia: W. B. Saunders Co., 2001.

PERIODICALS

Gines, P., and V. Arroyo. "Hepatorenal Syndrome." *Journal of the American Society of Nephrology* 10 (1999): 1833-9.

Hu, R. H. and P. H. Lee. "Salvaging Procedures for Dysfunctional Peritoneovenous Shunt." *Hepatogastroenterology* 48 (May-June 2001): 794-7.

Koike, T., S. Araki, H. Minakami, S. Ogawa, M. Sayama, H. Shibahara, and I. Sato. "Clinical Efficacy of Peritoneovenous Shunting for the Treatment of Severe Ovarian Hyperstimulation Syndrome." *Human Reproduction* 15 (2000): 113-17.

Orsi, F., R.F. Grasso, G. Bonomo, C. Monti, I. Marinucci and M. Bellomi. "Percutaneous Peritoneovenous Shunt

QUESTIONS TO ASK THE DOCTOR

- Is there any other treatment available for ascites?
- What are the risks associated with peritoneovenous shunting?
- How long will it take to recover from the surgery?
- How does the shunting mechanism work?
- How many peritoneovenous shunt procedures does the surgeon perform each year?
- Will further surgery be required?
- What happens if the shunt becomes blocked?

Positioning: Technique and Preliminary Results." *European Radiology* 12 (May 2002): 1188-92.

Wagayama, H., T. Tanaka, M. Shimomura, K. Ogura, and K. Shiraki. "Pancreatic Cancer with Chylous Ascites Demonstrated by Lymphoscintigraphy: Successful Treatment with Peritoneovenous Shunting." *Digestive Disturbance Science* 10 (August 2002): 1836-8.

ORGANIZATIONS

American Gastroenterological Association. 4930 Del Ray Avenue, Bethesda, MD 20814. (301) 654-2055. www.gastro.org.

Society for Vascular Surgery. 900 Cummings Center, Beverly, MA 01915-1314. (978) 927-8330. <svs.vasculaweb.org>.

OTHER

"Ascites." *Family Practice Notebook.*www.fpnotebook.com/GI35.htm.

Monique Laberge, Ph.D.

Permanent pacemakers *see* **Pacemakers**

PET scan *see* **Positron emission tomography (PET)**

pH monitoring

Definition

pH is a value that represents the balance of acidic and alkaline molecules in a given system. The human body requires a very precise balance between these in order to properly maintain homeostasis. Homeostasis, or physiological equilibrium, is the maintenance of stable conditions for bodily function. pH monitoring is the practice of keeping track of where the pH value lies in order to quickly diagnose and treat disorders that alter pH.

Description

pH monitoring is done to guard against physiological states in which the amount of acidic or alkaline molecules in the body is out of balance. Another term for acidic and alkaline is "acid and base". Acid is represented in the body as hydrogen ions. Base is represented in the body as hydroxide ions. Too much of either one can cause serious physical harm. A pH scale is designed with the number seven falling in the middle, defined as neutral. At a pH of seven the amount of acid and base present lies in balance. Any pH greater than seven is considered more alkaline or basic. Any pH less than seven is considered more acidic. Each area of the body has its own normal range for pH. Human blood normally lies between a pH of 7.34 to 7.45. Human stomach acid normally lies between a pH of 1.5 to 2.0. Human urine normally has a pH of approximately 6.0.

A physiological state where the blood is too acidic with a low pH is called acidosis. Acidosis is caused by an imbalance in hydrogen ions present in the blood, causing the pH to fall below 7.35. On the other side of the scale, alkalosis is a physiological state where the blood pH value rises above 7.45 due an imbalance in hydroxide, and becomes too basic. The farther the pH is altered from the normal range, the more serious the patient's condition. Even relatively small changes in blood pH can be life threatening. Blood pH values generally considered compatible with mammalian life lie between a pH of 6.8 to 7.8. For this reason, the body uses blood as a buffering system to maintain pH balance. Certain states of disease, disorders, or physical conditions sometimes overwhelm the body's buffering systems and medical assistance becomes necessary to maintain life. In these cases, pH monitoring is a critical tool in guarding against or treating drastic alterations in body chemistry.

Monitoring pH for Acidosis

Acidosis is physiological state of excessive acid in the blood. Acidosis can be caused by an increase in acid, or simply a decrease of base, causing what is known as metabolic acidosis. Acidosis can also be caused by abnormal respiratory function. Taking in too much carbon dioxide or too little oxygen through the lungs leads to increased amounts of carbon dioxide in the blood. Carbon dioxide in the blood is changed into multiple components, resulting in the release of hydrogen ions, causing acidosis. The type of acidosis originally caused by carbon dioxide and respiratory functioning is known as respiratory acidosis.

If an increase in acid or decrease in base occurs beyond the body's pH buffering capabilities, there are other compensatory mechanisms to restore equilibrium in pH. In response to a drop in blood pH, the brain causes a change in respiration for fast, deep breathing. This type of breathing causes an increased amount of carbon dioxide to be exhaled, drawing more and more carbon dioxide from the blood. The more carbon dioxide leaves the blood, the more hydrogen ions are removed, helping to correct acidosis. Additionally, the kidneys may increase excretion of hydrogen ions or decrease excretion of hydroxide ions in the urine. Even with these compensatory mechanisms, a severe state of acidosis often requires medical attention to correct, with pH monitoring as a critical tool for health management. Without proper medical attention the acidotic patient may experience nausea, vomiting, fatigue, confusion, weakness, shock, coma, or **death**. The treatment of acidosis is dependent on the cause of the disorder.

Conditions that Potentially Cause Acidosis and May Require pH Monitoring

- Ingestion of Wood Alcohol or Antifreeze (excessive acid)
- Aspirin Overdose (excessive acid)
- Poorly Controlled Diabetes (excessive acid)
- Kidney Dysfunction or Failure (cannot excrete acid normally)
- Lung Dysfunction (cannot expel carbon dioxide normally; e.g., severe pneumonia, emphysema, or asthma)
- Drugs that Disrupt Respiration (cannot expel carbon dioxide normally; e.g., narcotic pain-killer overdose)
- Ingestion of Acidic Poisons (excessive acid)
- Extreme Diarrhea (expel excessive base)

Monitoring pH for Alkalosis

Alkalosis is a physiological state of excessive base in the blood. Alkalosis can be caused by an increase in base, or a decrease of acid, causing what is known as metabolic alkalosis. Alkalosis can also be caused by abnormal respiratory function. Exhaling too much carbon dioxide leads to a decrease in carbon dioxide in the blood. A decrease in carbon dioxide in the blood leads to a decrease in hydrogen ions and a relative excess of hydroxide ions. This type of alkalosis is known as respiratory alkalosis. Respiratory alkalosis can be induced by hyperventilation, a type of breathing that is very rapid and deep and leads to expulsion of large amounts of carbon dioxide.

Acidosis—A pathological state in which there is a relative excess of hydrogen ions in the arterial blood.

Alkaline—A basic substance with pH above 7.0.

Alkalosis—A pathological state in which there is a relative excess of hydroxide ions in the arterial blood.

Anxiety Attack—A disorder in which sudden feelings of dread, fear, and apprehension of danger enter a person's mind in an overwhelming manner. Attacks may lead to a state of hyperventilation.

Arterial Blood—Blood from the arteries, the blood vessels that carry oxygen from the lungs to supply the body tissues.

Arterial Blood Gas (ABG)—A type of blood laboratory test done to check the blood for imbalances in pH or gases that affect pH.

Asthma—An inflammatory respiratory disorder in which the airway becomes obstructed and breathing is difficult.

Coronary Artery Bypass Surgery—A surgical procedure where arteries or veins from elsewhere in the patient's body grafted into the arteries of the heart as a way to bypass damaged or narrowed heart blood vessels. Heart blood vessels may have been damaged or narrowed from fat deposition and need to be bypassed to increase the blood supply and oxygen delivered to the heart.

Corticosteroid—A type of drug used to treat inflammatory conditions that also alters blood ions and affects pH.

Diuretic—A type of drug used to treat hypertension that also alters blood ions and affects pH.

Electrode—A device used to record an electric circuit or changes in ion concentrations.

Emphysema—Lung disease that causes damage to lung tissue and breathlessness.

Heart Lung Machine—A machine that temporarily takes over the function of the heart and lungs during surgical procedures in order to maintaining blood circulation and delivery of oxygen to body tissues while the heart is being operated on.

Heart Valve Replacement Surgery—Surgery performed to repair or replace the valves in the heart that control blood flow through the heart and are responsible for the audible heartbeat.

Homeostasis—The process of maintaining balance in the normal vital life functions of a living organism.

Hydrogen Ions—Ions that contain one hydrogen atom with a positive charge. Hydrogen ions cause blood to be acidic.

Hydroxide Ions—Ions that contain one oxygen and one hydrogen atom, with a negative charge. Hydroxide ions cause blood to be alkaline.

Ischemia—A state of decreased oxygen, where body tissues may experience damage due to oxygen deprivation.

Narcotic Pain Killer—A type of pain killer often used after surgical procedures that may alter blood pH.

Physiological—Pertaining to the normal vital life functions of a living organism.

Pneumonia—An inflammatory lung disease that affects the ability of the respiratory system to function.

Radial Artery—An artery present in the wrist that is convenient for drawing blood intended for laboratory testing.

Respiratory Function—The ability of the breathing structures of the body, including the lungs, to function.

Venous Blood—Blood that carries carbon dioxide from the tissues to the heart and then the lungs to be oxygenated.

If an increase in base or decrease in acid occurs beyond the body's pH buffering capabilities, compensatory mechanisms to restore equilibrium in pH include a change in respiration for slow, shallow breathing. This type of breathing causes a decreased amount of carbon dioxide to be exhaled, thereby increasing the amount of carbon dioxide and hydrogen ions in the blood. Additionally, the kidneys may increase excretion of hydroxide ions or decrease excretion of hydrogen ions in the urine. Similar to acidosis, a severe state of alkalosis often requires medical attention to correct, with pH monitoring as a critical tool for health management. Without proper medical attention the patient may experience irritability, muscle cramping, muscle spasms, seizures, delirium, and death. The treatment of alkalosis is dependent on the cause of the disorder.

Conditions that Potentially Cause Alkalosis and May Require pH Monitoring

- Prolonged Vomiting (loss of excessive acid)
- Ingestion of Alkaline Poisons (excessive base)
- Drugs that Cause Excessive Loss of Sodium or Potassium Ions (e.g., diuretics and corticosteroids)
- Severe Anxiety Attacks (hyperventilation)
- Pain and Fever (hyperventilation)
- Aspirin Overdose (Aspirin can cause both acidosis and alkalosis)

How pH is Monitored

pH is monitored through laboratory tests done on the blood drawn from an artery. Arterial blood is an accurate indicator of blood pH. Venous blood holds too much carbon dioxide taken from the tissues to be useful. Blood is usually taken from the radial artery located in the wrist. The blood is tested for pH, as well as levels of carbon dioxide and other pertinent blood components. The laboratory test is known as Arterial Blood Gas (**ABG**). It is very important that room air is not accidentally introduced into the sample of blood drawn, as the oxygen present would make the blood unsuitable for testing. If the patient's condition warrants it, the ABG test may be done several times a day.

pH Monitoring during Heart Surgery

Some types of heart surgery involve temporarily depriving parts of the heart of its blood supply during the procedure (while the patient is on a heart lung machine to maintain bodily function). Local blood deprivation results in decreased heart tissue oxygen (a condition called ischemia), increased tissue carbon dioxide levels, heart tissue acidosis, and possibly death of heart tissue. The level to which this actually occurs during the procedure varies from person to person. The severity of tissue acidosis has been shown to directly associate with the degree of ischemia that tissue is experiencing and consequent impact on long-term survival of the surgery patient.

Specific low pH values during different points in the surgical procedure have been identified as dangerous levels of acidosis. Allowing the heart tissue to fall below these values may be associated with post-operative heart failure and mortality. Purposefully raising the pH levels before these specific points in the procedure, prior to heart tissue ischemia and a drop in pH, may help keep the heart tissue pH above dangerous levels of acidosis and ischemia. Special intraoperative heart pH monitors have been designed to supervise the pH value of heart tissue during surgery and keep track of the surgeon's efforts in pH modification. Electrodes designed as sterile probes that detect pH are inserted directly into the heart and used as an early warning system for dangerous changes in pH. Surgical procedures that may be benefited by pH monitors include heart valve replacement surgery and coronary artery bypass surgery. pH monitoring is an important tool for surgeons to avoid or reverse acidosis and ischemia during heart surgery, thereby improving long-term patient survival.

Resources

BOOKS

Cecil Essentials of Medicine Sixth Edition. Saunders 2004.

Harrison's Principles of Internal Medicine Sixteenth Edition. McGraw-Hill 2005.

Merck Manual of Diagnosis and Therapy Eighteenth Edition 2006.

The Merck Manual Home Edition 2004.

PERIODICALS

Khuri SF, Healey NA, Hossain M, Birjiniuk V, Crittenden MD, Josa M, Treanor PR, Najjar SF, Kumbhani DJ, Henderson WG. "Intraoperative regional myocardial acidosis and reduction in long-term survival after cardiac surgery." *Journal of Thoracic and Cardiovascular Surgery* 129 (2005): 372-81.

Maria Basile, PhD

Phacoemulsification for cataracts

Definition

Phacoemulsification cataract surgery is a procedure in which an ultrasonic device is used to break up and then remove a cloudy lens, or cataract, from the eye to improve vision. The insertion of an intraocular lens (IOL) usually immediately follows phacoemulsification.

Purpose

Phacoemulsification, or phaco, as surgeons refer to it, is used to restore vision in patients whose vision has become cloudy from cataracts. In the first stages of a cataract, people may notice only a slight cloudiness as it affects only a small part of the lens, the part of the eye that focuses light on the retina. As the cataract grows, it blocks more light and vision becomes cloudier. As vision worsens, the surgeon will recommend cataract surgery, usually phaco, to restore clear vision. With advancements in cataract surgery such as the IOL patients can sometimes experience dramatic vision improvement.

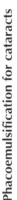
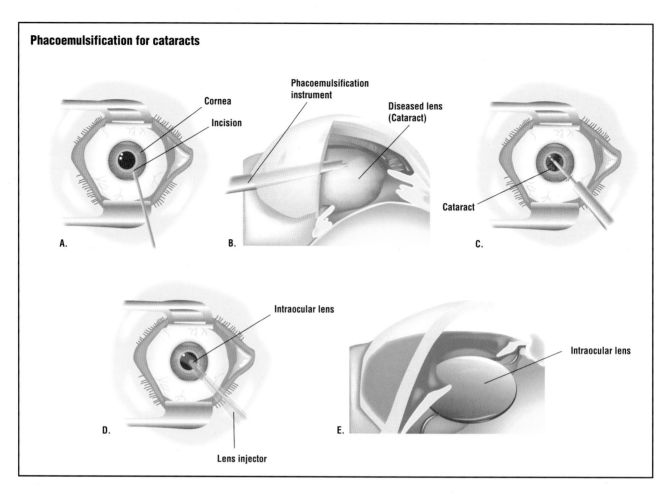

Phacoemulsification for cataracts

Cornea

Incision

Phacoemulsification instrument

Diseased lens (Cataract)

Cataract

A.

B.

C.

Intraocular lens

Intraocular lens

D.

E.

Lens injector

In a phacoemulsification procedure, an incision is first made in the cornea, the outer covering of the eye (A).
A phacoemulsification instrument uses ultrasonic waves to break up the cataract (B). Pieces of the cataract are then suctioned out (C). To repair the patient's vision, a folded intraocular lens is pushed through the same incision (D) and opened in place (E).
(Illustration by GGS Information Services. Cengage Learning, Gale.)

Demographics

As people age, cataracts are likely to form. The National Eye Institute (NEI) reports in a 2002 study that more than half of all United States residents 65 and older have a cataract. People who smoke are at a higher risk for cataracts. Increased exposure to sunlight or infrared radiation without eye protection may also be a cause.

Cataracts also can occur anytime because of injury, exposure to toxins, or such diseases as diabetes. Congenital cataracts are caused by genetic defects or developmental problems, or exposure to some contagious diseases during pregnancy.

However, the most common form of cataract in the United States is age-related. According to the NEI, cataracts are more common in women than in men, and Caucasians have cataracts more frequently than other races, especially as people grow older. People

who live close to the equator also are at higher risk for cataracts because of increased sunlight exposure. Heavy alcohol consumption is also a risk factor for cataract formation.

More than 2.5 million cataract surgeries are performed in the United States each year. The NEI reports that the federal government, through **Medicare**, spends more than $3.4 billion each year treating cataracts. Cataract surgery is one of the most common surgeries performed, and also one of the safest and most effective. Phaco is currently the most popular version of cataract surgery.

Description

Phacoemulsification is a variation of **extracapsular cataract extraction** (ECCE), a procedure in which the lens and the front portion of the capsule are removed. Formerly the most popular cataract surgery,

KEY TERMS

Astigmatism—Asymmetric vision defects due to irregularities in the cornea.

Capsulorrhexis—The creation of a continuous circular tear in the front portion of the lens capsule during cataract surgery to allow for removal of the lens nucleus.

Cornea—Clear, bowl-shaped structure at the front of the eye. It is located in front of the colored part of the eye (iris). The cornea lets light into the eye and partially focuses it.

Floaters—Spots in the field of vision.

Glaucoma—Disease of the eye characterized by increased pressure of the fluid inside the eye. Untreated, glaucoma can lead to blindness.

Lens (the crystalline lens)—A transparent structure in the eye that focuses light onto the retina.

Myopia—A refractive error that causes distant objects to appear blurry. Myopia results when light does not focus properly on the retina.

Retina—The inner light-sensitive layer of the eye containing rods and cones.

the older method of extracapsular extraction involves a longer incision, about 0.4 in (10 mm), or almost half the length of the eye. Recovery from the larger incision used for extracapsular extraction also requires almost a week-long hospital stay after surgery, and limited physical activity for weeks or even months.

Dr. Charles Kelman (1930–2004) introduced the technique of phacoemulsification in the late 1960s. He was inspired by his dentist's use of ultrasonic tools. His goal was to remove the cataract with a smaller incision, less pain, and shorter recovery time. He discovered that the cataract could be broken up, or emulsified, into small pieces using an **ultrasound** tip. At first, phaco was slow to catch on because of its high learning curve. With its success rate and shorter recovery period, surgeons slowly learned the technique. Over the past decades, surgeons have constantly refined phaco to make it even safer and more successful. Innovations in technology such as the foldable IOL also have helped improve outcomes by allowing surgeons to make smaller incisions.

During surgery, the patient will probably breathe through an oxygen tube because it might be difficult to breathe with the draping. The patient's blood pressure and heart rate also are likely to be monitored.

Before making the incision, the surgeon inserts a long needle, usually through the lower eyelid, to anesthetize the area behind the eyeball. The surgeon then puts pressure on the eyeball with his or her hand or a weight to see if there is any bleeding (possibly caused by inserting the anesthetic). The pressure will stop this bleeding. This force also decreases intraocular pressure (IOP), which lowers the chances of complications.

After applying the pressure, the surgeon looks through a microscope and makes an incision about 0.1 in (3 mm) on the side of the anesthetized cornea. As of 2003, surgeons are beginning to favor the temporal location for the incision because it has proved to be safer. The incision site also varies depending on the size and denseness of the cataract. Once the incision is made, a viscoelastic fluid is injected to reduce shock to the intraocular tissues. The surgeon then makes a microscopic circular incision in the membrane that surrounds the cataract; this part of the procedure is called capsulorrhexis. A water stream then frees the cataract from the cortex. The surgeon inserts a small titanium needle, or phaco tip, into the cornea. The ultrasound waves from the phaco tip emulsify the cataract so that it can be removed by suction. The surgeon first focuses on the cataract's central nucleus, which is denser than the rest of the cataract.

While the cataract is being emulsified, the machine simultaneously aspirates the cataract through a small hole in the tip of the phaco probe. The surgeon then removes the cortex of the lens, but leaves the posterior capsule, which is used to support the intraocular lens.

The folded IOL is inserted by an injector. The folded IOL means that a larger incision is not required. After the IOL is inserted into the capsular bag, the viscoelastic fluid is removed. No sutures are usually required after the surgery. Some surgeons may recommend that patients wear an eye shield immediately after the surgery.

The entire procedure takes between 15 and 20 minutes. The phaco procedure itself takes only a few minutes.

Most surgeons prefer a certain technique for the procedure, although they might vary due to the cataract's density and size. The variations on the phaco procedure lie mostly on what part of the nucleus the surgeon focuses on first, and how the cataract is emulsified. Some surgeons prefer a continuous "chop," while others divide the cataract into quadrants for removal. One procedure, called the "phaco flip," involves the surgeon inverting and then rotating the lens for removal. Advances in technology also may allow for even smaller incisions, some speculate as small as 0.05 in (1.4 mm).

Diagnosis/Preparation

People may have cataracts for years before vision is impaired enough to warrant surgery. Eye doctors may first suggest eyeglasses to temporarily help improve vision. But as the lens grows cloudier, vision deteriorates.

As cataracts develop and worsen, patients may notice these common symptoms:

- gradual (and painless) onset of blurry vision
- poor central vision
- frequent changes in prescription for corrective lenses
- increased glare from lights
- near-vision improvement to the point where reading glasses may no longer be needed
- poor vision in sunlight

Cataracts grow faster in younger people or in patients with diabetes, so doctors will recommend surgery more quickly in those cases. Surgery may also be recommended sooner if the patient suffers from such other eye diseases as age-related macular degeneration and the cataract interferes with complete eye examination.

When symptoms worsen to the point that everyday activities become problematic, surgery becomes necessary. A complete ocular exam will determine the severity of the cataract and what type of surgery the patient will receive. For some denser cataracts, the older method of extracapsular extraction is preferred.

The diagnostic examination should include measurement of visual acuity under both low and high illumination, microscopic examination of eye structures and pupil dilation, assessment of visual fields, and measurement of intraocular pressure (IOP).

If cataracts are detected in both eyes, each eye must be treated separately.

The patient's overall health must also be considered, and how it will affect the surgery's outcome. Surgeons may recommend a complete **physical examination** before surgery.

Although preoperative instructions may vary, patients are usually required not to eat or drink anything after midnight the day of the surgery. Patients must disclose all medications to determine if they must be discontinued before surgery. Patients taking **aspirin** for blood thinning usually are asked to stop for two weeks before surgery. Blood-thinning medications may put patients at risk for intraocular bleeding or hemorrhage. Coumadin, the prescription medicine for blood thinning, might still be taken if the risk for

stroke is high. People should consult with their eye doctor and internist to decide the best course of action.

An A-scan measurement, which determines the length of the eyeball, will be performed. This test helps to determine the refractive power of the IOL. Other pre-surgical testing such as a **chest x ray**, blood work, or **urinalysis** may be requested if other medical problems are an issue.

The surgeon may also request patients begin using antibiotic drops before the surgery to limit the chance of infection.

Cataract surgery is done on an outpatient basis, so patients must arrange for someone to take them home after surgery. On the day of the surgery, doctors will review the pre-surgical tests and insert dilating eye drops, antibiotic drops, and a corticosteroid or non-steroidal anti-inflammatory drop. Anesthetic eye drops will be given in both eyes to keep both eyes comfortable during surgery. A local anesthetic will be administered. Patients are awake for the surgery, but are kept in a relaxed state.

The patient's eye is scrubbed prior to surgery and sterile drapes are placed over the shoulders and head. The patient is required to lie still and focus on the light of the operating microscope. A speculum is inserted to keep the eyelids open.

Aftercare

Immediately following surgery, the patient is monitored in an outpatient recovery area. The patient is advised to rest for at least 24 hours, until he or she returns to the surgeon's office for follow-up. Only light meals are recommended on the day of surgery. The patient may still feel drowsy and may experience some eye pain or discomfort. Usually, over-the-counter medications are advised for pain relief, but patients should check with their doctors to see what is recommended. Such other side effects as severe pain, nausea, or vomiting should be reported to the surgeon immediately.

There will be some changes in the eye during recovery. Patients may see dark spots, which should disappear a few weeks after surgery. There also might be some discharge and itching of the eye. Patients may use a warm, moist cloth for 15 minutes at a time for relief and to loosen the discharge. All matter from the discharge should be gently cleared away with a tissue, not a fingertip. Pain and sensitivity to light are also experienced after surgery. Some patients may also have slight drooping or bruising of the eye which will improve as the eye heals.

Patients have their first postoperative visit the day after surgery. The surgeon will remove the eye shield and prescribe eye drops to prevent infections and control intraocular pressure. These eye drops are used for about a month after surgery.

Patients are advised to wear an eye shield while sleeping, and refrain from rubbing the eye for at least two weeks. During that time, the doctor will give the patient special tinted sunglasses or request that he or she wear current prescription eyeglasses to prevent possible eye trauma from accidental rubbing or bumping. Unlike other types of cataract extraction, patients can resume normal activity almost immediately after phaco.

Subsequent exams are usually at one week, three weeks, and six to eight weeks following surgery. This can change, however, depending on any complications or any unusual postoperative symptoms.

After the healing process, the patient will probably need new corrective lenses, at least for close vision. While IOLs can remove the need for myopic correction, patients will probably need new lenses for close work.

Risks

Complications are unlikely, but can occur. Patients may experience spontaneous bleeding from the wound and recurrent inflammation after surgery. Flashing, floaters, and double vision may also occur a few weeks after surgery. The surgeon should be notified immediately of these symptoms. Some can easily be treated, while floaters may be a sign of retinal detachment.

Retinal detachment is one possible serious complication. The retina can become detached by the surgery if there is any weakness in the retina at the time of surgery. This complication may not occur for weeks or even years; one study reported in 2006 that patients who have had cataracts removed by phaco have an increased risk of retinal detachment 20 years after surgery.

Infections are another potential complication, the most serious being endophthalmitis, which is an infection in the eyeball. This complication, once widely reported, is much more uncommon today because of newer surgery techniques and **antibiotics**.

Patients may also be concerned that their IOL might become displaced, but newer designs of IOLs also have limited reports of intraocular lens dislocation.

Other possible complications are the onset of glaucoma and, in very rare cases, blindness.

It is possible that a secondary cataract may develop in the remaining back portion of the capsule. This can occur for as long as one to two years after surgery. YAG capsulotomy, using a laser, is most often used for the secondary cataract. This outpatient procedure requires no incision. The laser makes a small opening in the remaining back part of the lens to allow light to penetrate.

Normal results

Most patients have restored visual acuity after surgery, and some will have the best vision of their lives after the insertion of IOLs. Some patients will no longer require the use of eyeglasses or contact lenses after cataract surgery. Patients will also have better color and depth perception and be able to resume normal activities they may have stopped because of impaired vision from the cataract, such as driving, reading, or sports.

Morbidity and mortality rates

Phacoemulsification has lowered the previous risks from cataract surgery, making it a much safer procedure. Before phacoemulsification, **death** after cataract surgery was still rare, but usually stemmed from the possible complications of **general anesthesia**. Phaco is performed under **local anesthesia**, eliminating the risk of general anesthetic use.

Other serious complications such as blindness also have been reduced with the widespread use of phaco. Newer antibiotics have enabled physicians to combat former debilitating infections that previously would have caused blindness.

Alternatives

Some older methods of cataract surgery may have to be used if the cataract is too large to remove with a small incision, including:

- Extracapsular cataract extraction (ECCE). While phaco is considered a type of extracapsular extraction, the older version of this technique requires a much larger incision and does not use the phaco machine. It is similar in that the lens and the front portion of the capsule are removed and the back part of the capsule remains. The surgeon might consider this technique if the patient has corneal disease or if the pupil becomes too small during the first stages of surgery. While standard ECCE and phacoemulsification have similar success rates and complication rates when performed by surgeons of comparable skill and length of experience, a meta-analysis of 17 trials of these two methods reported in 2006 that phacoemulsification gives a better long-term outcome than standard ECCE with sutures.

WHO PERFORMS THE
PROCEDURE AND WHERE IS IT
PERFORMED?

Ophthalmologists and optometrists may detect cataracts; however, only an ophthalmologist can perform cataract surgery. An anesthesiologist may be on hand during surgery to administer the local anesthetic. Surgical nurses will assist the ophthalmologist in the operating room and assist the patient preoperatively and postoperatively.

The outpatient surgery is performed in a hospital or surgery suite designed for ophthalmic surgery.

• Intracapsular cataract extraction (ICCE). This technique also requires a larger incision than phaco. It differs in that the lens and the entire capsule are removed. While ICCE is the easiest cataract surgery for the surgeon technically, this method carries an increased risk for the patient with increased potential for detachment of the retina and swelling after surgery. Recovery is long and most patients will have to use large "cataract glasses" to see.

Resources

BOOKS

Buettner, Helmut, ed. Mayo Clinic on Vision and Eye Health. Rochester, MN: Mayo Clinic Health Information, 2002.

Henderson, Bonnie An, ed. Essentials of Cataract Surgery. Thorofare, NJ: SLACK, 2007.

Malhotra, Raman, ed. Cataract: Assessment, Classification, and Management. New York: Elsevier, Butterworth Heinemann, 2007.

Slade, Stephen G., Richard N. Baker, and Dorothy Kay Brockman. The Complete Book of Laser Eye Surgery. Naperville, IL: Sourcebooks, Inc., 2000.

PERIODICALS

Erie, J. C., M. E. Raecker, K. H. Baratz, et al. "Risk of Retinal Detachment after Cataract Extraction, 1980–2004: A Population-based Study." Transactions of the American Ophthalmological Society 104 (2006): 167–175.

Riaz, Y., J. S. Mehta, R. Wormald, et al. "Surgical Interventions for Age-Related Cataract." Cochrane Database of Systematic Reviews, October 18, 2006: CD001323.

Shaw, A. D., G. S. Ang, and T. Eke. "Phacoemulsification Complication Rates." Ophthalmology 114 (November 2007): 2101–2102.

Smith, J. H. "Teaching Phacoemulsification in US Ophthalmology Residencies: Can the Quality Be Maintained?" Current Opinion in Ophthalmology 16 (February 2005): 27–32.

QUESTIONS TO ASK THE
DOCTOR

• Will Medicare pay for the surgery and my aftercare?

• If I have a cataract in the other eye, how long must I wait to have the other eye treated?

• Will I still need reading glasses after surgery? Will I still need eyeglasses to see far away even if you insert an intraocular lens?

• How many cataract surgeries have you performed? How many of these have been phacoemulsification?

• What precautions should I take to protect my eye after surgery?

• When can I resume my normal activities after surgery? Contact sports?

ORGANIZATIONS

American Academy of Ophthalmology. P.O. Box 7424, San Francisco, CA 94120-7424. (415) 561-8500. http://www.aao.org.

American Optometric Association. 243 North Lindbergh Blvd., St. Louis, MO 63141. (314) 991-4100. http://www.aoanet.org.

American Society of Cataract and Refractive Surgery. 4000 Legato Road, Suite 700, Fairfax, VA 22033-4055. (703) 591-2220. E-mail: <ascrs@ascrs.org>. http://www.ascrs.org.

National Eye Institute. 2020 Vision Place Bethesda, MD 20892-3655. (301) 496-5248. http://www.nei.nih.gov.

OTHER

"Cataract Surgery." EyeMdLink.com, [cited March 28, 2003]. http://www.eyemdlink.com/EyeProcedure.asp. EyeProcedureID = 19.

National Eye Institute (NEI). Cataract. Bethesda, MD: NEI, 2007. NIH Publication No. 03-201.

Samalonis, Lisa B. "Cataract Surgery Today." Eye World, February 2002 [cited March 28, 2003] http://www.eyeworld.org/feb02/0202p34.html.

Mary Bekker
Rebecca Frey, Ph.D.

Pharyngectomy

Definition

A pharyngectomy is the total or partial surgical removal of the pharynx, the cavity at the back of the mouth that opens into the esophagus at its lower end.

The pharynx is cone-shaped, has an average length of about 3 in (76 mm), and is lined with mucous membrane.

Purpose

A pharyngectomy procedure is performed to treat cancers of the pharynx that include:

- Throat cancer. Throat cancer occurs when cells in the pharynx or larynx (voice box) begin to divide abnormally and out of control. A total or partial pharyngectomy is usually performed for cancers of the hypopharynx (last part of the throat), in which all or part of the hypopharynx is removed.

- Hypopharyngeal carcinoma (HPC). A carcinoma is a form of cancerous tumor that may develop in the pharynx or adjacent locations and for which surgery may be indicated.

Description

Whether a pharyngectomy is performed in total or with only partial removal of the pharnyx depends on the localized amount of cancer found. The procedure may also involve removal of the larynx, in which case it is called a laryngopharyngectomy. Well-localized, early stage HPC tumors can be amenable to a partial pharyngectomy or a laryngopharyngectomy, but laryngopharyngectomy is more commonly performed for more advanced cancers. It can be total, involving removal of the entire larynx, or partial and may also involve removal of part of the esophagus (esophagectomy). Patients undergoing laryngopharyngectomy will lose some speaking ability and require special techniques or reconstructive procedures to regain the use of their voice.

Following a total or partial pharyngectomy, the surgeon may also need to reconstruct the throat so that the patient can swallow. A **tracheotomy** is used when the tumor is too large to remove. In this procedure, a hole is made in the neck to bypass the tumor and allow the patient to breathe.

For this type of surgery, patient positioning requires access to the lower part of the neck for the surgeon. This is conveniently achieved by placing the patient on a table fitted with a head holder, allowing the head to be bent back but well supported.

If a laryngopharyngectomy is performed, the surgeon starts with a curved horizontal neck skin incision. The **laryngectomy** incision is usually made from the breastbone to the lower most of the laryngeal cartilages, such that a 1–2 in (2.54–5.08 cm) bridge of skin is preserved. Once the incision is deepened, flaps are elevated until the larynx is exposed. The anterior jugular veins and strap muscles are left undisturbed. The

sternocleidomastoid muscle is then identified. The layer of cervical fibrous tissue is cut (incised) longitudinally from the hyoid (the bony arch that supports the tongue) above to the clavicle (collarbone) below. Part of the hyoid is then divided, which allows the surgeon to enter the loose compartment bounded by the sternomastoid muscle and carotid sheath (which covers the carotid artery) and by the pharynx and larynx in the neck. The pharyngectomy incisions and laryngeal removal are performed, and a view of the pharynx is then possible. Using scissors, the surgeon performs bilateral (on both sides), direct cuts, separating the pharynx from the larynx. If a preliminary tracheotomy has not been performed, the oral endotracheal tube is withdrawn from the tracheal stump and a new, cuffed, flexible tube inserted for connection to new anesthesia tubing. The wound is thoroughly irrigated (flushed); all clots are removed; and the wound is closed. The pharyngeal wall is closed in two layers. The muscle layer closure always tightens the opening to some extent and is usually left undone at points where narrowing may be excessive. In fact, studies show that a mucosal (inner layer) closure alone is sufficient for proper healing.

Diagnosis/Preparation

The initial **physical examination** for a pharyngectomy usually includes examination of the neck, mouth, pharynx, and larynx. A neurologic examination is sometimes also performed. Laryngoscopy is the examination of choice, performed with a long-handled mirror, or with a lighted tube called a laryngoscope. A local anesthetic might be used to ease discomfort. A MRI of the oral cavity and neck may also be performed.

If the physician suspects throat cancer, a biopsy will be performed—this involves removing tissue for examination in the laboratory under a microscope. Throat cancer can only be confirmed through a biopsy or using fine needle aspiration (FNA). The physician also may use an imaging test called a computed tomography (CT) scan. This is a special type of x ray that provides images of the body from different angles, allowing a cross-sectional view. A CT-scan can help to find the location of a tumor, to judge whether or not a tumor can be removed surgically, and to determine the cancer's stage of development.

Before surgery, the patient is also examined for nutritional assessment and supplementation, and careful staging of cancer, while surgical airway management is planned with the anesthesiologist such that a common agreement is reached with the surgeon concerning the timing of tracheotomy and intubation.

KEY TERMS

Anesthesia—A combination of drugs administered by a variety of techniques by trained professionals that provide sedation, amnesia, analgesia, and immobility adequate for the accomplishment of the surgical procedure with minimal discomfort, and without injury, to the patient.

Biopsy—Procedure that involves obtaining a tissue specimen for microscopic analysis to establish a precise diagnosis.

Carcinoma—A malignant growth that arises from epithelium, found in skin or, more commonly, the lining of body organs.

Computed tomography (CT) scan—An imaging technique that creates a series of pictures of areas inside the body, taken from different angles. The pictures are created by a computer linked to an x-ray machine.

Dysphagia—Difficulty in eating as a result of disruption in the swallowing process. Dysphagia can be a serious health threat because of the risk of aspiration pneumonia, malnutrition, dehydration, weight loss, and airway obstruction.

Esophagectomy—Surgical removal of the esophagus.

Esophagus—A long hollow muscular tube that connects the pharynx to the stomach.

Fine needle aspiration (FNA)—Technique that allows a biopsy of various bumps and lumps. It allows the

otolaryngologist to retrieve enough tissue for microscopic analysis and thus make an accurate diagnosis of a number of problems, such as inflammation or cancer.

Fistula—An abnormal passage or communication, usually between two internal organs or leading from an internal organ to the surface of the body.

Hypopharynx—The last part of the throat or the pharynx.

Laryngopharyngectomy—Surgical removal of both the larynx and the pharynx.

Laryngoscopy—The visualization of the larynx and vocal cords. This may be done directly with a fibreoptic scope (laryngoscope) or indirectly with mirrors.

Laryngectomy—Surgical removal of the larynx.

Larynx—Voice box.

Magnetic resonance imaging (MRI)—A procedure in which a magnet linked to a computer is used to create detailed pictures of areas inside the body.

Pharynx—The cavity at the back of the mouth. It is cone shaped and has an average length of about 3 in (76 mm) and is lined with mucous membrane. The pharynx opens into the esophagus at the lower end.

Tracheotomy—Opening of the trachea (windpipe) to the outside through a hole in the neck.

The anesthesiologist may elect to use an orotracheal (through the mouth and trachea) tube with anesthetic, which can be removed if a subsequent tracheotomy is planned.

Aftercare

After undergoing a pharyngectomy, special attention is given to the patient's pulmonary function and fluid/nutritional balance, as well as to local wound conditions in the neck, thorax, and abdomen. Regular postoperative checks of calcium, magnesium, and phosphorus levels are necessary; supplementation with calcium, magnesium, and 1,25-dihydroxycholecalciferol is usually required. A patient may be unable to take in enough food to maintain adequate nutrition and experience difficulty eating (dysphagia). Sometimes it may be necessary to have a feeding tube placed through the skin and muscle of the abdomen directly

into the stomach to provide extra nutrition. This procedure is called a **gastrostomy**.

Reconstructive surgery is also required to rebuild the throat after a pharyngectomy in order to help the patient with swallowing after the operation. Reconstructive surgeries represent a great challenge because of the complex properties of the tissues lining the throat and underlying muscle that are so vital to the proper functioning of this region. The primary goal is to re-establish the conduit connecting the oral cavity to the esophagus and thus retaining the continuity of the alimentary tract. Two main techniques are used:

- Myocutaneous flaps. Sometimes a muscle and area of skin may be rotated from an area close to the throat, such as the chest (pectoralis major flap), to reconstruct the throat.
- Free flaps. With the advances of microvascular surgery (sewing together small blood vessels under a microscope), surgeons have many more options to

WHO PERFORMS THE
PROCEDURE AND WHERE IS IT
PERFORMED?

A pharyngectomy is major surgery performed by a surgeon trained in otolaryngology. An anesthesiologist is responsible for administering anesthesia and the operation is performed in a hospital setting. Otolaryngology is the oldest medical specialty in the United States. Otolaryngologists are physicians trained in the medical and surgical management and treatment of patients with diseases and disorders of the ear, nose, throat (ENT), and related structures of the head and neck. They are commonly referred to as ENT physicians.

With cancer involved in pharyngectomy procedures, the otolaryngologist surgeon usually works with radiation and medical oncologists in a treatment team approach.

QUESTIONS TO ASK THE
DOCTOR

- How will the surgery affect my ability to swallow and to eat?
- What type of anesthesia will be used?
- How long will it take to recover from the surgery?
- When can I expect to return to work and/or resume normal activities?
- To what extent will my ability to speak be affected?
- What are the risks associated with a pharyngectomy?
- How many pharyngectomies do you perform in a year?

reconstruct the area of the throat affected by a pharyngectomy. Tissues from other areas of the patient's body such as a piece of intestine or a piece of arm muscle can be used to replace parts of the throat.

Risks

Potential risks associated with a pharyngectomy include those associated with any head and neck surgery, such as excessive bleeding, wound infection, wound slough, fistula (abnormal opening between organs or to the outside of the body), and, in rare cases, blood vessel rupture. Specifically, the surgery is associated with the following risks:

- Drain failure. Drains unable to hold a vacuum represent a serious threat to the surgical wound.
- Hematoma. Although rare, blood clot formation requires prompt intervention to avoid pressure separation of the pharyngeal repair and compression of the upper windpipe.
- Infection. A subcutaneous infection after total pharyngectomy is recognized by increasing redness and swelling of the skin flaps at the third to fifth postoperative day. Associated odor, fever, and elevated white blood cell count will occur.
- Pharyngocutaneous fistula. Patients with poor preoperative nutritional status are at significant risk for fistula development.
- Narrowing. More common at the lower, esophageal end of the pharyngeal reconstruction than in the

upper end, where the recipient lumen of the pharynx is wider.
- Functional swallowing problems. Dysphagia is also a risk which depends on the extent of the pharyngectomy.

Normal results

Oral intake is usually started on the seventh postoperative day, depending on whether the patient has had preoperative radiation therapy, in which case it may be delayed. Mechanical voice devices are sometimes useful in the early, post-operative phase, until the pharyngeal wall heals. Results are considered normal if there is no re-occurrence of the cancer at a later stage.

Morbidity and mortality rates

Smokers are at high risk of throat cancer. According to the Harvard Medical School, throat cancer also is associated closely with other cancers: 15% of throat-cancer patients also are diagnosed with cancer of the mouth, esophagus, or lung. Another 10–20% of throat-cancer patients develop these other cancers later. Other people at risk include those who drink a lot of alcohol, especially if they also smoke. Vitamin A deficiency and certain types of human papillomavirus (HPV) infection also have been associated with an increased risk of throat cancer.

Surgical treatment for hypopharyngeal carcinomas is difficult as most patients are diagnosed with advanced disease, and five-year disease specific survival is only 30%. Cure rates have been the highest with surgical resection followed by postoperative radiotherapy. Immediate reconstruction can be accomplished with regional and free tissue transfers. These techniques have greatly reduced morbidity, and allow most patients to successfully resume an oral diet.

Resources

BOOKS

Orlando, R. C., ed. *Esophagus and Pharynx.* London: Churchill Livingstone, 1997.

Pitman, K. T., J. L. Weissman, and J. T. Johnson. *The Parapharyngeal Space: Diagnosis and Management of Commonly Encountered Entities (Continuing Education Program (American Academy of Otolaryngology–Head and Neck Surgery Foundation).)* Alexandria, VA: American Academy of Otolaryngology, 1998.

Shin, L.M., L. M. Ross, and K. Bellenir, eds. *Ear, Nose, and Throat Disorders Sourcebook: Basic Information About Disorders of the Ears, Nose, Sinus Cavities, Pharynx, and Larynx Including Ear Infections, Tinnitus, Vestibular Disorders.* Holmes, PA: Omnigraphics Inc., 1998.

PERIODICALS

Chang, D. W., C. Hussussian, J. S. Lewin, et al. "Analysis of pharyngocutaneous fistula following free jejunal transfer for total laryngopharyngectomy." *Plastic and Reconstructive Surgery* 109 (April 2002): 1522–1527.

Ibrahim, H. Z., M. S. Moir, and W. W. Fee. "Nasopharyngectomy after failure of 2 courses of radiation therapy." *Archives of Otolaryngology - Head & Neck Surgery* 128 (October 2002): 1196–1197.

Iwai, H., H. Tsuji, T. Tachikawa, et al. "Neoglottic formation from posterior pharyngeal wall conserved in surgery for hypopharyngeal cancer." *Auris Nasus Larynx* 29 (April 2002): 153–157.

ORGANIZATIONS

American Academy of Otolaryngology. One Prince Street, Alexandria, VA 22314-3357. (703) 836-4444. http://www.entnet.org/

American Cancer Society (ACS). 1599 Clifton Rd. NE, Atlanta, GA 30329-4251. (800) 227-2345. http://www.cancer.org

OTHER

"Throat Cancer." Harvard Medical School. [cited May 31,2003] http://www.intelihealth.com/IH/ihtIH/WSIHW000/8987/29425/211361.html?d=dmtHealthAZ.

"Treatment of Laryngeal and Hypopharyngeal Cancers." American Cancer Society. [cited May 31, 2003]. http://www.cancer.org/docroot/CRI/content/CRI_2_2_4X_Treatment_of_laryngeal_and_hypopharyngeal_cancers_23.asp?sitearea=.

Monique Laberge, Ph.D.

Pharynx removal *see* **Pharyngectomy**

Phenobarbital *see* **Barbiturates**

Phlebectomy *see* **Vein ligation and stripping**

Phlebography

Definition

Phlebography is an x-ray test that provides an image of the leg veins after a contrast dye is injected into a vein in the patient's foot.

Purpose

Phlebography is primarily performed to diagnose deep vein thrombosis—a condition in which clots form in the veins of the leg. Pulmonary embolism can occur when those clots break off and travel to the lungs and pulmonary artery. Phlebography can also be used to evaluate congenital vein problems, assess the function of the deep leg vein valves, and identify a vein for arterial bypass grafting. **Ultrasound** has replaced phlebography in many cases; but phlebography is the "gold standard," or the best test by which others are judged, even though it is not used routinely.

Description

Phlebograph, (also called venography, ascending contrast phlebography, or contrast phlebography) is an invasive diagnostic test that provides a constant image of leg veins on a fluoroscope screen. Phlebography identifies the location and extent of blood clots, and enables the condition of the deep leg veins to be assessed. It is especially useful when there is a strong suspicion of deep vein thrombosis, after noninvasive tests have failed to identify the disease.

Phlebography is the most accurate test for detecting deep vein thrombosis. It is nearly 100% sensitive and specific in making this diagnosis. (Pulmonary embolism is diagnosed in other ways.) Accuracy is crucial since deep vein thrombosis can lead to pulmonary embolism, a potentially fatal condition.

Phlebography is not used often; however, because it is painful, expensive, time-consuming, exposes the patient to a fairly high dose of radiation, and can cause complications. In about 5% of cases, there are technical problems in conducting the test.

Phlebography takes 30–45 minutes, and can be done in a physician's office, a laboratory, or a hospital. During the procedure, the patient lies on a tilting x-ray table. The area where the catheter will be inserted is shaved, if necessary, and cleaned. In some cases, a local anesthetic is injected to numb the skin at the site of the insertion. A small incision may be required to make a point for insertion. The catheter is inserted and the contrast solution (or dye) is slowly

KEY TERMS

Contrast solution—A liquid dye injected into the body that allows structures, including veins, to be seen by x rays. Without the dye, the veins could not be seen on x rays.

Deep vein thrombosis—The development or presence of a blood clot in a vein deep within the leg. Deep vein thrombosis can lead to pulmonary embolism.

Invasive—A diagnostic test that invades healthy tissue; in the case of phlebography, through an incision in a healthy vein.

Pulmonary embolism—An obstruction of a blood vessel in the lungs, usually due to a blood clot that blocks a pulmonary artery. A pulmonary embolism can be very serious and in some cases is fatal.

injected. Injection of the dye causes a warm, flushing feeling in the leg that may spread through the body. The contrast solution may also cause slight nausea. Approximately 18% of patients experience discomfort from the contrast solution.

In order to fill the deep venous system with dye, a tight band (tourniquet) may be tied around the ankle or below the knee of the side into which the dye is injected, or the lower extremities may be tilted. The patient is asked to keep the leg still. The physician observes the movement of the solution through the vein with a fluoroscope. At the same time, a series of x rays is taken. When the test is finished, fluid is injected to clear the contrast from the veins, the catheter is removed, and a bandage is applied over the injection site.

Preparation

Fasting or drinking only clear liquids is necessary for four hours before the test, although the procedure may be done in an emergency even if the patient has eaten. The contrast solution contains iodine, to which some people are allergic. Patients should tell their physician if they have allergies or hay fever, or if they have had a reaction to a contrast solution.

Aftercare

Patients should drink large amounts of fluids to flush the remaining contrast solution from their bodies. The area around the incision will be sore for a few days. The physician should be notified if there is swelling, redness, pain, or fever. Pain medication is rarely needed. In most cases, the patient can resume normal activities the next day.

Risks

Phlebography can cause complications such as phlebitis, tissue damage, and the formation of deep vein thrombosis in a healthy leg. A rare side effect in up to 8% of cases is a severe allergic reaction to the dye. This usually happens within 30 minutes after injection of the dye, and requires medical attention.

Normal results

Normal phlebography results show proper blood flow through the leg veins.

Abnormal phlebography results show well-defined filling defects in veins. These findings confirm a diagnosis of deep vein thrombosis:

- blood clots
- consistent filling defects
- an abrupt end of a contrast column
- major deep veins that are unfilled
- dye flow that is diverted

Resources

BOOKS

Abeloff, MD et al. Clinical Oncology. 3rd ed. Philadelphia: Elsevier, 2004.

Grainger RG, et al. Grainger & Allison's Diagnostic Radiology: A Textbook of Medical Imaging. 4th ed. Philadelphia: Saunders, 2001.

Khatri, VP and JA Asensio. Operative Surgery Manual. 1st ed. Philadelphia: Saunders, 2003.

Mettler, FA. Essentials of Radiology. 2nd ed. Philadelphia: Saunders, 2005.

Townsend, CM et al. Sabiston Textbook of Surgery. 17th ed. Philadelphia: Saunders, 2004.

OTHER

"Lower-Limb Venography." Test Universe Website. 11 July 2001. http://www.testuniverse.com/mdx/MDX-2970.html.

Springhouse Corporation. "Catching Deep Vein Thrombosis in Time: Diagnostic Tests at a Glance." SpringNet. 2001. 11 July 2001. http://www.springnet.com/ce/p507bs4.htm.

Lee A. Shratter, M.D.
Lori De Milto
Stéphanie Islane Dionne

Phlebotomy

Definition

Phlebotomy is the act of drawing or removing blood from the circulatory system through a cut (incision) or puncture in order to obtain a sample for analysis and diagnosis. Phlebotomy is also done as part of the patient's treatment for certain blood disorders.

Purpose

Phlebotomy that is part of treatment (therapeutic phlebotomy) is performed to treat polycythemia vera, a condition that causes an elevated red blood cell volume (**hematocrit**). Phlebotomy is also prescribed for patients with disorders that increase the amount of iron in their blood to dangerous levels, such as hemochromatosis, hepatitis B, and hepatitis C. Patients with pulmonary edema may undergo phlebotomy procedures to decrease their total blood volume.

Phlebotomy is also used to remove blood from the body during **blood donation** and for analysis of the substances contained within it.

Description

Phlebotomy is performed by a nurse or a technician known as a phlebotomist. Blood is usually taken from a vein on the back of the hand or just below the elbow. Some blood tests, however, may require blood from an artery. The skin over the area is wiped with an antiseptic, and an elastic band is tied around the arm. The band acts as a tourniquet, retaining blood within the arm and making the veins more visible. The phlebotomy technician feels the veins in order to select an appropriate one. When a vein is selected, the technician inserts a needle

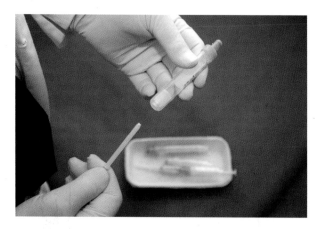

Preparing phlebotomy needles for withdrawal of blood samples. (*Pulse Picture Library/CMP Images/Phototake. Reproduced by Permission.*)

KEY TERMS

Finger stick—A technique for collecting a very small amount of blood from the fingertip area.

Hemochromatosis—A genetic disorder known as iron overload disease. Untreated hemochromatosis may cause osteoporosis, arthritis, cirrhosis, heart disease, or diabetes.

Thrombocytosis—A vascular condition characterized by high blood platelet counts.

Tourniquet—Any device that is used to compress a blood vessel to stop bleeding or as part of collecting a blood sample. Phlebotomists usually use an elastic band as a tourniquet.

into the vein and releases the elastic band. The appropriate amount of blood is drawn and the needle is withdrawn from the vein. The patient's pulse and blood pressure may be monitored during the procedure.

For some tests requiring very small amounts of blood for analysis, the technician uses a finger stick. A lance, or small needle, makes a small cut in the surface of the fingertip, and a small amount of blood is collected in a narrow glass tube. The fingertip may be squeezed to get additional blood to surface.

The amount of blood drawn depends on the purpose of the phlebotomy. Blood donors usually contribute a unit of blood (500 mL) in a session. The volume of blood needed for laboratory analysis varies widely with the type of test being conducted. Typically one or several small (5–10 mL) tubes are drawn. Therapeutic phlebotomy removes a larger amount of blood than donation and blood analysis require. Phlebotomy for treatment of hemochromatosis typically involves removing a unit of blood—250 mg of iron—once a week. Phlebotomy sessions are required until iron levels return to a consistently normal level, which may take several months to several years. Phlebotomy for polycythemia vera removes enough blood to keep the patient's hematocrit (proportion of red blood cells) below 45%. The frequency and duration of sessions depends on the patient's individual needs.

Diagnosis/Preparation

Patients having their blood drawn for analysis may be asked to discontinue medications or to avoid food (to fast) for a period of time before the blood test. Patients donating blood will be asked for a brief medical history, have their blood pressure taken, and have their hematocrit checked with a finger stick test prior to donation.

WHO PERFORMS THE
PROCEDURE AND WHERE IS IT
PERFORMED?

Phlebotomy is usually performed by a phlebotomy technician. Arterial collection may be performed by a physician. Collection occurs in the hospital or outpatient clinic.

Aftercare

After blood is drawn and the needle is removed, pressure is placed on the puncture site with a cotton ball to stop bleeding, and a bandage is applied. It is not uncommon for a patient to feel dizzy or nauseated during or after phlebotomy. The patient may be encouraged to rest for a short period once the procedure is completed. Patients are also instructed to drink plenty of fluids and eat regularly over the next 24 hours to replace lost blood volume. Patients who experience swelling of the puncture site or continued bleeding after phlebotomy should seek immediate medical treatment.

Risks

Most patients will have a small bruise or mild soreness at the puncture site for several days. Therapeutic phlebotomy may cause thrombocytosis and chronic iron deficiency (anemia) in some patients. As with any invasive procedure, infection is also a risk. This risk is minimized by the use of prepackaged sterilized equipment and careful attention to proper technique. There is no risk of HIV infection from phlebotomy, since all needles are disposed of after a single use. Arterial blood collection carries a higher risk than venous collection, and is performed by a physician or other specially trained professional. Patients who are anemic or have a history of cardiovascular disease may not be good candidates for phlebotomy.

Normal results

Normal results include obtaining the needed amount of blood with the minimum of discomfort to the patient.

Morbidity and mortality rates

Properly performed, phlebotomy does not carry the risk of mortality. It may cause temporary pain and bleeding, but these are usually easily managed.

Alternatives

Phlebotomy is a necessary medical procedure, and is required for a wide variety of other procedures.

QUESTIONS TO ASK THE
DOCTOR

• How many tubes of blood will you withdraw?

Resources

BOOKS

Hoffman R. et al. Hematology: Basic Principles and Practice. 4th ed. Philadelphia: Elsevier, 2005.
McPherson RA et al. Henry's Clinical Diagnosis and Management By Laboratory Methods. 21st ed. Philadelphia: Saunders, 2007.

Paula Anne Ford-Martin
Richard Robinson
Rosalyn Carson-DeWitt, MD

Photocoagulation therapy

Definition

Photocoagulation therapy is a method of treating detachments (tears) of the retina (the layer of light-sensitive cells at the back of the eye) with an argon laser. The high-intensity beam of light from the laser is converted into heat, which forces protein molecules in the affected tissue to condense and seal the tear.

Purpose

The purpose of photocoagulation therapy is to reattach a torn or detached portion of the retina and/or prevent further growth of abnormal blood vessels in the retina that can cause a detachment.

Demographics

The incidence of RD in the United States is about 0.3%, or one in 15,000 people.

The most common risk factors associated with RD are extreme nearsightedness (5% risk); cataract removal without lens implantation (2%); and cataract removal with loss of the vitreous body during surgery (10%). It is estimated that 15% of people with RD in one eye will eventually develop it in the other eye.

Males account for 60% and females for 40% of patients with RD below the age of 45. Above age 45, there is no significant gender difference.

With regard to racial or ethnic background, the incidence of RD is higher among Jews in the United

Choroid—The middle of the three tunicae or coats that surround the eyeball; the choroid lies between the retina and the sclera.

Coats' disease—A chronic and progressive disorder of the retina marked by exudative RD. It is named for George Coats (1876-1915), a British ophthalmologist. It occurs most frequently in preadolescent boys and young adults.

Cornea—The transparent front portion of the exterior cover of the eye.

Cryopexy—Reattachment of a detached retina by freezing the tissue behind the tear with nitrous oxide.

Diabetic retinopathy—Degeneration of the retina related to diabetes; both type 1 and type 2 diabetes can lead to diabetic retinopathy.

Eales disease—A disorder marked by recurrent hemorrhages into the retina and vitreous body. It occurs most often in males between the ages of 10 and 25.

Exudative RD—A type of retinal detachment caused by the accumulation of tissue fluid underneath the retina.

Floaters—Spots seen in front of the eyes, caused by clumping of the collagen fibers in the vitreous body.

Laser—A device that produces high-intensity, narrowly focused monochromatic light by exciting atoms and causing them to give off their energy in phase.

Laser in situ keratomileusis (LASIK)—A procedure in which the shape of the cornea is changed with an excimer laser in order to correct the patient's vision.

Macula—A small, yellowish depressed area on the retina that absorbs the shorter wave lengths of visible light and is responsible for fine detailed vision.

Marfan's syndrome—A hereditary disorder that affects the connective tissues of the body, the lens of the eye, and the cardiovascular system.

Ophthalmology—The branch of medicine that deals with the diagnosis and treatment of eye disorders.

Optometrist—A primary health care provider who examines eyes and diagnoses disorders of the eye as well as prescribing eyeglasses, contact lenses, and other vision aids.

Pneumatic retinopexy—Reattachment of a detached retina using an injected gas bubble to hold the retina against the back of the eye.

Pupil—The opening in the center of the iris of the eye that allows light to enter the eye.

Retina—The innermost of three layers of tissue surrounding the human eyeball. The retina surrounds the vitreous body and joins the optic nerve at the back of the eye.

Retinal detachment (RD)—A condition in which the inner layers of cells in the retina separate from the underlying pigmented layers of cells called the choroid.

Retinopathy of prematurity (ROP)—A disorder that occurs in premature infants in which blood vessels in the eye continue to grow in an abnormal pattern after delivery. It can lead to retinal detachment and blindness. ROP is also known as retrolental fibroplasia.

Sclera—The tough white outer tunica or coat of the eyeball.

Tunica (plural, tunicae)—The medical term for a membrane or piece of tissue that covers or lines a body part. The retina is the innermost of three tunicae that surround the eyeball.

Vitrectomy—Surgical removal of the vitreous body.

Vitreous body—The transparent gel that fills the inner portion of the eyeball between the lens and the retina. It is also called the vitreous humor or crystalline humor.

States than in the general population; the incidence of RD among African Americans is lower than average.

Description

Structure of the human eye

To fully understand how photocoagulation therapy works, it is helpful to have a basic picture of the structure of the human eye. The retina is the innermost tunica, or covering, of the posterior part of the eyeball. It is made of several layers of cells, one of which contains the rod and cone cells that are sensitive to light. Behind the retina are the other two tunicae of the eye, the choroid and the sclera. The sclera is a tough white layer of tissue that covers the exterior of the eyeball. At the front of the eye, the sclera is continuous with a transparent area of tissue known as the cornea.

At the back of the eye, the retina is continuous with the optic nerve. The macula, which is a yellowish oval-shaped area that is the central point of vision, lies in the center of the retina. In front of the retina is the vitreous body, which is also known as the vitreous humor, or simply the vitreous. The vitreous body is a clear gel that consists primarily of water and collagen fibers.

Types of retinal detachment (RD)

RHEGMATOGENOUS. A rhegmatogenous RD is the most common of the three types of retinal detachment. The word rhegmatogenous comes from a Greek word that means "tear." A rhegmatogenous RD typically occurs in older people. As the vitreous body in the center of the eyeball ages, it shrinks and pulls away from the retina. This separation is called a posterior vitreous detachment (PVD). A PVD is not the same thing as a retinal detachment, although it may slightly increase the risk of an RD. In places where the retina is still attached to the vitreous body, a small hole or tear can develop. Over time, fluid can seep into the area around the hole or tear and thus enlarge the area of detached tissue.

TRACTION. Traction RDs are most often found in adults with diabetic retinopathy or infants with retinopathy of prematurity (ROP). Diabetic retinopathy is a disorder that develops when the patient's diabetes affects the small blood vessels in the eye. Although diabetic retinopathy is more severe in patients with type 1 diabetes (insulin-dependent), it can also occur in patients with type 2. Retinal detachment is most likely to occur in a subtype of the disorder known as proliferative diabetic retinopathy. The term proliferative refers to the abnormal growth of new blood vessels along the surface of the vitreous body. These new blood vessels can bleed into the vitreous body and form scar tissue that pulls on the retina. Eventually, the scar tissue can exert enough pulling force to cause a retinal detachment.

In ROP, a traction RD can develop because premature birth interrupts the normal development of the blood vessels in the baby's eyes. After the baby is born, some of these blood vessels grow along the retina, bleed into the vitreous body, and form scar tissue similar to that found in diabetic retinopathy. Retinal detachment in ROP can be treated with photocoagulation.

EXUDATIVE. Exudative RDs occur when tissue fluid builds up in the space between the retina and the choroid underneath it. If enough fluid leaks into this space, it can push the retina away from the choroid and cause it to detach. Exudative RDs are associated with certain inflammatory disorders of the eye; tumors, including melanoma (cancer) of the choroid; and a congenital disorder known as Coats' disease, which affects the growth of the blood vessels in the retina.

Risk factors for retinal detachment

Retinal detachment is associated with a number of different factors and conditions, including:

- extreme nearsightedness
- genetic factors (retinal detachment tends to run in families)
- premature birth (the risk of ROP is highest in premature infants weighing less than 2.2 lb [1 kg] at birth)
- type 1 or type 2 diabetes
- cataract surgery
- sickle cell disease
- Coats' disease
- Eales' disease
- Marfan's syndrome
- breast cancer or melanoma
- leukemia
- history of previous retinal detachment
- age (Retinal detachment is most common in people between the ages of 40 and 70.)
- traumatic injury to the eye
- laser in-situ keratomileusis surgery (LASIK, a procedure done to correct vision and eliminate the need for glasses or contact lenses)

Photocoagulation therapy for retinal detachment is usually performed with an argon laser. A laser is a device that produces high-intensity, narrowly focused monochromatic light by exciting atoms and causing them to give off their energy in phases. The word laser comes from "light amplification by stimulated emission of radiation." An argon laser uses ionized argon to generate its light, which is in the blue-green portion of the visible light spectrum.

In a laser photocoagulation treatment, the patient is asked to sit in front of the instrument. After applying anesthetic eye drops, the ophthalmologist places a contact lens on the patient's eye and focuses the laser beam through it. He or she operates the laser by foot. The patient may see a brief burst of blue-green light. When the laser beam reaches the retina at the back of the eye, its light is absorbed by the pigment in the cells and converted to heat, which seals the edge of the retinal detachment against the underlying choroid. The procedure is short, taking about 10–30 minutes.

Diagnosis/Preparation

Diagnosis

The diagnosis of retinal detachment requires direct examination of the eye as well as taking the patient's medical history. The diagnosis may be made in some cases by an optometrist, who is a health professional qualified to examine the eye for diseases and disorders as well as taking measurements for corrective lenses. If the symptoms of RD appear suddenly, however, the patient is more likely to be diagnosed by an ophthalmologist, who is a physician specializing in treating disorders of the eye.

PATIENT HISTORY. Retinal detachment is not usually painful, and the patient's eye will look normal from the outside. In almost all cases, a patient with RD consults a doctor because he or she is having one or more of the following visual disturbances:

- blurring of vision that is not helped by blinking the eye
- a gray or black curtain or shade coming across the field of vision from one direction
- floaters, which appear as moving black spots in front of the eye (The sudden appearance of a large group, or "shower," of floaters is a serious symptom of RD.)
- flashes of light
- objects appearing wavy or distorted in shape
- blind spot in the visual field

The visual symptoms of retinal detachment may develop either gradually or suddenly. In a very small number of cases, a sudden retinal detachment may cause complete loss of vision in the affected eye.

Patients who have gone to a primary care physician or emergency room for these visual symptoms are referred to an ophthalmologist. Many ophthalmologists will give patients a piece of paper with a circle on it and ask them to draw what they are seeing on the circle in the area corresponding to the part of their visual field that is affected. In some cases, the location of the spots, light flashes, or shadows that a patient sees is a clue to the part of the retina that is detached.

The ophthalmologist will take a patient history, asking about a family history of eye disorders; previous diseases or disorders of the eye; other diseases or disorders that the patient may have, particularly diabetes or sickle cell disease; and a history of head trauma, direct blows to the eye, or surgical removal of a foreign body from the eye. If the patient suffered a head or eye injury within the past six months, the ophthalmologist will ask whether the visual disturbances started at the time of the injury or several months later.

EYE EXAMINATION. After taking the history, the ophthalmologist will examine the eye itself. This examination has several parts, including:

- A test of visual clarity or sharpness. This test is the same one used by an optometrist when fitting a patient for glasses or contact lenses.
- An external check for bleeding or any other signs of trauma to the eye.

- A test that measures the response of the pupil of the eye to changes in light intensity. One sign of RD is a difference in the pupillary reaction between the affected eye and the normal one. The pupil will not contract as far as it normally does when the doctor shines a light into the affected eye.
- A test that measures the amount of fluid pressure inside each eyeball. In RD, the affected eye typically has a lower pressure measurement than the other eye.
- Examination of the eye with a slit lamp, which is an instrument with a high-intensity light source that can be focused as a thin sliver of light. The examiner uses the slit lamp together with a binocular ophthalmoscope (an instrument that looks like a microscope with two eyepieces) in order to check first the front and then the back of the eye for any abnormalities. To check the front part, the doctor will touch the side of the eye with a strip of paper containing an orange dye. The dye stains the film of tear fluid on the outer surface of the eye, making it easier to see the structures in the front of the eye. Patients with RD usually have normal results for this part of the slit-lamp examination. In the second part, the doctor puts some drops in the patient's eye to make the pupil dilate. This procedure allows him or her to see the structures in the back of the eye. If the patient has RD, the doctor may see the retina lifted upward or forward, possibly moving back and forth. The retina will have a grayish color with darker blood vessels visible. It may have a pitted surface resembling an orange peel, and there may also be a line visible at the edge of the detachment.

LABORATORY AND IMAGING STUDIES. Today, there are no laboratory tests for retinal detachment. **Ultrasound**, however, can be used to diagnose retinal detachment if the doctor cannot see the retina with a slit lamp because of cataracts or blood seeping into the vitreous body. If the RD is exudative, ultrasound can be used to detect a tumor or hemorrhage underneath the retina.

Preparation

Treatment of RD follows as soon as possible after the diagnosis; however, an immediate procedure is not usually necessary since the time frame for treatment of a detached retina is several hours rather than only a few minutes.

If the patient has suffered a traumatic injury to the eye, the eye may be covered with a protective shield prior to treatment.

Preparation for photocoagulation therapy consists of eye drops that dilate the pupil of the eye and numb the eye itself. The laser treatment is painless, although some patients require additional anesthetic for sensitivity to the laser light.

Aftercare

Patients who have had photocoagulation therapy for retinal detachment are asked to have a friend or family member drive them home. The reason for this precaution is that the eye medication used to dilate the pupil of the patient's eye before the procedure takes several hours to wear off. During this period, the eye is unusually sensitive to light. The patient can go to work the next day with no restrictions on activity.

Risks

The most common risks of laser photocoagulation therapy are mild discomfort at the beginning of the procedure and the possibility that a second laser treatment will be needed to reattach the retina securely.

Normal results

Over 90% of retinal detachments can be repaired with prompt treatment, although sometimes a second procedure is needed. About 40% of patients treated for retinal detachment will have good vision within six months of surgery. The results are less favorable if the retina has been detached for a long time or if there is a large growth of fibrous tissue that has caused a traction detachment. These patients, however, will still have some degree of reading or traveling vision after the retina has been reattached. In a very small minority of patients, the surgeon cannot reattach the retina because of extensive growths of fibrous scar tissue on it.

Morbidity and mortality rates

The mortality rate for laser photocoagulation treatment of retinal detachment is extremely low; morbidity depends to a large extent on the cause of the RD. A study done in 2001 reported that laser therapy for rhegmatogenous RDs is as effective as pneumatic retinopexy or **scleral buckling**, but has the advantage of fewer complications after the procedure. In the treatment of ROP, laser photocoagulation has been found to be more effective than cryopexy in reducing the infant's risk of nearsightedness in later life.

Alternatives

Alternatives to laser photocoagulation as a treatment for RD depend on the location and size of the retinal detachment. Photocoagulation treatment works best on small tears in the retina. One alternative

WHO PERFORMS THE PROCEDURE AND WHERE IS IT PERFORMED?

Laser treatment of retinal detachment is performed by an ophthalmologist, who has specialized in the medical and surgical treatment of eye disorders. Ophthalmology is one of 24 specialties recognized by the American Board of Medical Specialties.

Photocoagulation therapy for retinal detachment is done as an outpatient procedure, either in the ophthalmologist's office or in an ambulatory surgery center.

for the treatment of small areas of detachment is cryopexy, which is performed as an outpatient procedure under **local anesthesia**. In cryopexy, the ophthalmologist uses nitrous oxide to freeze the tissue underneath the retinal tear. This procedure leads to the formation of scar tissue that seals the edges of the tear in place.

Pneumatic retinopexy is a procedure that can be used if the RD is located in the upper part of the eye. After numbing the patient's eye with a local anesthetic, the ophthalmologist injects a small bubble of gas into the vitreous body. The gas bubble rises and presses the torn part of the retina back against the underlying choroid. The bubble is slowly absorbed over the next two weeks. The ophthalmologist then uses either photocoagulation or cryopexy to complete the reattachment of the retina.

If the RD is large, the doctor may decide to perform a scleral buckle treatment or a vitrectomy. These procedures are more invasive than laser photocoagulation or cryopexy; however, they are still usually done as outpatient procedures. In a scleral buckle procedure, the doctor attaches a tiny silicon band to the sclera. The buckle, which remains in the eye permanently, puts pressure on the retina to hold it in place.

In a vitrectomy, the ophthalmologist removes the vitreous body and replaces it with air or a saline solution that puts pressure on the retina to hold it in place. Vitrectomies are usually performed if there is a very large tear in the retina; if the macula is involved; or if blood that has leaked into the vitreous body is interfering with diagnosis or treatment.

Resources

BOOKS

Marx, John A., et al. Rosen's Emergency Medicine. 6th ed. St. Louis, MO: Mosby, Inc., 2006.
Yanoff, M et al. Ophthalmology. 2nd ed. St. Louis: Mosby, 2004.

QUESTIONS TO ASK THE DOCTOR

- What are my chances of having normal vision after the laser therapy?
- What is the likelihood of my needing another laser treatment?
- Am I likely to develop retinal detachment in my other eye?
- How often should I schedule preventive eye examinations from now on?

PERIODICALS

Arevalo, J. Fernando, et al. "Retinal Detachment in Myopic Eyes after Laser in situ Keratomileusis." Journal of Refractive Surgery, 18 (November–December 2002): 708–714.

Dellone-Larkin, Gregory, and Cecilia A. Dellone. "Retinal Detachment." eMedicine, August 10, 2001 [March 21, 2003]. www.emedicine.com/emerg/topic504.htm.

El-Asrar, A. M., and S. A. Al-Kharashi. "Full Panretinal Photocoagulation and Early Vitrectomy Improve Prognosis of Retinal Vasculitis Associated with Tuberculoprotein Hypersensitivity (Eales' Disease)." British Journal of Ophthalmology, 86 (November 2002): 1248–1251.

Foroozan, R., B. P. Conolly, and W. S. Tasman. "Outcomes after Laser Therapy for Threshold Retinopathy of Prematurity." Ophthalmology, 108 (September 2001): 1644–1646.

Greenberg, P. B., and C. R. Baumal. "Laser Therapy for Rhegmatogenous Retinal Detachment." Current Opinion in Ophthalmology, 12 (June 2001): 171–174.

Lee, E. S., H. J. Koh, O. W. Kwon, and S. C. Lee. "Laser Photocoagulation Repair of Recurrent Macula-Sparing Retinal Detachments." Yonsei Medical Journal, 43 (August 2002): 446–450.

Vakili, Roya, Shachar Tauber, and Edward S. Lim. "Successful Management of Retinal Tear Post-Laser in situ Keratomileusis Retreatment." Yale Journal of Biology and Medicine, 75 (2002): 55–57.

van Meurs, J. C., et al. "Postoperative Laser Coagulation as Retinopexy in Patients with Rhegmatogenous Retinal Detachment Treated with Scleral Buckling Surgery: A Prospective Clinical Study." Retina, 22 (December 2002): 733–739.

Wu, Lihteh, and Carlos Cabezas. "Retinal Detachment, Exudative." eMedicine, June 28, 2001 [March 24, 2003]. www.emedicine.com/OPH/topic407.htm.

ORGANIZATIONS

American Academy of Ophthalmology. P. O. Box 7424, San Francisco, CA 94120-7424. (415) 561-8500. www.aao.org.

American Optometric Association. 243 North Lindbergh Blvd., St. Louis, MO 63141. (314) 991-4100. www.aoanet.org.

Canadian Ophthalmological Society (COS). 610-1525 Carling Avenue, Ottawa ON K1Z 8R9 Canada. www.eyesite.ca.

Diabetic Retinopathy Foundation. 350 North LaSalle, Suite 800, Chicago, IL 60610. www.retinopathy.org.

Wills Eye Hospital. 840 Walnut Street, Philadelphia, PA 19107. (215) 928-3000. www.willseye.org.

Rebecca Frey, PhD

Photorefractive keratectomy (PRK)

Definition

Photorefractive keratectomy (PRK) is a noninvasive refractive surgery in which the surgeon uses an excimer laser to reshape the cornea of the eye by removing the epithelium, the gel-like outer layer of the cornea.

Purpose

PRK, one of the first (and once the most popular) refractive surgeries, eliminates or reduces moderate nearsightedness (myopia), hyperopia (farsightedness), and astigmatism; it is most commonly used to treat myopia. Successfully treated PRK patients no longer require corrective lenses, and those who do still require correction, require much less.

PRK is an elective, **outpatient surgery**, and people choose the treatment for different reasons. Some simply no longer want to wear eyeglasses for cosmetic reasons. Sports enthusiasts may find eyeglasses or contact lenses troublesome during physical activities. Others may experience pain or dryness while wearing contact lenses, or have corneal ulcers that make wearing contact lenses painful. Firefighters and police officers may have trouble seeing in emergency situations when their contact lenses get dry or their eyeglasses fog up.

Demographics

There is no such thing as a typical PRK patient. Because it is an **elective surgery**, patients come from every age group and income bracket. PRK candidates, however, must be 18 or older; have myopia, hyperopia, or astigmatism; and have had stable vision for at least two years. While PRK is experiencing a slight resurgence in popularity, it lags behind the newer and less painful **laser in-situ keratomileusis (LASIK)**. The American Academy of Ophthalmology (AAO) estimates that 95% of all refractive surgeries are **LASIK**.

KEY TERMS

Ablation—The vaporization of eye tissue.

Astigmatism—Asymmetric vision defects due to irregularities in the cornea.

Cornea—The clear, curved tissue layer in front of the eye. It lies in front of the colored part of the eye (iris) and the black hole in the center of the iris (pupil).

Corneal topography—Mapping the cornea's surface with a specialized computer that illustrates corneal elevations.

Dry eye—Corneal dryness due to insufficient tear production.

Enhancement—A secondary refractive procedure performed in an attempt to achieve better visual acuity.

Excimer laser—An instrument that is used to vaporize tissue with a cold, coherent beam of light with a single wavelength in the ultraviolet range.

Hyperopia—The inability to see near objects as clearly as distant objects, and the need for accommodation to see objects clearly.

Myopia—A vision problem in which distant objects appear blurry. People who are myopic or near-sighted can usually see near objects clearly, but not far objects.

Presbyopia—A condition affecting people over the age of 40 in which the focusing of near objects fails to work because of age-related hardening of the lens of the eye.

The first PRK patients are sometimes referred to as "early adopters." These are people who are always interested in the latest technology and have the financial resources to take advantage of it. In the mid-1990s when PRK was first approved, patients were in their early 30s to mid-40s and financially stable. Prices have now stabilized at about $1,800 per eye for PRK.

While it has lost favor with the general public, PRK is the choice of the United States military. Military doctors prefer PRK over LASIK because the latter involves cutting a flap that doctors fear may loosen and become unhinged during combat.

Description

PRK was first performed in the 1980s and widely used in Europe and Canada in the early 1990s, but was not approved in the United States until 1995. PRK was the most popular refractive procedure until the creation of LASIK, which has a much shorter recovery time. PRK is still the preferred option for patients with thin corneas, corneal dystrophies, corneal scars, or recurrent corneal erosion.

PRK takes about 10 minutes to perform. Immediately before the procedure, the ophthalmologist may request corneal topography (a corneal map) to compare with previous maps to ensure the treatment plan is still correct. Ophthalmic personnel will perform a refraction to make sure the refractive correction the surgeon will program into the excimer laser is correct.

Patients may be given a sedative such as Valium to relax them before the surgery. Anesthetic drops will be applied to numb the eye and prevent pain during the procedure.

After the eye drops are inserted, the surgeon prepares the treated eye for surgery. If both eyes are being treated on the same day, the non-treated eye is patched. The surgeon inserts a speculum in the first eye to be treated to hold the eyelids apart and prevent movement. The patient stares at the blinking light of a laser microscope and must fixate his or her gaze on that light. The patient must remain still.

The surgeon double-checks the laser settings to make sure they are programmed correctly for the refractive error. With everything in place, the eye surgeon removes the surface corneal cells (epithelium) with a sponge, mechanical blade, or the excimer laser. With the epithelium completely removed, the surgeon will begin reshaping, or ablating, the cornea. This takes 15–45 seconds, and varies for refractive error; the stronger the error, the longer the ablation. Patients may worry that moving could cause irreversible eye damage, but they should know that, at the slightest movement, the doctor immediately stops the laser. When the ablation is completed, the surgeon places a bandage contact lens on the treated eye to protect it and allow the healing process to take place; it also eases some of the pain of the exposed cornea. The surgeon will also dispense anti-inflammatory and antibiotic eye drops to stop infection and reduce pain.

Diagnosis/Preparation

Patients should have a complete eye evaluation and medical history taken before surgery. Soft contact lens wearers should stop wearing their lenses at least one week before the initial exam. Gas-permeable lens wearers should not wear their lenses from three weeks to a month before the exam. Contact lens wear alters the cornea's shape, which should be allowed to return to its natural shape before the exam.

Patients should also disclose current medications. Allergy medications and birth control pills have been known to cause haze after surgery. Physicians will want to examine the potential risks involved with these medications.

Patients who have these conditions/history should not have the procedure, including:

- pregnant women or women who are breastfeeding
- patients with very small or very large refractive errors
- patients with scarred corneas or macular disease
- people with autoimmune diseases
- diabetics
- glaucoma patients
- patients with persistent blepharitis

Physicians will perform a baseline eye evaluation, including a manifest and cycloplegic refraction, measurement of intraocular pressure (to determine if the patient has glaucoma), slit-lamp biomicroscopy, tear film evaluation, corneal topography, evaluation of corneal thickness, dilated fundus examination, and measurement of scotopic pupil size.

If the patient is an appropriate candidate, he or she must sign an **informed consent** form that states he or she is aware of possible complications and outcomes of the procedure.

Presurgery preparations

The patient is advised to discontinue contact lens wear immediately and refrain from using creams, lotions, makeup, or perfume for at least two days before surgery. Patients may also be asked to scrub their eyelashes for a period of time to remove any debris.

Aftercare

Patients usually have follow-up appointments at 24 hours, four days, one week, one month, three months, six months, and then annually following PRK. More frequent visits may be necessary, if there are complications.

Patients should refrain from strenuous activity for at least one month after surgery. Creams, lotions, and makeup must also be avoided for at least two weeks.

The bandage contact lens is removed by the surgeon usually after four days (during the second visit). Patients must be diligent in using antibiotic drops and steroid drops. Because the epithelium is completely removed, there is a greater chance of infection and pain; the eye drops are needed to minimize these possible complications. The eye drops must be used for at least four months for some patients. The slow healing process is imperative to keeping the desired correction.

PRK has a long recovery rate, which is why LASIK gained popularity so quickly. Unlike LASIK, in which patients notice improved vision immediately and are back to normal routines the next day, PRK patients are advised to rest for at least two days. PRK patients also experience moderate pain the first few days of recovery, and may need pain relievers such as Demerol to ease the pain. Vision also fluctuates the first few weeks of recovery as the epithelium grows back. This can cause haze, and patients become concerned that the surgery was unsuccessful. PRK patients need to be aware that vision can fluctuate for as long as up to six months after surgery. Incorrect use of eye drops can cause regression.

Risks

PRK patients may experience glare, vision fluctuation, development of irregular astigmatism, vision distortion (even with corrective lenses), glaucoma, loss of best visual acuity, and, though extremely rare, total vision loss.

A more common side effect is long-term haze. Some patients who have aggressive healing processes can form corneal scars that can cause haze. With proper screening for this condition and with the use of eye drops, this risk can be lessened.

Complications associated with LASIK, such as photophobia, haloes, and dry eye, are not as common with PRK. However, The patient may be under-corrected or overcorrected, and enhancements might be needed to attain the best visual acuity.

Normal results

Most PRK patients achieve 20/40 vision, which means in most states they can legally drive a car without vision correction. Some patients will still need corrective lenses, but the lenses will not need to be as powerful.

There have been reports of regression after the PRK healing process is completed. Sometimes a patient will require an enhancement, and the surgeon must repeat the surgery. Patients should also be aware that with the onset of presbyopia after age 40, they will probably require vision correction for reading or close work.

Morbidity and mortality rates

Information about PRK mortality and morbidity is limited because the procedure is elective. Complications that can lead to more serious conditions, such as

WHO PERFORMS THE PROCEDURE AND WHERE IS IT PERFORMED?

An ophthalmologist performs PRK with the aid of ophthalmic technicians and nurses. The surgeon may have received specific refractive surgery training in medical school, but because it is a relatively new procedure, older surgeons may not have completed such training. Instead, these surgeons may have completed continuing medical education courses or may have had training provided by the laser companies.

Preparation and aftercare may be handled by an optometrist who works with the ophthalmologist on these cases. The optometrist usually establishes eligibility for PRK, and may also perform much of the follow-up, with the exception of the first post-PRK visit.

Hospitals are one setting for this surgery, but the most common location is an ambulatory surgery center or surgery suite. Surgeons at surgery centers owned by refractive surgery companies also perform PRK. These businesses hire support staff, optometrists and surgeons in a stand-alone surgery center or in a hospital.

infection, are treated with **topical antibiotics**. There is also a chance the patient could have a severe reaction to the **antibiotics** or steroids used in the healing process.

Alternatives

Because these patients only have mild to moderate myopia, hyperopia, or astigmatism, they can choose from most refractive surgeries and non-surgical procedures.

Surgical alternatives

- Laser in-situ keratomileusis (LASIK). The most popular refractive surgery, it is similar to PRK, but differs in how it reshapes the cornea. Instead of completely removing tissue, LASIK leaves a "flap" of tissue that the surgeon moves back into place after ablation. LASIK is less painful with a shorter recovery time. However, there are more complications associated with LASIK.
- Radial keratotomy (RK). RK was the first widely used surgical correction for mild to moderate

QUESTIONS TO ASK THE DOCTOR

- Why do you believe that PRK is the correct refractive surgery for me?
- How many PRK procedures have you performed?
- Is PRK your preferred procedure?
- How well will I see after the surgery?
- How many of your patients experience serious complications?
- Who will treat complications, if any, after the procedure?
- How long with the recovery process take? Do I need to limit my activities?

myopia. The surgeon alters the shape of the cornea without a laser. This is one of the oldest refractive procedures, and has proved successful on lower and moderate corrections.

- Astigmatic keratotomy (AK). AK is a variation of RK used to treat mild to moderate astigmatism. AK has proved successful if the errors are mild to moderate.

Non-surgical alternatives

Contact lenses and eyeglasses also can correct refractive errors. Improvements in contact lenses have made them easier to wear, and continuous-wear contact lenses, which a patient can sleep in for as long as 30 days, can provide a similar effect to PRK. A customized rigid gas-permeable contact lens is used for orthokeratology (Ortho-K), in which a patient wears the lens for a predetermined amount of time to reshape the cornea. After removing the lens, the patient's vision is improved and remains improved until the cornea returns to its natural shape. At that time, the patient repeats the process.

Resources

BOOKS

Yanoff, M., et al. *Ophthalmology.* 2nd ed. St. Louis: Mosby, 2004.

ORGANIZATIONS

American Academy of Ophthalmology. P.O. Box 7424, San Francisco, CA 94120-7424. (415) 561-8500. www.aao.org.

American Society of Cataract and Refractive Surgery. 4000 Legato Road, Suite 850, Fairfax, VA 22033-4055. (703) 591-2220. E-mail: ascrs@ascrs.org. www.ascrs.org.

Council for Refractive Surgery Quality Assurance. 8543
Everglade Drive, Sacramento, CA 95826-0769. (916)
381-0769. E-mail: info@usaeyes.org. www.usaeyes.org.

OTHER

Bethke, Walt. "Surface Procedures: The State of the Art."
Review of Ophthalmology, February 2003. http://www.
revophth.com/index.asp?page=1_283.htm (accessed
July 3, 2008).

Sabar, Ariel. "Laser Gives Kids Vision to Fly." The Baltimore Sun. February 27, 2003 [cited March 16, 2003].
www.sunspot.net/features/health/bal-te.ar.laser27
feb27,0,3705843.story?coll = bal-home-headlines.

Segre, Liz. "PRK: The Original Laser Eye Surgery." All
About Vision. www.allaboutvision.com/visionsurgery/
prk.htm (accessed July 3, 2008).

Mary Bekker

Physical examination

Definition

A physical examination is an evaluation of the
body and its functions using inspection, palpation
(feeling with the hands), percussion (tapping with the
fingers), and auscultation (listening). A complete
health assessment also includes gathering information
about a person's medical history and lifestyle, doing
laboratory tests, and screening for disease.

Purpose

The annual physical examination has been replaced
by the periodic health examination. How often this is
done depends on the patient's age, sex, and risk factors
for disease. The United States Preventative Services
Task Force (USPSTF) has developed guidelines for
preventative health examinations that health care professionals widely follow. Organizations that promote
detection and prevention of specific diseases, like the
American Cancer Society, generally recommend more
intensive or frequent examinations.

A comprehensive physical examination provides
an opportunity for the healthcare professional to
obtain baseline information about the patient for
future use, and to establish a relationship before problems happen. It provides an opportunity to answer
questions and teach good health practices. Detecting
a problem in its early stages can have good long-term
results.

Precautions

The patient should be comfortable and treated
with respect throughout the examination. As the examination proceeds, the examiner should explain what he
or she is doing and share any relevant findings.

Description

A complete physical examination usually starts at
the head and proceeds all the way to the toes. However, the exact procedure will vary according to the
needs of the patient and the preferences of the examiner. An average examination takes about 30 minutes.
The cost of the examination will depend on the charge
for the professional's time and any tests that are done.
Most health plans cover routine physical examinations including some tests.

The examination

First, the examiner will observe the patient's
appearance, general health, and behavior, along with
measuring height and weight. The vital signs—including
pulse, breathing rate, **body temperature**, and blood
pressure—are recorded.

With the patient sitting up, the following systems
are reviewed:

- Skin. The exposed areas of the skin are observed; the
size and shape of any lesions are noted.
- Head. The hair, scalp, skull, and face are examined.
- Eyes. The external structures are observed. The internal structures can be observed using an ophthalmoscope (a lighted instrument) in a darkened room.
- Ears. The external structures are inspected. A lighted
instrument called an otoscope may be used to inspect
internal structures.
- Nose and sinuses. The external nose is examined.
The nasal mucosa and internal structures can be
observed with the use of a penlight and a nasal
speculum.
- Mouth and pharynx. The lips, gums, teeth, roof of
the mouth, tongue, and pharynx are inspected.
- Neck. The lymph nodes on both sides of the neck and
the thyroid gland are palpated (examined by feeling
with the fingers).
- Back. The spine and muscles of the back are palpated
and checked for tenderness. The upper back, where
the lungs are located, is palpated on the right and left
sides and a stethoscope is used to listen for breath
sounds.

- Breasts and armpits. A woman's breasts are inspected with the arms relaxed and then raised. In both men and women, the lymph nodes in the armpits are felt with the examiner's hands. While the patient is still sitting, movement of the joints in the hands, arms, shoulders, neck, and jaw can be checked.

Then while the patient is lying down on the examining table, the examination includes:

- Breasts. The breasts are palpated and inspected for lumps.
- Front of chest and lungs. The area is inspected with the fingers, using palpation and percussion. A stethoscope is used to listen to the internal breath sounds.

The head should be slightly raised for:

- Heart. A stethoscope is used to listen to the heart's rate and rhythm. The blood vessels in the neck are observed and palpated.

The patient should lie flat for:

- Abdomen. Light and deep palpation is used on the abdomen to feel the outlines of internal organs including the liver, spleen, kidneys, and aorta, a large blood vessel.
- Rectum and anus. With the patient lying on the left side, the outside areas are observed. An internal digital examination (using a finger), is usually done if the patient is over 40 years old. In men, the prostate gland is also palpated.
- Reproductive organs. The external sex organs are inspected and the area is examined for hernias. In men, the scrotum is palpated. In women, a pelvic examination is done using a speculum and a Papanicolaou test (Pap test) may be taken.
- Legs. With the patient lying flat, the legs are inspected for swelling, and pulses in the knee, thigh, and foot area are found. The groin area is palpated for the presence of lymph nodes. The joints and muscles are observed.
- Musculoskeletal system. With the patient standing, the straightness of the spine and the alignment of the legs and feet is noted.
- Blood vessels. The presence of any abnormally enlarged veins (varicose), usually in the legs, is noted.

In addition to evaluating the patient's alertness and mental ability during the initial conversation, additional inspection of the nervous system may be indicated:

- Neurologic screen. The patient's ability to take a few steps, hop, and do deep knee bends is observed. The strength of the hand grip is felt. With the patient sitting down, the reflexes in the knees and feet can be tested with a small hammer. The sense of touch in the hands and feet can be evaluated by testing reaction to pain and vibration.
- Sometimes additional time is spent examining the 12 nerves in the head (cranial) that are connected directly to the brain. They control the sense of smell, strength of muscles in the head, reflexes in the eye, facial movements, gag reflex, and muscles in the jaw. General muscle tone and coordination, and the reaction of the abdominal area to stimulants like pain, temperature, and touch would also be evaluated.

Preparation

Before visiting the health care professional, the patient should write down important facts and dates about his or her own medical history, as well as those of family members. He or she should have a list of all medications with their doses or bring the actual bottles of medicine along. If there are specific concerns about anything, writing them down is a good idea.

Before the physical examination begins, the bladder should be emptied and a urine specimen can be collected in a small container. For some blood tests, the patient may be told ahead of time not to eat or drink after midnight.

The patient usually removes all clothing and puts on a loose-fitting hospital gown. An additional sheet is provided to keep the patient covered and comfortable during the examination.

Aftercare

Once the physical examination has been completed, the patient and the examiner should review what laboratory tests have been ordered and how the results will be shared with the patient. The medical professional should discuss any recommendations for treatment and follow-up visits. Special instructions should be put in writing. This is also an opportunity for the patient to ask any remaining questions about his or her own health concerns.

Risks

Other than discovering an unknown condition or health problem, which is the reason for performing a physical examination, there are no risks associated with the procedure.

Normal results

Normal results of a physical examination correspond to the healthy appearance and normal functioning of the body. For example, appropriate reflexes will be

KEY TERMS

Auscultation—The process of listening to sounds that are produced in the body. Direct auscultation uses the ear alone, such as when listening to the grating of a moving joint. Indirect auscultation involves the use of a stethoscope to amplify the sounds from within the body, like a heartbeat.

Hernia—The bulging of an organ, or part of an organ, through the tissues normally containing it; also called a rupture.

Inspection—The visual examination of the body using the eyes and a lighted instrument if needed. The sense of smell may also be used.

Ophthalmoscope—Lighted device for studying the interior of the eyeball.

Otoscope—An instrument with a light for examining the internal ear.

Palpation—The examination of the body using the sense of touch. There are two types: light and deep.

Percussion—An assessment method in which the surface of the body is struck with the fingertips to obtain sounds that can be heard or vibrations that can be felt. It can determine the position, size, and consistency of an internal organ. It is done over the chest to determine the presence of normal air content in the lungs, and over the abdomen to evaluate air in the loops of the intestine.

Reflex—An automatic response to a stimulus.

Speculum—An instrument for enlarging the opening of any canal or cavity in order to facilitate inspection of its interior.

Stethoscope—A Y-shaped instrument that amplifies body sounds such as heartbeat, breathing, and air in the intestine. Used in auscultation.

Varicose veins—The permanent enlargement and twisting of veins, usually in the legs. They are most often seen in people with occupations requiring long periods of standing, and in pregnant women.

present, no suspicious lumps or lesions will be found, and **vital signs** will be normal.

Abnormal results

Abnormal results of a physical examination include any findings that indicated the presence of a disorder, disease, or underlying condition. For example, the presence of lumps or lesions, fever, muscle weakness or lack of tone, poor reflex response, heart arhythmia, or swelling of lymph nodes will point to a possible health problem.

Resources

BOOKS

Bickley, L. S., and P. G. Szilagyi. *Bates' Guide to Physical Examination and History Taking.* 9th ed. Philadelphia: Lippincott Williams and Wilkins, 2007.

Jarvis, C. *Physical Examination and Health Assessment.* 5th ed. Philadelphia: Saunders, 2007.

Seidel. H. M., J. Ball, J. Dains, and W. Bennedict. *Mosby's Physical Examination Handbook.* 6th ed. St. Louis: MOsby, 2006.

Swartz, M. H. *Textbook of Physical Diagnosis: History and Examination.* 5th ed. Philadelphia: Saunders, 2005.

PERIODICALS

Corbett, E. C., D. M. Elnicki, and M. R. Conway. "When Should Students Learn Essential Physical Examination Skills? Views of Internal Medicine Clerkship Directors in North America." *Academic Medicine* 83, no. 1 (2008): 96–99.

Hatala, R., S. B. Issenberg, B. O. Kassen, G. Cole, C. M. Bacchus, and R. J. Scalese. "Assessing the relationship between cardiac physical examination technique and accurate bedside diagnosis during an objective structured clinical examination." *Academic Medicine* 82, no. 10 Suppl (2007): S26–S29.

Velez, N., P. Khera, and J. C. English. "Eyebrow loss: clinical review." *American Journal of Clinical Dermatology* 8, no. 6 (2007): 337–346.

Wu, E. H., M. J. Fagan, S. E. Reinert, and J. A. Diaz. " Self-confidence in and perceived utility of the physical examination: a comparison of medical students, residents, and faculty internists." *Journal of General Internal Medicine* 22, no. 12 (2007): 1725–1730.

ORGANIZATIONS

American Academy of Family Physicians. 11400 Tomahawk Creek Parkway, Leawood, KS 66211-2672. (913) 906-6000. E-mail: fp@aafp.org. http://www.aafp.org.

American Academy of Pediatrics. 141 Northwest Point Boulevard, Elk Grove Village, IL 60007-1098. (847) 434-4000; Fax: (847) 434-8000. E-mail: kidsdoc@aap.org. http://www.aap.org/default.htm.

American College of Physicians. 190 N Independence Mall West, Philadelphia, PA 19106-1572. (800) 523-1546, x2600, or (215) 351-2600. http://www.acponline.org.

American Medical Association. 515 N. State Street, Chicago, IL 60610. (312) 464-5000. http://www.ama-assn.org.

OTHER

Brown University School of Medicine. Information about Physical Examination. 2007 [cited December 30, 2007]. http://bms.brown.edu/curriculum/icm/ICMPhysicalExam.htm.

Loyola University Chicago Stritch School of Medicine. Information about Physical Examination. 2007 [cited

December 30, 2007]. http://www.meddean.luc.edu/
lumen/MedEd/MEDICINE/PULMONAR/PD/
Pdmenu.htm.

Medical Transcription Center. Information about Physical
Examination. 2007 [cited December 30, 2007]. http://
www.mtmonthly.com/.

National Library of Medicine. Information about Physical
Examination. 2007 [cited December 30, 2007]. http://
www.nlm.nih.gov/medlineplus/ency/article/
002274.htm .

L. Fleming Fallon, Jr, MD, DrPH

Pitocin *see* **Uterine stimulants**

Pituitary gland removal *see*
Hypophysectomy

▌ Planning a hospital stay

Definition

Planning a hospital stay includes determining what
hospitals or facilities are covered by the patient's insurance plan, evaluating the credentials of the health care
providers and the hospital, gathering information about
the hospital, including services offered, scheduling the
hospital stay, completing pre-admission testing, receiving and following all of the appropriate pre-admission
instructions, registering at the hospital upon arrival,
and completing an **informed consent** form.

Purpose

Patients are admitted to the hospital for a variety
of reasons, including scheduled tests, procedures, or
surgeries, emergency medical treatment, administration of medication, or to stabilize or monitor an existing medical condition.

Planning a hospital stay helps the patient understand what to expect before **admission to the hospital**
and ensures the patient is physically and psychologically ready.

Description

If the hospital stay was planned, some of the steps
involved in preparing for the hospital stay will take
place beginning one to two weeks before the patient is
admitted to the hospital. Many of these steps will not
apply if the hospital stay was unexpected or was the
result of an emergency.

Determining insurance coverage

Although there are many types of hospitals available to meet the needs of different patients, the
patient's choice of hospital may be limited by his or
her insurance plan. The patient should find out if the
selected hospital is approved by his or her plan. If the
patient receives care from a facility that is not
approved by the health care plan, the patient may be
responsible for paying for most or all of the medical
expenses related to the hospital stay.

Managed care insurance plans often require pre-
certification before any hospital stay, except for emergency hospital admissions. Usually, the patient's doctor has to authorize the hospital stay, and some types
of care provided in the hospital may require insurance
clearance.

If the patient has **Medicare** insurance (for patients
over age 65), a semiprivate room, meals, general nursing care, and other **hospital services** and supplies are
covered services. Those services not covered by Medicare include private duty nursing, a private room
(unless medically necessary), and television and telephone fees.

The patient may desire to seek a **second opinion**
to confirm the doctor's treatment recommendations.
The patient should check with his or her insurance
provider to determine if the second opinion consultation is covered.

FOR PATIENTS WITHOUT INSURANCE COVERAGE.
For patients who do not have insurance coverage,
other payment options and sources of financial aid
can be discussed. The patient should ask to speak
with the hospital's financial counselor for more
information.

Evaluating credentials

The patient should find out if the physicians who
will provide care in the hospital are board certified.
Even though board certification is not required for an
individual physician to practice medicine, most hospitals require that a certain percentage of their staff be
board certified. There are 24 certifying boards recognized by the American Board of Member Specialties
(ABMS) and the American Medical Association
(AMA). Most of the ABMS boards issue time-limited
certificates, valid for six to 10 years. This requires
physicians to become re-certified to maintain their
board certification—a process that includes a credential review, continuing education in the specialty, and
additional examinations.

KEY TERMS

Anesthesiologist—A specially trained physician who administers anesthesia.

Case manager—A health care professional who can provide assistance with a patient's needs beyond the hospital.

Catheter—A small, flexible tube used to deliver fluids or medications or used to drain fluid or urine from the body.

Clinical nurse specialists—Nurses with advanced training as well as a master's degree.

Discharge planner—A health care professional who helps patients arrange for health and home care needs after they go home from the hospital.

Electrocardiogram (ECG, EKG)—A test that records the electrical activity of the heart using small electrode patches attached to the skin on the chest.

General anesthesia—Anesthesia that makes the patient unconscious and not feel pain.

Guided imagery—A form of focused relaxation that coaches the patient to visualize calm, peaceful images.

Infectious disease team—A team of physicians who help control the hospital environment to protect patients against harmful sources of infection.

Informed consent—An educational process between health care providers and patients intended to instruct the patient about the nature and purpose of the procedure or treatment, the risks and benefits of the procedure, and alternatives, including the option of not proceeding with the test or treatment.

Inpatient surgery—Surgery that requires an overnight stay of one or more days in the hospital.

Local anesthesia—Anesthesia that numbs a localized area of the body.

NPO—A term that means "nothing by mouth." NPO refers to the time after which the patient is not allowed to eat or drink prior to a procedure or treatment.

Nurse manager—The nurse responsible for managing the nursing care on the nursing unit and also supervises all of the other personnel who work on the nursing unit.

Nursing unit—The floor or section of the hospital where patient rooms are located.

Outpatient surgery—Also called same-day or ambulatory surgery.

Pharmacologist—Medication specialist who checks patients' blood levels to monitor their response to immunosuppressive medications.

Regional anesthesia—Anesthesia that does not makes the patient unconscious; it works by blocking sensation in a region of the body.

Registered nurses—Specially trained nurses who provide care during the patient's hospital stay. Registered nurses provide medical care, medications, and education, as well as assess the patient's condition.

Social worker—A health care provider who can provide support to patients and families, including assistance with a patient's psychosocial adjustment needs and referrals for community support.

A physician's membership in professional societies is also an important consideration. Professional societies provide an independent forum for medical specialists to discuss issues of mutual interest and concern. They provide a place for doctors to discuss the latest practices and technologies, and to learn from eachothers' experiences of cases that went well or poorly. Examples of professional societies include the Society of Thoracic Surgeons (STS) and the American College of Physicians–American Society of Internal Medicine (ACP-ASIM).

To find information about a physician's qualifications, the patient can call a state or county medical association for assistance. A reference book is also available, *The Official ABMS Directory of Board-Certified Medical Specialists*, which lists all physicians who are certified by approved boards. This publication also contains brief information about each physician's medical education and training. The directory can be found in many hospital and university libraries, and in some local libraries.

Evaluating the health care team

Selecting a hospital that has a multi-disciplinary team of specialists is important. The medical team should include surgeons (as applicable), physicians who specialize in the patient's medical condition (such as cardiologists for heart disease and pulmonologists for lung disease), infectious disease specialists, pharmacologists, and advanced care registered nurses. Other medical team members may include fellows, residents, interns, clinical coordinators, physical therapists, occupational therapists, respiratory therapists, registered dietitians, social workers, and financial counselors.

Evaluating the hospital

The patient should find out if the hospital has been accredited by the Joint Commission on Accreditation of Healthcare Organizations, a professionally sponsored program that stimulates a high quality of patient care in health care facilities. Joint Commission accreditation means the hospital voluntarily sought accreditation and met national health and safety standards.

Here are some questions to consider when evaluating a hospital:

- Does the hospital offer treatment for the patient's specific condition? How experienced is the hospital staff in treating that condition?
- What is the hospital's success record in providing the specific medical treatment or procedure the patient needs?
- Does the hospital have experience treating other patients the same age as the potential patient?
- Does the hospital explain the patient's rights and responsibilities?
- Does the hospital have a written description of its services and fees?
- How much does the patient's type of treatment cost at the hospital?
- Is financial help available?
- Who will be responsible for the patient's specific care plan while he or she is in the hospital?
- If the hospital is far from the patient's home; will accommodations be provided for caregivers?
- What type of services are available during the patient's hospital stay?
- Will a discharge plan be developed before the patient goes home from the hospital?
- Does the hospital provide training to help the patient care for his or her condition at home?

Hospital services

Usually, the patient receives information about the hospital from the admitting office when the hospital stay is scheduled. This information should include directions to the hospital, parking information, lodging information if the patient is from out of town, types of rooms, and services offered.

Hospital services offered may include:

- Ethics consultation: Bioethics professionals are available at most hospitals to provide advice or help the

patient identify, analyze, and resolve ethical issues that may arise during the patient's care at the hospital.
- Barber or beautician: These services may incur a fee, in addition to the fees of the patient's hospital stay.
- Complementary techniques such as guided imagery and relaxation tapes, massage therapy, or aromatherapy (to reduce a patient's stress and anxiety).
- Home care: If home health services will be needed after the patient is discharged, they can be arranged by the social worker or nursing staff.
- Interpreter: An interpreter or other special services may be available to assist patients and family members who do not speak the language or are from out of the country.
- Nutrition therapy: Registered dietitians are available to provide comprehensive nutrition assessment, counseling, and education.
- Ombudsman: Health care personnel available to address concerns and problems about medical services that cannot be resolved by reporting these concerns to the nursing staff.
- Pastoral care: Clergy members are available at most hospitals to provide religious support and services to meet patients' spiritual needs. Many hospitals also have a small chapel that provides a quiet retreat for patients and family members of all religious backgrounds and faiths.
- Patient education: A variety of services are available to teach patients about their medical condition or to help them prepare for their scheduled tests or procedures. Patient education may include one-on-one instruction from a health care provider, educational sessions in a group setting, or self-guided learning videos or modules. Informative and instructional handouts are usually provided to explain specific medications, tests, or procedures.
- Pediatric services: Many hospitals have dedicated services and programs available to help children, teenagers, and their parents feel better prepared to cope more effectively with hospital stays, surgery, procedures, and other health-related events.
- Social work: Social workers are available to help patients manage the changes that may occur as a result of the patient's hospitalization. Social workers provide referrals to community resources and can help the family make arrangements for care in the home as necessary after the patient is discharged from the hospital.

Patient rights and responsibilities

All hospitals have a list of **patient rights** and responsibilities, established by the American Hospital

Association. These rights and responsibilities are usually published and posted throughout the hospital. By law, all patients have certain rights. Some patient rights include the right to:

- considerate and respectful care
- complete information about diagnosis, treatment, and expected recovery in terms the patient can understand
- knowledge of the name and function of any health care professional providing care
- informed consent
- the right to refuse treatment to the extent permitted by law and be informed of the medical consequences of refusing treatment

Each patient should obtain a list of his or her rights and responsibilities prior to a hospital admission.

Hospital environment

Most hospital rooms have a bed, bedside table, chair, telephone, television, and bathroom. Some hospitals charge a fee for use of the telephone or television; patients should be notified of these charges prior to their hospital admission. Each patient area has a call signal button so the patient can notify the nursing staff if help is needed. Most hospital rooms are doubles that are shared by two patients. In many cases a private room can be specifically requested in one is available. Some hospitals also have wards in which four or more patients stay in one room. Three nutritionally balanced meals are provided to the patient daily during a hospital stay; daily menus are usually provided for patients to select their food choices, as applicable. (Some patients have dietary restrictions so their food choices may be limited.)

Hospital caregivers

Sometimes, the patient's personal or family physician is not the attending physician who is in charge of the patient's overall care and treatment in the hospital. The attending physician may be a doctor on the hospital staff or a specialist. Fellows, residents, or interns may also provide care. Fellows are doctors who receive training in a special area of medicine after their residency training. Residents are doctors who have recently graduated from medical school and are training in a medical specialty. Interns are first-year residents.

Nurses work closely with doctors to supervise the care provided in the hospital. Nurses take the patient's **vital signs**, administer medications, provide treatments, and teach patients how to care for themselves. The head nurse, also called the clinical nurse manager, coordinates care for each patient on the nursing unit.

Other health care providers include medical technologists, radiographers, and nuclear medicine technicians who perform diagnostic tests, therapists such as physical therapists, occupational therapists, and speech therapists who provide specialized care as needed, and dietitians who provide nutrition counseling and nutrition assessments. There are several other health care providers who may assist patients during their hospital stay; patients should ask for more information about the types of providers they may be in contact with during the time they are in the hospital.

Information for visitors and family members

It may be helpful for the patient to select a spokesperson from the family to communicate with the health care providers. This may improve communication with the health care providers as well as with other family members. The patient should also communicate his or her wishes regarding the spokesperson's telephone communications to other family members.

Educational classes may be available for family members to learn more about the patient's condition and what to expect during the patient's **recovery at home**.

If a family member needs to contact the patient or the patient's other family members, the family member should call the hospital and ask for the nursing unit where the patient is staying. The nursing unit staff can connect the caller to the patient's room, take a message, or connect the caller to the patient's family members who are present. Since every hospital has **patient confidentiality** rules, some information may not be able to be disclosed over the telephone.

Most hospitals prohibit the use of cellular phones in patient care areas, as they interfere with the operation of medical equipment.

Most hospitals are smoke-free environments. There are usually designated outside areas where visitors can smoke.

Most hospitals have designated visiting hours that should be adhered to by family members and friends.

Most hospitals have on-site pharmacies where family members can fill the patient's prescriptions, gift shops, and a cafeteria. Usually a list of on-site and off-site dining options can be obtained from the hospital's information desk or social work department.

Preadmission testing

Preadmission testing includes a review of the patient's medical history, a complete **physical examination**, a variety of tests, patient education, and meetings with the health care team. The review of the patient's medical history includes an evaluation of the patient's previous and current medical conditions, surgeries and procedures, medications, and any other health conditions such as allergies that may impact the patient's hospital stay. Preadmission testing is generally scheduled for a few days before the hospital admission.

The patient may find it helpful to bring along a family member or friend to the preadmission testing appointments. This caregiver can help the patient remember important details to prepare for the hospital stay.

Preadmission instructions

Preadmission instructions include information about reserving blood products if necessary, taking or discontinuing medications, eating and drinking, **smoking cessation**, limiting activities, and preparing items to bring to the hospital.

Blood transfusions and blood donation

Blood transfusions may be necessary during surgery. A blood **transfusion** is the delivery of whole blood or blood components to replace blood lost through trauma, surgery, or disease. About one in three hospitalized patients will require a blood transfusion. The surgeon can provide an estimate of how much blood the patient's procedure may require.

To decrease the risk of infection and immunologic complications, some hospitals offer a **blood donation** program if surgery is scheduled or if it is known that blood products will be needed by the patient during his or her hospital stay. Autologous blood (from the patient) is the safest blood available for transfusion, since there is no risk of disease transmission. Methods of autologous donation or collection include:

- Intraoperative blood collection: The blood lost during surgery is processed, and the red blood cells are re-infused during or immediately after surgery.
- Preoperative donation: The patient donates blood once a week for about one to three weeks before surgery. The blood is separated and the blood components needed are re-infused during surgery.
- Immediate preoperative hemodilution: The patient donates blood immediately before surgery to decrease the loss of red blood cells during surgery. Immediately after donating, the patient receives fluids to compensate for the amount of blood removed. Since the blood is diluted, fewer red blood cells are lost from bleeding during surgery.
- Postoperative blood collection: Blood lost from the surgical site right after surgery is collected and re-infused after the surgical site has been closed.

The physician determines what type of blood collection process, if any, is appropriate.

Medication guidelines

Depending on the reason for the hospital stay, certain medications may be prescribed or restricted. The health care team will provide specific guidelines. If certain medications need to be restricted before the hospital stay, the patient will receive a complete list of the medications (including prescription, over-the-counter, and herbal medications) to avoid taking. The patient should not bring any medications to the hospital unless specifically instructed to by the hospital staff. In the majority of cases all necessary medications, as ordered by the doctor, will be provided in the hospital.

Eating and drinking guidelines

Before most procedures, the patient is advised not to eat or drink anything after midnight the evening before the surgery. This includes no smoking and no gum chewing. The patient should not drink any alcoholic beverages for at least 24 hours before being hospitalized, unless instructed otherwise.

Smoking cessation

Patients are encouraged to quit smoking and stop using tobacco products prior to their hospital admission and to make a commitment to be a nonsmoker. Quitting smoking will help the patient recover more quickly. There are usually several community-based smoking cessation programs available. Members of the hospital staff are more than happy to recommend a program to fit the patient's needs.

Activity

The patient should eat healthy foods, rest, and **exercise** as normal before a hospitalization, unless given other instructions. The patient should try to get enough sleep, although this can often be difficult if the patient is nervous or anxious about the upcoming hospital stay.

The patient should make arrangements ahead of time for someone to care for children and take care of any other necessary activities at home such as getting the mail or newspapers. The patient should inform family members about the scheduled hospital stay, so they can provide help and support.

Items to bring to the hospital

The patient should bring a list of current medications, allergies, and appropriate medical records upon admission to the hospital. The patient should also bring a prepared list of questions to ask.

The patient should not bring valuables such as jewelry, credit cards, checkbooks, or other such items. A small amount of cash (no more than $20) may be packed to purchase items such as newspapers or magazines. If necessary, patients can secure their personal belongings in the hospital cashier's office, safe, or vault for safekeeping until discharge. Most hospitals state in their policies that they are not responsible for lost or stolen personal items.

The patient should only pack what is needed. Some essential items include a toothbrush, toothpaste, comb or brush, deodorant, razor (not electric), slippers, robe, pajamas, and one change of comfortable clothes to wear when going home. The patient should also pack eyeglasses, hearing aids, and dentures, including their carrying cases, if applicable. These items should be labeled with the patient's name when not in use, should be stored in their carrying cases, and put in the bedside stand so they are not lost. They should never be placed on food trays because they may be forgotten and thrown out with the food garbage.

The patient should bring a list of family members' names and phone numbers to contact in an emergency. The patient may also want to pack a book or other personal item such as a family picture.

Personal electronic devices such as hair dryers, curling irons, electric razors, personal televisions, computers, and other electronic devices are not permitted in the hospital, since these devices may interfere with the hospital's medical equipment.

Transportation

The patient should arrange for transportation home, since the effects of certain medications given in the hospital make it unsafe to drive.

Hospital registration and admission

Upon arriving at the hospital, the patient first reports to the hospital registration or admitting area. The patient will be required to complete paperwork and show an insurance identification card, if insured. Often, a pre-registration process performed prior to the date of hospital admission helps make the registration process run smoothly. An identification bracelet that includes the patient's name and doctor's name will be placed on the patient's wrist.

If the patient is not feeling well upon arrival to the hospital, a family member or caregiver can help the patient complete the admitting process. Sometimes, a patient's illness may require that the hospital stay be rescheduled.

Informed consent

The health care provider will review the informed consent form and ask the patient to sign it. Informed consent is an educational process between health care providers and patients. Before any procedure is performed or any form of medical care is provided, the patient is asked to sign a consent form. Before signing the form, the patient should understand the nature and purpose of the procedure or treatment, the risks and benefits of the procedure, and alternatives, including the option of not proceeding with the procedure. Signing the informed consent form indicates that the patient understands and permits the surgery or procedure to be performed. During the discussion about the procedure, health care providers are available to answer the patient's questions about the consent form or procedure.

Advance directives

As part of the admissions process, the patient will be asked about advance directives. Advance directives are legal documents that increase a patient's control over medical decisions. A patient may decide medical treatment in advance, in the event that he or she becomes physically or mentally unable to communicate his or her wishes. Advance directives either state what kind of treatment the patient wants to receive (**living will**), or authorize another person to make medical decisions for the patient when he or she is unable to do so (durable **power of attorney**).

Advance directives are not required and may be changed or canceled at any time. Any change should be written, signed, and dated in accordance with state law, and copies should be given to the physician and to others who received original copies. Advance directives can be revoked either in writing or by destroying the document.

Advance directives are not do-not-resuscitate (DNR) orders. A **DNR order** indicates that a person—usually with a terminal illness or other serious medical condition—has decided not to have **cardiopulmonary resuscitation** (CPR) performed in the event that his or her heart or breathing stops.

Admission tests

Some routine tests will be performed, including blood pressure, temperature, pulse, and weight checks, blood tests, **urinalysis**; **chest x ray**, and **electrocardiogram** (ECG). A brief physical exam will be performed.

QUESTIONS TO ASK THE DOCTOR

- How can I prepare myself for the hospital stay?
- Who are the members of the health care team at this hospital?
- What types of questions should I ask my insurance provider to determine if the medical expenses of my hospital stay will be covered?
- What type of tests or procedures will be performed?
- What types of precautions must I follow before and after my hospital stay?
- Will I have to have blood transfusions during my hospital stay?
- Can I take my medications the day I am admitted to the hospital?
- Should I change my diet or eating habits before my hospital stay?
- How long will I have to stay in the hospital?
- What kind of pain or discomfort will I experience and what can I take to relieve it?
- What types of resources are available to me during my hospital stay, and during my recovery at home?
- After I go home from the hospital, how long will it take me to recover?
- What are the signs of infection, and what types of symptoms should I report to my doctor?
- What types of medications will I have to take? How long will I have to take them?
- When will I be able I resume my normal activities? When will I be able to drive? When will I be able to return to work?
- What lifestyle changes (including diet, weight management, exercise, and activity changes) are recommended to improve my condition?
- How often do I need to see my doctor for follow-up visits?

The health care team will ask several questions to evaluate the patient's condition. The patient should inform the health care team if he or she drinks alcohol on a daily basis so precautions can be taken to avoid complications.

Results

Patients who receive proper preparation for their hospital experience, including physical and psychological preparation, are less anxious and are more likely to make a quicker recovery at home, with fewer complications.

Resources

BOOKS

Buck, Jari Holland. *Hospital Stay Handbook: a Guide to Becoming a Patient Advocate for Your Loved Ones.* Woodbury, MN: Llewellyn Publications, 2007.

Wachter, Robert M., Lee Goldman, and Harry Hollander. *Hospital Medicine*, 2nd Ed. Philadelphia, PA: Lippincott Williams & Wilkins, 2005.

Williams, Mark V. et al, eds. *Comprehensive Hospital Medicine: an Evidence Based Approach.* Philadelphia : Saunders Elsevier, 2007.

PERIODICALS

Hume, Susan. "Six Tips for Hospital Survival." *The Exceptional Parent* 37.8 (August 2007): 35-37.

Rentsch, Denis, Christophe Luthy, Thomas V. Perneger and Anne-Francoise Allaz. "Hospitalisation Process Seen by Patients and Health Care Professionals." *Social Science and Medicine* 57.3 (August 2003): p.571-577.

ORGANIZATIONS

Agency for Health Care Policy and Research (AHCPR), Publications Clearinghouse. P.O. Box 8547, Silver Spring, MD, 20907. (800) 358-9295. <http://www/ahcpr.gov>.

American Association of Nurse Anesthetists (AANA). 222 South Prospect Avenue, Park Ridge, IL 60068-4001. (847) 692-7050. http://www.aana.com/.

American College of Surgeons. 633 N. Saint Clair Street, Chicago, IL 60611-3211. (312) 202-5000. http://www.facs.org/.

American Hospital Association. One North Franklin, Chicago, IL 60606. (312) 422-3000. http://www.hospitalconnect.com.

American Society of Anesthesiologists (ASA). 520 North Northwest Highway, Park Ridge, IL 60068-2573. (847) 825-5586. http://www.asahq.org/.

Joint Commission on Accreditation of Healthcare Organizations (JCAHO). One Renaissance Boulevard, Oakbrook Terrace, IL 60181. (630) 792-5800. http://www.jcaho.org.

National Heart, Lung and Blood Institute. Information Center. P.O. Box 30105, Bethesda, MD 20824-0105. (301) 251-2222. http://www.nhlbi.nih.gov .

National Institutes of Health. U.S. Department of Health and Human Services. 9000 Rockville Pike, Bethesda, MD 20892. (301) 496-4000. http://www.nih.gov.

Angela M. Costello
Robert Bockstiegel

Plastic, reconstructive, and cosmetic surgery

Definition

Plastic, reconstructive, and cosmetic surgery procedures are a variety of operations performed in order to repair or restore body parts to look normal, or to change a body part to look better. These types of surgery are highly specialized. They are characterized by careful preparation of a person's skin and tissues, by precise cutting and suturing techniques, and by care taken to minimize scarring. Recent advances in the development of miniaturized instruments, new materials for artificial limbs and body parts, and improved surgical techniques have expanded the range of plastic surgery procedures that can be performed.

Purpose

Although these three types of surgery share some common techniques and approaches, they have somewhat different emphases. Plastic surgery is usually performed to treat birth defects and to remove skin blemishes such as warts, acne scars, or birthmarks. Cosmetic surgery procedures are performed to make persons look younger or enhance their appearance in other ways. Reconstructive surgery is used to reattach body parts severed in combat or accidents, to perform skin grafts after severe burns, or to reconstruct parts of person's body that were missing at birth or removed by surgery. Reconstructive surgery is the oldest form of plastic surgery, having developed out of the need to treat wounded soldiers in wartime.

Demographics

The top 10 most commonly performed elective cosmetic surgeries in the United States include the following:

- liposuction
- breast augmentation
- eyelid surgery
- face lift
- tummy tuck
- collagen injections
- chemical peel
- laser skin resurfacing
- rhinoplasty
- forehead lift

There were approximately 31 million surgical procedures performed in the United States in 2006. Because many plastic and reconstructive surgical procedures are performed in private professional offices or as outpatient procedures, accurate statistics concerning the number of procedures performed are not available.

KEY TERMS

Blepharoplasty—Surgical reshaping of the eyelid.

Dermabrasion—A technique for removing the upper layers of skin with planing wheels powered by compressed air.

Face lift—Plastic surgery performed to remove sagging skin and wrinkles from an individual's face.

Liposuction—A surgical technique for removing fat from under the skin by vacuum suctioning.

Mammoplasty—Surgery performed to change the size or shape of breasts.

Rhinoplasty—Surgery performed to change the shape of the nose.

Description

Plastic surgery

Plastic surgery includes a number of different procedures that usually involve skin. Operations to remove excess fat from the abdomen ("tummy tucks"), **dermabrasion** to remove acne scars or tattoos, and reshaping the cartilage in children's ears (**otoplasty**) are common applications of plastic surgery.

Cosmetic surgery

Most cosmetic surgery is done on the face. It is intended either to correct disfigurement or to enhance a person's features. The most common cosmetic procedure for children is correction of a cleft lip or palate. In adults, the most common procedures are remodeling of the nose (**rhinoplasty**), removal of baggy skin around the eyelids (**blepharoplasty**), face lifts (rhytidectomy), or changing the size or shape of the breasts (mammoplasty). Although many people still think of cosmetic surgery as only for women, growing numbers of men are choosing to have face lifts and eyelid surgery, as well as hair transplants and "tummy tucks."

Reconstructive surgery

Reconstructive surgery is often performed on burn and accident victims. It may involve the rebuilding of severely fractured bones, as well as **skin grafting**. Reconstructive surgery includes such procedures as the reattachment of an amputated finger or toe, or implanting a prosthesis. Prostheses are artificial structures and materials that are used to replace missing limbs or teeth, or arthritic hip and knee joints.

Diagnosis/Preparation

General preparation

Preparation for nonemergency plastic or reconstructive surgery includes individual education, as well as medical considerations. Some operations, such as nose reshaping or the removal of warts, small birthmarks, and tattoos can be done as outpatient procedures under **local anesthesia**. Most plastic and reconstructive surgery, however, involves a stay in the hospital and **general anesthesia**.

Medical preparation

Preparation for plastic surgery includes the surgeon's detailed assessment of the parts of an individual's body that will be involved. Skin grafts require evaluating suitable areas of skin for the right color and texture to match the skin at the graft site. Face lifts and cosmetic surgery in the eye area require very close attention to the texture of the skin and the placement of surgical cuts (incisions).

Persons scheduled for plastic surgery under general anesthesia will be given a **physical examination**, blood and urine tests, and other tests to make sure that they do not have any previously undetected health problems or blood clotting disorders. The surgeon will check the list of prescription medications that the prospective patient may be taking to make sure that none of them will interfere with normal blood clotting or interact with the anesthetic.

Individuals are asked to avoid using **aspirin** or medications containing aspirin for a week to two weeks before surgery, because these drugs lengthen the time of blood clotting. Smokers are asked to stop smoking two weeks before surgery because smoking interferes with the healing process. For some types of plastic surgery, individuals may be asked to donate several units of their own blood before the procedure, in case a **transfusion** is needed during the operation. The prospective patient will be asked to sign a consent form before the operation.

Personal education

The surgeon will meet with the prospective patient before the operation is scheduled, in order to explain the procedure and to be sure that the individual is realistic about the expected results. This consideration is particularly important for people undergoing cosmetic surgery.

Medical considerations

Some people should not have plastic surgery because of certain medical risks. These groups include:

- persons recovering from a heart attack, severe infection (for example, pneumonia), or other serious illnesses
- people with infectious hepatitis or HIV infections
- individuals with cancer whose cancer might spread (metastasize)
- people who are extremely overweight (Individuals who are more than 30% overweight should not have liposuction.)
- persons with blood clotting disorders

Psychological

Plastic, cosmetic, and reconstructive surgeries have an important psychological dimension because of the high value placed on outward appearance in Western society. Many people who are born with visible deformities or disfigured by accidents later in life develop emotional problems related to social rejection. Other people work in fields such as acting, modeling, media journalism, and even politics, where their employment depends on how they look. Some people have unrealistic expectations of cosmetic surgery and think that it will solve all their life problems. It is important for anyone considering non-emergency plastic or cosmetic surgery to be realistic about its results. One type of psychiatric disorder, called body dysmorphic disorder, is characterized by an excessive preoccupation with imaginary or minor flaws in appearance. Persons with this disorder frequently seek unnecessary plastic surgery.

Aftercare

Medical

Medical aftercare following plastic surgery under general anesthesia includes bringing patients to a **recovery room**, monitoring their **vital signs**, and giving medications to relieve pain as necessary. Persons who have had fat removed from the abdomen may be kept in bed for as long as two weeks. Individuals who have had mammoplasties, **breast reconstruction**, and some types of facial surgery typically remain in the hospital for a week after the operation. Those who have had **liposuction** or eyelid surgery are usually sent home in a day or two.

People who have had outpatient procedures are usually given **antibiotics** to prevent infection and are sent home as soon as their vital signs are normal.

Psychological

Some individuals may need follow-up psychotherapy or counseling after plastic or reconstructive surgery. These people typically include children whose schooling and social relationships have been affected

WHO PERFORMS THE
PROCEDURE AND WHERE IS IT
PERFORMED?

Plastic, reconstructive, and cosmetic surgical procedures are performed by surgeons with specialized training in plastic and reconstructive surgery. Depending on the complexity of the procedures, they may be performed in hospitals as an inpatient, in outpatient facilities, or in private professional offices.

by birth defects, as well as persons of any age whose deformities or disfigurements were caused by trauma from accidents, war injuries, or violent crimes.

Risks

The risks associated with plastic, cosmetic, and reconstructive surgery include the postoperative complications that can occur with any surgical operation under anesthesia. These complications include wound infection, internal bleeding, pneumonia, and reactions to the anesthesia.

In addition to these general risks, some plastic, cosmetic, and reconstructive surgical procedures carry specific risks:

- formation of undesirable scar tissue
- development of persistent pain, redness, or swelling in the area of the surgery
- infection inside the body related to inserting a prosthesis (These infections can result from contamination at the time of surgery or from bacteria migrating into the area around the prosthesis at a later time.)
- anemia or fat embolisms from liposuction
- rejection of skin grafts or tissue transplants
- loss of normal feeling or function in the area of the operation (For example, it is not unusual for women who have had mammoplasties to lose sensation in their nipples.)
- complications resulting from unforeseen technological problems (The best-known example of this problem was the discovery in the mid-1990s that breast implants made with silicone gel could leak into the recipient's body.)

Normal results

Normal results include an individual's recovery from the surgery with satisfactory results and without complications.

QUESTIONS TO ASK THE
DOCTOR

- What will be the resulting appearance?
- Is the surgeon board certified in plastic and reconstructive surgery?
- How many similar procedures has the surgeon performed?
- What is the surgeon's complication rate?

Morbidity and mortality rates

Morbidity and mortality rates vary with the complexity and severity of different procedures. Mortality is similar to that associated with all surgical procedures. Morbidity is influenced by personal expectations. From a surgical perspective, most morbidity is due to errors associated with anesthesia, procedure, pain medications, and after care. From an individual's perspective, morbidity involves the degree to which actual results compared to expected outcomes. The latter distinction is very subjective.

Alternatives

Alternatives to plastic, reconstructive, and cosmetic surgical procedures include using various products that may be affixed to articles of clothing or the surface of the body.

Resources

BOOKS

Loftus, J. M. The Smart Woman's Guide to Plastic Surgery. 2nd ed. New York: McGraw-Hill, 2007.

Mendelson, R. The Chase for Beauty. Garden City, NY: Morgan James Publishing, 2008.

Papel, I. D. Facial Plastic and Reconstructive Surgery. 3rd ed. New York: Thieme Medical Publishers, 2008.

Shiffman, M. A., S. J. Mirrafati, S. M. Lam, and C. G. Cueteeaux. Simplified Facial Rejuvenation. New York: Springer, 2007.

Thorne, C. H., S. P. Bartlett, R. W. Beasley, S. J. Aston, and G. C. Gurtner. Grabb and Smith's Plastic Surgery. 6th ed. Philadelphia: Lippincott Williams and Wilkins, 2006.

PERIODICALS

Davison, S. P. "Essentials of plastic surgery." Plastic and Reconstructive Surgery 120, no. 7 (2007): 2112–2125.

Doer, T. D. "Lipoplasty of the face and neck." Current Opinions in Otolaryngology, Head and Neck Surgery 15, no. 4 (2007): 228–232.

Jose, R. M. "Plastic surgery: discipline defined by techniques." Plastic and Reconstructive Surgery 120, no. 2 (2007): 576–577.

Wallace, D. L., S, M. Jones, C. Milroy, and M. A. Pickford. "Telemedicine for acute plastic surgical trauma and burns." Journal of Plastic, Reconstructive and Aesthetic Surgery 61, no. 1 (2008): 31–36.

Whitaker, I. S., R. O. Karoo, G. Spyrou, and O. M. Fenton. "The birth of plastic surgery: the story of nasal reconstruction from the Edwin Smith Papyrus to the twenty-first century." Plastic and Reconstructive Surgery 120, no. 1 (2007): 327–336.

ORGANIZATIONS

American Academy of Facial Plastic and Reconstructive Surgery. 310 S. Henry Street, Alexandria, VA 22314. (703) 299-9291. http://www.aafprs.org/ .

American Board of Plastic Surgery. Seven Penn Center, Suite 400, 1635 Market Street, Philadelphia, PA 19103-2204. (215) 587-9322. http://www.abplsurg.org/.

American College of Surgeons. 633 North Saint Claire Street, Chicago, IL, 60611. (312) 202-5000. http://www.facs.org/.

American Society for Aesthetic Plastic Surgery. 11081 Winners Circle, Los Alamitos, California 90720. (888) 272-7711. http://www.surgery.org/.

American Society of Plastic Surgeons. 444 E. Algonquin Rd., Arlington Heights, IL 60005. (847) 228-9900. http://www.plasticsurgery.org/.

OTHER

American academy of Cosmetic Surgery. Information about Plastic and Reconstructive Surgery. 2007 [cited December 30, 2007]. http://www.cosmeticsurgery.org/Surgeons/education.asp.

American Board of Facial Plastic and Reconstructive Surgeryry. Information about Plastic and Reconstructive Surgery. 2007 [cited December 30, 2007]. http://www.abfprs.org/.

Canadian Society of Plastic Surgery. Information about Plastic and Reconstructive Surgery. 2007 [cited December 30, 2007]. http://www.plasticsurgery.ca/.

Mayo Clinic. Information about Plastic and Reconstructive Surgery. 2007 [cited December 30, 2007]. http://www.mayoclinic.org/plasticsurgery-rst/.

National Library of Medicine. Information about Plastic and Reconstructive Surgery. 2007 [cited December 30, 2007].http://www.nlm.nih.gov/medlineplus/plasticandcosmeticsurgery.html .

L. Fleming Fallon, Jr., MD, DrPH

Platelet count *see* **Complete blood count**

Pneumonectomy

Definition

Pneumonectomy is the medical term for the surgical removal of a lung.

Purpose

A pneumonectomy is most often used to treat lung cancer when less radical surgery cannot achieve satisfactory results. It may also be the most appropriate treatment for a tumor located near the center of the lung that affects the pulmonary artery or veins, which transport blood between the heart and lungs. In addition, pneumonectomy may be the treatment of choice when the patient has a traumatic chest injury that has damaged the main air passage (bronchus) or the lung's major blood vessels so severely that they cannot be repaired.

Demographics

Pneumonectomies are usually performed on patients with lung cancer, as well as patients with such noncancerous diseases as chronic obstructive pulmonary disease (COPD), which includes emphysema and chronic bronchitis. These diseases cause airway obstruction.

Approximately 342,000 Americans die of lung disease every year. Lung disease is responsible for one in seven deaths in the United States, according to the American Lung Association. This makes lung disease America's number three killer. More than 35 million Americans are now living with chronic lung disease.

Lung cancer

Lung cancer is the leading cause of cancer-related deaths in the United States. It is projected to claim more than nearly 158160,300 lives in 2007. Lung cancer kills more people than cancers of the breast, prostate, colon, and pancreas combined. Cigarette smoking accounts for nearly 90% of cases of lung cancer in the United States.

Lung cancer is the second most common cancer among both men and women and is the leading cause of **death** from cancer in both sexes. In addition to the use of tobacco as a major cause of lung cancer among smokers, second-hand smoke contributes to the development of lung cancer among nonsmokers. Exposure to asbestos and other hazardous substances is also known to cause lung cancer. Air pollution is also a probable cause, but makes a relatively small contribution to incidence and mortality rates. Indoor exposure to radon may also make a small contribution to the total incidence of lung cancer in certain geographic areas of the United States.

In each of the major racial/ethnic groups in the United States, the rates of lung cancer among men are about two to three times greater than the rates among women. Among men, age-adjusted lung cancer incidence

KEY TERMS

Bronchodilator—A drug that relaxes bronchial muscles resulting in expansion of the bronchial air passages.

Bronchopleural fistula—An abnormal connection between an air passage and the membrane that covers the lungs.

Corticosteroids—Any of various adrenal-cortex steroids used as anti-inflammatory agents.

Emphysema—A chronic disease characterized by loss of elasticity and abnormal accumulation of air in lung tissue.

Empyema—An accumulation of pus in the lung cavity, usually as a result of infection.

Malignant mesothelioma—A cancer of the pleura (the membrane lining the chest cavity and covering the lungs) that typically is related to asbestos exposure.

Pleural space—The small space between the two layers of the membrane that covers the lungs and lines the inner surface of the chest.

Pulmonary embolism—Blockage of a pulmonary artery by a blood clot or foreign matter.

Pulmonary rehabilitation—A program to treat COPD, which generally includes education and counseling, exercise, nutritional guidance, techniques to improve breathing, and emotional support.

rates (per 100,000) range from a low of about 14 among Native Americans to a high of 117 among African Americans, an eight-fold difference. For women, the rates range from approximately 15 per 100,000 among Japanese Americans to nearly 51 among Native Alaskans, only a three-fold difference.

Chronic obstructive pulmonary disease

The following are risk factors for COPD:

- current smoking or a long-term history of heavy smoking
- employment that requires working around dust and irritating fumes
- long-term exposure to second-hand smoke at home or in the workplace
- a productive cough (with phlegm or sputum) most of the time
- shortness of breath during vigorous activity
- shortness of breath that grows worse even at lower levels of activity
- a family history of early COPD (before age 45)

Diagnosis/Preparation

Diagnosis

In some cases, the diagnosis of a lung disorder is made when the patient consults a physician about chest pains or other symptoms. The symptoms of lung cancer vary somewhat according to the location of the tumor; they may include persistent coughing, coughing up blood, wheezing, fever, and weight loss. In cases involving direct trauma to the lung, the decision to perform a pneumonectomy may be made in the emergency room. Before scheduling a pneumonectomy, however, the surgeon reviews the patient's medical and surgical history and orders a number of tests to determine how successful the surgery is likely to be.

In the case of lung cancer, blood tests, a bone scan, and computed tomography scans of the head and abdomen indicate whether the cancer has spread beyond the lungs. **Positron emission tomography (PET)** scanning is also used to help stage the disease. Cardiac screening indicates how well the patient's heart will tolerate the procedure, and extensive pulmonary testing (e.g., breathing tests and quantitative ventilation/perfusion scans) predicts whether the remaining lung will be able to make up for the patient's diminished ability to breathe.

Preparation

A patient who smokes must stop as soon as a lung disease is diagnosed. Patients should not take **aspirin** or ibuprofen for seven to 10 days before surgery. Patients should also consult their physician about discontinuing any blood-thinning medications such as Coumadin or warfarin. The night before surgery, patients should not eat or drink anything after midnight.

Description

In a conventional pneumonectomy, the surgeon removes only the diseased lung itself. In a partial pneumonectomy, one or more lobes of a lung are removed. In an extrapleural pneumonectomy, the surgeon removes the lung, part of the membrane covering the heart (pericardium), part of the diaphragm, and the membrane lining the chest cavity (parietal pleura). Either operation is extensive, and require that the patient be given **general anesthesia**. An intravenous line inserted into one arm supplies fluids and medication throughout the operation, which usually lasts one to three hours.

The surgeon begins the operation by cutting a large opening on the same side of the chest as the diseased lung. This posterolateral **thoracotomy** incision extends from a point below the shoulder blade around the side of the patient's body along the curvature of the ribs at the front of the chest. Sometimes the surgeon removes part of the fifth rib in order to have a clearer view of the lung and greater ease in removing the diseased organ.

A surgeon performing a traditional pneumonectomy then:

- deflates (collapses) the diseased lung
- ties off the lung's major blood vessels to prevent bleeding into the chest cavity
- clamps the main bronchus to prevent fluid from entering the air passage
- cuts through the bronchus
- removes the lung
- staples or sutures the end of the bronchus that has been cut
- makes sure that air is not escaping from the bronchus
- inserts a temporary drainage tube between the layers of the pleura (pleural space) to draw air, fluid, and blood out of the surgical cavity
- closes the chest incision

Aftercare

Chest tubes drain fluid from the incision and a respirator helps the patient breathe for at least 24 hours after the operation. The patient may be fed and medicated intravenously. If no complications arise, the patient is transferred from the surgical **intensive care unit** to a regular hospital room within one to two days.

A patient who has had a conventional pneumonectomy will usually leave the hospital within 10 days. Aftercare during hospitalization is focused on:

- relieving pain
- monitoring the patient's blood oxygen levels
- encouraging the patient to walk in order to prevent formation of blood clots
- encouraging the patient to cough productively in order to clear accumulated lung secretions

If the patient cannot cough productively, the doctor uses a flexible tube (bronchoscope) to remove the lung secretions and fluids.

Recovery is usually a slow process, with the remaining lung gradually taking on the work of the lung that has been removed. The patient may gradually resume normal non-strenuous activities. A pneumonectomy patient who does not experience postoperative problems may be well enough within eight weeks to return to a job that is not physically demanding; however, 60% of all pneumonectomy patients continue to struggle with shortness of breath six months after having surgery.

Risks

The risks for any surgical procedure requiring anesthesia include reactions to the medications and breathing problems. The risks for any surgical procedure include bleeding and infection.

Between 40% and 60% of pneumonectomy patients experience such short-term postoperative difficulties as:

- prolonged need for a mechanical respirator
- abnormal heart rhythm (cardiac arrhythmia); heart attack (myocardial infarction); or other heart problem
- pneumonia
- infection at the site of the incision
- a blood clot in the remaining lung (pulmonary embolism)
- an abnormal connection between the stump of the cut bronchus and the pleural space due to a leak in the stump (bronchopleural fistula)
- accumulation of pus in the pleural space (empyema)
- kidney or other organ failure

Over time, the remaining organs in the patient's chest may move into the space left by the surgery. This condition is called postpneumonectomy syndrome; the surgeon can correct it by inserting a fluid-filled prosthesis into the space formerly occupied by the diseased lung.

Normal results

The doctor will probably advise the patient to refrain from strenuous activities for a few weeks after the operation. The patient's rib cage will remain sore for some time.

A patient whose lungs have been weakened by noncancerous diseases like emphysema or chronic bronchitis may experience long-term shortness of breath as a result of this surgery. On the other hand, a patient who develops a fever, chest pain, persistent cough, or shortness of breath, or whose incision bleeds or becomes inflamed, should notify his or her doctor immediately.

WHO PERFORMS THE SURGERY AND WHERE IS IT PERFORMED?

Pneumonectomies are performed in a hospital by a thoracic surgeon, who is a physician who specializes in chest, heart, and lung surgery. Thoracic surgeons may further specialize in one area, such as heart surgery or lung surgery. They are board-certified through the Board of Thoracic Surgery, which is recognized by the American Board of Medical Specialties. A doctor becomes board certified by completing training in a specialty area and passing a rigorous examination.

Morbidity and mortality rates

In the United States, the immediate survival rate from surgery for patients who have had the left lung removed is between 96% and 98%. Due to the greater risk of complications involving the stump of the cut bronchus in the right lung, between 88% and 90% of patients survive removal of this organ. Following lung volume reduction surgery, most investigators now report mortality rates of 5–9%.

Alternatives

Lung cancer

The treatment options for lung cancer are surgery, radiation therapy, and chemotherapy, either alone or in combination, depending on the stage of the cancer.

After the cancer is found and staged, the cancer care team discusses the treatment options with the patient. In choosing a treatment plan, the most significant factors to consider are the type of lung cancer (small cell or non-small cell) and the stage of the cancer. It is very important that the doctor order all the tests needed to determine the stage of the cancer. Other factors to consider include the patient's overall physical health; the likely side effects of the treatment; and the probability of curing the disease, extending the patient's life, or relieving his or her symptoms.

Chronic obstructive pulmonary disease

Although surgery is rarely used to treat COPD, it may be considered for people who have severe symptoms that have not improved with medication therapy. A significant number of patients with advanced COPD face a miserable existence and are at high risk of death, despite advances in medical technology. This

QUESTIONS TO ASK THE DOCTOR

- Why is it necessary to remove the whole lung?
- What benefits can I expect from a pneumonectomy?
- What are the risks of this operation?
- What are the normal results?
- How long will my recovery take?
- Are there any alternatives to this surgery?

group includes patients who remain symptomatic despite the following:

- smoking cessation
- use of inhaled bronchodilators
- treatment with antibiotics for acute bacterial infections, and inhaled or oral corticosteroids
- use of supplemental oxygen with rest or exertion
- pulmonary rehabilitation

After the severity of the patient's airflow obstruction has been evaluated, and the foregoing interventions implemented, a pulmonary disease specialist should examine him or her, with consideration given to surgical treatment.

Surgical options for treating COPD include laser therapy or the following procedures:

- Bullectomy. This procedure removes the part of the lung that has been damaged by the formation of large air-filled sacs called bullae.
- Lung volume reduction surgery. In this procedure, the surgeon removes a portion of one or both lungs, making room for the remaining lung tissue to work more efficiently. Its use is considered experimental, although it has been used in selected patients with severe emphysema.
- Lung transplant. In this procedure a healthy lung from a donor who has recently died is given to a person with COPD.

Resources

BOOKS

Argenziano, Michael, M.D., and Mark E. Ginsburg, M.D., eds. Lung Volume Reduction Surgery, 1st ed. Totowa, NJ: Humana Press, 2002.

Grann, Victor R., and Alfred I. Neugut. "Lung Cancer Screening at Any Price?" Journal of the American Medical Association289 (2003): 357-358.

Khatri, VP and JA Asensio. Operative Surgery Manual. 1st ed. Philadelphia: Saunders, 2003.

Mahadevia, Parthiv J., Lee A. Fleisher, Kevin D. Frick, et al. "Lung Cancer Screening with Helical Computed Tomography in Older Adult Smokers: A Decision and Cost-Effectiveness Analysis." Journal of the American Medical Association 289 (2003): 313-322.

Mason, RJ et al. Murray & Nadel's Textbook of Respiratory Medicine. 4th ed. Philadelphia: Saunders, 2007.

Pope, C. Arden III, Richard T. Burnett, Michael J. Thun, et al. "Lung Cancer, Cardiopulmonary Mortality, and Long-Term Exposure to Fine Particulate Air pollution." Journal of the American Medical Association287 (2002): 1132-1141.

Townsend, CM et al. Sabiston Textbook of Surgery. 17th ed. Philadelphia: Saunders, 2004.

ORGANIZATIONS

American Cancer Society. 1599 Clifton Road, N.E., Atlanta, GA 30329-4251. (800) 227-2345. www.cancer.org.

American Lung Association, National Office. 1740 Broadway, New York, NY 10019. (800) LUNG-USA. www.lungusa.org.

National Cancer Institute (NCI), Building 31, Room 10A03, 31 Center Drive, Bethesda, MD 20892-2580. Phone: (800) 4-CANCER. (301) 435-3848. www.nci.nih.gov.

National Comprehensive Cancer Network. 50 Huntingdon Pike, Suite 200, Rockledge, PA 19046. (215) 728-4788. Fax: (215) 728-3877. www.nccn.org/.

National Heart, Lung and Blood Institute (NHLBI). 6701 Rockledge Drive, P.O. Box 30105, Bethesda, MD 20824-0105. (301) 592-8573. www.nhlhi.nih.gov/.

OTHER

Aetna InteliHealth Inc. Lung Cancer. [cited May 17, 2003]. www.intelihealth.com..

American Cancer Society (ACS). Cancer Reference Information. <www3.cancer.org/cancerinfo>. [cited May 17, 2003].

Maureen Haggerty
Crystal H. Kaczkowski, M.Sc.
Rosalyn Carson-DeWitt, MD

Portacaval shunting *see* **Portal vein bypass**

Portal vein bypass

Definition

Portal vein bypass surgery diverts blood from the portal vein into another vein. It is performed when pressure in the portal vein is so high that it causes internal bleeding from blood vessels in the esophagus (the tube that brings food from the mouth to the stomach).

Purpose

The portal vein carries blood from the stomach and abdominal organs to the liver. It is a major vein that splits into many branches. In people with liver failure and cirrhosis, a chronic degenerative liver disease causing irreversible scarring of the liver, the liver is incapable of processing blood from the bowels. As a result, an abnormally high pressure develops in the veins that drain blood from the bowels as the body tries to form other channels for the blood to empty into the main circulation. These channels consist of fragile veins that surround the esophagus, stomach, or other areas of the digestive tract. Because of the fragility of these veins, they are prone to rupturing, which can result in massive amounts of bleeding. The abnormally high pressure within the veins draining into the liver, called portal hypertension, can also result in the formation of fluid seeping from the surface of the liver and collecting in large quantities in the abdominal cavity, a condition known as ascites.

Massive internal bleeding caused by portal hypertension occurs in about 40% of patients with cirrhosis. It is initially fatal in at least half of these patients. Patients who survive are likely to experience bleeding recurrence. Portal vein bypass, also called portacaval shunting, is performed on these surviving patients to control bleeding.

The purpose of portal vein bypass surgery is to lower portal hypertension by shunting blood away from the portal venous system and into the main venous system.

Demographics

Cirrhosis of the liver is caused by chronic liver disease. Common causes of chronic liver disease in the United States include hepatitis C infection and long-term alcohol abuse. Men and women are equally affected, but onset is earlier in men.

Description

Different portal vein bypass procedures are available. The surgery is usually performed under **general anesthesia**. The surgeon makes an abdominal incision and locates the portal vein. In portacaval shunting, blood from the portal vein is diverted into the inferior vena cava (one of the main veins leading back to the heart). This is the most common type of bypass. In splenorenal shunting, the splenic vein (a part of the portal vein) is connected to the renal (kidney) vein. A mesocaval shunt connects the superior mesenteric vein (another part of the portal vein) to the inferior vena cava.

Another procedure, called tranjugular intrahepatic portosystemic shunt (TIPS), has become the favored surgical approach. A TIPS is performed

Portal vein bypass (Portacaval shunt)

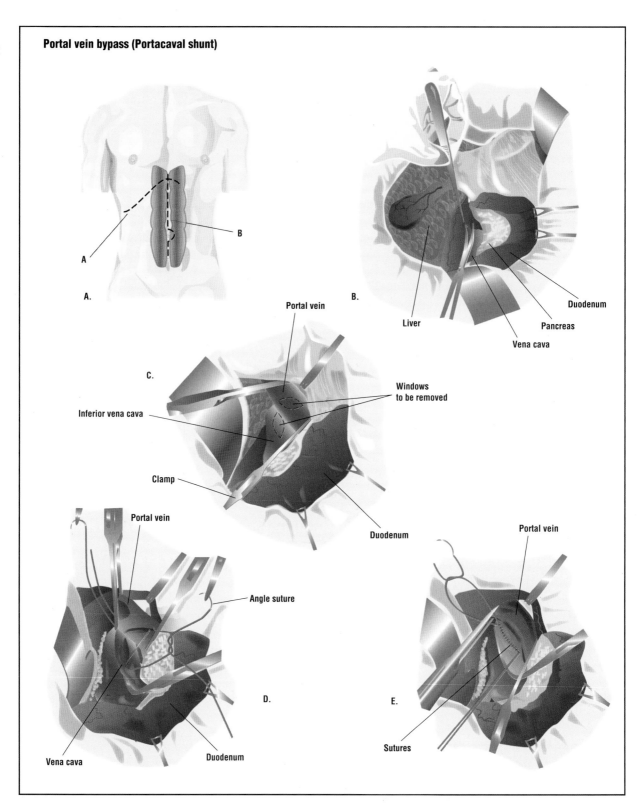

A.

B.

Liver

Duodenum

Pancreas

Vena cava

C.

Portal vein

Inferior vena cava

Windows
to be removed

Clamp

Duodenum

Portal vein

Angle suture

D.

E.

Portal vein

Vena cava

Duodenum

Sutures

Portal vein bypass can be achieved through one of two incisions (A). Once the abdomen is entered, the inferior vena cava is exposed (B). Further exposure reveals the portal vein. Both the portal vein and inferior vena cava are clamped (C). Windows are cut in both vessels (D), and the two are connected with sutures (E). *(Illustration by GGS Information Services. Cengage Learning, Gale.)*

KEY TERMS

Ascites—Fluid buildup in the abdominal cavity caused by fluid leaks from the surface of the liver and intestine.

Cirrhosis—A chronic degenerative liver disease causing irreversible scarring of the liver.

Inferior vena cava—A large vein that returns blood from the legs, pelvis, and abdomen to the heart.

Portal hypertension—Abnormally high pressure within the veins draining into the liver.

Portal vein—A large vein that carries blood from the stomach and intestines to the liver.

Varices—Uneven, permanent dilation of veins.

through a small nick in the skin, working through specialized instruments that are passed through the body using an x-ray camera for guidance. The TIPS procedure creates a shunt within the liver itself, by linking the portal vein with a vein draining away from the liver together with a device called a stent, which acts as a scaffold to support the connection between these two veins inside the liver.

Diagnosis/Preparation

A radiologist assesses patients for bypass surgery based on their medical history, **physical examination**, blood work, and liver imaging studies performed using computed tomography (CT) scans, ultrasounds, or **magnetic resonance imaging** (MRI) scans, and in consultation with the treating gastroenterologist, hepatologist, or surgeon.

Standard preoperative blood and urine tests are also performed. The heart and arterial blood pressure are monitored both during and after the operation.

Aftercare

The patient is connected to a heart monitor and fed through a nasogastric tube. Vital functions are monitored through blood and urine tests. Patients receive pain medication and **antibiotics**. Once released from the hospital, patients are expected to abstain from alcohol and to follow a diet and medication schedule designed to reduce the risks of bleeding.

Risks

Portal vein bypass surgery is high risk because it is performed on patients who are generally in poor

WHO PERFORMS THE PROCEDURE AND WHERE IS IT PERFORMED?

Portal vein bypass surgery is performed by a surgeon specialized in gastroenterology or hepatology in a hospital setting, very often as an emergency operation.

health. Those patients who survive the operation still face the risk of heart failure, brain disease due to a decrease in the liver's conversion of waste products (liver encephalopathy), hemorrhage, lung complications, infection, coma, and **death**.

Normal results

More than 90% of patients that undergo TIPS to prevent bleeding from varices will have a relief in their symptoms and experience little to no bleeding after surgery. When TIPS is performed for ascites, 60–80% of people will have relief in their ascites. The survival rate is directly related to the amount of liver damage patients have; the less damage, the more likely the patient is to recover. Cooperation with restrictions on alcohol and diet affect long-term survival.

Morbidity and mortality rates

Liver cirrhosis is a major medical problem worldwide and is associated with significant morbidity and mortality from its complications such as liver cell insufficiency and portal hypertension with ascites and gastrointestinal bleeding.

Alternatives

Before resorting to bypass surgery, physicians first attempt to treat portal hypertension with medications known as nonselective beta-blockers. These medications need to be taken daily to produce an effect and some patients may not be able to remain on beta-blocker therapy if they develop side effects. Other patients on beta-blocker therapy also remain at risk for bleeding from varices and from ascites.

Another approach is to seal off the veins to prevent rupturing. In sclerotherapy, a camera (endoscope) is passed down through the esophagus to inject the abnormal veins with substances that close them off. This can also be achieved with variceal band ligation, a procedure by which the abnormal veins are tied off with small rubber bands. Although sclerotherapy and variceal

QUESTIONS TO ASK THE
DOCTOR

• What are the possible complications involved in
  portal vein bypass surgery?
• Why is the surgery required?
• Are there any alternatives?
• What type of anesthesia will be used?
• How is the surgery performed?
• How long will I be in the hospital?
• How much portal vein bypass surgery do you
  perform in a year?

band ligation are very effective in targeting the abnormal and fragile veins around the esophagus, they do not lower the pressure of the blood inside the portal venous system. Thus, portal hypertension may still result in fluid accumulation inside the abdominal cavity, or in bleeding.

The best approach to relieve portal hypertension within a patient is by replacing their liver with a new one capable of filtering the blood. However, not many patients are suitable candidates for a liver transplant.

Resources

BOOKS

Feldman, M, et al.. Sleisenger & Fordtran's Gastrointestinal and Liver Disease. 8th ed. St. Louis: Mosby, 2005.

Khatri, VP and JA Asensio. Operative Surgery Manual. 1st ed. Philadelphia: Saunders, 2003.

Townsend, CM et al. Sabiston Textbook of Surgery. 17th ed. Philadelphia: Saunders, 2004.

PERIODICALS

Fuchs, J., et al. "Mesenterico-left Portal Vein Bypass in Children with Congenital Extrahepatic Portal Vein Thrombosis: A Unique Curative Approach." Journal of Pediatric Gastroenterology and Nutrition 36 (February 2003): 213–216.

ORGANIZATIONS

American College of Surgeons. 633 N. Saint Clair St., Chicago, IL 60611. (312) 202-5000. http://www.faacs.org.

Society for Vascular Surgery. 900 Cummings Center, Beverly, MA 01915-1314. (978) 927-8330. <http://svs.vasculaweb.org>.

OTHER

"Cirrhosis and Portal Hypertension." Family Doctor. <http://familydoctor.org/handouts/188.html>.

Tish Davidson, AM
Monique Laberge, PhD

Positron emission tomography (PET)

Definition

Positron emission tomography (PET) is a noninvasive scanning technique that utilizes small amounts of radioactive positrons (positively charged particles) to visualize body function and metabolism.

Purpose

PET is the fastest growing nuclear medicine tool in terms of increasing acceptance and applications. It is useful in the diagnosis, staging, and treatment of cancer because it provides information that cannot be obtained by other techniques such as computed tomography (CT) and **magnetic resonance imaging** (MRI).

PET scans are performed at medical centers equipped with a small cyclotron. Smaller cyclotrons and increasing availability of certain radiopharmaceuticals are making PET a more widely used imaging modality.

Physicians first used PET to obtain information about brain function, and to study brain activity in various neurological diseases and disorders including stroke, epilepsy, Alzheimer's disease, Parkinson's disease, and Huntington's disease; and in psychiatric disorders such as schizophrenia, depression, obsessive-compulsive disorder, attention deficit hyperactivity disorder (ADHD), and Tourette syndrome. PET is now used to evaluate patients for these cancers: head and neck, lymphoma, melanoma, lung, colorectal, breast, and esophageal. PET also is used to evaluate heart muscle function in patients with coronary artery disease or cardiomyopathy.

Description

PET involves injecting a patient with a radiopharmaceutical similar to glucose. An hour after injection of this tracer, a PET scanner images a specific metabolic function by measuring the concentration and distribution of the tracer throughout the body.

When it enters the body, the tracer courses through the bloodstream to the target organ, where it emits positrons. The positively charged positrons collide with negatively charged electrons, producing gamma rays. The gamma rays are detected by photomultiplier-scintillator combinations positioned on opposite sides of the patient. These signals are processed by the computer and images are generated.

Shreve, P. "Pitfalls in Oncologic Diagnosis with FDG PET Imaging: Physiologic and Benign Variants." *Radiographics* 62 (January/February 1999).

"Studies Argue for Wider Use of PET for Cancer Patients." *Cancer Weekly Plus* 15 (December 1997): 9.

OTHER

Di Carli, M. F. "Positron Emission Tomography (PET)." *1st Virtual Congress of Cardiology.* October 4, 1999. http://www.fac.org.

Madden Yee, Kate. "Start-up Enters Breast Imaging Arena with Scintimammography, PET Offerings." *Radiology News.* March 14, 2001. http://www.auntminnie.com.

"Nycomed Amersham and the Medical Research Council: Major Collaboration in World Leading Imaging Technology." *Medical Research Center* 2001. http://www.mrc.ac.uk/whats_new/press_releases/PR_2001/mrc_02_01.html.

Dan Harvey
Lee A. Shratter, M.D.

KEY TERMS

Electron—One of the small particles that make up an atom. An electron has the same mass and amount of charge as a positron, but the electron has a negative charge.

Gamma ray—A high-energy photon emitted by radioactive substances.

Half-life—The time required for half of the atoms in a radioactive substance to disintegrate.

Photon—A light particle.

Positron—One of the small particles that make up an atom. A positron has the same mass and amount of charge as an electron, but the positron has a positive charge.

PET provides an advantage over CT and MRI because it can determine if a lesion is malignant. The two other modalities provide images of anatomical structures, but often cannot provide a determination of malignancy. CT and MRI show structure, while PET shows function. PET has been used in combination with CT and MRI to identify abnormalities with more precision and indicate areas of most active metabolism. This additional information allows for more accurate evaluation of cancer treatment and management.

Resources

BOOKS

Bares, R., and G. Lucignani. *Clinical PET.* Kluwer Academic Publishers, 1996.

Gulyas, Balazs, and Hans Muller-Gartner. *Positron Emission Tomography: A Critical Assessment of Recent Trends.* Kluwer Academic Publishers, 1996.

Kevles, Bettyann Holtzmann. *Medical Imaging in the Twentieth Century.* Rutgers University Press, 1996.

PERIODICALS

"Brain Imaging and Psychiatry: Part 1." *Harvard Mental Health Letter* 13 (Jan. 1997): 1.

"Brain Imaging and Psychiatry: Part 2." *Harvard Mental Health Letter* 13 (February 1997): 1403.

Goerres, G. "Position Emission Tomography and PET CT of the Head and Neck: FDG Uptake in Normal Anatomy, in Benign Lesions, and Changes Resulting from Treatment." *American Journal of Roentgenology* (November 2002): 1337.

Kostakoglu, L. "Clinical Role of FDG PET in Evaluation of Cancer Patients." *Radiographics* (March-April 2003): 315.

Post-surgical infections

Definition

Post-surgical infections are any kind of infection that occurs in the immediate post-operative period. They are an extremely common complication of any type of surgical procedure, striking about 600,000 of the 30 million individuals who undergo surgery annually.

Description

A mnemonic called the three W's is often used to remember the most common targets of post-surgical infection:

- Wind—Infections of the respiratory system
- Water—Infections of the urinary system
- Wound—Infections involving the incision and surgical site

Other areas prone to infection after surgery include the intravenous site or the site of any other type of port.

There are several reasons why there is a high risk of respiratory infection following surgery:

- The use of **general anesthesia** suppresses the functioning of the mucociliary ladder, allowing mucus and organisms to accumulate
- Suppression of the gag reflex may allow aspiration of saliva into the respiratory tract

- Intubation may inadvertently introduce organisms into the respiratory tract
- Pain following surgery may interfere with an individual's ability to breathe deeply and to cough in order to clear their respiratory tract of excess secretions
- Pain medications further suppress an individual's tendency to breathe deeply

Respiratory infections usually manifest themselves through fever, cough, sputum production, shortness of breath, low blood oxygen. Suspected respiratory infections may be diagnosed through **chest x ray** and sputum culture.

Urinary tract infections are common because of the frequent use of a catheter during surgery, or through the post-operative period. **Post-surgical pain** and the side effects of anesthesia and pain medications may also result in urinary retention, requiring repeated in-and-out catheterization, increasing the risk of urinary tract infection.

Urinary tract infections usually manifest themselves through painful, frequent urine. Urine may appear bloody or cloudy. Suspected urinary tract infections may be diagnosed through **urinalysis** or **urine culture**.

About 2-5% of all surgical patients develop infections at the site of their operation. The following factors increase the risk of wound infection after surgery:

- Patient's age (elderly and newborns have higher risk)
- Weakened immune system
- Skin disease
- Malnutrition
- Co-existing diseases (such as diabetes, cancer)
- Operations involving areas that are already infected
- Transplants
- Implants
- Inadequate **bowel preparation**
- Lengthy surgery
- Use of drains
- Hemorrhage or hematoma during surgery
- Unintentional nick in bowel
- Use of blood transfusion
- Inappropriate use of **antibiotics**
- Poor sterile technique

Wound, incision, or surgical site infections usually manifest themselves as increased pain and tenderness at the site, redness, swelling, pus production, bleeding, and poor wound healing. Diagnosis is often made by swabbing the area and culturing the pus to identify the specific organism.

Antibiotics are chosen based on either presumptive knowledge of the most common type of organism to cause infection in a given post-surgical setting, or based on the results of cultures of infected material. Antibiotics may be given orally or intravenously, and multiple antibiotics may be required, depending on the organism types and the severity of the infection.

Resources

BOOKS

Cohen, J., et al. *Infectious Diseases.* 2nd ed. St. Louis: Mosby, 2004.
Gershon, A. A., et al. *Infectious Diseases of Children.* 11th ed. St. Louis: Mosby, 2004.
Khatri, V. P., and J. A. Asensio. *Operative Surgery Manual.* 1st ed. Philadelphia: Saunders, 2003.
Long, S. S., et al. *Principles and Practice of Pediatric Infectious Diseases.* 2nd ed. London: Churchill Livingstone, 2003.
Mandell, G. L., et al. *Principles and Practice of Infectious Diseases.* 6th ed. London: Churchill Livingstone, 2005.
Townsend, C. M., et al. *Sabiston Textbook of Surgery.* 17th ed. Philadelphia: Saunders, 2004.

Rosalyn Carson-DeWitt, MD

Post-surgical pain

Definition

Post-surgical pain is a complex response to tissue trauma during surgery that stimulates hypersensitivity of the central nervous system. The result is pain in areas not directly affected by the surgical procedure. Post-operative pain may be experienced by an inpatient or outpatient. It can be felt after any surgical procedure, whether it is minor dental surgery or a triple-bypass heart operation.

Purpose

Postoperative pain increases the possibility of post-surgical complications, raises the cost of medical care, and most importantly, interferes with recovery and return to normal activities of daily living. Management of post-surgical pain is a basic patient right. When pain is controlled or removed, a patient is better able to participate in activities such as walking or eating, which will encourage his or her recovery. Patients will also sleep better, which aids the healing process.

Description

Pain is recognized in two different forms: physiologic pain and clinical pain. Physiologic pain comes and goes, and is the result of experiencing a high-intensity sensation. It often acts as a safety mechanism to warn individuals of danger (e.g., a burn, animal scratch, or broken glass). Clinical pain, in contrast, is marked by hypersensitivity to painful stimuli around a localized site, and also is felt in non-injured areas nearby. When a patient undergoes surgery, tissues and nerve endings are traumatized, resulting in incision pain. This trauma overloads the pain receptors that send messages to the spinal cord, which becomes overstimulated. The resultant central sensitization is a type of posttraumatic stress to the spinal cord, which interprets any stimulation—painful or otherwise—as unpleasant. That is why a patient may feel pain in movement or physical touch in locations far from the surgical site.

Patients handle post-operative pain in highly individualized ways. Health care professionals have observed that some patients report that they are in extreme pain after surgery, demanding large doses of pain medications while others seem to do well with much less medication. Several theories have been put forth to account for this discrepancy. For example, differences in body size seemed to require differing amounts of medication, but this theory did not explain differences in pain perception among patients of the same build. Emotional well-being was considered a better indicator of the ability to tolerate pain. It has been theorized that patients with stronger support systems and better attitudes actually perceive less pain than others. Some health care professionals have even speculated that extreme pain was not real in many cases, but was a way to seek attention.

Clear biological evidence proving that individuals are born with varying thresholds of pain perception was only recently discovered. Psychiatrist and radiologist Jon-Kar Zubieta, from the Mental Health Research Institute at the University of Michigan, found that variations in an amino acid in a newly discovered gene, which codes for an enzyme that accesses neurotransmitters in the brain, produce different levels of pain perception. Only three combinations produce the variation. One individual may be able to fully access and metabolize the opioid neurotransmitters that reduce the sensation of pain. This person would have a higher threshold of pain tolerance and a lower level of pain perception. Another might not be able to do so at all, and that individual would experience more intense pain from the same stimulus. A third person might be able to tolerate a moderate amount of pain.

KEY TERMS

Epidural catheter—A thin plastic tube, through which pain medication is delivered, inserted into the patient's back before surgery.

Intubation—Placing a tube in the patient's airway to maintain adequate oxygen intake.

Opioids—Narcotic pain medications.

NSAIDs—Nonsteroidal anti-inflammatory drugs, popular over-the-counter pain relievers.

Patient-controlled analgesia (PCA)—The patient administers a dose of pain medication by pressing a button on a pump, which delivers the medication through a tube attached to either an IV or an epidural catheter.

Subcutaneous—Under the skin.

This variation in genes not only shows that individuals do indeed experience pain at different levels, but it also points to differences in how people behave toward other stressors. Genetic variation may be a factor in the impact of long-term illness and depression that often accompanies chronic pain.

Since pain perception is highly subjective, it is important for the health care team to be aware of pain sensitivity differences in patients, and to value patient self-reports as reliable tools for pain assessment. The most common self-report system in use is the pain intensity scale. The patient is asked to identify where the pain falls on a scale of 0 "no pain at all" to 10 "the worst pain in the world." This scale, however, does have limitations. The Short-Form McGill Questionnaire, which uses sensory words or synonyms, may allow the patient to communicate more accurate, descriptive information about pain and may be a better tool in planning **pain management** strategies.

It is clear that there is a real need for providing different approaches to post-surgical pain management. A variety of interventions may be used before, during, and after surgery. Most of these methods involve medications given orally, intravenously, intramuscularly, or topically (via the skin). Some must be administered by a health care professional, others can be administered by the patient.

Pain management methods

Presurgery pain management

The goal of post-surgical pain management is to reduce the amount pain a patient experiences after surgery. New research has suggested that preventing the nervous system from being overtaxed by pain from the trauma of surgery may lead to a less painful postoperative experience. Pretreated patients may require less post-surgical medications, and they may recover more quickly, possibly experiencing pain-free days far sooner than patients who have used traditional post-surgical pain methods.

Also, in view of improved, less-invasive surgical techniques and the insurance industry's attempts to trim rising medical costs by reducing the length of hospital stays, many patients have no longer been required to remain in the hospital overnight after a surgery. Recently, outpatient (also called ambulatory) surgery has become the procedure of choice for many complex surgeries, such as **hysterectomy** and prostatectomy. After ambulatory surgery the must be made comfortable enough to return home and given tools to manage his or her own pain.

Preemptive analgesia introduces anesthetic drugs near the spinal cord or, sometimes, in nerve blocks in specific regions of the body. An epidural catheter, a thin plastic tube through which pain medication is delivered, is inserted into the patient's back before surgery. The patient may also receive **general anesthesia** and post-surgical pain medications as needed. Sometimes, the epidural catheter remains in place for several hours or days after surgery, and is attached to a pump so the patient can administer medication on demand.

In other cases, peripheral nerve blocks are used to limit sensation in specific regions of the body. By injecting local anesthetic near a nerve or nerve plexus that supplies the area where the surgery will be performed, all sensation is blunted and the affected area is numbed and feels "asleep." Some patients remain awake, but sedated, during surgery; others are given general anesthesia. Two important advantages to the use of peripheral nerve blocks in patients who are awake during surgery is the avoidance of the side effects of general anesthesia (nausea and vomiting) and complications that could occur during intubation, the placement of a tube in the patient's airway. The use of peripheral nerve blocks alone may be best suited to surgical procedures involving the arms, legs, and shoulders.

Pain management during surgery

General anesthesia is the standard for pain management during surgery. Topical local anesthetics are also sometimes used to numb the surgical site before any incisions are made. This is the method used frequently with laparoscopic procedures. In a **laparoscopy**, the surgeon inserts a laparascope (an instrument that has a tiny video camera attached) through a small incision. Other small incisions are made into which the surgeon inserts **surgical instruments**, and in this way the surgeon repairs or removes diseased or damaged tissues. Local anesthetics minimize pain trauma to the surgical site and the central nervous system.

Post-surgery pain management

In most hospitals during the past century, post-surgical pain management consisted only of the administration of **analgesics** and narcotics immediately after surgery. These drugs were usually given by intravenous or intramuscular injection, or by mouth. This is still the most common method for managing post-operative pain.

Management of these drugs, nevertheless, has variant applications. Some hospitals insist on a routine of scheduled medications, rather than giving medications as needed. The health care staff in these instances state that when patients take medications before the pain appears, the body does not over-react to the pain stimulus. Therefore, staying ahead of the pain is critical.

Other hospitals advocate continuous around-the-clock dosing through the use of a pump-type device that immediately delivers medication into the veins (intravenously, the most common method), under the skin (subcutaneously), or between the dura mater and the skull (epidurally). A health care provider programs the device with the specific dosage to deliver at each request made by the patient, as well as the total permitted during the time for which the device is set (commonly eight hours, sometimes 12, especially if the health care providers are working 12-hour shifts). Some of these devices are very sophisticated and even monitor themselves, ringing an alarm bell if there is an indication that they might be malfunctioning. The patient administers the dose by pushing a button, and is encouraged to keep a steady supply of medication within his or her system. This is called **patient-controlled analgesia** (PCA).

PCA provides pain medication at the patient's need. However, because opium-like pain-relievers (opioids) are the medications these pumps deliver, there has been some concern about possible narcotic addiction. The pumps are calibrated to a maximum dosage, and are limited to a maximum dose every eight (or twelve) hours. The health care staff checks the equipment regularly, and records the number of times the patient pushed the pump button during the previous period. If the patient has pushed the button more times than allowed, the pump refuses to administer more medication. The patient should notify the health care staff if a specific medication is ineffective. In some cases, the patient needs encouragement to use the pump more, if necessary.

Nonsteroid anti-inflammatory analgesics (NSAIDs) are best used for continuous around-the-clock pain relief. This prevents the extremes in pain perception that occur with on-demand dosing; sometimes the patient feels no pain and extreme pain at other times. Opioids are best given on a schedule or in a computerized pump, which can prevent overdoses.

Another method used post-surgically is the On-Q or the "pain relief ball." It is a balloon-type device that administers non-narcotic medication to the incision site through a small catheter. When the incision site is closed, the catheter is attached to the surgical site and the balloon or pump is either taped to the patient's skin, carried in a pocket or pouch, or attached to the patient's clothing. The pump numbs the incision site by flooding it with anesthetic. Recent tests show that On-Q reduces narcotic use by 40% in cesarean patients, and eliminates all narcotics in 43% of hysterectomy patients.

Alternative non-medical methods

Some non-medical methods can help reduce postoperative pain. Patient education about the surgical procedure and the expected after-care necessary can help reduce stress, which can affect the perception of pain. Education, like visualization, prepares the mind for surgery and recovery. The patient knows what to expect, thereby removing fear of the unknown. Education also enlists the patient's cooperation and may encourage a feeling of control and empowerment, which reduces stress, fear, and helplessness. These factors can contribute to less perceived pain. Therefore, both education and visualization can be helpful in minimizing pain perception and encouraging a positive attitude after surgery, which can promote healing.

Meditation and deep breathing techniques also can reduce stress. These techniques can lower blood pressure and increase oxygen levels, which are critical to a healthy recovery. Hypnosis before and after surgery may calm the mind and emotions, and mute the perception of pain.

Multiple methods

Multimodal analgesia uses more than one method of pain management. Multiple methods can actually reduce the amount of medications necessary to relieve pain, and can minimize uncomfortable side effects. Using presurgical, surgical, and post-surgical techniques allows the patient to come out of surgery with the pain already under control. He or she does not have to experience the shock of intense pain at the incision site or elsewhere in the body. Some pain is probable; however, a patient should not be in intense pain after surgery. Pain management should occur before pain appears rather than in reaction to pain.

Further knowledge about multimodal pain management will be necessary as more outpatient and office-based surgery is done. Finding the right combination of methods for an individual patient is the challenge and responsibility of the health care team.

Opioid-tolerant patients

Of great concern to health-care professionals is how to provide post-operative pain management to patients who are opioid tolerant. These patients require higher and more frequent doses of narcotics for pain relief. They may also need to stay on the narcotics longer, and gradually step back down to their presurgery levels.

Patients who are opioid tolerant are not necessarily illegal drug users, but may be taking medications in combination with a narcotic, such as oxycodone/acetaminophen or acetaminophen/codeine. Patients who take opioid medications regularly may be treating pain for conditions like cancer, fibromyalgia, arthritis, or traumatic physical injuries.

It is important for anesthesiologists to aggressively treat pain for opioid-tolerant patients in the **recovery room**, where they can be closely monitored. Patient-controlled pain administration or continuous infusion, either in an IV or in an epidural catheter, has the best chance of controlling post-surgical pain together with the pain caused by preexisting conditions. When the patient is able to take medications orally, NSAIDs can supplement the use of opioid analgesia, sometimes reducing the total amount of opioids used. Newer, COX-2 inhibitors have proven effective in reducing pain without many of the side effects that NSAIDs possess (liver complications, kidney impairment, intestinal tract irritation, and bleeding), and seem to be a good fit for many opioid-tolerant patients.

Preparation

Before having any surgery, the patient should talk with the physician, surgeon, and if possible, the anesthesiologist in order to gain a full understanding of the procedure and what to expect immediately following surgery. It is important to develop a pain management plan with the health care team, and for the patient to be open about medication use, including opioids. Usually the patient will meet the anesthesiologist the day of the surgery to discuss pain management options for the operation. Being informed about the surgical procedure and anesthesia options will give the patient an opportunity to ask questions and respond accurately to those asked by the anesthesiologist.

The physician should take a complete medical history, and order tests to determine the patient's current liver and kidney functions. The patient should not eat or drink before surgery. This helps minimize the side effects of general anesthesia and pain medications, such as nausea and vomiting. If the patient cannot reach a comfort level with the prescribed medication regime, he or she should discuss this with the health-care staff and physician.

Normal results

After surgery, a patient should not have to endure severe pain. A reasonable comfort level can be reached in most cases. Prudent pain management will allow the patient to eat, sleep, move, and begin doing normal activities even while in the hospital, and especially when returning home. Recovery may take several weeks after surgery; however, the patient should be made comfortable as possible with a regime of oral pain medications.

Risks

Pain medications may have unpleasant side effects. In many people, narcotics cause nausea, vomiting, and impaired mental functioning. NSAIDs can cause kidney failure, intestinal bleeding, and liver dysfunction, although these side-effects are not common with short-term use. The NSAID ketorolac has been associated with acute renal (kidney) failure even when given for minor oral surgery in an outpatient setting. Early screening for kidney problems and close monitoring for kidney failure or dehydration can prevent most of these problems.

There are adequate safeguards in place, especially in patient-controlled analgesic pumps, to prevent addiction to narcotics; however, some patients do become addicted.

Resources

BOOKS

Brunicardi, F. Charles et al, eds. *Schwartz's Principles of Surgery*, 8th Ed. New York: McGraw-Hill, Health Pub. Division, 2005.

Hatfield, Anthea and Michael Tronson. *The Complete Recovery Room Book*, 3rd Ed. New York: Oxford University Press, 2002.

Rawlinson, Nigel and Derek Alderson. *Surgery: Diagnosis and Management*, 4th Ed. Malden, MA: Blackwell Pub., 2009.

PERIODICALS

"Many Think the Worst Part of Recovering from Surgery is Getting Over the General Anaesthetic." *British Medical Journal* 328.7443 (April 3, 2004): 844-845.

Doering, Lynn V., Anthony W. McGuire and Darlene Rourke. "Recovering from Cardiac Surgery: What Patients Want You to Know." *American Journal of Critical Care* 11.4 (July 2002): 333-344.

Hume, Susan. "Six Tips for Hospital Survival." *The Exceptional Parent* 37.8 (August 2007): 35-37.

ORGANIZATIONS

American Association of Nurse Anesthetists (AANA). 222 S. Prospect Ave., Park Ridge, IL 60068-4001. (847) 692-7050. www.aana.com.

Association of Perioperative Registered Nurses (AORN). 2170 S. Parker Rd., Suite 300, Denver, CO 80231. (800) 755-2676 or (303) 755-6304. www.aorn.org.

Janie Franz
Robert Bockstiegel

Postoperative care

Definition

Postoperative care is the management of a patient after surgery. This includes care given during the immediate postoperative period, both in the **operating room** and postanesthesia care unit (PACU), as well as during the days following surgery.

Purpose

The goal of postoperative care is to prevent complications such as infection, to promote healing of the surgical incision, and to return the patient to a state of health.

Description

Postoperative care involves assessment, diagnosis, planning, intervention, and outcome evaluation. The extent of postoperative care required depends on the individual's presurgical health status, type of surgery, and whether the surgery was performed in a day-surgery setting or in the hospital. Patients who have procedures done in a day-surgery center usually require only a few hours of care by health care professionals before they are discharged to go home. If postanesthesia or postoperative complications occur within these hours, the patient must be admitted to the hospital. Patients who are admitted to the hospital may require days or weeks of postoperative care by hospital staff before they are discharged.

Postanesthesia care unit (PACU)

The patient is transferred to the PACU after the surgical procedure, anesthesia reversal, and extubation (if it was necessary). The amount of time the patient spends in the PACU depends on the length of surgery, type of surgery, status of regional anesthesia (e.g., spinal anesthesia), and the patient's level of consciousness. Rather than being sent to the PACU, some patients may be transferred directly to the critical care unit. For example, patients who have had coronary artery bypass grafting are sent directly to the critical care unit.

In the PACU, the anesthesiologist or the nurse anesthetist reports on the patient's condition, type of surgery performed, type of anesthesia given, estimated blood loss, and total input of fluids and output of urine during surgery. The PACU nurse should also be made aware of any complications during surgery, including variations in hemodynamic (blood circulation) stability.

Assessment of the patient's airway patency (openness of the airway), **vital signs**, and level of consciousness are the first priorities upon admission to the PACU. The following is a list of other assessment categories:

- surgical site (intact dressings with no signs of overt bleeding)
- patency (proper opening) of drainage tubes/drains
- body temperature (hypothermia/hyperthermia)
- patency/rate of intravenous (IV) fluids
- circulation/sensation in extremities after vascular or orthopedic surgery
- level of sensation after regional anesthesia
- pain status
- nausea/vomiting

The patient is discharged from the PACU when he or she meets established criteria for discharge, as determined by a scale. One example is the Aldrete scale, which scores the patient's mobility, respiratory status, circulation, consciousness, and pulse oximetry. Depending on the type of surgery and the patient's condition, the patient may be admitted to either a general surgical floor or the **intensive care unit**. Since the patient may still be sedated from anesthesia, safety is a primary goal. The patient's call light should be in the hand and side rails up. Patients in a day surgery setting are either discharged from the PACU to the unit, or are directly discharged home after they

---

KEY TERMS

Ambulate—To move from place to place (walk).

Auscultation—The act of listening to sounds arising within organs as an aid to diagnosis and treatment.

Catheter—A tubular medical device inserted into canals, vessels, passageways, or body cavities to permit injection or withdrawal of fluids, or to keep a passage open.

Deep vein thrombosis—Potentially life-threatening blood clot in one of the deep veins of the body, and often in the legs secondary to immobility after surgery. Symptoms include pain, warmth, swelling, and redness.

Dehiscence— Separation of a surgical incision or rupture of a wound closure.

Ileus—Obstruction in or immobility of the intestines. Symptoms include nausea and vomiting, absent bowel sounds, abdominal pain, and abdominal distension.

Incentive spirometer—Device that is used postoperatively to prevent lung collapse and promote maximum inspiration. The patient inhales until a preset volume is reached, then sustains the volume by holding his or her breath for three to five seconds.

Oximetry—Measuring the degree of oxygen saturation of circulating blood.

PACU—The postanesthesia care unit, where the patient is cared for after surgery.

Patency—The quality or state of being open or unobstructed.

Patient-controlled analgesia pump—A pump that the patient uses to self-administer medication to control pain.

Pulmonary embolism—Potentially life-threatening blockage of a pulmonary artery by fat, air, or a blood clot that originated elsewhere in the body. Symptoms include acute shortness of breath and sudden chest pain.

---

have urinated, gotten out of bed, and tolerated a small amount of oral intake.

First 24 hours

After the hospitalized patient transfers from the PACU, the nurse taking over his or her care should assess the patient again, using the same previously mentioned categories. If the patient reports "hearing" or feeling pain during surgery (under anesthesia) the observation should not be discounted. The anesthesiologist or nurse anesthetist should discuss the possibility of an episode of awareness under anesthesia with the patient. Vital signs, respiratory status, pain status, the incision, and any drainage tubes should be monitored every one to two hours for at least the first eight hours. **Body temperature** must be monitored, since patients are often hypothermic after surgery, and may need a warming blanket or warmed IV fluids. Respiratory status should be assessed frequently, including assessment of lung sounds (auscultation) and chest excursion, and presence of an adequate cough. Fluid intake and urine output should be monitored every one to two hours. If the patient does not have a urinary catheter, the bladder should be assessed for distension, and the patient monitored for inability to urinate. The physician should be notified if the patient has not urinated six to eight hours after surgery. If the patient had a vascular or neurological procedure performed, circulatory status or neurological status should be assessed as ordered by the surgeon, usually every one to two hours. The patient may require medication for nausea or vomiting, as well as pain.

Patients with a **patient-controlled analgesia** pump may need to be reminded how to use it. If the patient is too sedated immediately after the surgery, the nurse may push the button to deliver pain medication. The patient should be asked to rate his or her pain level on a pain scale in order to determine his or her acceptable level of pain. Controlling pain is crucial so that the patient may perform coughing, deep breathing exercises, and may be able to turn in bed, sit up, and, eventually, walk.

Effective preoperative teaching has a positive impact on the first 24 hours after surgery. If patients understand that they must perform respiratory exercises to prevent pneumonia; and that movement is imperative for preventing blood clots, encouraging circulation to the extremities, and keeping the lungs clear; they will be much more likely to perform these tasks. Understanding the need for movement and respiratory exercises also underscores the importance of keeping pain under control. Respiratory exercises (coughing, deep breathing, and incentive spirometry) should be done every two hours. The patient should be turned every two hours, and should at least be sitting on the edge of the bed by eight hours after surgery, unless contraindicated (e.g., after **hip replacement**). Patients who are not able to sit up in bed due to their surgery will have sequential compression devices on their legs until they are able to move about. These are stockings that inflate with air in order to simulate the effect of walking on the calf muscles, and return blood to the heart. The patient should be encouraged to splint any chest and abdominal incisions with a pillow to decrease the pain caused by coughing and moving. Patients should be kept NPO (nothing by mouth) if ordered by the surgeon, at least until their cough and gag reflexes have returned. Patients often have a dry mouth following surgery, which can be relieved with oral sponges dipped in ice water or lemon ginger mouth swabs.

Patients who are discharged home after a day surgery procedure are given prescriptions for their pain medications, and are responsible for their own pain control and respiratory exercises. Their families (or caregivers) should be included in preoperative teaching so that they can assist the patient at home. The patient should be reminded to call his or her physician if any complications or uncontrolled pain arise. These patients are often managed at home on a follow-up basis by a hospital-connected visiting nurse or **home care** service.

After 24 hours

After the initial 24 hours, vital signs can be monitored every four to eight hours if the patient is stable. The incision and dressing should be monitored for the amount of drainage and signs of infection. The surgeon may order a dressing change during the first postoperative day; this should be done using sterile technique. For home-care patients this technique must be emphasized.

The hospitalized patient should be sitting up in a chair at the bedside and ambulating (walking) with assistance by this time. Respiratory exercises are still be performed every two hours, and incentive spirometry values should improve. Bowel sounds are monitored, and the patient's diet gradually increased as tolerated, depending on the type of surgery and the physician's orders.

The patient should be monitored for any evidence of potential complications, such as leg edema, redness, and pain (deep vein thrombosis), shortness of breath (pulmonary embolism), dehiscence (separation) of the incision, or ileus (intestinal obstruction). The surgeon should be notified immediately if any of these occur. If dehiscence occurs, sterile saline-soaked dressing packs should be placed on the wound.

Preparation

Patients receive a great deal of information on postoperative care. They may be offered pain medication in preparation for any procedure that is likely to cause discomfort. Patients may receive educational materials such as handouts and video tapes, so that they will have a clear understanding of what to expect postoperatively.

Aftercare

Aftercare includes ensuring that patients are comfortable, either in bed or chair, and that they have their call lights accessible. After dressing changes, blood-soaked **dressings** should be properly disposed of in a biohazard container. Pain medication should be offered before any procedure that might cause discomfort. Patients should be given the opportunity to ask questions. In some cases, they may ask the nurse to demonstrate certain techniques so that they can perform them properly once they return home.

Normal results

The goal of postoperative care is to ensure that patients have good outcomes after surgical procedures. A good outcome includes recovery without complications and adequate **pain management**. Another objective of postoperative care is to assist patients in taking responsibility for regaining optimum health.

Resources

BOOKS

Khatri, VP and JA Asensio. Operative Surgery Manual. 1st ed. Philadelphia: Saunders, 2003.

Townsend, CM et al. Sabiston Textbook of Surgery. 17th ed. Philadelphia: Saunders, 2004.

PERIODICALS

Barone, C.P., M. L. Lightfoot, and G. W. Barone. "The Postanesthesia Care of an Adult Renal Transplant Recipient." Journal of PeriAnesthesia Nursing 18, no.1 (February 2003): 32-41.

Smykowski, L., and W. Rodriguez. "The Post Anesthesia Care Unit Experience: A Family-centered Approach." Journal of Nursing Care Quality 18, no. 1 (January-March 2003): 5-15.

Wills, L. "Managing Change Through Audit: Post-operative Pain in Ambulatory Care." Paediatric Nursing 14, no.9 (November 2002): 35-8.

ORGANIZATIONS

National Institutes of Health. 9000 Rockville Pike, Bethesda, MD 20892. (301) 496-4000. Email: NIHInfo @OD.NIH.GOV. http://www.nih.gov/

Abby Wojahn, R.N., B.S.N, C.C.R.N.
Crystal H. Kaczkowski, MSc.
Rosalyn Carson-DeWitt, MD

Potassium test *see* **Electrolyte tests**

Power of attorney

Definition

Power of attorney, also known as durable medical power of attorney, is a legal mechanism that empowers a designated person to make medical decisions for a patient should the patient be unable to make the decisions due to incapacitation.

Purpose

Power of attorney assures that a patient's wishes are acknowledged in the medical setting. Along with other legal documents such as a **living will** and a **do not resuscitate (DNR) order**, the power of attorney designates the agent or person who is legally authorized to act for the patient in the medical setting. All three mechanisms are a part of what is known as advanced medical directives. The purpose of advanced directives is to have the patient's wishes for medical care carried out even when the patient is incapacitated and can no longer make his or her wishes known.

Description

The patient's agent is the person appointed by the patient to represent him or her in medical situations where decisions must be made. This surrogate, through the power of attorney authorization, has all of the rights that the patient has with respect to deciding on medical procedures. These include the rights to refuse treatment, to agree to treatment, or to have treatment withdrawn.

Guided by a living will, which is a document developed in advance that reflects the patient's wishes, the agent acts on behalf of the patient with providers, administrators, and other legal agents. In most states, surrogates can act for the patient on any medical procedure, including a decision to refuse life support procedures such as resuscitation. States differ, however, on whether health agents can invoke a **DNR order**.

In the difficult times that families experience with a seriously ill or terminally ill family member, health agents play a major role in making decisions and stipulating what the patient's wishes are with respect to his or her treatment or palliative care needs. Health agents can work with or without a living will. The crucial feature of the power of attorney is that it empowers the patient's agent to respond to changes in the patient's health and to make flexible decisions. It is the health agent, rather than the patient, who must be apprised of all medical options, weigh the risk and benefits, and make a decision based on the specific situation.

KEY TERMS

Advanced medical directives—Documents prepared in advance of medical care that reflect the wishes of patients for or against medical procedures should they become incapacitated.

Health care agent—Also known as the surrogate or patient representative, this is the person who has power of attorney to have the patient's wishes carried out if the patient is incapacitated.

Living will—A document that is usually included in advanced medical directives containing explicit medical procedures that patients' wishes to have or to refuse should they become incapacitated.

Preparation

The person who has the medical power of attorney for a patient is only as good as his or her level of understanding of the patient and level of respect for the patient's wishes. There are some specific steps that can be taken to prepare the health care agent for power of attorney responsibilities. These steps include:

- The patient must think about medical treatments he or she would or would not like to have in different medical situations such as accidents, acute and life-threatening injuries, nursing home care, etc.

- If possible, the patient should write down his or her medical wishes and have these developed into a living will.

- The patient will want to convey these medical wishes to family and friends, as well as the identity of the person who will have power of attorney.

- Whether a written document is drafted or not, it is important that the patient have discussions with the designated agent so that his or her wishes can be carried out if the need arises. Not all elements of the medical decisions required can be known in advance. Hence, it is very important that the health agent knows the patient, knows the patient's wishes and rationale, and understands fully what is of value to the patient. Family and health providers should also be informed of the patient's wishes.

Medical decisions likely to be faced in severe health emergencies include options for **cardiopulmonary resuscitation** (CPR), diagnostic tests, administration of drugs, surgery, the use of life-supporting technologies, and organ and tissue use. However, there are also other decisions that can may require decisions from the agent. These may include family members, and how much say they will have in decision making, issues of visitation, and other issues only somewhat related to the medical care. It is important that the agent understand and honor the wishes of the patient in all of these areas.

Once the initial steps for the advanced instructions are in place, an official medical power of attorney form for the state of residence or health care must be filled out. These may be two different states. It is important to have a medical power of attorney for any and all states in which medical care might be provided.

Normal results

All medical directives, whether the living will, power of attorney, or **do not resuscitate order**, are respected by all health personnel in whatever medical setting the chosen state stipulates. These generally include hospitals, emergency rooms, emergency vehicles, and short- or long-term care facilities such as **hospice** care. Many states also include the home. The medical directives become a part of the patient's medical record and must be honored by any and all health personnel involved in the patient's treatment or care.

Resources

BOOKS

Cebuhar, Jo Kline. *Last Things First, Just in Case... : the Practical Guide to Living Wills and Durable Powers of Attorney for Health Care.* West Des Moines, IA: Murphy Pub., 2006.

Doukas, David John and William Reichel. *Planning for Uncertainty: Living Wills and Other Advance Directives for You and Your Family*, 2nd Ed. Baltimore, MD: Johns Hopkins University Press, 2007.

Haman, Edward A. *Power of Attorney Handbook*, 5th Ed. Naperville, IL: Sphinx Pub., 2004.

PERIODICALS

"Make Medical and Financial Preparations." *USA Today* 136.2749 (Oct 2007): 11-12.

Stephenson, Correy E. "Caution: Use Power of Attorney Wisely." *Minnesota Lawyer* (Jan 21, 2008).

Nancy McKenzie, PhD
Robert Bockstiegel

Prednisone *see* **Corticosteroids**

Preoperative autologous blood donation *see* Autologous **blood donation**

Preoperative care

Definition

Preoperative care is the preparation and management of a patient prior to surgery. It includes both physical and psychological preparation.

Purpose

Patients who are physically and psychologically prepared for surgery tend to have better surgical outcomes. Preoperative teaching meets the patient's need for information regarding the surgical experience, which in turn may alleviate most of his or her fears. Patients who are more knowledgeable about what to expect after surgery, and who have an opportunity to express their goals and opinions, often cope better with postoperative pain and decreased mobility. Preoperative care is extremely important prior to any invasive procedure, regardless of whether the procedure is minimally invasive or a form of major surgery.

Preoperative teaching must be individualized for each patient. Some people want as much information as possible, while others prefer only minimal information because too much knowledge may increase their anxiety. Patients have different abilities to comprehend medical procedures; some prefer printed information, while others learn more from oral presentations. It is important for the patient to ask questions during preoperative teaching sessions.

Description

Preoperative care involves many components, and may be done the day before surgery in the hospital, or during the weeks before surgery on an outpatient basis. Many surgical procedures are now performed in a day surgery setting, and the patient is never admitted to the hospital.

Physical preparation

Physical preparation may consist of a complete medical history and physical exam, including the patient's surgical and anesthesia background. The patient should inform the physician and hospital staff if he or she has ever had an adverse reaction to anesthesia (such as anaphylactic shock), or if there is a family history of malignant hyperthermia. Laboratory tests may include **complete blood count**, electrolytes, **prothrombin time**, activated **partial thromboplastin time**, and **urinalysis**. The patient will most likely have an **electrocardiogram** (EKG) if he or she has a history of cardiac disease, or is over 50 years of age. A

KEY TERMS

Activated partial thromboplastin time (APTT)—A lab test that detects coagulation defects in the intrinsic clotting cascade. Used to regulate heparin dosing.

Ambulate—Move from place to place (walk).

Anaphylactic shock—A systemic reaction that is often severe and occasionally fatal due to a second exposure to a specific antigen (i.e., wasp venom or penicillin) after previous sensitization that results in symptoms (particularly respiratory symptoms, fainting, itching, and hives).

Anesthesia—A safe and effective means of alleviating pain during a medical procedure.

Complete blood count (CBC)—A lab test that determines the number of red and white blood cells per cubic millimeter of blood.

Electrocardiogram (EKG)—A graphic record showing the electrical activity of the heart.

Incentive spirometer—Device that is used postoperatively to prevent lung collapse and promote maximum inspiration. The patient inhales until a preset volume is reached, then sustains the volume by holding the breath for three to five seconds.

Patient-controlled analgesia pump—A pump that the patient uses to self-administer medication to control pain.

Prothrombin time (PT)—A lab test that detects coagulation defects in the extrinsic clotting cascade. Used to regulate coumadin dosing.

chest x ray is done if the patient has a history of respiratory disease. Part of the preparation includes assessment for risk factors that might impair healing, such as nutritional deficiencies, steroid use, radiation or chemotherapy, drug or alcohol abuse, or metabolic diseases such as diabetes. The patient should also provide a list of all medications, vitamins, and herbal or food supplements that he or she uses. Supplements are often overlooked, but may cause adverse effects when used with general anesthetics (e.g., St. John's wort, valerian root). Some supplements can prolong bleeding time (e.g., garlic, gingko biloba).

Latex allergy has become a public health concern. Latex is found in most sterile surgical gloves, and is a common component in other medical supplies including **general anesthesia** masks, tubing, and multi-dose medication vials. It is estimated that 1–6% of the

---

general population and 8–17% of health care workers have this allergy. Children with disabilities are particularly susceptible. This includes children with spina bifida, congenital urological abnormalities, cerebral palsy, and Dandy-Walker syndrome. At least 50% of children with spina bifida are latex-sensitive as a result of early, frequent surgical exposure. There is currently no cure available for latex allergy, and research has found that the allergy accounts for up to 19% of all anaphylactic reactions during surgery. The best treatment is prevention, but immediate symptomatic treatment is required if the allergic response occurs. Every patient should be assessed for a potential latex reaction. Patients with latex sensitivity should have their chart flagged with a caution label. Latex-free gloves and supplies must be used for anyone with a documented latex allergy.

Bowel clearance may be ordered if the patient is having surgery of the lower gastrointestinal tract. The patient should start the bowel preparation early the evening before surgery to prevent interrupted sleep during the night. Some patients may benefit from a sleeping pill the night before surgery.

The night before surgery, skin preparation is often ordered, which can take the form of scrubbing with a special soap (i.e., Hibiclens), or possibly hair removal from the surgical area. Shaving hair is no longer recommended because studies show that this practice may increase the chance of infection. Instead, adhesive barrier drapes can contain hair growth on the skin around the incision.

Psychological preparation

Patients are often fearful or anxious about having surgery. It is often helpful for them to express their concerns to health care workers. This can be especially beneficial for patients who are critically ill, or who are having a high-risk procedure. The family needs to be included in psychological preoperative care. Pastoral care is usually offered in the hospital. If the patient has a fear of **dying** during surgery, this concern should be expressed, and the surgeon notified. In some cases, the procedure may be postponed until the patient feels more secure.

Children may be especially fearful. They should be allowed to have a parent with them as much as possible, as long as the parent is not demonstrably fearful and contributing to the child's apprehension. Children should be encouraged to bring a favorite toy or blanket to the hospital on the day of surgery.

Patients and families who are prepared psychologically tend to cope better with the patient's postoperative

course. Preparation leads to superior outcomes since the goals of recovery are known ahead of time, and the patient is able to manage postoperative pain more effectively.

Informed consent

The patient's or guardian's written consent for the surgery is a vital portion of preoperative care. By law, the physician who will perform the procedure must explain the risks and benefits of the surgery, along with other treatment options. However, the nurse is often the person who actually witnesses the patient's signature on the consent form. It is important that the patient understands everything he or she has been told. Sometimes, patients are asked to explain what they were told so that the health care professional can determine how much is understood.

Patients who are mentally impaired, heavily sedated, or critically ill are not considered legally able to give consent. In this situation, the next of kin (spouse, adult child, adult sibling, or person with medical **power of attorney**) may act as a surrogate and sign the consent form. Children under age 18 must have a parent or guardian sign.

Preoperative teaching

Preoperative teaching includes instruction about the preoperative period, the surgery itself, and the postoperative period.

Instruction about the preoperative period deals primarily with the arrival time, where the patient should go on the day of surgery, and how to prepare for surgery. For example, patients should be told how long they should be NPO (nothing by mouth), which medications to take prior to surgery, and the medications that should be brought with them (such as inhalers for patients with asthma).

Instruction about the surgery itself includes informing the patient about what will be done during the surgery, and how long the procedure is expected to take. The patient should be told where the incision will be. Children having surgery should be allowed to "practice" on a doll or stuffed animal. It may be helpful to demonstrate procedures on the doll prior to performing them on the child. It is also important for family members (or other concerned parties) to know where to wait during surgery, when they can expect progress information, and how long it will be before they can see the patient.

Knowledge about what to expect during the postoperative period is one of the best ways to improve the patient's outcome. Instruction about expected activities can also increase compliance and help prevent complications. This includes the opportunity for the patient to practice coughing and deep breathing exercises, use an incentive spirometer, and practice splinting the incision. Additionally, the patient should be informed about early ambulation (getting out of bed). The patient should also be taught that the respiratory interventions decrease the occurrence of pneumonia, and that early leg exercises and ambulation decrease the risk of blood clots.

Patients hospitalized postoperatively should be informed about the tubes and equipment that they will have. These may include multiple intravenous lines, drainage tubes, **dressings**, and monitoring devices. In addition, they may have sequential compression stockings on their legs to prevent blood clots until they start ambulating.

Pain management is the primary concern for many patients having surgery. Preoperative instruction should include information about the pain management method that they will utilize postoperatively. Patients should be encouraged to ask for or take pain medication before the pain becomes unbearable, and should be taught how to rate their discomfort on a pain scale. This instruction allows the patients, and others who may be assessing them, to evaluate the pain consistently. If they will be using a **patient-controlled analgesia** pump, instruction should take place during the preoperative period. Use of alternative methods of pain control (distraction, imagery, positioning, mindfulness meditation, music therapy) may also be presented.

Finally, the patient should understand long-term goals such as when he or she will be able to eat solid food, go home, drive a car, and return to work.

Preparation

It is important to allow adequate time for preparation prior to surgery. The patient should understand that he or she has the right to add or strike out items on the generic consent form that do not pertain to the specific surgery. For example, a patient who is about to undergo a **tonsillectomy** might choose to strike out (and initial) an item that indicates sterility might be a complication of the operation.

Normal results

The anticipated outcome of preoperative care is a patient who is informed about the surgical course, and copes with it successfully. The goal is to decrease complications and promote recovery.

Resources

BOOKS

Khatri, VP and JA Asensio. Operative Surgery Manual. 1st ed. Philadelphia: Saunders, 2003.

Townsend, CM et al. Sabiston Textbook of Surgery. 17th ed. Philadelphia: Saunders, 2004.

PERIODICALS

Dean, A., and T. Fawcett. "Nurses' use of evidence in preoperative fasting." Nursing Standard 17, no.12 (December 2002): 33-7.

ORGANIZATIONS

National Institutes of Health. 9000 Rockville Pike, Bethesda, MD 20892. (301) 496-4000. Email: NIHInfo @OD.NIH.GOV. http://www.nih.gov/.

Abby Wojahn, R.N., B.S.N., C.C.R.N.
Crystal H. Kaczkowski, M.Sc.
Rosalyn Carson-DeWitt, MD

Preparing for surgery

Definition

Preparing for a planned surgery (also called **elective surgery**) includes selecting a surgery center and surgeon to perform the procedure, scheduling the surgery, undergoing **presurgical testing**, meeting with health-care professionals and the **surgical team**, receiving education about the procedure, receiving and following all of the appropriate preoperative instructions, and signing a consent form.

Purpose

Preparing for surgery helps the patient understand what to expect before surgery and ensures the patient is physically and psychologically ready for the surgery.

Description

Most patients go to the surgery center or hospital the same day as the scheduled surgery; thus, many of the steps involved in preparing for surgery will take place from one to four weeks before the scheduled surgery. Many surgeries are performed on an outpatient basis, which means that the patient goes home the same day as the surgery.

Selecting a surgeon and surgery center

SURGEON. A surgeon, along with a multi-disciplinary team of surgical specialists, will perform the surgery.

The surgeon should be board certified by the American Board of Surgery, as well as certified by the medical specialty board or boards related to the type of surgery performed. Certification from a medical specialty board means that the surgeon has completed an approved educational training program (including three to seven years of full-time training in an accredited residency program). Certification also includes an evaluation, including an examination that assessed the surgeon's knowledge, skills, and experience necessary to perform high-quality patient care in that specialty.

There are 24 certifying boards recognized by the American Board of Member Specialties (ABMS) and the American Medical Association (AMA). Most of the ABMS boards issue time-limited certificates, valid for six to 10 years. This requires physicians to become re-certified to maintain their board certification—a process that includes a credential review, continuing education in the specialty, and additional examinations. Even though board certification is not required for an individual physician to practice medicine, most hospitals require that a certain percentage of their staff be board certified.

The letters FACS (Fellow of the American College of Surgeons) after a surgeon's name are a further indication of a surgeon's qualifications. Those who become Fellows of the American College of Surgeons have passed a comprehensive evaluation of their **surgical training** and skills; they also have demonstrated their commitment to high standards of ethical conduct. This evaluation is conducted according to national standards that were established to ensure that patients receive the best possible surgical care.

A surgeon's membership in professional societies is also an important consideration. Professional societies provide an independent forum for medical specialists to discuss issues of national interest and mutual concern. Examples of professional societies include the Society of Thoracic Surgeons (STS) and the American College of Physicians–American Society of Internal Medicine (ACP-ASIM).

To find information about a surgeon's qualifications, the patient can call a state or county medical association for assistance. A reference book is also available: *The Official ABMS Directory of Board Certified Medical Specialists* that lists all surgeons who are certified by approved boards. This publication also contains brief information about each surgeon's medical education and training, and it can be found in many libraries.

SURGERY CENTER. The surgeon will arrange for the procedure to be performed in a hospital where he or

KEY TERMS

Case manager—A health-care professional who can provide assistance with a patient's needs beyond the hospital.

Discharge planner—A health-care professional who helps patients arrange for health and home care needs after they go home from the hospital.

Electrocardiogram (ECG, EKG)—A test that records the electrical activity of the heart using small electrode patches attached to the skin on the chest.

Infectious disease team—A team of physicians who help control the hospital environment to protect patients against harmful sources of infection.

Informed consent—An educational process between health-care providers and patients intended to instruct the patient about the nature and purpose of the procedure or treatment, the risks and benefits of the procedure, and alternatives, including the option of not proceeding with the test or treatment.

Inpatient surgery—Surgery that requires an overnight stay of one or more days in the hospital.

NPO—A term that means nothing by mouth. NPO refers to the time after which the patient is not allowed to eat or drink prior to a procedure or treatment.

Outpatient surgery—Also called same-day or ambulatory surgery. The patient arrives for surgery and returns home on the same day.

she has staff privileges. The patient should make sure the hospital has been accredited by the Joint Commission on Accreditation of Healthcare Organizations, a professionally sponsored program that stimulates a high quality of patient care in health-care facilities. Joint Commission accreditation means the hospital voluntarily sought accreditation and met national health and safety standards. There is also an accreditation option that is available for **ambulatory surgery centers**.

Selecting a surgery center that has a multidisciplinary team of specialists is important. The surgery team should include surgeons, infectious disease specialists, pharmacologists, and advanced care registered nurses. Other surgical team members may include fellows and residents, clinical coordinators, physical therapists, respiratory therapists, registered dietitians, social workers, and financial counselors.

Choosing a surgery center with experience is important. Some questions to consider when choosing a surgery center or hospital include:

- How many surgeries are performed annually and what are the outcomes/survival rates of those surgeries?

- How do the surgery center's outcomes compare with the national average?

- Does the surgery center offer treatment for a patient's specific condition? How experienced is the staff in treating that condition?

- What is the center's success record in providing the specific medical treatment or procedure?

- Does the surgery center have experience treating patients the same age as the inquiring patient?

- Does the surgery center explain the patient's rights and responsibilities?

- Does the surgery center have a written description of its services and fees?

- How much does the patient's type of treatment cost at this surgery center?

- Is financial help available?

- Who will be responsible for the patient's specific care plan while he or she is in the hospital?

- If the center is far from the patient's home, will accommodations be provided for caregivers?

- What type of services are available during the patient's hospital stay?

- Will a discharge plan be developed before the patient goes home from the hospital?

- Does the hospital provide training to help the patient care for his or her condition at home?

Scheduling the surgery

Depending on the nature of the surgery, it may be scheduled within days or weeks after the surgery is determined to be the appropriate treatment option for the patient. The patient's surgery time may not be determined until the business day before the scheduled surgery. The patient may be instructed to call the surgical center to find out the time of the scheduled surgery.

The time the patient is told to report to the surgery center (arrival time) is not the time when the surgery will take place. Patients are told to arrive at the surgery center far enough in advance (usually about two hours prior to the scheduled surgery time) so they can be properly prepared for surgery. In some cases, the patient's surgery may need to be rescheduled if another patient requires **emergency surgery** at the patient's scheduled time.

The patient should ask the health-care providers if the scheduled surgery will be performed on an outpatient or inpatient basis. Outpatient means the patient goes home the same day as the surgery; inpatient means a hospital stay is required.

Presurgical testing

Presurgical testing, also called preoperative testing or surgical consultation, includes a review of the patient's medical history, a complete **physical examination**, a variety of tests, patient education, and meetings with the health-care team. The review of the patient's medical history includes an evaluation of the patient's previous and current medical conditions, surgeries and procedures, medications, and any other health conditions such as allergies that may impact the surgery. Presurgical testing is generally scheduled within one week before the surgery.

The patient may find it helpful to bring along a family member or friend to the presurgical testing appointments. This caregiver can help the patient remember important details to prepare for surgery.

After attending the surgical consultation, the patient may desire to seek a **second opinion** to confirm the first doctor's treatment recommendations. The patient should check with his or her insurance provider to determine if the second opinion consultation is covered.

Meeting with the surgical team

During the surgical consultation, the patient meets with the surgeon or a member of the surgeon's health-care team to discuss the surgery and other potential treatment options for the patient's medical condition. At some time before the surgery, the patient will meet with other health-care providers, including the anesthesiologist, nurse clinicians, and sometimes a dietitian, social worker, or rehabilitation specialist.

Patient education

The surgical team will ensure that the patient understands the potential benefits and risks of the procedure as well as what to expect before the procedure and during the recovery. Patient education may include one-on-one instruction from a health-care provider, educational sessions in a group setting, or self-guided learning videos or modules. Informative and instructional handouts are usually provided to explain specific presurgical requirements.

Some surgery centers offer services such as guided imagery and relaxation tapes, massage therapy, aromatherapy, or other complementary techniques to reduce a patient's level of stress and anxiety before a surgical procedure. Guided imagery is a form of focused relaxation that coaches the patient to visualize calm, peaceful images. Several research studies have proven that guided imagery can significantly reduce stress and anxiety before and after surgical and medical procedures and help the patient recover more rapidly. Guided imagery and relaxation tapes are available at many major bookstores and from some surgery centers. The patient may be able to listen to the tapes during the procedure, depending on the type of procedure being performed.

Preoperative instructions

Preoperative instructions include information about reserving blood products for surgery, taking or discontinuing medications before the surgery, eating and drinking before surgery, quitting smoking, limiting activities before surgery, and preparing items to bring to the hospital the day of surgery.

BLOOD TRANSFUSIONS AND BLOOD DONATION. Blood transfusions may be necessary during surgery. A blood **transfusion** is the delivery of whole blood or blood components to replace blood lost through trauma, surgery, or disease. About one in three hospitalized patients will require a blood transfusion. The surgeon can provide an estimate of how much blood the patient's procedure may require.

To decrease the risk of infection and immunologic complications, some surgery centers offer a preoperative **blood donation** program. Autologous blood (from the patient) is the safest blood available for transfusion, since there is no risk of disease transmission. Methods of autologous donation or collection include:

- Intraoperative blood collection: the blood lost during surgery is processed, and the red blood cells are re-infused during or immediately after surgery.
- Preoperative donation: the patient donates blood once a week for one to three weeks before surgery. The blood is separated and the blood components needed are re-infused during surgery.
- Immediate preoperative hemodilution: the patient donates blood immediately before surgery to decrease the loss of red blood cells during surgery. Immediately after donating, the patient receives fluids to compensate for the amount of blood removed. Since the blood is diluted, fewer red blood cells are lost from bleeding during surgery.
- Postoperative blood collection: blood lost from the surgical site right after surgery is collected and re-infused after the surgical site has been closed.

The surgeon determines what type of blood collection process, if any, is appropriate.

MEDICATION GUIDELINES. Depending on the type of surgery scheduled, certain medications may be prescribed or restricted before the surgery. The health-care team will provide specific guidelines. If certain medications need to be restricted before surgery, the patient will receive a complete list of the medications (including prescription, over-the-counter, and herbal medications) to avoid taking before the scheduled surgery.

If the physician advises the patient to take prescribed medication within 12 hours before surgery, it should be taken with small sips of water.

The patient should not bring any medications to the hospital; all necessary medications, as ordered by the doctor, will be provided in the hospital.

EATING AND DRINKING BEFORE SURGERY. Before most surgeries, the patient is advised not to eat or drink anything after midnight the evening before the surgery. This includes no smoking and no gum chewing. The patient should not drink any alcoholic beverages for at least 24 hours before surgery, unless instructed otherwise. If the patient has diabetes or if the surgery is to be performed on a child, the patient should ask the health-care team for specific guidelines about eating and drinking before surgery.

Smoking cessation

Patients who will undergo any surgical procedure are encouraged to quit smoking and stop using tobacco products at least two weeks before the procedure, and to make a commitment to be a nonsmoker after the procedure. Ideally, the patient should quit smoking at least eight weeks prior to surgery. Quitting smoking before surgery helps the patient recover more quickly from surgery. There are several **smoking cessation** programs available in the community. The patient should ask a health-care provider for more information if he or she needs help quitting smoking.

Activity before surgery

The patient should eat right, rest, and **exercise** as normal before surgery, unless given other instructions. The patient should try to get enough sleep to build up energy for the surgery. The health-care team may advise the patient to scrub the planned surgical site with a special disinfecting soap the evening before the surgery.

MAKING PLANS FOR HOME AND WORK. The patient should make arrangements ahead of time for someone to care for children and take care of any other necessary activities at home such as getting the mail or newspapers. The patient should inform family members about the scheduled surgery in advance, so they can provide help and support before, during, and after surgery.

The patient should ask the health-care team what supplies may be needed after surgery during **recovery at home** so these items can be purchased or rented ahead of time. Some supplies that may be needed include an adaptive chair for the toilet or bathtub, or supplies for changing the wound dressing at home. Ask the health care providers if **home care** assistance (in which a visiting nurse visits the home to provide medical care) will be needed after surgery.

Items to bring to the hospital

The patient should bring a list of current medications, allergies, and appropriate medical records upon admission to the surgery center. The patient should also bring a prepared list of questions to ask.

The patient should not bring valuables such as jewelry, credit cards or other items. A small amount of cash (no more than $20) may be packed to purchase items such as newspapers or magazines.

Women should not wear nail polish or makeup the day of surgery.

If a hospital stay is expected after surgery, the patient should only pack what is needed. Some essential items include a toothbrush, toothpaste, comb or brush, deodorant, razor, eyeglasses (if applicable), slippers, robe, pajamas, and one change of comfortable clothes to wear when going home. The patient should also bring a list of family members' names and phone numbers to contact in an emergency.

Transportation

The patient should arrange for transportation home, since the effects of anesthesia and other medications given before surgery make it unsafe to drive.

Preoperative preparation

Upon arriving at the hospital or surgery center, the patient will be required to complete paperwork and show an insurance identification card, if insured. An identification bracelet that includes the patient's name and doctor's name will be placed on the patient's wrist.

INFORMED CONSENT. The health-care provider will review the **informed consent** form and ask the patient to sign it. Informed consent is an educational process between health-care providers and patients. Before any procedure is performed, the patient is asked to sign a consent form. Before signing the form, the patient should understand the nature and purpose of the procedure or treatment, the risks and benefits of the procedure, and alternatives, including the option of not proceeding with the procedure. Signing the informed consent form indicates that the patient permits the surgery or procedure to be performed. During the discussion about the procedure, the health-care providers are available to answer the patient's questions about the consent form or procedure.

ADVANCED DIRECTIVES. The health-care provider will ask the patient if he or she has any advance directives to be included in the patient's file. Advance directives are legal documents that increase a patient's control over medical decisions. A patient may decide medical treatment in advance, in the event that he or she becomes physically or mentally unable to communicate his or her wishes. Advance directives either state what kind of treatment the patient wants to receive (**living will**), or authorize another person to make medical decisions for the patient when he or she is unable to do so (durable **power of attorney**). Advance directives are not required and may be changed or canceled at any time. Any change should be written, signed and dated in accordance with state law, and copies should be given to the physician and to others who received original copies. Advance directives can be revoked either in writing or by destroying the document. Advance directives are not do-not-resuscitate (DNR) orders. A **DNR order** indicates that a person—usually with a terminal illness or other serious medical condition—has decided not to have **cardiopulmonary resuscitation** (CPR) performed in the event that his or her heart or breathing stops.

TESTS AND PREOPERATIVE EVALUATION. Some routine tests will be performed, including blood pressure, temperature, pulse, and weight checks; blood tests; **urinalysis**; **chest x ray**; and **electrocardiogram** (ECG). A brief physical exam will be performed. In some cases, an enema may be required. The health-care team will ask several questions to evaluate the patient's condition and to complete the final preparations for surgery. The patient should inform the health-care team if he or she drinks alcohol on a daily basis so precautions can be taken to avoid complications during and after surgery.

FINAL SURGICAL PREPARATION. Preoperative preparation generally includes these steps:

- The patient changes into a hospital gown.
- The patient removes (as applicable) contact lenses and glasses, dentures, hearing aids, nail polish, and jewelry.
- The patient empties his or her bladder.
- The health-care providers clean and possibly shave the area on the body where the surgery will be performed.
- The patient may receive medication to aid relaxation.

- An intravenous catheter will be placed in a vein in the patient's arm to deliver fluids, medications, or blood during surgery.
- In some hospitals, the patient may wait in an area called a holding area until the operating room and surgical team are ready. Depending on the hospital's policy, one or two of the patient's family members may wait with the patient.
- The patient is taken to the operating room in a wheelchair or on a bed (also called a gurney) where monitors are placed to evaluate the patient's condition during surgery.
- Anesthesia is administered; the type of anesthesia administered will depend upon the procedure, the patient's general health, and medications.
- A catheter may be placed in the patient's bladder to drain urine.
- The patient's vital signs, including the blood oxygen level, electrical activity of the heart, blood pressure, pulse, temperature, breathing, mental status, and level of consciousness, are continuously monitored during and after the surgery.

Information for families

While the patient is in surgery, the family members wait in a designated waiting area. Some hospitals or surgery centers offer a pager to the patient's family so they can be contacted for updates about the progress of the surgery. It may be helpful for the patient to select a spokesperson from the family to communicate with the health-care providers. This may improve communication with the health-care providers as well as to other family members. The patient should also communicate his or her wishes regarding the spokesperson's telephone communications to other family members.

Educational classes may be available for family members to learn more about the patient's surgery and what to expect during the recovery.

When the surgery is complete, the surgeon usually contacts the family members to provide information about the surgery. If a problem or complication occurs during surgery, the family members are notified immediately.

Normal results

Patients who receive proper preparation for surgery, including physical and psychological preparation, experience less anxiety and are more likely to make a quicker recovery at home, with fewer complications. Patients who perceive their surgical and

QUESTIONS TO ASK THE DOCTOR

- Will I have to have blood transfusions during the surgery?
- Do I take my medications the day of the surgery?
- Can I eat or drink the day of the surgery? If not, how long before the surgery should I stop eating and drinking?
- How long does my type of surgery typically last?
- How long will I have to stay in the hospital after surgery?
- What kind of pain or discomfort will I experience after the surgery and what can I take to I relieve it? What type of bruising, swelling, scarring, or pain should be expected after surgery?
- What types of resources are available to me during my hospital stay, and during my recovery at home?
- After I go home from the hospital, how long will it take me to recover?
- What are the signs of infection, and what types of symptoms should I report to my doctor?
- How should I care for my incision?
- What types of medications will I have to take after surgery? How long will I have to take them?
- When will I be able I resume my normal activities? When will I be able to drive? When will I be able to return to work?
- What lifestyle changes (including diet, weight management, exercise, and activity changes) are recommended after the surgery to improve my condition?
- How often do I need to see my doctor or surgeon for follow-up visits after surgery?
- Can I receive follow-up care from my primary physician, or do I need to have follow-up visits with the surgeon?

postoperative experiences as positive report that they had minimal pain and nausea, were relaxed, had confidence in the skills of their health-care team, felt they had some control over their care, and returned to their normal activities within the expected timeframe.

Resources

BOOKS

Huddleston, Peggy. *Prepare for Surgery, Heal Faster.* Cambridge, MA: Angel River Press, 2002.

Lichtenberg, Maggie. *The Open Heart Companion: Preparation and Guidance for Open-Heart Surgery Recovery.* Sante Fe, NM: Open Heart Pub., 2006.

PERIODICALS

Callery, Peter. "Preparing Children for Surgery." *Pediatric Nursing* 17.3 (April 2005): 12-13.

Larson, Heather. "Pre-Op Jitters: Preparing for Surgery." *Whole Life Times* (Jan 2002): 22-24.

Lucas, Brian. "Preparing Patients for Hip and Knee Replacement Surgery." *Nursing Standard* 22.2 (Sept 19, 2007): 50-58.

ORGANIZATIONS

Agency for Health Care Policy and Research (AHCPR), Publications Clearinghouse. P.O. Box 8547, Silver Spring, MD, 20907. (800) 358-9295. <http://www/ahcpr.gov>.

American Board of Surgery. 1617 John F. Kennedy Boulevard, Suite 860, Philadelphia, PA 19103. (215) 568-4000. http://www.absurgery.org/.

American Association of Nurse Anesthetists (AANA). 222 South Prospect Avenue, Park Ridge, IL 60068-4001. (847) 692-7050. http://www.aana.com/.

American College of Surgeons. 633 N. Saint Clair Street, Chicago, IL 60611-3211. (312) 202-5000. http://www.facs.org/.

American Society of Anesthesiologists (ASA). 520 North Northwest Highway, Park Ridge, IL 60068-2573. (847) 825-5586. <http://http://www.asahq.org/.

National Heart, Lung and Blood Institute. Information Center. P.O. Box 30105, Bethesda, MD 20824-0105. (301) 251-2222. http://www.nhlbi.nih.gov.

Angela M. Costello
Robert Bockstiegel

Pressure sores *see* **Bedsores**

Presurgical testing

Definition

Presurgical or preoperative testing refers to the preparation and management of a patient before surgery.

Purpose

Presurgical testing, sometimes called preoperative testing, prepares a patient for surgery psychologically and physically.

Demographics

The U.S. Department of Health and Human Services' National Center for Health Statistics reported more than 44.9 million inpatient surgical procedures (requiring an overnight hospital stay) performed in the United States in 2005. About 50 million outpatient surgical procedures (in which the patient goes home the same day of surgery) were performed in that year.

Obstetrical, cardiovascular, digestive, musculoskeletal, and neurological surgeries are among the majority of the inpatient surgical procedures performed. The majority of outpatient surgeries were performed on the digestive system, eyes, musculoskeletal system, female reproductive organs, and urinary system.

In recent years there has been a change in attitude toward routine presurgical testing. In the years following World War II, administering routine laboratory tests to patients before surgery became part of normal clinical procedure. It was thought that such testing would help doctors to detect abnormalities before surgery that might lead to complications during or after the operation. Until the 1980s few surgeons evaluated either the clinical or the cost-effectiveness of these tests. In the mid-1980s, however, some researchers began to publish papers showing that preoperative testing was not only expensive but also did not necessarily benefit patients. One study published in the *Journal of the American Medical Association* in 1985 noted that 60% of a sample group of 2000 patients had had laboratory tests ordered for no apparent reason. Of the abnormal test findings, only 0.22% influenced preoperative management of the patients.

Newer recommendations for presurgical testing of healthy patients undergoing **elective surgery** are as follows:

- Consider a complete patient history and thorough physical examination the most important part of preoperative testing.

- The patient's hemoglobin level should be tested before for major surgery with significant expected blood loss or CBC count if the cost is not substantially increased.

- Serum creatinine level (a blood test) should be tested in people older than 40 years.

- Electrocardiogram (ECG or EKG) for patients over 40.

- Chest x-ray for patients older than 60.

- It is not necessary to repeat any laboratory test if the results were normal within 4 months of the scheduled surgery and if there has been no change in the patient's health.

Patients with heart disease or lung disease, or undergoing **emergency surgery**, require more complete evaluation.

KEY TERMS

Biopsy—The removal of a small sample of tissue for analysis to determine a diagnosis.

Bone densitometry test—A test that quickly and accurately measures the density of bone.

Catheter—A small, flexible tube used to deliver fluids or medications.

Chest x ray—A diagnostic procedure in which a small amount of radiation is used to produce an image of the structures of the chest (heart, lungs, and bones) on film.

Echocardiogram—An imaging procedure used to create a picture of the heart's movement, valves and chambers. The test uses high-frequency sound waves that come from a hand wand placed on the chest. Echocardiogram may be used in combination with Doppler ultrasound to evaluate the blood flow across the heart's valves.

Electrocardiogram (ECG, EKG)—A test that records the electrical activity of the heart using small electrode patches attached to the skin on the chest.

Pulmonary function test—A test that measures the capacity and function of the lungs, as well as the blood's ability to carry oxygen. During the test, patient breathes into a device called a spirometer.

Description

A planned surgery usually involves a surgical consultation, presurgical testing, the surgery itself, and **recovery at home**.

During the surgical consultation, the patient meets with the surgeon or a member of the surgeon's health-care team to discuss the surgery and other potential treatment options for the patient's medical condition. A thorough review of the patient's medical history and a complete physical exam are performed at this time. The medical review includes an evaluation of the patient's previous and current medical conditions, surgeries and procedures, medications, and any other health conditions, such as allergies, that may impact the surgery.

The **surgical team** will ensure that the patient understands the potential benefits and risks of the procedure. Patient education may include one-on-one instruction from a health care provider, educational sessions in a group setting, or self-guided learning videos or modules. Informative and instructional handouts are usually provided to explain specific pre-surgical requirements.

After attending the surgical consultation, the patient may desire a **second opinion** to confirm the first doctor's treatment recommendations.

Diagnosis/Preparation

Presurgical testing includes a variety of tests, patient education, and meetings with the health care team to inform the patient about what to expect before the procedure and during the recovery. Presurgical testing is generally scheduled within one week before the surgery.

Several tests are performed before surgery to provide complete information about the patient's overall health, to prepare the patient for anesthesia (as applicable), and to identify and treat any potential problems ahead of time. Each surgery patient does not have the same presurgery tests. In addition to checking the patient's **vital signs** (temperature, blood pressure, and pulse), more common tests include:

- blood tests
- urine tests
- chest x rays
- pulmonary function tests
- computed tomography scan (CT or CAT scan)
- heart function tests that may include an electrocardiogram or echocardiogram

If the patient recently had these tests performed (within the past six months), he or she can request the test results be forwarded to the surgical center.

Before some surgical procedures, such as valve surgery, a complete dental exam is needed to reduce the risk of infection. Other precautions will be taken before the surgery to reduce the patient's risk of infection.

Informed consent is an educational process between health-care providers and patients. Before any procedure is performed, the patient is asked to sign a consent form. Before signing the form, the patient should understand the nature and purpose of the diagnostic procedure or treatment, the risks and benefits of the procedure, and alternatives, including the option of not proceeding with the test or treatment. During the discussion about the procedure, the health-care providers are available to answer the patient's questions about the consent form or procedure.

Advance directives are legal documents that increase a patient's control over medical decisions. A patient may decide medical treatment in advance, in the event that he or she becomes physically or mentally unable to communicate his or her wishes. Advance directives either state what kind of treatment the patient wants to receive (**living will**), or authorize another person to make medical decisions for the patient when he or she is unable to do so (durable **power of attorney**).

Advance directives are not required and may be changed or canceled at any time. Any change should be written, signed, and dated in accordance with state law, and copies should be given to the physician and to others who received original copies. Advance directives can be revoked either in writing or by destroying the document.

Advance directives are not a do-not-resuscitate (DNR) order, which indicates that a person—usually with a terminal illness or other serious medical condition—has decided not to have **cardiopulmonary resuscitation** (CPR) performed in the event that his or her heart or breathing stops.

Patients who will undergo any surgical procedure are encouraged to quit smoking and stop using tobacco products at least two weeks before the procedure, and to make a commitment to be a nonsmoker after the procedure. Quitting smoking before surgery helps the patient recover more quickly from surgery. There are several **smoking cessation** programs available in the community. The patient should ask a health-care provider for more information if he or she needs help quitting smoking.

The presurgical evaluation may include meetings with the anesthesiologist, surgeon, nurse clinicians, and other health-care providers who will manage the patient's care during and after surgery, such as a dietitian, social worker, or rehabilitation specialist.

The patient's surgery time may not be determined until the business day before the scheduled surgery. The patient may be instructed to call the surgical center to find out the time of the scheduled surgery.

Patients are told to come to the surgery center far enough in advance (usually about two hours prior to the scheduled surgery time) so they can be properly prepared for surgery. In some cases, the patient's surgery may need to be rescheduled if another patient requires emergency surgery at the patient's scheduled time.

Some surgery centers offer services such as guided imagery and relaxation tapes, massage therapy, or other complementary techniques to reduce a patient's level of stress and anxiety before a surgical procedure.

Guided imagery is a form of focused relaxation that coaches the patient to visualize calm, peaceful images. Several research studies have proven that guided imagery can significantly reduce stress and anxiety before and after surgical and medical procedures and help the patient recover more rapidly. Guided imagery tapes are available at many major bookstores and from some surgery centers. The patient listens to the guided imagery tapes on his or her own CD or tape player before and after the surgery. The patient may even be able to continue listening to the tapes during the procedure, depending on the type of procedure being performed.

Blood transfusions may be necessary during surgery. A blood **transfusion** is the delivery of whole blood or blood components to replace blood lost through trauma, surgery, or disease. About one in three hospitalized patients will require a blood transfusion. The surgeon can provide an estimate of how much blood the patient's procedure may require.

To decrease the risk of infection and immunologic complications, some surgery centers offer a preoperative **blood donation** program. Autologous blood (blood taken from the patient) is the safest blood available for transfusion, since there is no risk of disease transmission. Methods of autologous donation or collection include:

- Intraoperative blood collection: The blood lost during surgery is processed and the red blood cells are reinfused during or immediately after surgery.
- Preoperative donation: The patient donates blood once a week for about one to three weeks before surgery. The blood is separated, and the blood components needed are reinfused during surgery.
- Immediate preoperative hemodilution: The patient donates blood immediately before surgery to decrease the loss of red blood cells during surgery. After donating, the patient receives fluids to compensate for the amount of blood removed. Since the blood is diluted, fewer red blood cells are lost from bleeding during surgery.
- Postoperative blood collection: Blood lost from the surgical site right after surgery is collected and reinfused after the surgical site has been closed.

The surgeon determines what type of blood collection process, if any, is appropriate.

Depending on the type of surgery scheduled, certain medications may be prescribed or restricted before the surgery. The health-care team will provide specific guidelines. If certain medications need to be restricted before surgery, the patient will receive a complete list of the medications (including prescription, over-the-counter, and herbal medications) to avoid taking before the scheduled surgery.

Prescribed medications that need to be taken within 12 hours before surgery should be swallowed with small sips of water.

Before most surgeries, the patient is advised not to eat or drink anything after midnight the evening before the surgery. This fast includes no smoking and no gum chewing. The patient should not drink any alcoholic beverages for at least 24 hours before surgery, unless instructed otherwise.

Most patients are admitted to the surgery center or hospital the same day as the scheduled surgery. The patient should bring a list of current medications, allergies, and appropriate medical records upon admission to the surgery center.

The patient should arrange for transportation home, since the effects of anesthesia and other medications given before surgery make it unsafe to drive.

Resources

BOOKS

[No authors listed.] *Diagnostic Tests*. Philadelphia: Lippincott Williams and Wilkins, 2007.

Kee, Joyce LeFever. *Handbook of Laboratory and Diagnostic Tests: with Nursing Implications.* Upper Saddle River, NJ: Pearson/Prentice Hall, 2008.

Newman, Mark, Lee Fleisher, and Mitchell Fink, eds. *Perioperative Medicine: Managing for Outcome.* Philadelphia: Saunders Elsevier, 2008.

"Preoperative Care." In *Mosby's Medical, Nursing and Allied Health Dictionary,* 5th ed. Edited by Kenneth Anderson, Lois E. Anderson, and Walter D. Glanze. B.C. Decker, 1998.

PERIODICALS

Fattahi, T. "Perioperative Laboratory and Diagnostic Testing: What Is Needed and When?" *Oral and Maxillofacial Surgery Clinics of North America* 18 (February 2006): 1–6.

Froehlich, J. B., D. Karavite, P. L. Russman, et al. "American College of Cardiology/American Heart Association Preoperative Assessment Guidelines Reduce Resource Utilization before Aortic Surgery." *Journal of Vascular Surgery* 36 (October 2002): 758–763.

Hoeks, S. C., et al. "Preoperative Cardiac Testing before Major Vascular Surgery." *Journal of Nuclear Cardiology* 14 (November-December 2007): 885–891.

Kaplan, E. B., L. B. Sheiner, and A. J. Boeckmann. "The Usefulness of Preoperative Laboratory Screening." *Journal of the American Medical Association* 253 (June 28, 1985): 3576–3581.

Meding, J. B., M. Klay, A. Healy, et al. "The Prescreening History and Physical in Elective Total Joint Arthroplasty." *Journal of Arthroplasty* 22 (September 2007): 21–23.

"Recommended Practices for Managing the Patient Receiving Anesthesia." *AORN Journal* 75, no. 4 (April 2002): 849.

ORGANIZATIONS

American Board of Surgery. 1617 John F. Kennedy Boulevard, Suite 860, Philadelphia, PA 19103. (215) 568-4000. http://www.absurgery.org/.

American College of Surgeons. 633 N. Saint Clair Street, Chicago, IL 60611-3211. (312) 202-5000. http://www.facs.org/.

American Hospital Association (AHA). One North Franklin, Chicago, IL 60606-3421. (312) 422-3000. http://www.aha.org/aha_app/index.jsp.

National Heart, Lung and Blood Institute. Information Center. P.O. Box 30105, Bethesda, MD 20824-0105. (301) 592-8573. http://www.nhlbi.nih.gov .

OTHER

Reports of the Surgeon General. National Library of Medicine. http://sgreports.nlm.nih.gov/NN/.

Sharma, Gyanendra. "Preoperative Testing." eMedicine, March 15, 2007. http://www.emedicine.com/med/topic3172.htm [cited January 11, 2008].

SurgeryLinx. MDLinx, Inc. 1025 Vermont Avenue, NW, Suite 810, Washington, DC 20005. (202) 543-6544. http://sgreports.nlm.nih.gov/NN/.

Surgical Procedures, Operative. http://www.mic.ki.se/Diseases/e4.html.

Angela M. Costello
Rebecca Frey, Ph.D.

Private insurance plans

Definition

Private insurance plans include all forms of health insurance that are not funded by the government.

Purpose

These plans are intended to protect their beneficiaries from the high costs that may be incurred for health care. Most private insurance plans in the United States are employment-based.

Of the nearly 243 million Americans who are covered by private health insurance, approximately nine in 10 (215 million, or 88%) are enrolled in employment-based plans.

Description

Private health insurance plans may be purchased on an individual or group basis. Most group plans are offered by large employers, although some are available through voluntary associations. Individual policies are usually more expensive than group policies. Furthermore, they may have additional coverage restrictions.

KEY TERMS

Co-insurance—The percentage of health care charges that an insurance company pays after the beneficiary pays the deductible. Most co-insurance percentages are 70–90%.

Deductible—An amount of money that an insured person is required to pay on each claim made on an insurance policy.

Indemnity—Protection, as by insurance, against damage or loss.

Indemnity plans—Private health insurance plans that allow the policyholder to choose any physician or hospital when health care is needed.

Long-term care (LTC) insurance—A type of private health insurance intended to cover the cost of long-term nursing home or home health care.

Medigap—A group of 10 standardized private health insurance policies intended to cover the coinsurance and deductible costs not covered by Medicare.

Portability—A feature that allows employees to transfer health insurance coverage or other benefits from one employer to another when they change jobs.

Preferred provider organizations (PPOs)—Private health insurance plans that require beneficiaries to select their health care providers from a list approved by the insurance company.

Premium—The amount paid by an insurance policyholder for insurance coverage. Most health insurance policy premiums are payable on a monthly basis.

There are several major categories of private health insurance in the United States.

Indemnity plans

Indemnity plans are private insurance plans that allow beneficiaries to choose any physician or hospital when they need medical care. Most indemnity plans have a deductible, or amount that the policyholder must pay before the plan will cover any costs. After the deductible has been satisfied, indemnity plans pay a co-insurance percentage, most often 70–90% of the charges. The beneficiary pays the remainder of the bill.

Preferred provider organization (PPO) plans

PPO plans are similar to indemnity plans in that they usually have both a deductible and a co-insurance percentage. Unlike indemnity plans, PPOs offer a list of physicians and hospitals from which enrollees must select in order to receive the plan's maximum benefit. PPOs tend to be less expensive than indemnity plans because health care providers are often willing to reduce their fees in order to participate in these plans. Many large companies have moved their insured employees into PPOs because of their cost effectiveness.

A person enrolled in a PPO can choose to seek care from a non-network provider. This is called going out of network. Some people find this beneficial because it allows continuity of care from an existing provider. Enrollees may also propose their physician for membership in the PPO so that continuity of service may be provided.

Health maintenance organization (HMO) plans

HMOs usually have no deductible. Beneficiaries are charged a small co-payment, typically between $5 and $25 per visit, and the plan covers all other charges. The list of preferred providers is generally smaller than that of a PPO. In most HMOs, each beneficiary selects a primary care physician who is responsible for all health care needs. Referrals to specialists must be made through the primary care physician. Like PPOs, HMOs are usually able to charge lower premiums because their participating health care providers agree to accept substantially reduced fees.

Long-term care (LTC) insurance

Long-term care insurance, or LTC, is a type of private health insurance intended to cover the cost of custodial or nursing **home care**. It can be very expensive, and persons considering this form of insurance should not purchase it if the premiums cause financial hardship in the present.

Medigap insurance plans

Medicare does not offer complete health insurance protection. Medigap insurance is a type of plan intended to supplement Medicare coverage. There are 10 standard Medigap benefit packages. These are identified by the letters A through J, and are available in most states, United States territories, and the District of Columbia. Medigap policies pay most or all of the co-insurance amounts charged by Medicare. Some Medigap policies cover Medicare deductibles.

Medical savings accounts (MSAs)

Medical savings accounts are not health insurance plans in the strict sense, but offer a partial alternative to expensive individual private insurance plans. MSAs are similar to Individual Retirement Accounts (IRAs), and have been considered a significant tax break for self-employed individuals. They were created as a four-year pilot project by the Health Insurance Portability and Accountability Act (HIPAA) of 1996. Effective December 31, 2000, the federal government issued an extension on these accounts for two years. The extension is currently renewed every year.

An MSA must be combined with a qualified high-deductible private health plan. Without an MSA, a self-employed individual can deduct qualified medical expenses only under the itemized deductions of a 1040 tax form, and the expenses must exceed 7.5% of the adjusted gross income.

The cost of health insurance

The cost of private health insurance has risen steadily over the past two decades, largely because of the rising cost of health care in the United States. Between 1980 and 1995, the total amount spent on health care in the United States each year rose from $247.2 billion to $1.04 trillion, more than a 400% increase. Between 1995 and 2006, the amount doubled again, to more than $2 trillion per year. The reasons for the escalating costs include the following:

- Increased longevity. The life expectancy of most Americans is approximately 76 years. When older people join an insured group, the entire group's health care risks and costs rise.
- Advances in medical technology. New technology is often expensive.

The rising costs of health insurance over the past 30 years have caused many employers to curtail or drop health insurance as an employee benefit. The cost of health insurance premiums increased from $16.8 billion in 1970 to $310 billion in 1995. By 2006, employers were spending $11,400 per year to insure a family of four. Many employers have increased the amount of money employees are expected to contribute toward their health care. Others, particularly smaller businesses, do not offer health insurance at all. A 1997 study found that only 34% of workers in smaller businesses were covered through their employers, whereas 82% of employees in the largest companies were covered. Experts feel that this trend will continue. Workers in large-employer health insurance plans generally have policies that cover more health services, have lower deductibles, and offer more opportunities to enroll in HMOs.

Uninsured persons

The U.S. Census Bureau reported in 1997 that 43.4 million people in the United States, or 16.1% of the population, had no health insurance coverage. Between 1998 and 1999, both the number and proportion of uninsured Americans declined slightly, to 42.6 million and 15.5% respectively. As of 2005, the federal government estimated that nearly 47 million Americans, or 16 percent of the population, were without health insurance.

Some workers do not have health insurance because they cannot afford it. In the 1950s, employer-based health insurance served most American families reasonably well because many workers were employed by large firms and remained with them for life. The trend over the past two decades is employment by small firms that do not offer health insurance as a benefit, and a tendency to change employers every few years. Most uninsured workers are self-employed, work only part-time, or hold low-wage jobs that do not give them access to lower-cost employer-sponsored group plans. Workers in these three categories do not qualify for coverage by government programs for low-income people.

The other major category of uninsured people includes those who cannot purchase private insurance at affordable rates because they are likely to need expensive medical services. Those who have a high risk of developing cancer or are HIV-positive may not be able to obtain coverage from any insurance company. As early as the 1980s, some insurance companies began introducing clauses that excluded or restricted benefits for persons with pre-existing conditions. These clauses denied private insurance to anyone already diagnosed with a serious medical condition. One of the goals of the Health Insurance Portability and Accountability Act (HIPPA) of 1996 was to help workers who could not change jobs because they had family members with serious health problems. In the past, they would have been denied health insurance by the preexisting condition clauses in the new employer's plan. HIPAA requires employer-sponsored insurance plans to accept transfers from other plans without imposing preexisting condition clauses.

An individual private health insurance plan can be expensive and restrictive. It may, however, be the only choice for a consumer who is not employed; self-employed; or is a new hire at a company and must wait several months or more before the company's coverage takes effect.

Tax credit proposals

One approach to the rising costs of private health insurance that is gaining bipartisan political support is to offer tax credits that would allow more Americans to purchase health insurance. The present federal tax code favors workers who already have employer-sponsored health insurance. Supporters of the tax credit approach maintain that it would give workers a wider choice of health plans, create greater portability of health insurance, and encourage groups other than employment-based populations (e.g., church groups, unions, fraternal organizations) to sponsor insurance plans for their members.

See also Long-term insurance.

Resources

BOOKS

Green, M. A., and J. A. Rowell. Understanding Health Insurance. 9th ed. Florence, KY: CENGAGE Delmar Learning, 2007.

Murray, J. E. Origins of American Health Insurance: A History of Industrial Sickness Funds. New Haven, CT: Yale University Press, 2007.

Parker, P. M. The 2007-2012 World Outlook for Private Health Insurance Carriers. San Diego, CA: ICON Group International, 2006.

Preker, A. S., R. M. Scheffler, and M. C. Bassett. Private Voluntary Health Insurance in Development: Friend or Foe? Washington, DC: World Bank Publications, 2006.

Stevens, R. A., C. E. Rosenberg, and L. R. Burns. History And Health Policy in the United States: Putting the Past Back in. New Brunswick, NJ: Rutgers University Press, 2006.

van Boom, W. H., and M. Faure. Shifts in Compensation between Private and Public Systems. New York: Springer, 2007.

PERIODICALS

Danis, M., S. D. Goold, C. Parise, and M. Ginsberg. "Enhancing employee capacity to prioritize health insurance benefits." Health Expectations 10, no. 3 (2007): 236–247.

Gould, E. "Health insurance eroding for working families: employer-provided coverage declines for fifth consecutive year." International Journal of Health Services 37, no. 3 (2007): 441–467.

Levy, P., R. Nocerini, and K. Grazier. "Paying for disease management." Disease Management 10, no. 4 (2007): 235–244.

Molinari, N. A., M. Kolasa, M. L. Messonnier, and R. A, Schieber. "Out-of-pocket costs of childhood immunizations: a comparison by type of insurance plan." Pediatrics 120, no. 5 (2007): e1148–e1156.

O'Donnell, T. P., and M. K. Fendler. "Prescription or proscription? The general failure of attempts to litigate and legislate against PBMS as "fiduciaries," and the role of market forces allowing PBMS to contain private-sector prescription drug prices.." Journal of Health Law 40, no. 2 (2007): 205–240.

ORGANIZATIONS

America's Health Insurance Plans, 601 Pennsylvania Avenue, NW, South Building, Suite 500, Washington, DC 20004, Phone: (202) 778-3200, Fax: (202) 331-7487. http://www.ahip.org/.

American Association of Retired Persons (AARP). 601 E. Street NW, Washington, DC 20049. (800) 424-3410, http://www.aarp.org/.

American College of Healthcare Executives. One North Franklin, Suite 1700, Chicago, IL 60606-4425. (312) 424-2800. Fax: 312-424-0023. http://www.ache.org/.

American Medical Association. 515 N. State Street, Chicago, IL 60610. (312) 464-5000. http://www.ama-assn.org.

United States Department of Health and Human Services. 200 Independence Avenue SW, Washington, DC 20201. http://www.hhs.gov.

OTHER

American Society of Cosmetic Breast Surgery. Information about Private Health Insurance Plans. 2007 [cited December 31, 2007]. http://www.ahcpr.gov/consumer/insuranceqa/.

Association of Health Insurance Advisors. Information about Private Health Insurance Plans. 2007 [cited December 31, 2007]. http://www.ahia.net/.

Council for Affordable Health Insurance. Information about Private Health Insurance Plans. 2007 [cited December 31, 2007]. http://cahionline.org/cahi_index.shtml.

Georgetown University Health Policy Institute. Information about Private Health Insurance Plans. 2007 [cited December 31, 2007]. http://www.healthinsuranceinfo.net/.

Health Insurance Information, Counseling & Assistance Program of New York State. Information about Private Health Insurance Plans. 2007 [cited December 31, 2007]. http://hiicap.state.ny.us/.

L. Fleming Fallon, Jr., MD, DrPH

PRK *see* **Photorefractive keratectomy (PRK)**
Proctosigmoidoscopy *see* **Sigmoidoscopy**

Prophylaxis, antibiotic

Definition

A prophylaxis is a measure taken to maintain health and prevent the spread of disease. Antibiotic prophylaxis is the focus of this article and refers to the use of **antibiotics** to prevent infections.

Purpose

Antibiotics are well known for their ability to treat infections. But some antibiotics also are prescribed to prevent infections. This usually is done only in certain situations or for people with particular medical problems.

For example, people with abnormal heart valves have a high risk of developing heart valve infections even after only minor surgery. This happens because bacteria from other parts of the body get into the bloodstream during surgery and travel to the heart valves. To prevent these infections, people with heart valve problems often take antibiotics before having any kind of surgery, including dental surgery.

Antibiotics also may be prescribed to prevent infections in people with weakened immune systems such as those with AIDS or people who are having chemotherapy treatments for cancer. But even healthy people with strong immune systems may occasionally be given preventive antibiotics—if they are having certain kinds of surgery that carry a high risk of infection, or if they are traveling to parts of the world where they are likely to get an infection that causes diarrhea, for example.

In all of these situations, a physician should be the one to decide whether antibiotics are necessary. Unless a physician says to do so, it is not a good idea to take antibiotics to prevent ordinary infections.

Because the overuse of antibiotics can lead to resistance, drugs taken to prevent infection should be used only for a short time.

Description

Among the drugs used for antibiotic prophylaxis are amoxicillin (a type of penicillin) and **fluoroquinolones** such as ciprofloxacin (Cipro) and trovafloxacin (Trovan). These drugs are available only with a physician's prescription and come in tablet, capsule, liquid, and injectable forms.

For surgical prophylaxis, the cephalosporin antibiotics are usually preferred. This class includes cefazolin (Ancef, Kefzol), cefamandole (Mandol), cefotaxime (Claforan), and others. The choice of drug depends on its spectrum and the type of bacteria that are most likely to be encountered. For example, surgery on the intestines, which have many anaerobic bacteria, might call for cefoxitin (Mefoxin), while in heart surgery, where there are no anaerobes, cefazolin might be preferred.

Recommended dosage

The recommended dosage depends on the type of antibiotic prescribed and the reason it is being used. For the correct dosage, the patient is advised to check with the physician or dentist who prescribed the medicine or the pharmacist who filled the prescription. The patient is recommended to be sure to take the medicine

KEY TERMS

AIDS—Acquired immunodeficiency syndrome. A disease caused by infection with the human immunodeficiency virus (HIV). In people with this disease, the immune system breaks down, opening the door to other infections and some types of cancer.

Antibiotic—A medicine used to treat infections.

Chemotherapy—Treatment of an illness with chemical agents. The term is typically used to describe the treatment of cancer with drugs.

Immune system—The body's natural defenses against disease and infection.

exactly as prescribed, and not to take more or less than directed, and to take the medicine only for as long as the physician or dentist says to take it.

The recommended dose of prophylactic antibiotic for surgery has varied with studies. At one time, it was common to give a dose of antibiotic when the patient was called to the **operating room**, and to continue the drug for 48 hours after surgery. More recent studies indicate that a single antibiotic dose, given immediately before the start of surgery, may be just as effective in preventing infection, while reducing the risk of drug side effects.

Precautions

The warnings listed below refer primarily to the effects of the drugs when taken in multiple doses. When prophylactic antibiotics are used as a single dose, adverse effects are very unlikely. The only exceptions are for people who are allergic to the antibiotic used. Since **cephalosporins** are closely related to penicillins, people who are allergic to penicillins should avoid cephalosporin antibiotics.

If the medicine causes nausea, vomiting, or diarrhea, the patient is advised to check with the physician or dentist who prescribed it as soon as possible. Patients who are taking antibiotics before surgery should not wait until the day of the surgery to report problems with the medicine. The physician or dentist needs to know right away if problems occur.

For other specific precautions, the patient is advised to see the entry on the type of drug prescribed such as penicillins or fluoroquinolones.

Side effects

Antibiotics may cause a number of side effects. For details, the patient is advised to see entries on specific types of antibiotics. Anyone who has unusual or disturbing symptoms after taking antibiotics should get in contact with the prescribing physician.

Interactions

Whether used to treat or to prevent infection, antibiotics may interact with other medicines. When this happens, the effects of one or both of the drugs may change or the risk of side effects may be greater. Anyone who takes antibiotics for any reason should inform the physician about all the other medicines he or she is taking and should ask whether any possible interactions may interfere with drugs' effects. For details of drug interactions, the candidate is advised to see entries on specific types of antibiotics.

Resources

BOOKS

Khatri, VP and JA Asensio. Operative Surgery Manual. 1st ed. Philadelphia: Saunders, 2003.
Libby, P. et al. Braunwald's Heart Disease. 8th ed. Philadelphia: Saunders, 2007.
Townsend, CM et al. Sabiston Textbook of Surgery. 17th ed. Philadelphia: Saunders, 2004.

PERIODICALS

Guthrie, P. "Doctors, Patients Must Act Together to Save Antibiotics' Potency, Experts Say." Atlanta Journal-Constitution (March 19, 2003).

Nancy Ross-Flanigan
Sam Uretsky, PharmD

Prostaglandins *see* **Uterine stimulants**

Prostate-specific antigen test *see* **Tumor marker tests**

Prostate resection *see* **Transurethral resection of the prostate**

Prostatectomy, open *see* **Open prostatectomy**

▋ Prothrombin time

Definition

The prothrombin time test belongs to a group of blood tests that assess the clotting ability of blood. The test is also known as the pro time or PT test.

Purpose

The PT test is used to monitor patients taking certain medications as well as to help diagnose clotting disorders.

Diagnosis

Patients who have problems with delayed blood clotting are given a number of tests to determine the cause of the problem. The prothrombin test specifically evaluates the presence of factors VIIa, V, and X, prothrombin, and fibrinogen. Prothrombin is a protein in the liquid part of blood (plasma) that is converted to thrombin as part of the clotting process. Fibrinogen is a type of blood protein called a globulin; it is converted to fibrin during the clotting process. A drop in the concentration of any of these factors will cause the blood to take longer to clot. The PT test is used in combination with the **partial thromboplastin time** (PTT) test to screen for hemophilia and other hereditary clotting disorders.

Monitoring

The PT test is also used to monitor the condition of patients who are taking warfarin (Coumadin). Warfarin is a drug that is given to prevent clots in the deep veins of the legs and to treat pulmonary embolism. It interferes with blood clotting by lowering the liver's production of certain clotting factors.

Description

A sample of the patient's blood is obtained by venipuncture. The blood is collected in a tube that contains sodium citrate to prevent the clotting process from starting before the test. The blood cells are separated from the liquid part of blood (plasma). The PT test is performed by adding the patient's plasma to a protein in the blood (thromboplastin) that converts prothrombin to thrombin. The mixture is then kept in a warm water bath at 37°C for one to two minutes. Calcium chloride is added to the mixture in order to counteract the sodium citrate and allow clotting to proceed. The test is timed from the addition of the calcium chloride until the plasma clots. This time is called the prothrombin time.

Preparation

The doctor should check to see if the patient is taking any medications that may affect test results. This precaution is particularly important if the patient is taking warfarin, because there are a number of

KEY TERMS

Disseminated intravascular coagulation (DIC)—A condition in which spontaneous bleeding and clot formation occur throughout the circulatory system. DIC can be caused by transfusion reactions and a number of serious illnesses.

Fibrin—The protein formed as the end product of the blood clotting process when fibrinogen interacts with thrombin.

Fibrinogen—A type of blood protein called a globulin that interacts with thrombin to form fibrin.

Plasma—The liquid part of blood, as distinct from blood cells.

Prothrombin—A protein in blood plasma that is converted to thrombin during the clotting process.

Thrombin—An enzyme in blood plasma that helps to convert fibrinogen to fibrin during the last stage of the clotting process.

Thromboplastin—A protein in blood that converts prothrombin to thrombin.

Warfarin—A drug given to control the formation of blood clots. The PT test can be used to monitor patients being treated with warfarin.

medications that can interact with warfarin to increase or decrease the PT time.

Aftercare

Aftercare consists of routine care of the area around the puncture site. Pressure is applied for a few seconds and the wound is covered with a bandage.

Risks

The primary risk is mild dizziness and the possibility of a bruise or swelling in the area where the blood was drawn. The patient can apply moist warm compresses.

Normal results

The normal prothrombin time is 11–15 seconds, although there is some variation depending on the source of the thromboplastin used in the test. (For this reason, laboratories report a normal control value along with patient results.) A prothrombin time within this range indicates that the patient has normal amounts of clotting factors VII and X.

Abnormal results

A prolonged PT time is considered abnormal. The prothrombin time will be prolonged if the concentration of any of the tested factors is 10% or more below normal plasma values. A prolonged prothrombin time indicates a deficiency in any of factors VII, X, V, prothrombin, or fibrinogen. It may mean that the patient has a vitamin K deficiency, a liver disease, or disseminated intravascular coagulation (DIC). The prothrombin time of patients receiving warfarin therapy will also be prolonged—usually in the range of one and one half to two times the normal PT time. A PT time that exceeds approximately two and a half times the control value (usually 30 seconds or longer) is grounds for concern, as abnormal bleeding may occur.

Morbidity and mortality rates

Morbidity rates are excessively miniscule. The most common problems are minor bleeding and bruising. Since neither are reportable events, morbidity can only be estimated. Mortality is essentially zero.

Alternatives Resources

There are no alternatives to a prothrombin time.

Precautions

The only precaution needed is to clean the venipuncture site with alcohol.

Side effects

The most common side effects of a prothrombin time test are minor bleeding and bruising.

Resources

BOOKS

Fischbach, F. T. and M. B. Dunning. A Manual of Laboratory and Diagnostic Tests. 8th ed. Philadelphia: Lippincott Williams & Wilkins, 2008.

McGhee, M. A Guide to Laboratory Investigations. 5th ed. Oxford, UK: Radcliffe Publishing Ltd, 2008.

Price, C. P. Evidence-Based Laboratory Medicine: Principles, Practice, and Outcomes. 2nd ed. Washington, DC: AACC Press, 2007.

Scott, M.G., A. M. Gronowski, and C. S. Eby. Tietz's Applied Laboratory Medicine. 2nd ed. New York: Wiley-Liss, 2007.

Springhouse, A. M.. Diagnostic Tests Made Incredibly Easy!. 2nd ed. Philadelphia: Lippincott Williams & Wilkins, 2008.

PERIODICALS

Aksungar, F. B., A. E. Topkaya, Z. Yildiz, S. Sahin, and U. Turk. "Coagulation status and biochemical and inflammatory markers in multiple sclerosis." Journal of Clinical Neuroscience 15, no. 4 (2008): 393–397.

Awan, M. S., M. Iqbal, and S. Z. Imam. "Epistaxis: when are coagulation studies justified?" Emergency Medicine Journal 25, no. 3 (2008): 156–157.

Mueck, W., B. I. Eriksson, K. A. Bauer et al. "Population pharmacokinetics and pharmacodynamics of rivaroxaban - an oral, direct factor Xa inhibitor - in patients undergoing major orthopaedic surgery." Clinical Pharmacokinetics 47, no. 3 (2008): 203–216.

Rosenkrantz, A., M. Hinden, B. Leschmik, et al. "Calibrated automated thrombin generation in normal uncomplicated pregnancy." Thrombosis and Hemostasis 99, no. 2 (2008): 331–337.

ORGANIZATIONS

American Association for Clinical Chemistry. http://www.aacc.org/AACC/.

American Society for Clinical Laboratory Science. http://www.ascls.org/.

American Society of Clinical Pathologists. http://www.ascp.org/.

College of American Pathologists. http://www.cap.org/apps/cap.portal.

OTHER

American Clinical Laboratory Association. Information about clinical chemistry. 2008 [cited February 24, 2008]. http://www.clinical-labs.org/.

Clinical Laboratory Management Association. Information about clinical chemistry. 2008 [cited February 22, 2008]. http://www.clma.org/.

Lab Tests On Line. Information about lab tests. 2008 [cited February 24, 2008]. http://www.labtestsonline.org/.

National Accreditation Agency for Clinical Laboratory Sciences. Information about laboratory tests. 2008 [cited February 25, 2008]. http://www.naacls.org/.

L. Fleming Fallon, Jr, MD, DrPH

Proton pump inhibitors

Definition

The proton pump inhibitors are a group of drugs that reduce the secretion of gastric (stomach) acid. They act by binding with the enzyme $H+$, $K(+)$-*ATPase, hydrogen/potassium adenosine triphosphatase*, which is sometimes referred to as the proton pump. This enzyme causes parietal cells of the stomach lining to produce acid.

Although they perform much the same functions as the histamine H-2 receptor blockers, the proton pump inhibitors reduce stomach acid more and over a longer period.

Purpose

Proton pump inhibitors are used to treat ulcers; gastroesophageal reflux disease (GERD), a condition in which backward flow of acid from the stomach causes heartburn and injury of the food pipe (esophagus); and conditions in which the stomach produces too much acid, such as Zollinger-Ellison syndrome. Omeprazole is used in combination with other medications to treat recurrent ulcers caused by helicobacter pylori infections.

Two of the proton pump inhibitors, lansoprazole and omeprazole, have been used to improve pancreatic enzyme absorption in cystic fibrosis patients with intestinal malabsorption.

Proton pump inhibitors may be used to protect against the ulcerogenic effects of non-steroidal anti-inflammatory drugs and to help heal ulcers caused by these drugs.

Description

There are five drugs in this class: esomeprazole (Nexium), lansoprazole (Prevacid), omeprazole (Prilosec), pantoprazole (Protonix), and rabeprazole (AcipHex). They act in a similar manner, and their cautions and adverse effects are similar.

The products are generally formulated as enteric-coated granules. Absorption does not start until the granules have left the stomach and reached the intestine, so the onset of action is delayed about an hour, subject to gastric emptying time. Since they act slowly, proton pump inhibitors are not a suitable alternative to antacids which have a rapid effect.

Although these drugs are eliminated from the body relatively quickly, usually within 90 minutes of absorption, they all work for over 24 hours after a dose. This is because the factor that determines duration of action is how long it takes the body to replace the $H+$, $K(+)$-ATPase. There is some build up over time. For example, a single dose of lansoprazole reduces stomach acid by 71%, but after a week of regular dosing, the acid reduction rises to 80%.

For treatment of recurrent ulcers, the proton pump inhibitors are part of combination therapy that uses an antibiotic (occasionally two **antibiotics**) and proton pump inhibitor. There are a number of regimens, and while they may vary in the selection of specific drugs, or even types of drugs used, usually they include a proton pump inhibitor. The cure rates are all within similar ranges for these regimens.

Recommended dosage

Dose varies with the indication. The following are commonly prescribed doses:

- Esomeprazole: 20 to 40 mg once a day.
- Lansoprazole: 15 to 30 mg once a day.
- Omeprazole: 20 to 40 mg once a day.
- Pantoprazole: 40 mg once or twice a day.
- Rabeprazole: 20 mg once a day. In hypersecretory conditions, doses as high as 60 mg twice daily have been reported.

In the above examples, the lower dose is usually adequate for GERD, while the higher dose may be required for ulcer therapy or hypersecretory conditions.

Precautions

Proton pump inhibitors should not be given to any patient who has shown a reaction to any of the components of the drug or a related drug. Proton pump inhibitors should also not be given to patients with severe liver disease.

Omeprazole is pregnancy category C, while esomeprazole, lansoprazole, rabeprazole, and pantoprazole are category B. As of 2008, there are no adequate and well-controlled studies concerning the effects of these drugs on pregnant women. These drugs should be used during pregnancy only if the potential benefit justifies the risk to the fetus. Because the proton pump inhibitors are excreted into breast milk, they should not be used by women who are breastfeeding their babies.

The proton pump inhibitors may mask the symptoms of stomach cancer.

Side effects

The proton pump inhibitors are relatively safe drugs. The most commonly observed adverse effects are constipation, diarrhea, dizziness, headache, skin itch, and skin rash. Less often, the following adverse effects have been reported: abdominal pain with cramps, appetite changes, and nausea.

The following adverse effects are extremely rare but have been reported with this class of drugs:

- acute pancreatitis
- anxiety
- cough
- depression
- drug toxin-related hepatitis
- erythema multiforme

KEY TERMS

Antacid—A substance that counteracts or neutralizes acidity, usually of the stomach. Antacids have a rapid onset of action compared to histamine H-2 receptor blockers and proton pump inhibitors, but they have a short duration of action and require frequent dosing.

Cystic fibrosis—A hereditary disease that appears in early childhood, involves functional disorder of digestive glands, and is marked especially by faulty digestion due to a deficiency of pancreatic enzymes, by difficulty in breathing due to mucus accumulation in airways, and by excessive loss of salt in the sweat.

Enteric coat—A coating put on some tablets or capsules to prevent their disintegration in the stomach. The contents of coated tablets or capsules will be released only when the dose reaches the intestine. This may be done to protect the drug from stomach acid, to protect the stomach from drug irritation, or to delay the onset of action of the drug.

GERD—A chronic condition in which the lower esophageal sphincter allows gastric acids to reflux into the esophagus, causing heartburn, acid indigestion, and possible injury to the esophageal lining.

Malabsorption—Defective or inadequate absorption of nutrients from the intestinal tract.

Parietal cells—Cells of the gastric glands that secret hydrochloric acid.

Recurrent ulcer—Stomach ulcers that return after apparently complete healing. These ulcers appear to be caused by helicobacter pylori infections and can generally be successfully treated with a combination of antibiotics and gastric acid reducing compounds, particularly the proton pump inhibitors.

- flu-like symptoms
- myalgia
- Stevens-Johnson syndrome
- thrombocytopenia
- toxic epidermal necrolysis
- ulcerative colitis
- upper respiratory hypersensitivity reaction
- upper respiratory infection
- vomiting

Interactions

Proton pump inhibitors should not be used in conjunctions with the anti-retroviral (anti-AIDS) drug atazanavir (Rayataz). The conjunction may reduce the effectiveness of the atazanavir. Proton pump inhibitors should not be used in combination with the anti-fungal drugs itraconazole or ketoconazole. This combination may reduce the effectiveness of the anti-fungal drugs.

Resources

BOOKS

Atkinson, A. J., D. R. Abernathy, C. E. Daniels, R. Dedrick, and S. P. Markey. Basic & Clinical Pharmacology. 2nd ed. New York: Academic Press, 2006.

Edmunds, M. W. Introduction to Clinical Pharmacology. 5th ed St. Louis: Mosby, 2005.

Katzung, B. G. Basic & Clinical Pharmacology. 10th ed. New York: McGraw-Hill, 2006.

Roach, S., S., and S. M. Ford. Introductory Clinical Pharmacology. 8th ed. Philadelphia: Lippincott Williams & Wilkins, 2006.

PERIODICALS

Dharmarajan, T. S., M. R. Kanagala, P. Murakonda, A. S. Lebelt, and E. P. Norkus. "Do Acid-lowering agents affect vitamin B12 status in older adults?." Journal of the American Medical Directors Association 9, no. 3 (2008): 162–167.

Freeman, H. J. "Proton pump inhibitors and an emerging epidemic of gastric fundic gland polyposis." World Journal of Gastroenterology 14, no. 9 (2008): 1318–1320.

Sheiman, J. M. "Prevention of NSAID-Induced Ulcers." Current Treatment Options in Gastroenterology 11, no. 2 (2008): 125–134.

Wright, M. J., D. D. Proctor, K. L. Insogna, and J. E. Kerstetter. "Proton pump-inhibiting drugs, calcium homeostasis, and bone health." Nutrition Review 66, no. 2 (2008): 103–108.

ORGANIZATIONS

American College of Clinical Pharmacy. http://www.accp.com/.

American College of Clinical Pharmacology. http://www.accp1.org .

American College of Physicians. 190 N Independence Mall West, Philadelphia, PA 19106-1572. (800) 523-1546, x2600, or (215) 351-2600. http://www.acponline.org.

American Medical Association. 515 N. State Street, Chicago, IL 60610. (312) 464-5000. http://www.ama-assn.org.

OTHER

Drug Information Association. Information about prescription drugs. 2008 [cited February 25, 2008]. http://www.diahome.org/DIAHome/.

Mayo Clinic. Information about prescription drugs. 2008 [cited February 24, 2008]. http://www.mayoclinic.com/health/drug-information/DrugHerbIndex.

National Library of Medicine. Information about prescription drugs. 2008 [cited February 24, 2008]. http://www.nlm.nih.gov/medlineplus/druginformation.html/.

Physician's Drug Reference. Information about prescription drugs. 2008 [cited February 22, 2008]. http://www.pdr.net/drug-information/?engine = adwords !8815&keyword = %2Adrug + information %2A&match_type = &gclid = CMztjYHjgJICFQrAaAodKE339g.

L. Fleming Fallon, Jr, MD, DrPH

PSA test *see* **Tumor marker tests**

Psyllium *see* **Laxatives**

Pubo-vaginal sling *see* **Sling procedure**

Pulmonary embolism *see* **Venous thrombosis prevention**

Pulse oximeter

Definition

The pulse oximeter is a photoelectric instrument for measuring oxygen saturation of blood.

Purpose

A pulse oximeter measures the amount of oxygen present in blood by registering pulsations within an arteriolar bed (an area between arteries and capillaries). It is a noninvasive method widely used in hospitals on newborns, persons with pulmonary disorders, and individuals undergoing pulmonary and cardiac procedures. Oxygen levels can be estimated during **exercise**, surgery, or other medical procedures, or while a person is asleep.

Description

The oximeter consists of a light-emitting diode (LED), a photodetector probe containing a permanent or disposable sensor, alarms for pulse rate and oxygen levels, a display screen, and cables. The device works by emitting beams of red and infrared light that are passed through a pulsating arteriolar bed. Sensors detect the amount of light absorbed by oxyhemoglobin and deoxyhemoglobin in the red blood cells. The ratio of red to infrared light measured by the photodetector indicates the amount of oxygen present in the

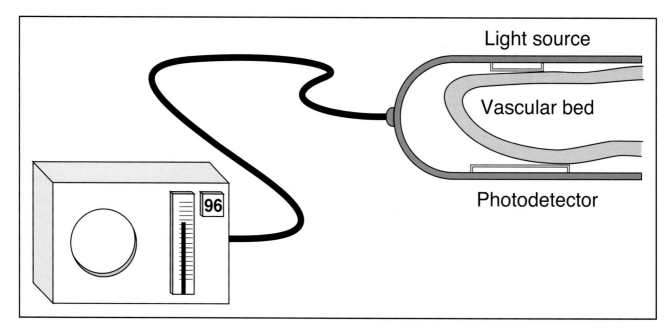

Light source

Vascular bed

Photodetector

A pulse oximeter uses infrared light and a photo sensor to detect the amount of oxygen in a patient's blood. *(Illustration by Argosy. Cengage Learning, Gale.)*

KEY TERMS

Arteriolar bed—An area in which arterioles cluster between arteries and capillaries.

Arterioles—The smallest branches of arteries.

Capillaries—Tiny blood vessels with a diameter of a red blood cell through which a single layer of cells flows.

Deoxyhemoglobin—Hemoglobin with oxygen removed.

Hemoglobin—The iron-containing protein in the blood that transports oxygen from the lungs to all parts of the body.

Oxyhemoglobin—Hemoglobin combined with oxygen.

blood. The sensor is attached to the body over the arteriolar area in the ear, the fingertip, the big toe, or across the bridge of the nose. Clip sensors can be used on fingers or the earlobe.

The pulse oximeter is widely used in most hospitals and in research laboratories that study pulmonary function. Oximeters are used in hospital settings such as intensive care units, pulmonary units, and in health care centers. Portable hand-held devices are available,

and are used to spot check patients and for in-home use under the supervision of a physician.

Usage

Several steps can be taken to improve the accuracy of readings. If possible, the patient should not smoke 24 hours prior to pulse oximetry. Fingernail polish should be removed if the oximeter will be attached to the finger. For people with poor circulation, hands should be slowly warmed with warm towels before attaching the oximeter. Abnormally high or low temperatures, as well as reduced hemoglobin, can influence the amount of oxygen adhering to the hemoglobin within the red blood cells, altering the reading. The sensor should be wrapped securely around the finger to prevent outside light from interfering with the reading, which could render it invalid. The device must not be used near flammable anesthetics.

Resources

BOOKS

West, John B. *Pulmonary Pathophysiology: The Essentials,* 6th ed. Philadelphia: Lippincott Williams & Wilkins, 2008.

ORGANIZATIONS

American Academy of Family Physicians. P. O. Box 11210, Shawnee Mission, KS 66207. (913)906-6000. *http://www.aafp.org.*

American Academy of Pediatrics. 141 Northwest Point Boulevard, Elk Grove Village, IL 60007-1098. (847) 434-4000. http://www.aap.org.

American College of Physicians. 190 N Independence Mall West, Philadelphia, PA 19106-1572. (800) 523-1546 or (215) 351-2600. http://www.acponline.org.

OTHER

Hill, Chris. "Introduction to Pulse Oximetry." *PulseOx.Info.* November 19, 2007 [cited February 12, 2008]. http://www.pulseox.info.

Hill, E. and M. D. Stoneham "Practical Applications of Pulse Oximetry" *World Federation of Societies of Anaesthesiologists.* 2000 [cited February 12, 2008]. http://www.nda.ox.ac.uk/wfsa/html/u11/u1104_01.htm.

"Principles of Pulse Oximetery Technology." *Oximetry.org.*September 10, 2002 [cited February 12, 2008]. http://www.oximetry.org/pulseox/principles.htm.

L. Fleming Fallon, Jr., M.D., Ph. D.
Tish Davidson, A. M.

Pyloroplasty

Definition

Pyloroplasty is a surgical procedure in which the pylorus valve at the lower portion of the stomach is cut and resutured, relaxing and widening its muscular opening (pyloric sphincter) into the duodenum (first part of the small intestine). Pyloroplasty is a treatment for patients at high risk for gastric or peptic ulcer disease (PUD).

Purpose

Pyloroplasty surgery enlarges the opening through which stomach contents are emptied into the intestine, allowing the stomach to empty more quickly. A pyloroplasty is performed to treat the complications of PUD or when medical treatment has not been able to control PUD in high-risk patients.

Demographics

Nearly four million people in the United States have PUD; about five adults in 100,000 will develop an ulcer. About 1.7% of children being treated in general pediatric practices are diagnosed with PUD. The presence of ulcer-causing *Helicobacter pylori* bacteria occurs in 10% of the population in industrialized countries and is believed to cause 80–90% of primary ulcers. In the United States, *H. pylori* infection occurs more frequently in black and Hispanic populations than in white. The frequency of secondary ulcers (caused by other existing conditions) is not known as it depends on the frequency of other illnesses, chronic diseases, and drug use. Primary and secondary PUD can occur in patients of all ages. Primary PUD is rare in children under age 10, increasing during adolescence. Secondary PUD is more prevalent in children under age six.

Description

Peptic ulcer disease develops when there is an imbalance between normal conditions that protect the lining (mucosa) of the stomach and the intestines and conditions that disrupt normal functioning of the lining. Protective factors include the water-soluble mucosal gel layer, the production of bicarbonate in the lining to balance acidity, the regulation of gastric acid (stomach acid) secretion, and blood flow in the lining. The aggressive factors that work against this protective gastric-wall system are excessive acid production, *H. pylori* bacterial infection, and a reduced blood flow (ischemia) in the mucosal lining. These aggressive factors can cause inflammation and ulcer development. A peptic ulcer is a type of sore or hole (perforation) that forms on the lining of the stomach (gastric ulcer) or intestine (duodenal ulcer), when the lining has been eaten away by stomach acid and digestive juices. Peptic ulcers can be primary, caused by *H. pylori* infection, or secondary, caused by excess acid production, stress, use of medications, and other underlying conditions that disrupt the gastric environment. Although *H. pylori* is believed to cause the majority of all ulcers, not all people infected with it develop ulcers. In high-risk individuals, the bacteria more readily disturb the balance between good factors and destructive factors, upsetting the protective function of the stomach and intestine lining. An ulcer develops when the lining can no longer protect the organs. Secondary ulcers are usually found in the stomach; primary ulcers can be in the stomach or intestine.

Other factors that contribute to mucosal inflammation and ulceration include:

• alcohol and caffeine use
• non-steroidal anti-inflammatory drugs (NSAIDs)
• aspirin
• cigarette smoking
• exposure to certain irritating chemicals
• emotional disturbances and prolonged stress
• traumatic injuries and burns

Pyloroplasty

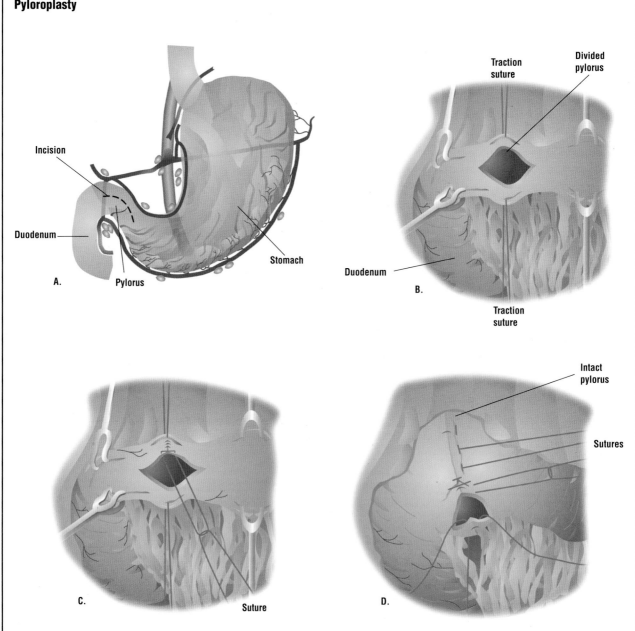

In a pyloroplasty, an incision is made in the area that connects the stomach to the duodenum (small intestine), called they pylorus (A). The pylorus is divided laterally (B), and then stitched longitudinally (C and D), allowing for a larger connection. *(Illustration by GGS Information Services. Cengage Learning, Gale.)*

- respiratory failure
- blood poisoning
- critical illnesses that create imbalances in body chemistry

Symptoms of gastric or peptic ulcer include burning pain, nausea, vomiting, loss of appetite, bloating, burping, and losing weight.

When PUD is diagnosed or high risk established, medical treatment will begin to treat *H. pylori* infection if present and to restore balanced conditions in the mucosal lining. Any underlying condition may be treated simultaneously, including respiratory disorders, fluid imbalance, or stomach and digestive disorders. Medications may be prescribed to help correct gastric disturbances and control gastric acid secretion.

KEY TERMS

Gastric (or peptic) ulcer—An ulcer (sore or hole) in the stomach lining, duodenum, or other part of the gastrointestinal system.

Pyloric sphincter—A broad band of muscle in the pylorus valve at the bottom end of the stomach.

Pylorus—The valve at the bottom end of the stomach that releases food from the stomach into the intestines.

Vagotomy—A surgical procedure in which the nerves that stimulate stomach acid production and gastric motility (movement) are cut.

- heart rate, pulse, and blood pressure
- chest examination and x ray, if necessary
- palpation (pressing with the hands) of the abdomen
- rectal examination and stool testing
- pelvic examination in sexually active females
- examination of testicles and inguinal (groin) area in males
- testing for the presence of *Helicobacter pylori*
- complete blood count and blood chemistry profile
- urinalysis
- imaging studies of gastrointestinal system (x ray, other types of scans)
- biopsy of stomach lining using a tube-like telescopic instrument (endoscope)

Preparation

Before surgery, standard preoperative blood and urine tests will be performed and various x rays may be ordered. The patient will not be permitted to eat or drink anything after midnight the night before the procedure. When the patient is admitted to the hospital, cleansing enemas may be ordered to empty the intestine. If nausea or vomiting are present, a suction tube may be used to empty the stomach.

Aftercare

The patient will spend several hours in a recovery area after surgery where blood pressure, pulse, respiration, and temperature will be monitored. The patient's breathing may be shallower than normal because of the effect of anesthesia and the patient's reluctance to breathe deeply and experience pain at the site of the surgical incision. The patient will be shown how to support the site while breathing deeply or coughing, and will be given pain medication as needed. Fluid intake and output will be measured. The operative site will be observed for any sign of redness, swelling, or wound drainage. Intravenous fluids are usually given for 24–48 hours until the patient is gradually permitted to eat a special light diet and as bowel activity resumes. About eight hours after surgery, the patient may be allowed to walk a little, increasing movement gradually over the next few days. The average hospital stay, dependent upon the patient's overall recovery status and any underlying conditions, ranges from six to eight days.

Risks

Potential complications of this abdominal surgery include excessive bleeding, surgical wound infection, incisional hernia, recurrence of gastric ulcer, chronic

Certain drugs that are prescribed for other conditions, especially NSAIDs, may be discontinued if they are known to cause inflammation. Adult patients may be advised to discontinue alcohol and caffeine use and to stop smoking.

When medical treatment alone is not able to improve the conditions that cause PUD, a pyloroplasty procedure may be recommended, particularly for patients with stress ulcers, perforation of the mucosal wall, and gastric outlet obstruction. The surgery involves cutting the pylorus lengthwise and resuturing it at a right angle across the cut to relax the muscle and create a larger opening from the stomach into the intestine. The enlarged opening allows the stomach to empty more quickly. A pyloroplasty is sometimes done in conjunction with a **vagotomy** procedure in which the vagus nerves that stimulate stomach acid production and gastric motility (movement) are cut. This may delay gastric emptying and pyloroplasty will help correct that effect.

Diagnosis

Diagnosis begins with an accurate history of prior illnesses and existing medical conditions as well as a family history of ulcers or other gastrointestinal (stomach and intestines) disorders. A complete history and comprehensive diagnostic testing may include:

- location, frequency, duration, and severity of pain
- vomiting and description of gastric material
- bowel habits and description of stool
- all medications, including over-the-counter products
- appetite, typical diet, and weight changes
- family and social stressors
- alcohol consumption and smoking habits

WHO PERFORMS THE PROCEDURE AND WHERE IS IT PERFORMED?

A pyloroplasty surgery is performed by a general surgeon in a hospital or medical center operating room.

diarrhea, and malnutrition. After the surgery, the surgeon should be informed of an increase in pain, and of any swelling, redness, drainage, or bleeding in the surgical area. The development of headache, muscle aches, dizziness, fever, abdominal pain or swelling, constipation, nausea or vomiting, rectal bleeding, or black stools should also be reported.

Normal results

Complete healing is expected without complications. Recovery and a return to normal activities should take from four to six weeks.

Morbidity and mortality rates

Successful treatment of *Helicobacter pylori* has improved morbidity and mortality rates, and the prognosis for PUD, with proper treatment and avoidance of causative factors, is excellent. Pyloroplasty is rarely performed in primary ulcer disease. Morbidity and mortality are higher in patients with secondary ulcers because of underlying illness that complicates both PUD and surgical treatment.

Resources

BOOKS

Monahan, Frances. *Medical-Surgical Nursing.* Philadelphia: W. B. Saunders Co., 1998.

QUESTIONS TO ASK THE DOCTOR

- How will this surgery be performed?
- What is your experience with this procedure? How often do you perform this procedure?
- Why must I have the surgery?
- What are my options if I opt not have the surgery?
- How can I expect to feel after surgery?
- What are the risks involved in having this surgery?
- How quickly will I recover? When can I return to school or work?
- What are my chances of getting this condition again?
- What can I do to avoid getting this condition again?

ORGANIZATIONS

American Gastroenterological Association. 7910 Woodmont Ave., Seventh Floor, Bethesda, MD 20814. (301) 654-2055. http://www.gastro.org.
National Institute of Diabetes and Digestive and Kidney Disorders. 31 Center Drive, Bethesda, MD 20892. (301) 496-7422. http://www.niddk.nih.gov.

OTHER

"Peptic Ulcer Surgery." *Mayo Clinic Online.* March 5, 1998. http://www.mayohealth.org.
"Peptic Ulcer Disease." Harvard Medical School and Aetna Consumer Health Information. *InteliHealth.* March 6, 2001. http://www.intelihealth.com.

Kathleen D. Wright, RN
L. Lee Culvert

Pylorus repair *see* **Pyloroplasty**

TECHNICAL COLLEGE OF THE LOWCOUNTRY
LEARNING RESOURCES CENTER
POST OFFICE BOX 1288
BEAUFORT, SOUTH CAROLINA 29901-1288